Fundamentals of
FOOT
SURGERY

Fundamentals of
FOOT SURGERY

EDITOR

E. DALTON McGLAMRY
D.P.M., D.Sc. (Hon.)

Diplomat ABPS
Peachtree Podiatry Group, P.C.
Past President, American Podiatric Medical Association
Former Editor, Journal of the American Podiatry Association
National Consultant in Podiatry, Office of the Surgeon General, U.S.A.F.
Founder and Secretary-Treasurer of the Doctors Hospital Podiatric Education and Research Institute
Podiatric Surgical Staff-Doctors Hospital, Tucker, Georgia
Faculty, Doctors Hospital Podiatry Institute

Author's editor
REBEKAH McGLAMRY, B.A.

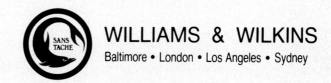

WILLIAMS & WILKINS
Baltimore • London • Los Angeles • Sydney

Editor: Jonathan N. Pine, Jr.
Associate Editor: Carol Eckhart
Copy Editor: CRACOM Corporation
Design: JoAnne Janowiak
Illustration Planning: Lorraine Wrzosek
Production: Anne G. Seitz

Copyright © 1987
Williams & Wilkins
428 East Preston Street
Baltimore, MD 21202, U.S.A.

Printed in the United States of America

Library of Congress Cataloging-in-Publication Data

Fundamentals of foot surgery.

Includes index.
  1. Foot—Surgery. I. McGlamry, E. Dalton.
[DNLM: 1. Foot—surgery. WE 880 F981]
RD563.F88   1987   617'.585059   86-13288

Composed and printed at the
Waverly Press, Inc.   87 88 89 90 91   10 9 8 7 6 5 4 3 2 1

Foreword

The science of foot surgery is reaching new levels of sophistication. The complexity of foot anatomy and its intrinsic relationship with biomechanical foot function call for more exacting criteria in choice of procedures and delicate execution of surgical techniques in achieving maximum functional restoration of the disordered foot. In response to this striving for excellence there is an evident need for a text to restudy and update basic anatomical, biomechanical, surgical, and management principles. E. Dalton McGlamry has accepted the challenge and has made a very important contribution by producing this intriguing text, *Fundamentals of Foot Surgery*. The book invites the experienced practitioner as well as the newcomer to examine discriminating approaches to basic subjects that should yield great dividends.

Dr. McGlamry, the editor, and his contributors address many pertinent subjects in this extremely well-illustrated textbook of three sections and 22 chapters. It is interesting to highlight some of the issues that make this book impressive.

Too often, too little undergraduate time is spent on the intricacies of foot anatomy. An enlightening presentation of developmental, microscopic, and cross-sectional foot anatomy updates this subject and puts it into useful perspective. Biomechanics of the foot is comprehensively explained. Radiology of the foot reemphasizes studies of the weight-supporting foot in assessing functional derangements. The full gamut of scanning and imaging techniques is helpfully surveyed. The utterly precise attention to surgical principles portrays the finesse required in foot surgery. The management of a selected group of foot disorders associated with classical conditions and disease processes is covered in a satisfying manner. Special con-

siderations of limb salvage, reflex sympathetic dystrophy management, and choice of proper prosthetic appliances vital to long-range postsurgical rehabilitation are added subjects that make this book of inestimable value.

Dr. McGlamry has outstanding qualifications for preparing this textbook. He is a practicing foot surgeon with a reputation for discriminating surgical judgment and impeccable surgical techniques. The following are a few of his accomplishments: Diplomate and former Director, American Board of Podiatric Surgery; director of a three-year residency program in foot surgery for 15 years; author of numerous papers and monographs on foot surgery; producer of many instructional films, including a National Medical Education award winner; conductor of college-based postgraduate seminars. He has also served as Review Editor of the *Journal of Foot Surgery*, 1965–1970, and Editor of the *Journal of the American Podiatry Association*, 1972–1984. He is past president of the American Podiatry Association.

Characteristically, Dr. McGlamry has called upon colleagues to contribute their expertise in this book, and they have generously responded. It is a privilege for the reader to visit with each of these surgeons through the viewpoints of their offerings. The years of dedication to this effort are acknowledged with appreciation for this worthy endeavor. Thank you all for a fine contribution to the science of foot surgery.

Felton O. Gamble, D.P.M.
Associate in Surgery (Podiatry)
College of Medicine
The University of Arizona
Tucson, Arizona

Preface

The purpose of the book is to provide in one volume the background information that should be a fundamental part of the knowledge of every surgeon who treats the foot and leg. The book is divided into three sections.

Section I covers fundamentals and principles. Chapter 1 details the precise surgical anatomy of the foot and leg. Chapter 2 presents surgically applicable biomechanics. Additional chapters cover radiology, surgical principles, sutures and wound closure, materials, instrumentation, internal fixation, postoperative considerations and anesthesia.

Section II includes nine chapters and is devoted entirely to surgical patients with special medical considerations. Such patients include those with neuromuscular disease, diabetes mellitus, rheumatoid disorders, and other medical problems affecting the foot.

Section III deals with special considerations and includes chapters on limb salvage, reflex sympathetic dystrophy, and prosthetics in the lower extremity.

In preparing *Fundamentals of Foot Surgery* we have involved authors from a wide cross-section of the country. The material they present includes both the historical as well as the current state of the art. I am indebted to each of the contributing authors for their contributions to the book.

Special thanks are due to many people who contributed to the preparation of the book. The staff of Williams & Wilkins contributed in many ways. Rodney Ruch and Michael McGlamry served as our medical photographers. The podiatry residents of Doctors Hospital, Tucker, GA assisted with much of the research and proof reading. The Atlanta Slide Arts Production Company did most of the tables and charts as well as converting color slides to black and white prints for the book.

For planning the book content I am indebted to John Ruch, D.P.M., dean of faculty, Doctors Hospital Podiatry Institute and to Kieran Mahan, D.P.M., Vice President for Clinical Sciences at Pennsylvania College of Podiatric Medicine.

Rebekah McGlamry, B.A., served as author's editor for every author. In addition, her work as computer specialist made the book and its two companion volumes possible.

It is my hope that *Fundamentals of Foot Surgery* along with the two-volume *Comprehensive Textbook of Foot Surgery* will be of assistance to podiatric medical students, residents, and practitioners of podiatric surgery.

E. Dalton McGlamry, D.P.M., D.Sc.(hon)

Contributors

Alan S. Banks, D.P.M.
Doctors Hospital
Tucker, Georgia
  D.P.M., Pennsylvania College of Podiatric Medicine, 1984;
  Bachelor of Science Degree, Mercer University, Macon, Georgia;
  Third-year Resident, Doctors Hospital, Tucker, Georgia;
  Faculty, Doctors Hospital Podiatric Education and Research Institute

Robert E. Bergman, D.O.
Anesthesiologist
Tucker, Georgia
  Chairman, Department of Anesthesia, Doctors Hospital, Tucker, Georgia;
  Director, Anesthesia Training, Podiatry Residents, Doctors Hospital, Tucker, Georgia;
  Member, Advisory Board and Instructor for Emergency Medical Technicians, Dekalb County, Georgia;
  Member, American College of Osteopathic Anesthesiologists;
  Member, American Society of Anesthesiologists

Steven J. Berlin, D.P.M.
Private Practice
Bel Air, Maryland
  Chief, Podiatry Services, Fallston General Hospital, Fallston, Maryland;
  Clinical Director, Maryland Podiatry Residency Program, Bon Secours Hospital, Baltimore, Maryland;
  Diplomate, American Board Podiatric Surgeons;
  Fellow, American College Foot Surgeons;
  Speical Editor, Oncology, *Journal of the American Podiatry Medical Association*;
  President, Podiatric Pathology Laboratories, Inc.;
  Fellow, American Society of Podiatric Dermatology

Marc Bernbach, D.P.M.
Doctors Hospital
Tucker, Georgia
  D.P.M., Pennsylvania College of Podiatric Medicine, Philadelphia, Pennsylvania—Degree of Doctor of Podiatric Medicine, 1985;

Second-year Resident, Doctors Hospital, Tucker, Georgia

Jeffrey Boberg, D.P.M.
Private Practice
Livingstone, New Jersey
  D.P.M., Pennsylvania College of Podiatric Medicine, Philadelphia, Pennsylvania, 1981;
  Completed three years of Podiatric Residency, Doctors Hospital, Tucker, Georgia;
  Fellow, American College of Foot Surgeons;
  Academic Coordinator, Residency Training Committee, West Essex General Hospital, Livingston, New Jersey;
  Attending Staff, Columbus Hospital, Newark, New Jersey; West Essex General Hospital, Livingston, New Jersey; Kennedy Memorial Hospitals, Saddle Brook, New Jersey; Roseland Surgical Center, Roseland, New Jersey

James L. Bouchard, D.P.M.
Private Practice
Roswell, Georgia
  Board Certified, American Board of Podiatric Surgery;
  Chairman, Department of Podiatry, Doctors Hospital, Tucker, Georgia;
  Faculty, Doctors Hospital Podiatric Education and Research Institute;
  Podiatry Consultant, Veterans Administration Hospital, Atlanta, Georgia;
  First-year Residency, University of Texas Health Science Center, San Antonio, Texas;
  Second and third years of Podiatric Residency, Doctors Hospital, Tucker, Georgia

John M. Buckholz, D.P.M.
Private Practice
New Town Square, Pennsylvania
  Director, Podiatric Residency, St. Joseph's Hospital, Philadelphia, Pennsylvania;
  Diplomate, American Board of Podiatric Surgery;
  Professor, Podiatric Surgery, Pennsylvania College of Podiatric Medicine;
  AO/ASIF Course Chairman;
  Member, American College of Foot Surgeons;

Member, American Society of Bone and Mineral Research;

Former Vice-president, Clinical Education, Pennsylvania College of Podiatric Medicine

Michael J. Burns, D.P.M.
Private Practice
Ft. Collins, Colorado

Diplomate, American Board of Podiatric Surgery;

Diplomate, American Board of Podiatric Orthopedics;

Fellow, American Academy of Podiatric Sports Medicine;

Fellow, American College of Foot Orthopedists;

Fellow, American College of Foot Surgeons;

Faculty Affiliate, Colorado State University, Ft. Collins, Colorado;

Editor, *Journal of the American Podiatric Medical Association*

Tom Cain, D.P.M.
Private Practice
Lilburn, Georgia

D.P.M., Pennsylvania College of Podiatric Medicine, Philadelphia, Pennsylvania—Degree of Doctor of Podiatric Medicine, 1982;

Three-year residency in Podiatric Surgery, Doctors Hospital, Tucker, Georgia;

Faculty, Doctors Hospital Podiatric Education and Research Institute;

Active Staff, Doctors Hospital, Tucker, Georgia;

Fellow, American College of Foot Surgeons

Raymond G. Cavaliere, D.P.M.
Private Practice
Howard Beach, New York

Three-year residency in Podiatric Surgery, Doctors Hospital, Tucker, Georgia;

Faculty, Doctors Hospital Podiatric Education and Research Institute;

Fellow, American College of Foot Surgeons, 1985;

D.P.M., New York College of Podiatric Medicine, New York, New York;

Clinical Assistant Professor of Podiatric Medicine, College of Podiatric Medicine and Surgery, University of Osteopathic Medicine and Health Sciences, Des Moines, Iowa;

Assistant Professor of Surgical Sciences, New York College of Podiatric Medicine, New York, New York

D. Richard DiNapoli, D.P.M.
Doctors Hospital
Tucker, Georgia

Second-year resident, Doctors Hospital, Tucker, Georgia;

D.P.M., Pennsylvania College Pennsylvania College of Podiatric Medicine, Philadelphia, Pennsylvania, 1985

Bruce Dobbs, D.P.M.
California College of Podiatric Medicine
San Francisco, California

Diplomate, American Board of Podiatric Surgery;

Professor of Surgery, California College of Podiatric Medicine, San Francisco, California;

Chief, Division of Podiatry, Seton Medical, Daly City, California;

Fellow, American College of Foot Surgeons;

General Editor, *Journal of the American Podiatric Medical Association*

Gary L. Dockery, D.P.M.
Private Practice
Seattle, Washington

Fellow, American College of Foot Surgeons;

Diplomate, American Board of Podiatric Surgery;

Diplomate, American Board of Podiatric Orthopedics;

Director, Podiatric Education and Residency Training, Waldo General Hospital, Seattle, Washington, 1979–1985;

Director, and Chairman of Board, Northwest Podiatric Foundation for Research and Education;

Private Practice, Seattle Foot and Ankle Clinic, Seattle, Washington

Michael S. Downey, D.P.M.
Pennsylvania College of Podiatric Medicine
Philadelphia, Pennsylvania

Three Year Residency, Podiatric Surgery, Doctors Hospital, Tucker, Georgia, 1986;

Faculty, Doctors Hospital Podiatric Education and Research Institute;

D.P.M., Pennsylvania College of Podiatric Medicine, Doctor of Podiatric Medicine, 1983;

Assistant Professor, Department of Podiatric Surgery, Pennsylvania College of Podiatric Medicine

Gordon E. Duggar, B.S. (Pharm), D.P.M.
Decatur, Georgia

Diplomate, American Board of Podiatric Surgery;

Surgical Staff, Doctors Hospital, Tucker, Georgia;

Surgical Staff, Atlanta Hospital, Atlanta, Georgia

Charles F. Fenton, III, D.P.M.
Private Practice
Atlanta, Georgia

Diplomate, American Board of Podiatric Surgery;

Fellow, American College of Foot Surgeons;

Atlanta Hospital and Medical Center;

Staff, Doctors Hospital, Tucker, Georgia

Joshua Gerbert, D.P.M.
California College of Podiatric Medicine
San Francisco, California

Chairman and Professor, Department of Podiatric Surgery, California College of Podiatric Medicine;

Surgical Editor, *Journal of the American Podiatric Medical Association*;

Diplomate, American Board of Podiatric Surgery;

Staff, Pacific Coast Hospital

Donald R. Green, D.P.M.
Private Practice
San Diego, California

Clinical Professor, California College of Podiatric Medicine;

Clinical Professor, California College of Podiatric Medicine;
Clinical Professor, Ohio College of Podiatric Medicine;
Clinical Professor, College of Podiatric Medicine and Surgery, University of Osteopathic Medicine and Health Sciences, Des Moines, Iowa;
Former Chairman and Professor, Surgery Department, Pennsylvania College of Podiatric Medicine;
Diplomate, American Board of Podiatric Surgery;
Podiatric Residency Director, Hillside Hospital, San Diego;
Faculty, Doctors Hospital Podiatric Education and Research Institute;
Hospital Affiliations—Mercy Hospital and Medical Center, San Diego; Hillside Hospital, San Diego;
Second- and third-year residency in Podiatric Surgery, Doctors Hospital, Tucker, Georgia;
First-year residency, Jewish Memorial Hospital, New York, New York

Grace M. Guastella, D.P.M.
Private Practice
Jonesboro, Georgia

George Gumann, D.P.M.
Private Practice
Columbus, Georgia
Diplomate, American Board of Podiatric Surgery;
Staff Podiatrist, Martin Army Hospital, Ft. Benning, Georgia;
Clinical Faculty, Pennsylvania College of Podiatric Medicine;
Clinical Faculty, Scholl College of Podiatric Medicine

Vincent J. Hetherington, D.P.M.
University of Osteopathic Medicine and Health Sciences
Des Moines, Iowa
Associate Professor of Podiatric Medicine;
Associate Dean for Clinical Affairs, University of Osteopathic Medicine and Health Sciences, College of Podiatric Medicine and Surgery;
Diplomate, American Board of Podiatric Surgery;
Staff, Des Moines General Hospital

Kinley W. Howard, D.P.M.
Private Practice
Valdosta, Georgia
D.P.M., Ohio College of Podiatric Medicine, 1984;
Two-Year Resident, Atlanta Hospital, Atlanta, Georgia;
Certified Registered Nurse Anesthetist;
Private Practice, Valdosta, Georgia

Allen Mark Jacobs, D.P.M.
Private Practice
St. Louis, Missouri
Diplomate, American Board of Podiatric Surgery;
Chairperson, Department of Podiatric Medicine and Surgery, Lindell Hospital, St. Louis, Missouri;
Contributing Editor, *Journal of Foot Surgery*

Marla Jassen, D.P.M.
Private Practice
Towson, Maryland
Residency, Doctors Hospital, Tucker, Georgia;
Member, Podiatry Examination Committee, Virginia State Board of Medicine;
Lecturer, Maryland Podiatry Residency Program;
Staff, Howard County General Hospital, Inc., Columbia, Maryland;
Staff, Fallston General Hospital, Fallston, Maryland;
Staff, Bon Secours Hospital, Baltimore, Maryland

A. Louis Jimenez, D.P.M.
Private Practice
Snellville, Georgia
First-year Podiatric Residency, Harrison Community Hospital, Mt. Clemens, Michigan
Second- and Third-year Podiatric Residency, Doctors Hospital, Tucker, Georgia;
Faculty, Doctors Hospital Podiatric Education and Research Institute;
Active Staff, Doctors Hospital, Tucker, Georgia

Stanley R. Kalish, D.P.M.
Private Practice
Jonesboro, Georgia
Second- and Third-year Residency, Doctors Hospital, Tucker, Georgia;
Diplomate, American Board of Podiatric Surgery;
Faculty, Doctors Hospital Podiatric Education and Research Institute;
Staff, Doctors Hospital, Tucker, Georgia

Gary M. Lepow, D.P.M.
Private Practice
Houston, Texas
Certified, American Board of Podiatric Surgery;
Board of Directors, Council of Teaching Hospitals;
Board Member, National Board of Podiatric Medical Examiners;
Instructor, Harris County Podiatric Medical Residency Program;
Chairman, Committee on Residency Training, Council on Podiatric Medical Education, American Podiatric Medical Association;
Attending Podiatrist, St. Luke's Episcopal Hospital and Texas Heart Institute, Houston, Texas

Kieran T. Mahan, D.P.M.
Pennsylvania College of Podiatric Medicine
Philadelphia, Pennsylvania
Vice President, Clinical Education, Pennsylvania College of Podiatric Medicine;
Diplomate, American Board of Podiatric Surgery;
Associate Professor, Department of Surgery, Pennsylvania College of Podiatric Medicine;
Faculty, Doctors Hospital Podiatric Education and Research Institute;
Director of Continuing Education, Department of Podiatric Surgery, Pennsylvania College of Podiatric Medicine;
Three-year Residency in Podiatric Surgery, Doctors Hospital, Tucker, Georgia;

Member, Podiatric Trauma Team, St. Joseph's
Hospital, Philadelphia, Pennsylvania

D. Scot Malay, D.P.M.
Pennsylvania College of Podiatric Medicine
Philadelphia, Pennsylvania
  Three-year Residency, Doctors Hospital, Tucker,
    Georgia;
  D.P.M., Pennsylvania College of Podiatric Medi-
    cine;
  Faculty, Doctors Hospital Podiatric Education and
    Research Institute;
  Assistant Professor, Department of Podiatric Sur-
    gery, Pennsylvania College of Podiatric Medicine

David E. Marcinko, D.P.M.
Private Practice
Atlanta, Georgia
  Adjunct Clinical Assistant Professor, Scholl College
    of Podiatric Medicine;
  Assistant Director, Podiatric Surgical Residency
    Training Program, Atlanta Hospital, Atlanta,
    Georgia;
  Diplomate, American Board of Podiatric Surgery
  Three-year Residency, Atlanta Hospital, Atlanta,
    Georgia;
  Private Practice, Peachtree Podiatry Group, At-
    lanta, Georgia;
  Active Staff, Atlanta Hospital, Atlanta, Georgia;
  Active Staff, Doctors Hospital, Tucker, Georgia

Jerry R. Maxwell, D.P.M.
Private Practice
Edmond, Oklahoma
  Three-year Residency in Podiatric Surgery, Doctors
    Hospital, Tucker, Georgia;
  Board eligible, American Board of Podiatric Sur-
    gery;
  Staff, Edmond Memorial Hospital, Edmon, Okla-
    homa;
  Staff, Doctors General Hospital, Oklahoma City,
    Oklahoma

Daniel J. McCarthy, D.P.M., Ph.D.
Baltimore, Maryland
  Chief, Podiatric Section, Surgical Service, Veter-
    ans Administration Medical Center, Baltimore,
    Maryland;
  Adjunct Clinical Professor, New York, Ohio, and
    Pennsylvania Colleges of Podiatric Medicine;
  Distinguished Practitioner, National Academy of
    Practice;
  Fellow, Past President and Trustee, American So-
    ciety of Podiatric Dermatology;
  Special Editor for Pathology, *Journal of the Amer-
    ican Podiatric Medical Association*;
  Formerly Professor and Chairman, Department of
    Anatomy, Pennsylvania College of Podiatric
    Medicine

E. Dalton McGlamry, D.P.M.
Peachtree Podiatry Group, PC
Atlanta, Georgia

  Diplomate, American Board of Podiatric Surgery;
  Secretary-Treasurer, Doctors Hospital Podiatric
    Education and Research Institute, Tucker, Geor-
    gia;
  Faculty, Doctors Hospital Podiatric Education and
    Research Institute;
  Attending Staff, Doctors Hospital, Tucker, Georgia;
  Former Editor, *Journal of the American Podiatric
    Medical Association*;
  Past President, American Podiatric Medical Asso-
    ciation

Thomas J. Merrill, D.P.M.
Doctors Hospital
Tucker, Georgia
  D.P.M., Scholl College of Podiatric Medicine, 1984;
  Third-year Resident, Doctors Hospital, Tucker,
    Georgia;
  Faculty, Doctors Hospital Podiatric Education and
    Research Institute

Stephen J. Miller, D.P.M.
Private Practice
Anacortes, Washington
  Diplomate, American Board of Podiatric Surgery;
  Faculty, Doctors Hospital Podiatric Education and
    Research Institute;
  Staff Podiatrist and Residency Instructor, Island
    Hospital, Anacortes, Washington;
  Staff Podiatrist, Waldo General Hospital, Seattle,
    Washington;
  Special Editor, *Journal of the American Podiatric
    Medical Association*;
  Trustee, Northwest Podiatric Foundation, Seattle,
    Washington;
  Three-year Residency, Podiatric Surgery, Doctors
    Hospital, Tucker, Georgia

Chester A. Nava, Jr., D.P.M.
Private Practice
Louisville, Kentucky
  D.P.M., Scholl College of Podiatric Medicine, Phil-
    adelphia, Pennsylvania, 1985;
  First-year Resident, James C. Giuffre Medical Cen-
    ter, Philadelphia, Pennsylvania;
  Member and Contributor, Cell Kinetics Society of
    North America

Robert G. O'Keefe, D.P.M.
Private Practice
Chicago, Illinois
  Associate Professor, Department of Surgery, Scholl
    College of Podiatric Medicine, Chicago, Illinois;
  Attending Staff, St. Anne's West Hospital, North-
    lake, Illinois;
  Consulting Staff, Columbus Hospital, Chicago, Illi-
    nois;
  Diplomate, American Board of Podiatric Surgery

Lawrence M. Oloff, D.P.M.
California College of Podiatric Medicine
San Francisco, California
  Associate Professor, Departments of Podiatric Med-
    icine and Surgery, California College of Podiatric
    Medicine, San Francisco, California;

Diplomate, American Board of Podiatric Surgery;
Former Co-Director, Residency Training, Lindell Hospital, St. Louis, Missouri;
Contributing Editor, *Journal of Foot Surgery*

Louis G. Pack, D.P.M.
Private Practice
Atlanta, Georgia
Diplomate, American Board of Podiatric Surgery;
Former Clinical Instructor, Emory University School of Medicine;
Former Director, Residency Training and Postgraduate Education, Atlanta Hospital and Medical Center;
Past Chairman of Board, American Diabetes Association, Atlanta Chapter

Irving Pikscher, D.P.M.
Private Practice
Chicago, Illinois
Associate Professor, Department of Podiatric Medicine, Scholl College of Podiatric Medicine, Chicago, Illinois;
Chairman, Podiatry Section, Central Community Hospital, Chicago, Illinois;
Diplomate, American Board of Podiatric Surgery

Howard R. Reinherz, D.P.M.
Private Practice
Kenosha, Wisconsin
Certified Orthotist;
Past President, American Board of Podiatric Surgery;
Past President, American College of Foot Surgeons;
Diplomate, American Board of Podiatric Surgery;
Chief, Podiatry Department and Secretary of Medical Staff, American International Hospital, Zion, Illinois;
Staff, American International Hospital, Zion, Illinois

Richard P. Reinherz, D.P.M.
Private Practice
Kenosha, Wisconsin
Editor, *Journal of Foot Surgery*;
Diplomate, American Board of Podiatric Surgery;
Director, Postgraduate Residency Training, American International Hospital, Zion, Illinois;
Clinical Instructor, Southeastern Wisconsin Family Practice Residency Program, Medical College of Wisconsin;
Past Chairman, Kenosha, Wisconsin Board of Health;
Staff, American International Hospital, Zion, Illinois;
Staff, St. Catherine's and Kenosha Memorial Hospitals, Kenosha, Wisconsin

Barry N. Rodgveller, D.P.M.
Private Practice
San Pedro, California
Diplomate, American Board of Podiatric Surgery;
Director, Baja Project for Crippled Children, Mexicali, B.C., Mexico;

Clinical Associate Professor, California College of Podiatric Medicine, San Francisco, California;
Clinical Instructor, Southern California Podiatric Medical Center, Los Angeles, California;
Attending Staff, University of Southern California Medical Center, Los Angeles, California;
Attending Staff, San Pedro Peninsula Hospital, San Pedro, California;
Attending Staff, Memorial Hospital of Gardena, Gardena, California;
Attending Staff, Memorial Hospital of Hawthorne, Hawthorne, California

Richard D. Roth, D.P.M.
Private Practice
Jupiter-Tequesta, Florida
Visiting Assistant Professor, Pennsylvania College of Podiatric Medicine, Philadelphia, Pennsylvania;
Former Fellow in Rheumatology, Arthritis Center, Albert Einstein Medical Center, Northern Division, Philadelphia, Pennsylvania;
Attending Staff and Former Chairman, Podiatry Section, Humana Hospital Palm Beaches, West Palm Beach, Florida;
Staff Member, Palm Beach-Martin County Medical Center and Palm Beach Gardens Medical Center

John A. Ruch, D.P.M.
Private Practice
Tucker, Georgia
Director, Podiatric Residency Program, Doctors Hospital, Tucker, Georgia;
Second- and Third-year Residency, Doctors Hospital, Tucker, Georgia;
Faculty, Doctors Hospital Podiatric Education and Research Institute;
Diplomate, American Board of Podiatric Surgery

Barbara S. Schlefman, D.P.M.
Private Practice
Tucker, Georgia
Faculty, Doctors Hospital Podiatric Education and Research Institute;
General Editor, *Journal of the American Podiatric Medical Associations*;
Attending Staff, Doctors Hospital, Tucker, Georgia and Atlanta Hospital, Atlanta, Georgia;
D.P.M.—Illinois College of Podiatric Medicine, Chicago, Illinois, 1980;
Fellow, American College of Foot Surgeons;
Diplomate, American Board of Podiatric Surgery (Board Certified);
President, American Association of Women Podiatrists

John M. Schuberth, D.P.M.
Kaiser Foundation Hospital
Department of Podiatry/Orthopedics
San Francisco, California
Diplomate, American Board of Podiatric Surgery;
Attending Staff, Department of Podiatry/Orthopedics, Kaiser Foundation Hospital, San Francisco, California;

Fellow, American College of Foot Surgeons;
Advisor, Northwest Podiatric Foundation

Nathan H. Schwartz, D.P.M.
Private Practice
Atlanta, Georgia
    Director, Residency Program, Atlanta Hospital, Atlanta, Georgia;
    Diplomate, American Board of Podiatric Surgery;
    Staff, Atlanta Hospital, Atlanta, Georgia;
    Staff, Windy Hill Hospital, Marietta, Georgia;
    Former Associate Professor of Surgery, Ohio College of Podiatric Medicine

Barry L. Scurran, D.P.M.
Kaiser-Permanente Medical Center
Hayward, California
    Chief, Podiatric Surgery, Kaiser Permanente Medical Center, Hayward, California;
    Diplomate, American Board of Podiatric Surgery;
    Clinical Associate Professor of Surgery, California College of Podiatric Medicine

Stephen Silvani, D.P.M.
Kaiser-Permanente Medical Center
Hayward, California
    Diplomate, American Board of Podiatric Surgery;
    Clinical Assistant Professor of Surgery, California College of Podiatric Medicine;
    Attending Podiatrist, Second-year Surgical Residency Program, Permanente Medical Group, Hayward and Fremont, California;
    Staff Podiatrist, Kaiser Permanente Medical Center at Hayward and Ambulatory Surgical Center at Fremont, California

Thomas F. Smith, D.P.M.
Private Practice
Augusta, Georgia
    Clinical Instructor, Department of Surgery, Pennsylvania College of Podiatric Medicine;
    Special Editor, *Journal of the American Podiatric Medical Association*;
    Faculty, Doctors Hospital Podiatric Education and Research Institute, Tucker, Georgia;
    Private Practitioner, Augusta, Georgia;
    Attending Staff, Doctors Hospital, Tucker, Georgia;
    Attending Staff, University Hospital, Augusta, Georgia

John A. Vanore, D.P.M.
Private Practice
Chicago, Illinois
    Podiatry Residency Director, Central Community Hospital, Chicago, Illinois;
    Diplomate, American Board of Podiatric Surgery;
    Adjunct Clinical Professor, Scholl College of Podiatric Medicine, Chicago, Illinois

Harold W. Vogler, D.P.M.
Pennsylvania College of Podiatric Medicine
Philadelphia, Pennsylvania
    Professor, Department of Surgery, Pennsylvania College of Podiatric Medicine;
    Diplomate, American Board of Podiatric Surgery;
    Member, Resident Training Committee in Reconstructive and Traumatological Surgery of the Foot and Ankle, St. Joseph's Hospital, Philadelphia, Pennsylvania;
    Senior Attending Staff, Department of Surgery, St. Joseph's Hospital, Philadelphia, Pennsylvania

George F. Wallace, D.P.M.
Private Practice
Hasbrouck, New Jersey
    Clinical Instructor, Department of Surgery, Pennsylvania College of Podiatric Medicine;
    Clinical Assistant, Department of Orthopedic and Traumatic Surgery, Podiatry Section, Hackensack Medical Center, Hackensack, New Jersey;
    Staff, South Bergen Hospital, Hasbrouck Heights, New Jersey;
    Staff, Kennedy Memorial Hospital at Saddle Brook, Saddle Brook, New York

Kim Weeber, D.P.M.
Private Practice
Colorado Foot and Ankle Clinic
Englewood, Colorado
    Two Years of Residency, Atlanta Hospital, Atlanta, Georgia;
    Staff, Highlands Center Hospital, Denver, Colorado;
    Staff, Pulse Medical Staff, Englewood, Colorado

Edwin W. Wolf, D.P.M.
Private Practice
New York, New York
    Diplomate, American Board of Podiatric Surgery;
    Director of Residency and Podiatric Medical Education, Parsons Hospital, Queens, New York;
    Attending Surgeon, St. Clare's Hospital, New York, New York;
    Consultant, Veterans Administration Hospital, St. Albans, Queens, New York

Gerard V. Yu, D.P.M.
Private Practice
Euclid, Ohio
    Associate Professor and Chairman, Department of Surgery, Ohio College of Podiatric Medicine;
    Three Years of Residency, Doctors Hospital, Tucker, Georgia;
    Member, Dow Corning Implant Advisory Panel;
    Staff, Huron Road Hospital, Cleveland, Ohio;
    Faculty, Doctors Hospital Podiatric Education and Research Institute, Tucker, Georgia

Contents

SECTION 1

Fundamentals and Principles

SECTION **2**

Surgical Patients with Special Medical Considerations

SECTION 1

Fundamentals and Principles

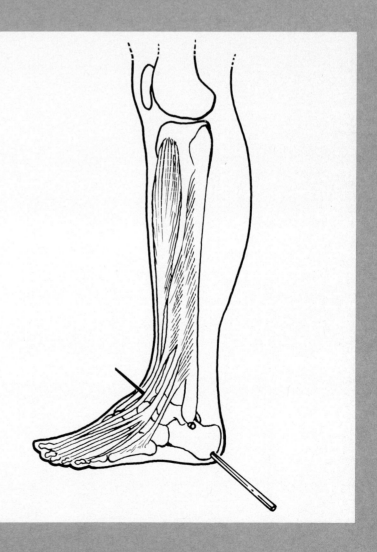

CHAPTER 1

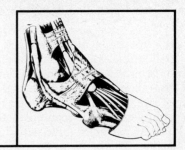

Anatomy

Daniel J. McCarthy, D.P.M., Ph.D.

Developmental Anatomy of the Lower Extremity

The art and science of surgery can be viewed as an exercise in applied anatomy. In this sense, anatomical considerations become important to the podiatric surgeon and an understanding of normal and abnormal morphology becomes pivotal to the outcome of operative procedures.

The anatomical discipline can be reduced into three divisions: the developmental, the microscopic, and the gross applications. The present discussion will touch on the morphogenetic events relative to the ontogeny of the lower extremities. The intent is to survey the topic rather than to be encyclopedic. The reader is referred to such works as that of Sarrafian for a more complete discourse on developmental anatomy.

The initial indication of development of the lower extremities of human embryos occurs in the third week of gestation as a diminutive blastemic bud lateral to the fifth lumbar and first sacral myotomes (1). Once begun, the prospective anlage of the extremity develops fairly rapidly from the fourth fetal week.

The primordial blastema is convex dorsally and flat ventrally. Early growth extends the part perpendicular to the trunk in a lateral direction. Initially, the proximal portion is cylindrical but it becomes tapered towards its end. The four-week-old embryo demonstrates the anlage of prospective thigh and leg and the prospective foot appears as a distally disposed disc in the seventh week (2) (Fig. 1.1).

Important morphogenetic changes occur almost daily and relationships may be somewhat confusing because the embryo is arched with the prospective head region facing caudally and complex rotations of parts are occurring.

Early on the prospective plantar surface is directed cephalad in a manner similar to that of a palms up position of one's hand in which the thumbs are laterally disposed.

As the sixth embryonic week ensues, 90% of inward rotation occurs. The left foot disc rotates counterclockwise and the right moves clockwise (3). Consequently, the plantar surfaces of the feet along with the posterior leg surfaces are directed toward the mid sagittal plane of the body. While the plantar surfaces of the feet face one another during the sixth fetal week, the dorsal surfaces of the developing feet face laterally along with the future anterior leg surfaces.

The prospective tibial border of the foot and leg are oriented cephalad, while the fibular border is caudally directed.

The digits of the human foot originate as a slight cleavage from the distal convexity of the foot disc (4). The third toe forms an apex and is the longest member initially. The second toe is next to develop to be followed by the first, fourth, and finally fifth digits. This occurrence can be expressed as the digital formula $3 > 2 > 1 > 4 > 5$. There is considerable variation of digital formulations until the usual adult formula $1 > 2 > 3 > 4 > 5$ is attained late in the sixth fetal week (3) (Fig. 1.2).

The metatarsal length formula again demonstrates the third as the longest early in the sixth fetal week. Like the digits, it is expressed $3 > 2 > 1 > 4 > 5$. During the last trimester of pregnancy the adult metatarsal length formula is reached as $3 > 1 > 3 > 4 > 5$.

Yet another interesting modification of the six-week-old human embryo is the appearance of the plantar pads. These are aggregations of fat and connective tissues occurring at the regions of prospective interdigital spaces. Additional tibial and fibular pads form.

As the eighth fetal week approaches, the fibular pad is lost while the tibial and first interdigital pad merge (3,5). Although the plantar (walking) pads appear to regress during the fetal period, perhaps because of swelling, the hallucal and remaining three interdigital pads can be seen postnatally.

As the embryonic period closes, the toes are well delineated, the great toe is oriented on the tibial border of the foot, and all digits are fanned out and well separated. The foot shows no angulation and is in equinus relative to the leg. The lower extremity viewed in its entirety is in external rotation (6).

As the fetal period begins with the close of the eighth embryonic week, the foot is in 90° of equinus and is adducted. The foot becomes supinated and is externally rotated relative to the leg. Bohm states that dorsiflexion of the foot on the ankle occurs in the middle of the third month of gestation. Marked pedal supination with adductus of the first metatarsal, as well as a small amount of equinus, persist, however (3).

The foot pronates into a position of midsupination early in the fourth month. Equinus is not now present but mild metatarsus adductus can be observed. Pronatory changes continue through the fetal period, but some degree of supination may persist after birth.

Failure of the foot and leg to undergo the rotational and morphogenetic changes just described results in a variety of congenital deformities including talipes equino varus (3,7).

DIFFERENTIATION

The differentiation of tissues has been studied in humans by observation and by experimentation in animals. Urodele amphibians have the ability to regenerate whole limbs, tails, and eye parts (8). It has been shown that induction of tissues and organs requires interaction between mesoderm and ectoderm and that innervation plays a crucial role in organ development.

Regenerating limbs in experimental animals develop from a blastema in much the same way as has been observed in embryonic human limbs. The limb primordium in the human is blastemic and is first heralded by lateral ectodermal ridges. Differentiation occurs in a proximodistal direction (1).

The human skeleton appears first as a condensation of mesenchyme that subsequently undergoes chondrification and ossification (Fig. 1.3). In the six-week-old embryo, the mesenchymal anlage of metatarsals and phalanges are widely spread apart with a thick web separating them (9).

The intermetatarsal angle between the first and second metatarsals is about 32° in the second month of gestation. As the eighth month is approached, the adult angulation of 60° is established. During this period, the first metatarsal demonstrates rapid growth

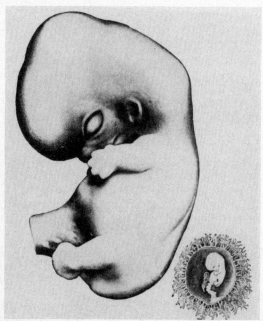

Figure 1.1. Limb position and embryonic curvature of human fetus at age of seven weeks. (Reprinted with permission from Corliss CE: *Patten's Human Embryology*. New York, McGraw-Hill Book Co, 1976.)

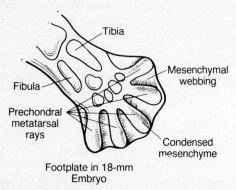

Footplate in 18-mm Embryo

Figure 1.2. Skeletal development of human foot during sixth embryonic week. Prechondral metatarsal rays are in place and condensed; mesenchyme webs interdigital regions. (Modified from Bardeen CR: Studies of the development of the human skeleton. *Am J Anat* 4:265, 1905.

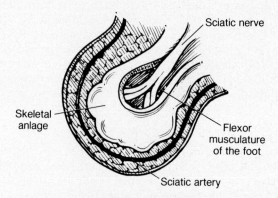

Limb bud in 11-mm Embryo

Figure 1.3. Development of flexor musculature of human foot in relation to tibial nerve as it proceeds distally from sciatic nerve in five-week-old embryos. (Modified from Sarrafian SK: *Anatomy of the Foot and Ankle*. Philadelphia, JB Lippincott Co, 1983.)

to established adult relationships with the lesser metatarsals. During the third month of gestation, metatarsal II angles at 13° in cross section to incline toward the first metatarsal, which angles 25° toward the second. This angulation decreases with growth so that the second metatarsal inclines at a 5° angle and the first metatarsal rotation toward the second decreases to 13° (Fig. 1.4). These adult relationships are established during the eighth month of gestation (3).

The chronological sequence of chondrification in the foot in the human embryo is summarized in Figure 1.5. The middle three metatarsals are first to appear, whereas the distal phalanx of the fifth digit is the last to chondrify.

OSSEOUS MORPHOGENESIS

The tridactylic fanlike characteristic of the evolving discount foot has already been mentioned. The median ray, destined to become the third metatarsal and its associated phalanges, is the principal member and two other ray rudiments appear on either side of it. When the fetus is six weeks old, all five rays may be identified (Fig. 1.6).

Those condensations of mesenchyme destined to become bones must undergo division to form joints. Such activities are heralded by the division of single homogenous interzones. This is the condition that exists as the fetal period ends in the eighth week of gestation (Fig. 1.7).

Cavitations develop within the matrix in locations of the prospective joint structure. The interzones are no longer homogenous as three layered interzones of mesenchyme form. The processes of chondrification and ossification of the mesenchymal models of bone will be briefly reviewed in the histological study, which will shortly follow.

Interesting developmental changes occur in the relationships of individual foot bones, particularly those of the tarsal bones. A slit occurs in the central mesenchymal condensation of the leg as the prospective tibia and fibula evolve. This event tends to separate the developing foot into cephalad and caudal components. The prospective tibia relates to the developing talus, navicular, cuneiforms, and metatarsals I and II. The fibula extends to relate to the calcaneus, cuboid, and metatarsals III, IV, and V.

As early as the sixth embryonic week the prospective talar element is wedged between the distal extremities of the developing tibia and fibula.

In six-week-old embryos, the tibial malleolus projects more distally than the fibular malleolus. However, the obliquity of the distal tibia is corrected so that by the end of the eighth week the fibular malleolus assumes the adult relationship and is situated distal to the medial. The distal extremities of tibia and fibula now make contact.

The calcaneus and fibula are in direct contact at the end of the sixth week of gestation. The talus and calcaneus lie side by side at this early period with the talus overlapping the calcaneus slightly on its medial flank (10). As the seventh embryonic week closes with the appearance of the sustentaculum tali, the talus narrows and elongates and moves to a position superior to the calcaneus. Complex positional and rotational alterations occur in the bones making up the greater tarsus. The medially directed talar neck angulates about 33° at four months of gestation (3). A correction of this angle is accomplished as growth proceeds so that the postnatal condition demonstrates an average 22° of inward angulation relative to the trochlea of the talus.

The calcaneus is initially relatively short: its posterior aspect grows more rapidly than does the anterior as the adult shape is assumed. The marked embryonic varus torsion of the calcaneus decreases over time from 32° to 6° or less at birth.

The medial cuneiform, cuboid, and navicular are identifiable during the middle of the sixth week of gestation. The middle and lateral cuneiforms delay their appearance until the seventh week of embryogeny (3).

Symphalangia (fusion of the phalanges) is common between the middle and distal phalanges of the fifth toe and represents a failure of the joint to form. Other developmentally relevant fusions involve osseous or cartilaginous talocalcaneal coalitions, particularly bridges between the sustentaculum tali and contiguous portions of the talus. Connections between calcaneus and navicular, as well as calcaneus and cuboid, can develop. Fusions between the cuboid and metatarsal IV or metatarsal III with the third cuneiform may also occur.

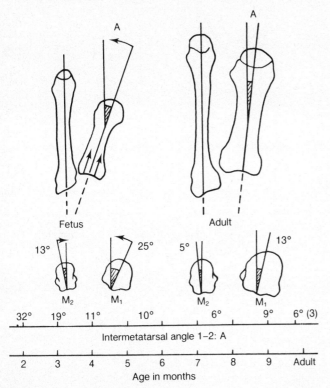

Figure 1.4. Rotation and angulation of metatarsals during growth. (Modified from Sarrafian SK: *Anatomy of the Foot and Ankle.* Philadelphia, JB Lippincott Co, 1983.)

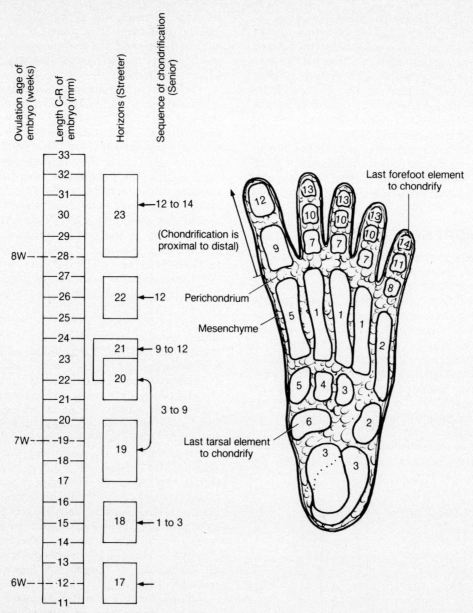

Figure 1.5. Chronological sequence of chondrification of embryonic foot. (Modified from Sarrafian SK: *Anatomy of the Foot and Ankle*. Philadelphia, JB Lippincott Co, 1983.)

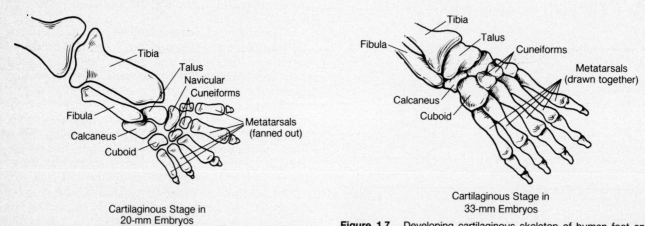

Cartilaginous Stage in
20-mm Embryos

Figure 1.6. Cartilaginous arrangement of skeleton of human fetal foot at end of sixth fetal week. (Modified from Bardeen CR: Studies of the development of the human skeleton. *Am J Anat* 4:265, 1905.)

Cartilaginous Stage in
33-mm Embryos

Figure 1.7. Developing cartilaginous skeleton of human foot and leg in early fetal period (eighth week). (Modified from Bardeen CR: Studies of the development of the human skeleton. *Am J Anat* 4:265, 1905.)

Ligaments and tendon sheaths usually differentiate in a proximodistal orientation. The fibrous interconnections known as ligaments make their appearance before the appearance of their continguous joint spaces. No useful purpose would be served in describing the appearance of the dozens of ligaments that form in the human foot in fetuses of 33 to 85 mm long.

The posterior talofibular ligament transversely bridges the region between the posterior aspect of the fibular malleolus and the posterolateral border of the talus. It is among the first ligaments to appear in the fetal human feet of 33-mm fetuses. Among the last to appear is the talocalcaneal interosseous ligament in the sinus tarsi of fetuses measuring 85 mm.

It is important to recognize the appearance of several ligamentous and ligament-like structures that profoundly affect the function of other structures governing the foot (3).

Consider the anterior annular ligament, perhaps better described as the extensor retinaculum, because the structure is not a true ligament. In the adult foot it contains the extensor and invertor muscles of the foot. It consists of superior and divided inferior bands. The superior part of the extensor retinaculum appears first in fetuses 30 mm long, transversely attaching the distal portions of tibia and fibula. As growth proceeds to the 40 mm stage, the inferior band of the extensor retinaculum takes the vague form of a medially directed Y. Its upper wing is modified as the frondiform ligament to enclose the four tendons of m. extensor digitorum longus. This tunnellike structural plan next involves the tendon of m. extensor hallucis longus, which lies adjacent to the extensor digitorum longus tendon.

Finally, in fetuses 65 mm long, a tunnel forms to enclose the tendon of m. tibialis anterior. At this time the lower limb of the inferior extensor retinaculum is in place. These structures become intimately involved with the deep fascia enclosing the foot and leg (Figs. 1.8, 1.9, 1.10). Blood vessels and nerves are directed deep to the extensor retinaculum in a groove between the tendons of m. extensor hallucis longus and m. tibialis anterior (3).

The peroneal retinaculum in the adult foot demonstrates superior and inferior bands that contain the muscles peroneus longus et brevis. Three structural levels are apparent developmentally. Initially, the canal for the peroneal muscle anlage posterior to the fibular malleolus is closed by a semiannular lamina of connective tissue. The formation of this single tunnel occurs early on in 23-mm long fetuses.

The superior and inferior peroneal retinaculum arise as separate encirclements of the longus and brevis tendons, each having a thin wall of connective tissue about their respective sheaths. These ringlike structures begin and end with the posteriorlateral aspect of the calcaneal apophysis. They will make connections with the peroneal tubercle of the calcaneus.

Additionally, the tendon of m. peroneus longus grooves the inferolateral aspect of the cuboid to cross-

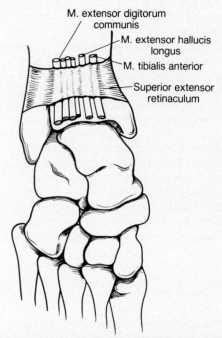

Extensor Retinaculum in 30-mm embryo

Figure 1.8. Development of extensor retinaculum occurs initially by formation of superior band (1). Tunnels of extrinsic extensor muscles of foot follow: that for m. extensor hallucis longus is first, m. tibialis anterior last. These events characterize the 30-mm long embryo.

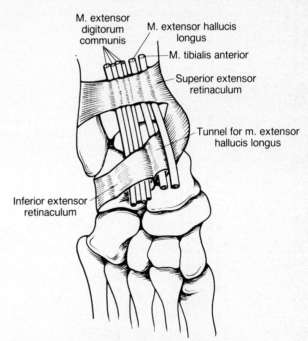

Extensor Retinaculum in 40-mm fetus

Figure 1.9. Frondiform ligament and inferior extensor retinaculum develops in 40-mm long fetuses in relation to tendons of m. extensor digitorum longus (2,3). Tendons of m. extensor hallucis longus and m. tibialis anterior are well formed at this time.

brace the foot by changing direction to insert on the inferolateral border of the first metatarsal and medial cuneiform. This requires the formation of a more or less dense sheath of connective tissue for the peroneus longus. It extends from the cuboid proximal to the groove for peroneus longus to the base of the fifth metatarsal (3).

Continuity is established between the several cavities enclosing the peroneal tendons. The plantar segment just mentioned begins the process, to be followed by the double ringed portion more proximally, and the retromalleolar peroneal tunnel completes the process.

The flexor retinaculum develops about the medial aspect of the ankle joint and contains the tendons of the extrinsic musculature for plantarflexion and inversion of the foot. It, like the anterior compartment, has been incorrectly called the lacinate and medial annular ligament.

The initiating developmental event is the formation of fibrous sheaths forming tunnels for the tendons of m. tibialis posterior, flexor digitorum longus, and flexor hallucis longus in order from anterior to posterior. The flexor retinaculum is formed secondarily as connective tissue slips pass superfically between the tunnels formed for tibialis posterior and flexor digitorum and extend distally to incorporate fibers of origin of m. abductor hallucis (3). The posterior tibial nerve, artery, and vein pass through a third compartment of the flexor retinaculum, and the tendon of m. flexor hallucis longus forms the fourth compartment.

These structural events cover the tarsal tunnel, and the fibers of the flexor retinaculum unite with those of the extensor retinaculum.

The cuneocuboidometatarsal interosseous ligaments present an interesting morphogenesis in that mesenchymal connective tissues form a homogenous lamina. This structure fills the interspaces between adjacent sides of all metatarsals, all cuneiforms, and between the lateral cuneiform and cuboid. Ultimately, by a process of absorption, only oblique transverse interosseous bands persist. The medial cuneiform attaches to the medial aspect of the base of the second metatarsal. The lateral aspect of the second metatarsal has interosseous attachment to the lateral cuneiform. The lateral cuneiform makes interosseous attachment to the medial aspect of the base of the fourth metatarsal. No attachments remain between the bases of the first and second metatarsals. No interosseous ligamentous attachments persist between the fourth and fifth metatarsals and the cuboid (3).

The deep transverse intermetatarsal ligament is important both to podiatric surgery and to orthopedics. Its development occurs slowly in 23-mm long fetuses and its morphogenesis may extend to the 110 mm stage. Connective tissue slips extend from the plantar capsules of the metatarsophalangeal joints. All five joints are involved and development consists of a thickening of the fibrous structures. The long and short flexor tendons are superficial to the deep transverse metatarsal ligaments except in the regions of the first and fifth metatarsal joints, where the structure is not present.

The long plantar ligament attaches anteriorly to the bases of the second, third, fourth, and frequently to the fifth metatarsals, as well as to the plantar tuberosity of the cuboid. Posteriorly it is anchored to both medial and lateral processes of the inferior surface of the calcaneus, as well as to the anterior calcaneal tubercle. Connective tissue fibers of the ligamentous anlage form in association with the plantar calcaneocuboid joint and the inferior surface of the sheath of peroneus longus. However, all of these structures retain their identity even before the sixth month of development. Eventually the long plantar ligament will form a compartment for the deep passage of the tendon of m. peroneus longus (3).

MYOGENESIS

There is evidence that condensations of mesenchyme destined to differentiate into muscles do so in response to inductive influences of nerves. Very early in ontogeny, myoblasts and scleroblastema, the precursor tissues of muscle and bone, respectively, cannot be distinguished one from the other.

Initially, cavitations that indicate the locations of future intermuscular spaces appear and nerves destined to supply these regions extend distally into the spaces.

Anlages of prospective muscle groups of the foot and leg begin to organize in situ and nerves infiltrate these masses at about the 12-mm stage (11). The muscles of the anterior compartment destined to become the extensors of the foot on the leg differentiate in relation to the peroneal nerve (Fig. 1.11). M. tibialis anterior is identified in relationship to a broad flat tendon contiguous to the medial cuneiform and base of the first metatarsal.

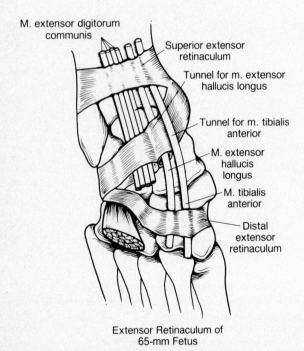

M. extensor digitorum communis

Superior extensor retinaculum

Tunnel for m. extensor hallucis longus

Tunnel for m. tibialis anterior

M. extensor hallucis longus

M. tibialis anterior

Distal extensor retinaculum

Extensor Retinaculum of 65-mm Fetus

Figure 1.10. Inferior extensor retinaculum is well formed in 65-mm long fetuses. Tendinous sheaths for m. tibialis anterior and m. extensor digitorum longus are well demonstrated. The tendons proper of extensor hallucis longus and tibialis posterior can be identified as they emerge from beneath retinaculum. (Modified from Sarrafian SK: *Anatomy of the Foot and Ankle.* Philadelphia, JB Lippincott Co, 1983).

M. extensor hallucis longus and m. extensor digitorum longus undergo cleavage from a single myogenous anlage. Originally the prospective extensor tendon plate cannot be distinguished from the scleroblastema, but bone and tendon eventually undergo separation and individual tendons organize in relation to the metatarsal rays they will serve.

As this segmentation occurs, the belly of m. extensor digitorum et hallucis brevis organizes.

The peroneal musculature develops in close proximity to the anlage of the anterior compartment, but a clear separation is established very early (3). Initially, both peroneus longus and brevis tendons relate to the base of the fifth metatarsal. The crossbrace extension of the tendon of peroneus longus does not appear until the end of the eighth week. At this time, it grooves the cuboid bone to attach to the medial cuneiform. It is initially tightly attached to the scleroblastema of the foot.

The musculature of the superficial compartment of the posterior leg unites with the posterior surface of the calcaneus; m. gastrocnemius and m. soleus become separate muscle masses and the tendo achillis becomes well differentiated.

The musculature of the deep compartment of the posterior leg terminates on a flattened flexor tendon plate (Fig. 1.3). M. flexor hallucis longus becomes distinct fibularly to be followed by the more tibially oriented m. flexor digitorum longus. These last named muscles become bound in a common sheath as they cross the inferior tarsal surface during the eighth week. M. tibialis posterior emerges from a more deeply oriented tibially situated anlage: its tendinous plate will attach to the navicular anlage, but will fan out deeply to involve the inferior surfaces of all of the tarsal bones except the talus.

The intrinsic muscles of the foot are at first indistinct relative to the more precocious extrinsic

musculature of the foot (11). M. flexor accessorious (quadratus plantae) and m. abductor digiti quinti are the first muscle masses to be observed within the foot itself. The intrinsic musculature of the fifth ray precedes the seven interossei and four lumbricales in development.

Superficially on the flexor surface of the developing foot, m. flexor digitorum brevis emerges as a somewhat fan-shaped structure that will undergo cleavage distally to form four tendons inserting on the lesser digits (11).

Adductor hallucis develops from a single anlage deep to the flexor plate of the developing foot. The anlage divides to form transverse and oblique heads. The more superficially situated intrinsic muscles investing the first ray emerge as distinct entities as the eighth embryonic week closes. Flexor hallucis brevis separates into medial and lateral segments. It becomes tendinous distally to attach to the tibial and fibular aspects of the plantar surface of the proximal hallucal phalanx. The fibular tendinous slip associates with that of m. adductor hallucis which is well formed at this time (3). The tibial tendinous slip associates with the less well-formed abductor hallucis that marks the medial border of the developing foot.

As the third trimester is approached the musculature of the lower extremity is definitively developed and all muscle groups are identifiable (Fig. 1.12). The foot remains in marked adductus at this time (Fig. 1.13). The condition may persist after birth.

ANGIOGENESIS

The development of the blood supply to the lower extremities is part of the process known as angiogenesis. These morphogenetic events involve only the mesodermal germ layer. Angioblastic tissues originally

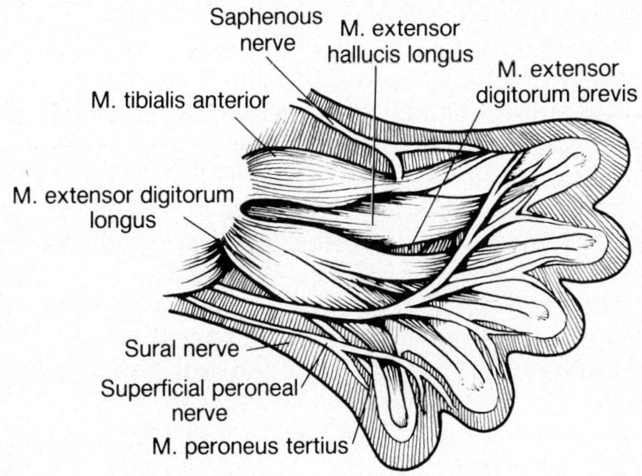

Saphenous nerve
M. extensor hallucis longus
M. extensor digitorum brevis
M. tibialis anterior
M. extensor digitorum longus
Sural nerve
Superficial peroneal nerve
M. peroneus tertius

Foot in 20-mm Embryo

Figure 1.11. Differentiation of m. extensor digitorum brevis et longus, m. extensor hallucis longus, m. tibialis anterior, and m. peroneus longus et brevis in relationship to sural nerve laterally and to superficial peroneal nerve tibially in seven-week-old human embryo. (Modified from Sarrafian SK: *Anatomy of the Foot and Ankle.* Philadelphia, JB Lippincott Co, 1983.)

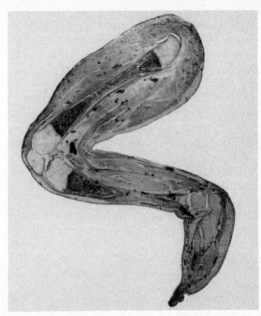

Figure 1.12. Cryomicrotomy midsagittal section of full limb of fetus entering third trimester. All muscle groups can be identified at this time.

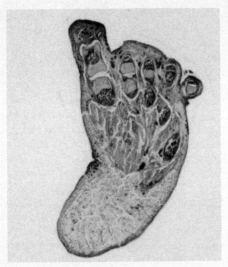

Figure 1.13.   Cryomicrotomy section of foot of fetus entering third trimester. Typical developmental condition of adductus is obvious.

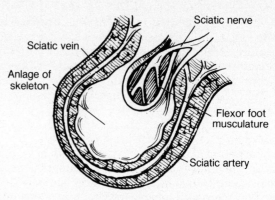

Flexor Surface in Limb Bud of 11-mm Embryo

Figure 1.14.   Vascularization of foot disc via sciatic artery on extensor surface of five-week-old embryo. Sciatic vein lies on flexor surface. (Modified from Sarrafian SK: *Anatomy of the Foot and Ankle.* Philadelphia, JB Lippincott Co, 1983.)

appear as isolated solid masses and cords that hollow out leaving flattened lining cells, the endothelium.

A complete description of angiogenesis is beyond the scope of this discussion. It is a complex event in which extraembryonic vessels are important early on. Vitelline and umbilical vessels are responsible for nourishment and excretion of the rapidly growing embryo. However, it is characteristic for the embryo to lay down complicated networks of small vessels and to select from vessels that will persist (12). Frequently, vessels important in the embryonic stage diminish to be replaced by permanent structures that will persist in the adult form. The developmental pattern of the aortic arches is an excellent example of this phenomenon.

In the development of the arterial supply to the human lower extremity, the principle vessel is known as the sciatic artery (Fig. 1.14). It is given off as one of the branches very early in embryogenesis: the foot plexus forms the termination of the sciatic artery of the umbilical artery. The umbilical artery persists in the adult body as the internal iliac artery.

In 9-mm long embryos, the external iliac artery is diminutive, but it extends as the femoral artery as embryonic growth proceeds. The femoral artery becomes dominant, while the sciatic artery is fragmented and its remaining sections are annexed by the femoral artery to form the popliteal and peroneal arteries. The inferior gluteal artery of the adult marks the proximal vestige of the original sciatic artery.

The popliteal and distal femoral arteries unite to form the adult posterior tibial artery, which extends into the plantar foot vessels that terminate as plantar digital arteries (13).

The popliteal artery gives off another sprout that will extend along the extensor surface of the leg as the anterior tibial artery. The anterior tibial artery extends to join the vessels of the dorsal plexus of the foot, and eventually tarsal, metatarsal, and dorsal digital arteries are formed.

VEINS

Early in embryogenesis the extraembryonic umbilical and vitelline veins communicate with the cardinal veins within the embryo itself. Paired precardinal veins extend cranial while the two postcardinal veins proceed caudad. The latter vessels fuse as the iliac anastomosis of the postcardinals. Complex additions and deletions of embryonic veinous systems occur in a manner similar to those events characteristic of the development of arteries (12).

Veins tend to form superficial rebate to the more deeply situated arteries. The limb blastema demonstrates a peripheral border vein that drains into the iliac anastomosis of the postcardinal system. The primitive tibial border vein is destined to regress, but the fibular section will persist to a degree in the adult. The fibular portion of the border vein is annexed at the level of the knee by the great saphenous vein that arises separately from the embryonic postcardinal vein. In addition, the great saphenous vein gives off posterior tibial and femoral tributaries.

The fibular border vein persists in the adult as the inferior gluteal vein. The small saphenous vein and the anterior tibial vein are also remnants of the border vein on the fibular aspect of the developing limb bud.

Principal veins are interlaced by complex networks of interconnecting veins. Of these, some persist in the adult form, possibly in response to oxygen gradient factors. Others are destined to regress and disappear. The endothelial lining of veins is peculiar in forming flaps that prevent retrograde flow of venous blood.

LYMPHATICS

Lymphatics develop as more or less discrete mesenchymal cavitations. These link into continuous channels that continue to ramify into a unidirectional system for the return of tissue fluid.

Embryonically, six lymphatic sacs develop (3). The last of these are the caudally situated and paired sciatic sacs that are in place as the second embryonic month closes. The general plan of development is initiated cranially and it proceeds caudally. During the sixth week, paired jugular sacs appear to be followed by a single retroperitoneal.

The cisterna chyli is also unpaired and appears at the end of the second month. It receives tissue fluid from the two posterior sacs, which in turn drain the lymphatics of the feet and leg (12).

Lymph sacs, including the posterior sacs, disintegrate to form networks that will form lymph nodes in a chainlike organization.

Histologically, lymphatics are lined with flattened endothelial cells. They resemble thin-walled veins, and like veins, have systems of valves to prevent retrograde flow of tissue fluid (12).

PERIPHERAL NERVES

The development of the central nervous system, consisting of the brain and spinal cord, is a complex issue beyond the scope of this discussion. The development of peripheral nerves is also complicated and much of what is known or suspected has been the result of animal experimentation. For example, it has been shown that the presence of peripheral nerve tissue is required to induce blastema. Urodele amphibians are capable of regenerating amputated limbs and tails as adult animals. However, it has been shown that the experimental removal of and its presumed inductive control of peripheral nerve tissue in the region of the blastema can prevent the normally expected limb bud regeneration (8).

Sensory and motor spinal nerves innervate the lower extremities: these are classified as somatic afferent and somatic efferent, respectively. The arrangement of spinal nerves to the lower extremities is segmental, but this organization is established in response to the development of myotomes (12). It is not inherently metameric relative to the morphogenesis of the neural tube and neural crest as such.

As the fourth embryonic week closes, developing spinal ganglia are represented as localized enlargements contiguous to the ganglionic crest. At this time, ventral root fibers can be seen extending from the ventrolateral wall of the developing spinal cord. These fibers will eventually organize into motor tracts. Dorsal root fibers emerge from the adjacent spinal ganglia where their cell bodies are situated. These elements are destined to form the sensory tracts. As development proceeds, centrally directed dorsal fibers enter the marginal zone of the spinal cord. Peripheral processes join fibers of the ventral root and the elements of a simple reflex arc are in place.

Early in development, the spinal ganglia are interconnected by cellular bridges of the neural crest. These attachments become disassociated in 10-mm long embryos, and the dorsal and ventral rami become identifiable. Ventral and lateral terminal divisions subsequently form from the ramus communicans, which has developed from a medial projection off the ventral ramus (3).

Nerve plexuses arise as interconnecting loops of nerve tissue and extend from one spinal nerve to adjacent nerves in series (12). Regions where the muscles serving the limbs are contiguous to the musculature of the trunk appear to attract the formation of nerve plexuses. The lumbosacral plexus is evident in embryos of six weeks, an event that follows the appearance of the brachial plexus.

The lumbosacral plexus bifurcates to form a ventral division destined to supply the flexor musculature, while a dorsal division innervates the extensor muscles. Ingrowing nerve fibers are guided toward their terminal points by chemotaxis and a directive-oriented ultrastructure. The attraction for the ingrowth of nerves is initially nonspecific and is in response to increased metabolic activity in a part (3).

Initially, the lumbosacral plexus is represented by a flat plate of developing nerve cells. From this plate, nerve cords extend into the intermuscular spaces to end in the premuscle masses. These developmental activities are recapitulated whenever nerves regenerate.

The flattened plate of the developing lumbosacral plexus bifurcates into paired medial and lateral trunks. This separation is enhanced by the physical presence of the anlage of pelvis and the femur. The medial trunks are ventrally situated in the embryo: its cranial component develops into the adult obturator nerve while the caudal component becomes the tibial nerve (3).

The lateral trunks are dorsally situated in the embryo: its cranial component develops into the adult femoral nerve while the caudal component becomes the peroneal nerve. The adult sciatic nerve is comprised of the caudal pair (11).

The limb bud receives contributions from the

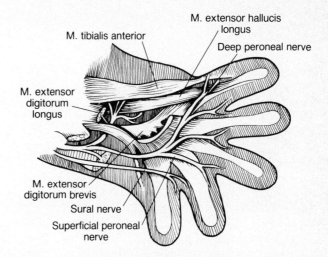

Deep Layer, Extensor Surface
in 20-mm Embryo

Figure 1.15. Neurogenesis in seven-week-old embryo: Anterior tibial nerve, sural nerve, superficial peroneal nerve, and deep peroneal nerve. Muscle masses differentiating include m. tibialis anterior, m. extensor hallucis longus, m. extensor digitorum longus et brevis. (Modified from Sarrafian SK: *Anatomy of the Foot and Ankle*. Philadelphia, JB Lippincott Co, 1983.)

sciatic nerve that can be easily identified in seven-week-old embryos. Included are the saphenous, sural, anterior tibial, deep, and superficial peroneal nerves (Fig. 1.15). Muscles develop in concert with the developing nerve supply, the latter apparently in part inducing this developmental event.

References

1. O'Rahilly R, Gardner E, Bray DJ: The ectodermal thickening and ridge in the limbs of staged human embryos. *J Embryol Exp Morphol* 256, 1956.
2. Streeter GL: Developmental horizons in human embryos. In *Contributions to Embryology*, Washington DC, Carnegie Institution of Washington, vols 21, 32, 34, 1945, 1948, 1951.
3. Sarrafian SK: *Anatomy of the Foot and Ankle*. Philadelphia, JB Lippincott Co, 1983.
4. Bardeen CR, Lewis WH: Development of the limbs, body, wall and back in man. *Am J Anat* 1:1, 1901–1902.
5. Straus WL Jr.: Growth of the human foot and its evolutionary significance. *Contrib Embryol* 19:95, 1927.
6. Corliss CE: *Patten's Human Embryology*. New York, McGraw-Hill Book Co, 1978.
7. Gardner E, Gray DJ, O'Rahilly R: The prenatal development of the skeleton and joints of the human foot. *J Bone Joint Surg*(Am) 41:5, 847, 1959.
8. Stone LS: Regeneration. In Thornton CS (ed):*Vertebrate Regeneration*. Chicago, University of Chicago Press, 1956.
9. Bardeen CR. Studies of the development of the human skeleton. *Am J Anat* 4:265, 1905.
10. Barlow TE: Some observations on the development of the human foot. Thesis. University of Manchester, Manchester, 1943.
11. Bardeen CR: Development and variations of the nerves and musculature of the inferior extremity and of the neighboring regions of the trunk of man. *Am J Anat* 6:263, 1906–1907.
12. Arey LB: *Developmental Anatomy*, ed 7. Philadelphia, WB Saunders Co, 1974.
13. Senior HO: The development of the arteries of the human lower extremities. *Am J Anat* 25:55, 1919.

Microscopic Anatomy

THE SKIN

The human skin is the largest organ of the human body and has many complex functions (1). It is divisible into an outer epidermis of ectodermal origin and an underlying dermis of mesodermal origin. The two layers are fused at the epidermal-dermal junction where rete ridges of the epidermis interdigitate with the dermal papillae. Inductive influences are interchanged at this point and for this reason the skin has considerable ability to regenerate.

The epidermis is divisible into four cellular strata (Fig. 1.16). Some authorities recognize a fifth layer, the stratum lucidum, situated between the stratum corneum and stratum granulosum; this layer, however, is doubtless an artifact of fixation at the light microscopic level.

The deepest of the epidermal layers is the stratum basale, which lies on a basement membrane to which hemidesmosomes are afixed. The basal cell is the least differentiated of all epidermal cells: it is a high cuboidal cell with a large nucleus; the surrounding cyto-plasm is relatively attenuated with few organelles. Depending on the inductive influences operable, the cell may replicate itself or enter into the biosynthetic pathway of keratinization (2). Under other circumstances it may form adnexa (hair follicles, nails, or sebaceous or sudiferous glands). In wound healing, cells of the germinativum have been observed to be migratory and phagocytic (3).

The stratum spinosum is of variable thickness depending on its location throughout the body. The term "spinosum" indicates the occurrence of apparent bridges between cells. In actuality bridging does not exist: Electron microscopy has identified "tight junctions" at those points where hemidesmosomes of adjacent cells are present (2). Spinosal cells begin a process of flattening out in parallel to the free surface of the skin and the nuclei become progressively smaller. The cells' cytoplasm becomes more dominant and rich in organelles such as rough endoplasmic reticulum, Golgi apparatus, free ribosomes, membrane coating granules, and tonofilaments; all of these structures are important to the processes of keratinization (4).

The stratum granulosum also varies in thickness and constitutes the third layer of skin. It is deeply basophilic because of the presence of keratohyaline granules that grow, coalesce, and mesh with tonofilaments. Clearly these three layers of epidermis are involved in the dynamic process of keratinization. It is incorrect to view the skin as having a viable basal layer, but that subsequent layers of cells pushing upward toward the free surface of skin are in various stages of necrosis (2).

The stratum corneum is the outermost layer of the human skin. These cells, having passed through the granular layer, do not normally demonstrate even remnants of nuclei or subcellular organelles. Such cells are flattened and elongated relative to the free surface of the skin and their plasma membranes are markedly widened. A para-aminosalicylic acid (PAS) positive substance occupies the intercellular spaces and provides intercellular cohesion. Cells of the stratum corneum are normally arranged in a basket-weave formation.

The Dermis

The dermis underlies the epidermis and consists of a mucopolysaccharide matrix in which collagenic and reticular fibers are found (Fig. 1.17). The predominant cell is the fibroblast (Fig. 1.18). It is of stellate shape and has a large flattened deeply basophilic nucleus. Its cytoplasm is rich in rough endoplasmic reticulum and Golgi apparatus indicating its high level of biosynthetic activity. It produces the dermal matrix and the collagenic fibers that characterize the dermis (2). Pinocytotic vesicles are common to the fibroblast because they extrude precursor products of dermal

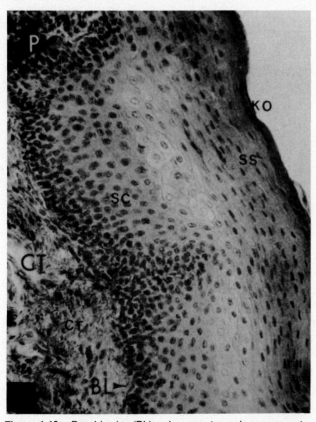

Figure 1.16. Basal lamina (BL) or basement membrane separates dermis from epidermis. Basal cells resting on membrane are high cuboidal. Stratum spinosum (SC) demonstrates gradual flattening of cells and are especially squamous or flat in form (SS) as stratum granulosum is approached. Keratinous layer of stratum corneum (KO), connective tissue of dermis (CT), and papillae (P) Light microscopy (LM) × 175. (From Matthews JL, Martin JH: *Atlas of Human Histology and Ultrastructure.* Philadelphia, Lea and Febiger, 1971.)

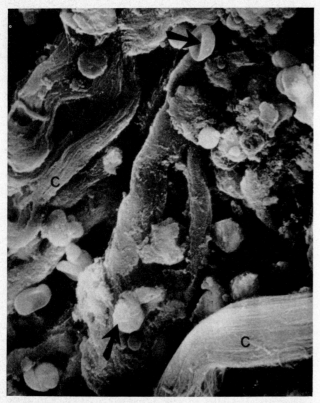

Figure 1.17.   Dermis is interlaced with collagenic (C) and reticular fibers among which red and white blood cells are found (arrows). Scanning electron microscopy (SEM).

structures into the surrounding tissues. The dermis is supplied with small caliber blood vessels and nerves. The epidermis does not ordinarily demonstrate the presence of blood vessels. Migratory cells including neutrophiles, eosinophiles, basophiles, lymphocytes, plasma cells, and histiocytes may invade the dermis.

The epidermal-dermal interface also demonstrates migratory cells.

Regenerative Ability

The skin has excellent powers for regeneration (1). When wounded, hemorrhage fills the defect and a fibrin meshwork occurs. Cells of the stratum basale become migratory following mitotic bursts at the periphery of the wound. Polymorphonuclear leukocytes followed by lymphocytes debride the wound predictably. Migratory basal cells proceed over the contiguous dermis beneath the clot until they meet cells of like type from the opposite direction (3). Eventually the defect is closed and cells proliferate upward to reconstitute the stratification normal to the epidermis. A reserve of relatively undifferentiated epidermal cells can also be recruited from adnexa in the immediate region of the wound to assist in the reconstitution of the epidermis. Fibroblasts enter the dermis and synthesize new matrix, collagenic, and reticular fibers. Blood vessels reconstitute the region of the wound by budding into the dermis. Initially, an interlacing network is formed from which the most useful are selected to persist while others atrophy.

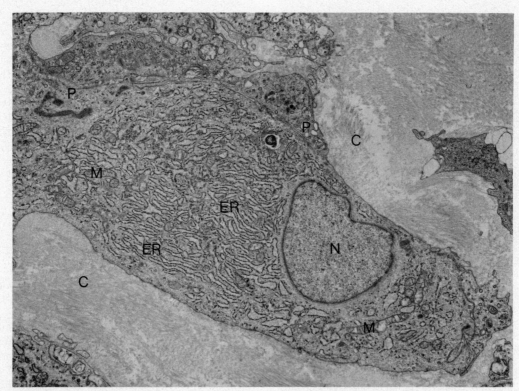

Figure 1.18.   Fibroblast is biosynthetic cell of dermis that provides matrix, collagenic, and reticular fibers to region. It is cell rich in subcellular organelles: Endoplasmic reticulum (ER), pinocytotic ves- cicles (P), collagen (C), nucleus (N), mitochondria (M). Transmission electron microscopy × 11,400 (TEM).

The adnexa are important features of the integumentary system. These structures include the hair (Fig. 1.19), glands (Fig. 1.20), and nails (Fig. 1.21). Their structural detail is discussed in relation to the respective illustrations shown here.

BONE

Bone is made up of several tissue types so as to provide form, stability, and support for the body. Each individual bone, therefore, is to be regarded as an organ.

Externally, bone is invested by the periosteum, which is a sheath of dense fibrous connective tissue: it contains blood vessels and nerves. That portion of the periosteum contiguous to bone contains multipotent cells capable of forming osteoblasts that are necessary to bone growth and repair. The periosteum is made adherent to bone by perforating or Sharpey's fibers (5).

The organization of bone substance may be characterized as compact or spongy. Both organic and inorganic constituents are present. The organic content is mainly ossein or bone collagen in a matrix or in gelatinous substances. The inorganic residues contain 85% calcium phosphate, 10% calcium carbonate, and 5% other assorted materials (5).

Compact bone demonstrates a system of interconnecting canals. Haversian canals generally traverse the long axis of long bones (Fig. 1.22). Their arrangement is less orderly in irregular bones such as the talus. Haversian canals are lined with multipotent cells capable of osteogenesis. Additionally, they conduct bloodvessels, nerves, and lymphatics. Volkmann's canals pass vertically or at an angle towards haversian canals and interconnect these channels. Compact bone is characterized by the haversian systems or osteons just described. Osteons are the structural unit in which the haversian canal is central and concentric haversian lamella, which may number up to 40 rings, surround the canal to an average thickness of 5 microns (5).

Spongy bone is characterized by loosely organized trabeculae, plates, tubules, and globular shells that are formed beneath an investment of compact bone (Fig. 1.23). Interspaces are occupied by a well vascularized marrow.

An inner endosteum is a delicate lining of marrow cavities somewhat analogous to the external periosteum.

The principle cells of bone include osteoblasts, osteocytes, and osteoclasts. Osteoblasts are specialized bone forming cells differentiated from mesenchymal precursor cells. They are positioned on the surface areas of bone and are variable in shape. Such cells have eccentric nuclei and are rich in endoplasmic

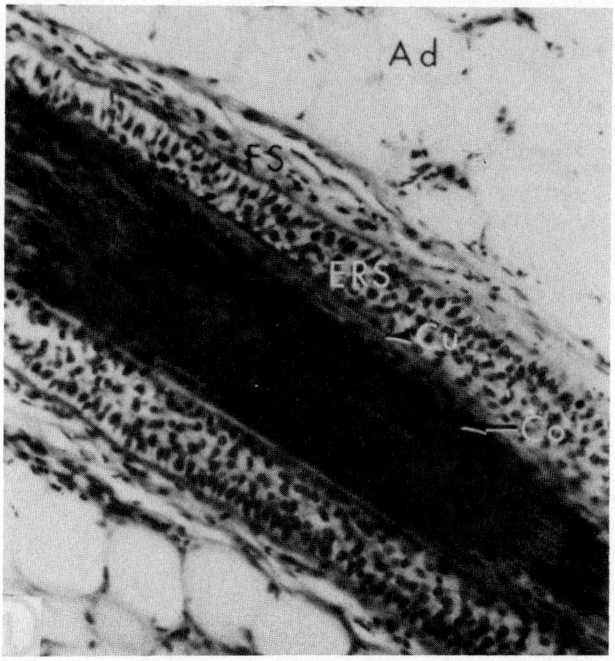

Figure 1.19. Developmentally, hair forms as result of invagination and evagination of ectodermal cells. Adipose tissue (Ad) surrounds hair follicle structure. Hair itself is surrounded by fibrous sheath (FS). External root sheath (ERS) forms outermost layer of hair that is continuous with surface epithelium. Internal root sheath arises from epithelial cells of follicle and is reflected toward free surface between external root sheath and cuticle (Cu). The cuticle and cortex (Co) consist of keratinized cells and surround narrow medulla. Hair follicles are associated with sebaceous glands and smooth muscle cells. × 200. (From Matthews JL, Martin JH: Atlas of Human Histology and Ultrastructure. Philadelphia, Lea and Febiger, 1971.)

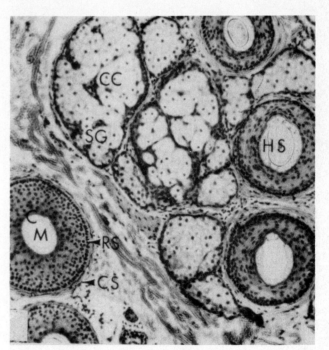

Figure 1.20. Glands of skin are of several types including sebaceous and sudiferous types. Sebaceous glands (Sg) elaborate oily substances into hair follicle about hair shaft (HS). These spherical glands are encapsulated with connective tissue. Stratified squamous cells line ducts in continuity with outer root sheath. Alveoli are filled with epithelial secretory cells that contribute to holocrine system in which cellular components degrade to make up secretion. Pyknotic nuclei are common in the cells of the central portion of the gland. (CC) LM × 350. (From Matthews JL, Martin JH: Atlas of Human Histology and Ultrastructure. Philadelphia, Lea and Febiger, 1971.)

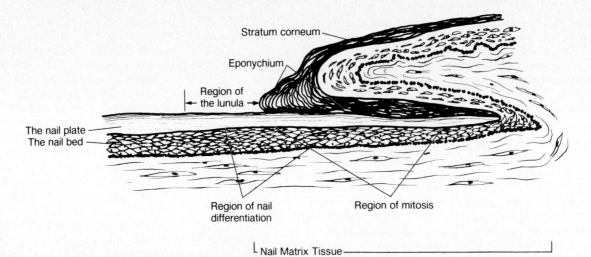

Figure 1.21.   Nails are keratinous plates developed from matrix or germinal region located proximal to nail itself and in close relationship to contiguous dorsal surface of ungual phalanx. Lateral margins are folds of skin termed the ungualabia.

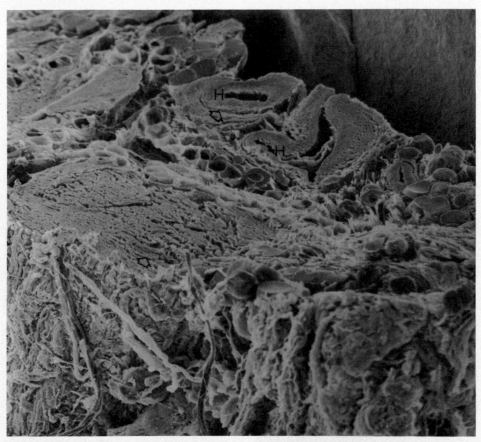

Figure 1.22.   Compact bone is characterized by haversian canals (H) surrounded by concentric matrix rings or lamellae (arrows). Volk-mann's canals intersect haversian systems and canaliculi are still smaller canals receiving bone cell processes. SEM. × 120.

reticulum for the synthesis and deposition of osteoid (Fig. 1.24). Osteoblasts possess extensive cytoplasmic processes that communicate with other like cells (6).

With the progressive deposition of bone matrix, osteoblasts become entrapped and eventually become mature osteocytes. The interconnecting cytoplasmic processes persist within channels called canaliculi. Cell bodies are resident with lacunae.

The osteoclast responsible for bone resorption is formed in part by the coalescence of osteoblasts (5). Such cells are large, plemorphic, and multinucleated. They resemble giant cells and have from 3 to 15 nuclei. The cytoplasm of osteoclasts is rich in rough endoplasmic reticulum indicating that its principal activity is to form osteolytic enzymes and to modulate the pH of bone tissue. It demonstrates a fimbriated border,

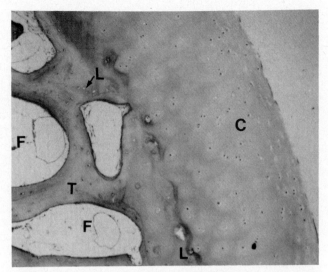

Figure 1.23. Cancellous bone is characterized by trabeculae through which vascularity is provided for internal aspect of bone. Marrow and fat also occupy deep central internal spaces. Trabeculae (T), cartilage (C), lacunae (L), fat of marrow (F). LMO. × 80.

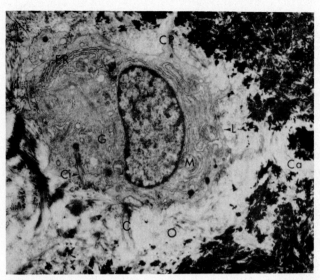

Figure 1.24. Cell processes (CP) extend into canaliculi (Ca), which extend from lacunar space (L) in which bone cell body is situated. Gradually, maturing osteocyte becomes entrapped within matrix and its osteoid (O). (G) Golgi complex. (ER) rough endoplasmic reticulum. (M) Mitochondria. (C) cilium. TEM × 5100.

Figure 1.25. Bone resorption and remodeling of bone is accomplished by osteoclasts (O). These giantlike cells are probably formed by fusion of many osteoblasts and are multinucleated. Consequently, they are pleomorphic. They demonstrate only limited ability for mobility by virtue of their fimbriated borders (arrows) and are not phagocytic. SEM × 200.

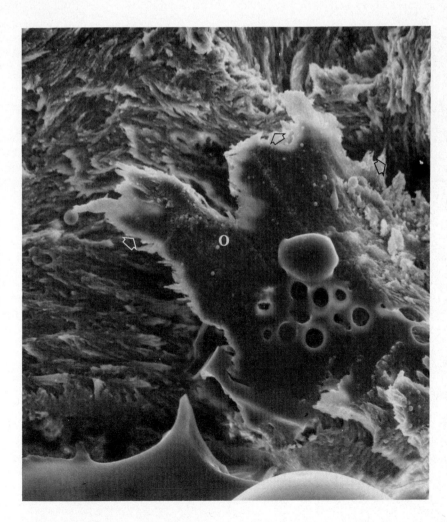

but it is not actively mobile or phagocytic (Fig. 1.25). Osteoclasts are resident in depressions on bony surfaces called Howship's lacunae.

Bone forms using intramembranous and intracartilaginous modes of development. Bones of the lower extremities develop by intracartilaginous processes, but bone healing may employ certain features of intramembranous methods.

Intracartilaginous bone development proceeds from a cartilaginous model formed from mesenchymal anlage. Primary centers of ossification located in the diaphysis of bone appear as early as the second fetal month. Secondary epiphyseal centers occur at later dates.

In brief, the growth of bones relates to a primary center of ossification and a series of stages or zones can be defined (7). The process is dynamic and the zones change morphologically with maturation of the bone. Beginning with the extremity of the cartilaginous model and moving toward the ossification center, the following levels of development are definable.

Farthest removed from the center is a reserve zone of primitive hyaline cartilage. Beneath is a proliferative zone of mitotic cartilaginous cells that arrange in definitive rows oriented in the long axis of the model. A third zone that does not demonstrate mitosis of its cells but interstitial growth occurs by the addition of matrix and enlargement of individual cells and their lacunae. This is the maturation zone. A fourth zone, that of calcification, is relatively narrow and represents the completion of the osteogenic cell life cycle. A fifth and final stage involving chondrogenic activities in bone formation involves necrosis and dissolution (5). Both chondrocytes and matrix in the zone of regression are involved, but hardier portions of matrix and calcified elements persist along with lacunae (Fig. 1.26). At this time mesenchymal cells of the area differentiate into osteoblasts.

A zone of ossification forms the sixth of eight formative strata. This is the result of osteoblastic aggregations along the exposed plates of calcified cartilage. Osteoblasts form new matrix and differentiate into osteocytes as a calcifying matrix is formed entrapping the maturing cells. This seventh stage, forming an osseous zone, extends to the center of ossification.

The zone of resorption compensates for the extension of the osseous zone. Resorption progressively lengthens the marrow cavity. It occurs at the oldest central portion of the bony mass.

Regenerative Ability

Interruptions in the continuity of bone cannot be repaired by the injured osseous tissue itself. Initially, a procallus develops about the damaged site from granulation tissue that organizes from clotted blood into which blood vessels and fibroblasts have proliferated.

Temporary callus forms a strong union as cartilage invades the area that subsequently undergoes a degree of calcification. These events essentially reca-

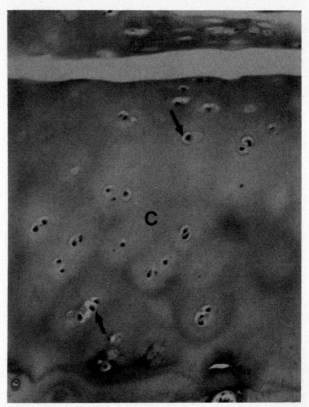

Figure 1.26. Cartilage (C) presents homogeneous matrix in which young chondroblasts are biosynthetically active: eventually more mature chondrocytes become entrapped in essentially avascular cartilage (arrows). LM. LM × 360.

pitulate those of endochondral ossification as healing proceeds (5).

The periosteum and endosteum of bone are reservoirs for mesenchymal cells that differentiate into osteoblasts, which in turn form matrix. Bony callus is at first spongy then becomes compact as maturation is completed. Osteoclasts are active in the processes of resorption and remodeling and the original form of bone is restored (5).

It has been shown that low oxygen tension results in the formation of cartilage whereas high oxygen tension favors the development of bone. Consequently, poorly united bone may attempt healing by a mixture of chondrification and ossification. Nonunion or pseudarthrosis represent failures in bone healing. It is common for poorly united bone fragments to have repeated hemorrhages and multiple reattempts at healing.

NERVES

Nerve cells or neurons arise from precursor cells termed neuroblasts (5). Special cell types that are morphologically unipolar or bipolar are to be seen in the central nervous system. Most neurons, however, are multipolar, indicating they have many dendrons.

Dendrons conduct impulses towards the nerve cell bodies, while a single process, the axon, conducts impulses away. Axons and dendrons may appear morphologically similar (8).

Nerve cell bodies are plemorphic and of variable size. A nerve cell body has a centrally situated nucleus, a prominent basophilic nucleolus, and the chromation is in the active uncoiled state (Fig. 1.20). Aggregations of nerve cell bodies are called ganglia.

The perikaryon (cytoplasm of the nerve cell) is a dynamic, apparently homogeneous substance, but transmission electron microscopy reveals many subcellular organelles. Neurofibrils occur in the cell body, as well as in the nerve processes. Mitochondria and diffuse Golgi apparatus can be observed along with stacks of flat, rough, endoplasmic reticulum and free ribosomes (Fig. 1.21). Deeply basophilic Nissl bodies are characteristic of neuroplasm (5).

A variety of inclusions including lipid, vesicles, granules, and occasionally pigment are identified in the perikaryon (9).

Nerve fibers are classified as myelinated and unmyelinated. Each may or may not possess a neurolemma (Fig. 1.27).

The general plan of organization for peripheral nerve fibers demonstrates an axis cylinder or axon in the central position. This is surrounded by as many as 50 layers of myelin sheath that give a cross-sectional appearance similar to a jelly roll. The myelin sheath may be considered as a modified plasma membrane or neurolemma composed of lipid and protein.

Nodes of Ranvier are constrictions occuring at regular intervals along interruptions that subdivide the myelin sheath into myelin segments (Fig. 1.27). Internodal segments occur between individual nodes of Ranvier (5).

Externally, myelinated fibers are covered by the neurolemmal sheath of Schwann, which provides a somewhat rigid and tough investment (Fig. 1.28). This sheath is made up of a series of flattened cells situated between contiguous nodes where it dips to make connection with the axon itself. Ultrastructural examination demonstrates an external plasma membrane with a basal lamina. Cell nuclei are flattened and oval in appearance.

Nerves are composed of a variety of tissues organized to perform a specific function and are therefore organs. Individual nerve fibers are contained by an investing layer of connective tissue, the endoneurium. Henle's sheath is the gelatinous portion most closely adherent to the axon itself (5).

Nerve fibers collectively organized into cablelike structures are termed nerve funiculi or fascicles, which are encased by perineuri that give off perineural septae.

The epineurium is a more loosely organized investment of nerve fascicles making up the nerve trunk itself. Peripheral nerves are mixed nerves and contain myelinated and unmyelinated fibers.

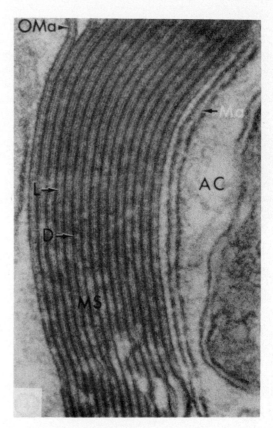

Figure 1.28. Cross section of axis cylinder (AC) surrounded by concentrically layered myelin sheath (MS), which demonstrates its typically "jelly roll" configuration. Plasma membranes originating from Schwann's cells invest each layer and form alternating dark (D) and light (L) bands spaced at intervals of 11 to 16 μm. Inner mesaxonal investment (Ma), outer mesonal axon investment (OMa). TEM × 110,000. (From Matthews JL, Martin JH: *Atlas of Human Histology and Ultrastructure.* Philadelphia, Lea and Febiger, 1971.)

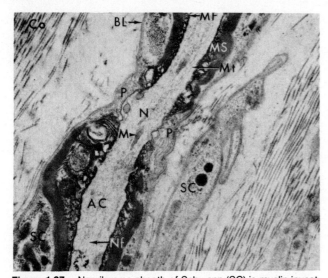

Figure 1.27. Neurilemma sheath of Schwann (SC) is myelin investment of axis cylinder made up of many axons (AC). Nodes of Ranvier (N) occur wherever myelin sheath (MS) terminates on either side of node. Schwann's cell extends cytoplasmic processes (P) across nodal regions devoid of myelin. Schwann's cell membrane folds (MF), neurofilaments (NF), microtubules (MT), mitochondria (M), basal lamina (BL), collagenic fibers of the interstitial connective tissues (C). TEM. TEM × 11,000. (From Matthews JL, Martin JH: *Atlas of Human Histology and Ultrastructure.* Philadelphia, Lea and Febiger, 1971.)

NERVOUS TISSUE

The epineurium provides entrances for blood vessels, lymphatics, and vasomotor nerves (nervi nervorum) (8).

Regenerative Ability

The degree to which injured nerves regenerate depends on the degree of injury, the approximation of injured parts, and the continuity of sheath cells that tend to guide regenerating axons.

Following trauma, peripheral nerve fibers undergo primary and secondary degeneration. Primary degeneration occurs immediately at the injury site. It proceeds toward the cell body over approximately two internodal segments. Secondary or wallerian degeneration is more extensive and involves the portion of the nerve that has been separated from the nerve cell body. Such axonal segments become edematous and fragmented and are phagocytosed by macrophages (5).

Within two weeks of injury axonal debris is cleared and at the end of the first week, proliferation by a neurolemmal sheath of Schwann's cells becomes evident. Sheath cells are crucial for the successful regeneration of nerves because they guide the regrowth of axons (5).

Recent studies show that the living proximal segment of the axon vigorously sprouts numerous fine nerve filaments from its tip. If this activity is properly guided, nerve regeneration can become successful as it is guided through the endoneural tube. If, however, scar tissue blocks regeneration, the process is aborted. Occasionally, the wrong structure is innervated by a regenerating nerve. Regenerating nerves grow at an optimal rate of 4 mm daily (5). It is important to understand that nerve fiber regeneration is a formidable process because it is related to the size of the nerve cell body. In the leg, a single regenerating fiber must produce a cytoplasmic volume equal to 250 times that of the nerve cell body.

Patency of the nerve cell body is pivotal to the regeneration of its axon. Restitution may require several months. Consequently, axonal regeneration can be adversely affected. Nerve cell bodies, when injured, are poorly stained with analine dyes. This is the result of chromatolipes of the normally deeply basophilic Nissl bodies: such changes are referred to as the axon reaction. At the same time, the cell nucleus is displaced peripherally, the cell body becomes edematous, and subcellular organelles are disrupted (5).

MUSCLE TISSUE

The muscular tissues are comprised of voluntary or skeletal, involuntary cardiac, and smooth types. Each of the three kinds are distinctive in their structure. Because this discussion is surgically oriented, voluntary or skeletal muscle will be emphasized. Cardiac muscle will not be discussed.

Smooth muscle is nonstriated and involuntary: its innervation is by elements of the autonomic nervous system (10). Such muscle tissue frequently lines hollow organs in which contractions occur with wavelike motions.

Individual smooth muscle fibers are of variable length with an elongated, tapering, and spindle shape (Fig. 1.29). Smooth muscles have a central pale staining nucleus. The contractile elements are composed of actin and myosin and are resolvable under the electron microscope as myofilaments. Myofibrils are seen at the light microscopic level, but these are artifactual because they are produced by clumping during tissue preparation. In the lower extremities, smooth muscle is encountered in blood vessels and about hair follicles and glands.

Skeletal muscles make up the fleshy structure of the lower extremities, as well as throughout the body. Such muscles are under voluntary control. Skeletal muscle fibers are cross striated and multinucleated because they are formed by the fusion of a number of muscle cells. Individual fibers are cylindrical and tapered at the ends although the latter often bifurcate or branch.

The investing membrane of a striated muscle cell or fiber is the sarcolemma, near which the numerous elongated nuclei are peripherally situated. Like smooth muscle, contractile myofibrils are contained within the sarcoplasm. Fibrils may bunch artifactually as bundles called Kolliker's columns, which in cross section are referred to as Cohnheim's areas.

The organization of actin and myosin in voluntary muscle is responsible for the characteristic light and dark cross banding of the organ. Reciprocal actions of these two substances provides for a rachetlike movement that provides contraction and relaxation of muscle fibers. Mitochondria are situated between fi-

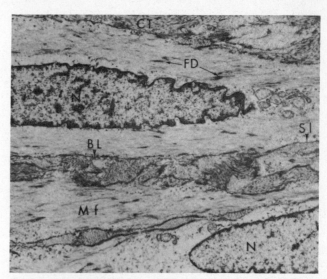

Figure 1.29. Involuntary or smooth muscle cells respond to impulses from autonomic nervous system. They are associated with such structures as blood vessels, erector apparatus of hair, and glands. Such cells are tapered and range in length from 20 μm to 0.5 mm. Nuclei (N) are more or less centrally located and are elongated. Myofilaments (Mf) are mainly actin. Fusiform densities (FD), sarcolemma (SI), basal lamina (BL), interstitial connective tissue stroma (CT). TEM × 5,100. (From Matthews JL, Martin JH: *Atlas of Human Histology and Ultrastructure.* Philadelphia, Lea and Febiger, 1971.)

bers, and a smooth sarcoplasmic reticulum with dilated terminal cisterna are identified.

A poorly refractile isotropic (I) band constitutes the light zone composed of the actin component. I bands are bisected by somewhat darker Z bands (11).

An anisotropic (A) band is dark and doubly refractile. It is composed of the myosin component. The A bands have evenly spaced spines. They overlap the thinner actin filaments in a regularly geometricalal fashion mechanically presumably to engage the I band.

The fundamental unit of structure of skeletal muscle is termed a sarcomere and represents the area between two contiguous Z bands. It contains half of an I band at either end and an A band (Fig. 1.30).

Muscle as an organ is composed of muscle fiber bundles or fascicles that are interlaced by a delicate connective tissue endomysium. Fascicles in turn are surrounded by connective tissue investment, the perimysium. An epimysium invests the muscle in toto.

Blood vessels and lymphatics richly invest muscle tissue. Motor endplates innervate each muscle and each muscle fiber receives a twig from the innervating nerve (5).

A harnesslike confluence of endomysium, perimysium, and epimysium joins in a continuous connective tissue structure that fixes the muscle as a whole on bone as an aponeurosis or tendon. Growth occurs here at the muscle-tendon junction by the addition of sarcomeres (12).

Regenerative Ability

Injured muscle fibers have a limited ability to regenerate if the tissues have nuclei. However, substantial injuries including surgical trauma are more likely to heal by fibrogenesis and a connective tissue scar across the defect. Such activity is made possible by fibroblasts in the area and is not an activity of the muscle fiber cell (5).

BLOOD VESSELS

Arteries, veins, and, to a certain extent, lymphatics share certain morphological characteristics, but variability relative to size makes for differences. The podiatric surgeon is most likely to encounter small- and medium-sized vessels.

Medium-sized arteries and, indeed, all vessels have an inner elongated endothelium, the tunica intima. A fenestrated internal elastic membrane invests it separating it from the more prominent middle layer, the tunica media (13).

The most external layer of vessels is the tunica adventitia which is equal or thinner in girth relative to the media. The adventitia is composed of collagenous fibers in a matrix (Fig. 1.31).

Veins are similarly constructed, but the tunica media is relatively diminutive and the adventitia is relatively thicker (Fig. 1.32). Valves formed by local foldings of the tunica intima are characteristic of veins and they prevent retrograde flow of blood (14). Lymphatics also possess valves. They demonstrate a tunica intima, a tunica media with an inner circular and outer longitudinal layer of smooth muscle, and an

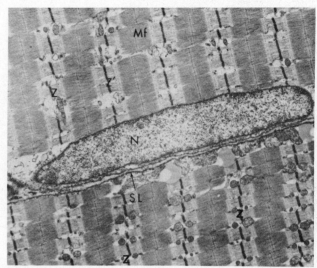

Figure 1.30. Sarcolemma of voluntary muscle invests cell with its eccentrically located nucleus (N) in close relationship to periphery. Myofilaments (Mf) are closely packed in regular array within cell. Z (Z) lines demarcate limits of sarcomere unit. A bands are dark, H zones are light. TEM × 7,000. (From Matthews JL, Martin JH: *Atlas of Human Histology and Ultrastructure.* Philadelphia, Lea and Febiger, 1971.)

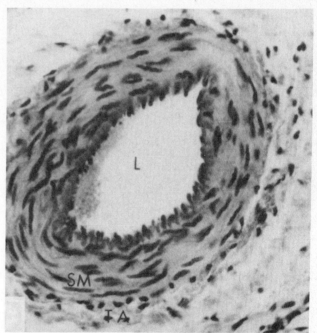

Figure 1.31. Blood vessel lumen (L) is surrounded by lining of endothelial cells that rest on a basal lamina. Internal and external elastic lamina may invest circularly arranged bands of smooth muscle fibers (SM). Tunica adventitia (TA) surrounds whole vessel and is made up of collagenic fibers, matrix, and fibroblasts. This dense investment of blood vessel is supported by stroma of more loosely organized interstitial connective tissue. LM × 200. (From Matthews JL, Martin JH: *Atlas of Human Histology and Ultrastructure.* Philadelphia, Lea and Febiger, 1971.)

adventitia in which longitudinal smooth muscle fibers may occur (15).

Vessels become progressively smaller as they proceed distally. Terminal arterioles and venules are interconnected by endothelial tubes, the capillaries.

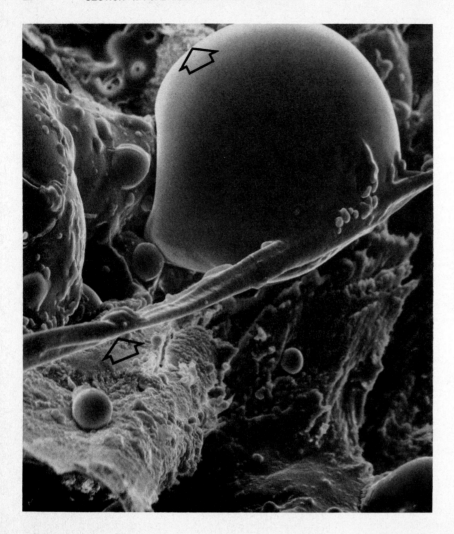

Figure 1.32. Veins are larger in diameter, but thinner walled than their respective accompanying arteries. They are smooth externally and often intersect demonstrating ballooned out structure at these points of junction (arrows). SEM. × 200.

Regenerative Ability

Severed blood vessels and lymphatics repair traumas that interrupt their continuity. These events recapitulate embryogeny to a degree. Solid endothelial sprouts emerge from patent portions of both of the injured ends probably in response to a low oxygen gradient. They usually form a network from which a single vessel is selected to persist as the endothelial tube hollows out (5). Mesenchymal-like cells subsequently differentiate into myoblasts and fibroblasts that produce tunica media and tunica adventitia, respectively.

CONNECTIVE TISSUES

The term "connective tissue" covers a wide variety of structural entities. It includes such specialized tissues as blood in which the matrix is the plasma portion and the formed elements are the cellular constituents. Hematology is a highly specialized field and is beyond the scope of this discussion. Connective tissues are of mesodermal origin and are developed through the differentiation of mesenchymal tissue of the embryo. Such tissues have a matrix or ground substance that is initially a coagulable fluid, which later organizes embryonically as mucous tissue. The cellular component is composed of pleuripotential cells appropriately termed mesenchymal cells (5). Such cells are morphologically stellate- or star-shaped and have a scanty cytoplasm from which numerous cell processes may be formed. On differentiation they become precursors to the adult formative "blast" cells. In general connective tissues can be grouped as being of loose or dense types. Primitive mesenchymal like cells persist in the adult scattered throughout both loose and dense connective tissue (4). This is especially important to the regenerative capability of connective tissues because these cells are "multipotent" and can differentiate along several lines to allow for repair of a variety of tissues. Cells of the reticuloendothelial system composed of macrophages are derived from this source (5).

LOOSE CONNECTIVE TISSUE
Reticular Tissue

Reticular tissues are loosely organized throughout many organs and are important in lymphoid organs, bone marrow, and the liver. The primary cellular constituent is the fibroblast and phagocytic reticular cells that are part of the reticuloendothelial system just mentioned (5).

Areolar Tissue

Areolar tissue is perhaps the most widespread of the connective tissues and is composed of minute open regions within its matrix. It provides a stroma for body organs, binding down muscle, blood vessels, and nerves, membranes, and skin components.

Adipose Tissue

Fat or adipose tissue varies quantitatively according to the individual's nutritional state. A panniculus adiposus is especially abundant in the human foot about the plantar heel and metatarsophalangeal regions. Age produces qualitative changes of these and other body regions (5). Specialized fat cells are morphologically atypical. Scanning electron microscopy demonstrates them as ovoid, smooth-surfaced, balloonlike structures of variable size dependent on the amounts of lipid contained (Fig. 1.33).

Stellate lipoblasts differentiate from mesenchymal cells and become rounded as they accumulate lipid droplets (13). Fat droplets coalesce forcing the nucleus into a compressed peripheral position along with a severely attenuated cytoplasm. This provides the cell with the characteristic "signet ring" appearance (Fig. 1.34).

Regenerative Ability

Adipose (as well as all loose connective tissues) tissues regenerate well. Clearly individual adipose tissue cells are incapable of regeneration. However, there is an abundant reservoir of mesenchymal-like cells available within the syncytium to differentiate into cells capable of fully regenerating adipose tissues, as well as all other loose connective tissues (5).

Dense Connective Tissues

Dense connective tissues are characterized by a greater abundance of coarser fibers more compactly arranged than occurs in loose connective tissues. The matrix of dense connective tissues varies considerably among tissues and organs. Septae and trabeculae, which partition structures, demonstrate an irregularity of collagenous fibers. These fibrillar tissue constituents are arranged in direct proportion to the density of the connective tissues.

Collagen is the protein component of the principle fibrillar constituent of dense connective tissue (13). It

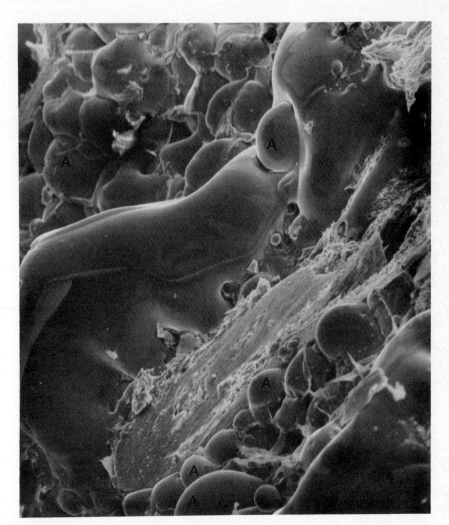

Figure 1.33. Adipose (fat) cells vary in amount of lipid accumulated and are varied in terms of size. Adipocytes (A) are ovoid in shape and smooth walled. SEM. × 80.

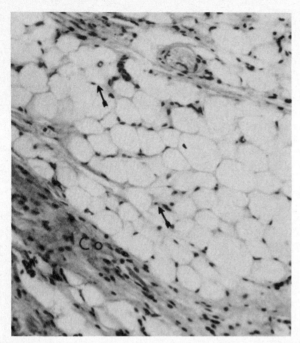

Figure 1.34. Fat cells demonstrate signet ring configuration (arrow) as accumulated fat forces cell nucleus toward periphery. Amount of fat varies between cells. Aggregates of fat cells are supported by stroma of connective tissue rich in collagenic fibers (Co). Fibroblasts are plentiful within stroma. LM × 150. (From Matthews JL, Martin JH: *Atlas of Human Histology and Ultrastructure.* Philadelphia, Lea and Febiger, 1971.)

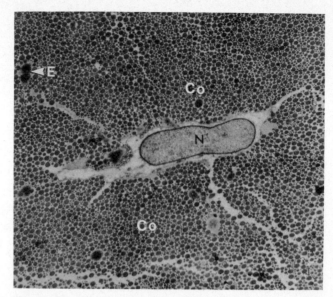

Figure 1.35. Tendons are representative of dense connective tissues. Biosynthetic cells are fibroblasts that characteristically demonstrate prominent nucleus (N) relative to reduced amount of cytoplasm. Collagenic fibers (Co) give structure strength and resiliance. Elastic fibers (E) are scattered throughout collagenic structure. TEM × 10,000. (From Matthews JL, Martin JH: *Atlas of Human Histology and Ultrastructure.* Philadelphia, Lea and Febiger, 1971.)

is immediately recognizable as eosinophilic wavy fibrils that neither branch nor unite. They are adhered one to another by cementing substance. They are synthesized by fibroblasts as tropocollagen. Collagenous fibers come together in bundles that normally range from 1 to 12 μm in thickness (Fig. 1.35). In poorly healing fibrotic situations, so-called "super collagenic fibers" are common: they, however, are coarse and frayed. Transmission electron microscopy reveals periodic cross banding that repeats every 0.064 μm. This phenomenon is the result of tropocollagen macromolecules measuring 0.28 by 0.0014 μm being side by side (4).

Fascia and Membranes

Fascias, membranes, and similar structures are dense connective tissues demonstrating interwoven irregularly arranged characteristics. Periosteum of bone is such a structure.

Tendons, Ligaments, and Aponeurosis

Tendons, ligaments, and aponeurosis are dense connective tissues that contain the greatest concentrations of collagen in orderly, regular arrangements. Tendons show the highest degree of order as do aponeurosis, which are expansions of the tendinous structure (13). Primary tendon bundles constitute the structural unit that contains fine fibrils gathered into a large collagenous fiber measuring about 30 μm. Fibroblasts orient along the long axis of primary bundles. Primary bundles aggregate forming a tendon

fascicle. Tendons, which fix muscle to bone, are formed by fascicles organized into cablelike structures. Fascicles are ensheathed within loose connective tissue called endotendineum. Peritendineum compartmentalizes groups of fascicles by radiating outward from a central region. Epitendineum encases the tendon as an organ; it represents the most dense expression of the tendon's stroma (5).

Regenerative Ability

Dense regular connective tissues are found as tough sheets, bands, and cords that respond to mechanical demands. Injuries to these structures and organs repair with comparative ease. Contiguous connective tissues are not involved; rather, fibroblasts invade the traumatized region. They synthesize matrix and fine collagenous fibers in a proper lengthwise orientation. As the fault repairs, the fine fibers aggregate in more coarse bundles with great tensile strength. Blood vessels and nerves regenerate about the part in the usual way (5).

JOINTS

Diarthrotic or freely movable joints are of importance to the podiatric surgeon. Articular hyaline cartilages are formed disclike at the opposing surfaces of contiguous bones with a joint cavity between. Hyaline cartilage is avascular and demonstrates a glassy, translucent bluish appearance (16). The matrix or ground substance is chondromucoprotein. Chondroblasts and chondrocytes frequently are found to aggregate in cell nests. Occasionally they orient in rows. Spaces in which cells are situated are called lacunae.

Cartilage is invested by a more cellular perichondrium that consists of densely packed collagenous fibers. Its deeper cells are multipotent and may differentiate as chondroblasts.

Joint capsules form collarlike investments for two opposing articular surfaces. Two layers are of importance. The outermost layer is of dense fibrous connective tissue rich in collagenic fibers. It is structurally similar to the periosteum of contiguous bone (17). The innermost layer is a synovial membrane. Fibroblast-like cells are identifiable along with a vascular network. The region presents an epithelioid appearance and may evaginate as synovial villi. Synovial fluid, which is an extract of lymph and blood plasma, bathes the surfaces within the joint space (5).

Regenerative Ability

Hyaline cartilage does not repair injuries. The tissue is avascular and its cells are locked within their lacunae. The perichondrium has multipotent cells that may form chondroblasts capable of forming matrix in regions near the perichondrium (5). Mature cartilage, if fractured, may undergo fibrosis from deeper regions, and calcification of such repair is common.

References

1. Pinkus H, Mehregan AH: *A Guide to Dermatohistopathology.* New York, Appleton-Century-Crofts, 1969.
2. Odland GF, Reed TH: Keratinization. In Zelickson AS(ed): *Ultrastructure of Normal and Abnormal Skin.* Philadelphia, Lea and Febiger, 1967.
3. Ross R: Wound healing. *Sci Am* 220:40–50, 1969.
4. Ham AW: *Histology,* ed 7. Philadelphia, JB Lippincott Co, 1969.
5. Arey LB: *Human Histology,* ed 4. Philadelphia, WB Saunders Co, 1974.
6. Hancock NM: *Biology of Bones.* New York, Cambridge University Press, 1972.
7. Weinmann JB, Sicher H: *Bone and Bones: Fundamentals of Bone Biology,* ed 2. St Louis, The CV Mosby Co, 1955.
8. Bourne GH(ed): *Structure and Function of Nervous Tissue,* vols 4, 5. New York, Academic Press, 1972.
9. Peters A, Palay SL, Webster HT: *The Fine Structure of Nervous System: The Cells and Their Processes.* New York, Harper and Row, 1970.
10. Gabella G: Fine structure of smooth muscle. *Proc Trans Roy Soc Lond* (B) 265:7, 1973.
11. Knappeis GG, Carlsen F: The ultrastructure of the Z disc in skeletal muscle. *J Cell Biol* 13:323, 1962.
12. Sandow A: Skeletal muscle. *Ann Rev Physiol* 32:87, 1970.
13. Mathews LL, Martin JH: *Atlas of Human Histology and Ultrastructure.* Philadelphia, Lea & Febiger, 1971.
14. Franklin KJ: *A Monograph on Veins.* Springfield, Ill, Charles C Thomas, 1937.
15. Abramson DI(ed): *Blood Vessels and Lymphatics.* New York, Academic Press, 1962.
16. Barnett CH, Davies DV, McConaill MA: *Synovial Joints.* London, Longmans Green and Co, 1961.
17. Davies DV: The anatomy and physiology of joints. In *Copemans' Textbook of the Rheumatic Diseases,* ed 2. Edinburg, E & S Livingston, 1955.

Osteology of the Lower Extremities

OSTEOLOGY

It will be the intent of this study on the osteology of the lower extremity to emphasize the bones of the foot. However, it will also be necessary to survey briefly the bones constituting the thigh and leg as well because they give origin to the extrinsic musculature of the foot.

FEMUR

The femur is the longest and strongest bone of the human body (1). It articulates proximally with the os innominatum at the acetabulum and distally with the tibia and patella. Proximally it presents a head and neck that terminates with the greater and lesser trochanters. The shaft (body) of the bone is somewhat cylindrical and presents three borders and three surfaces. The posterior surface demonstrates a prominent ridge or border having a medial and lateral lip. This ridge, the linea aspera, which terminates distally by divergence of the two ridges, delineates a triangular area known as the popliteal surface and the two lines terminate at the medial and lateral condyles of the femur. The medial supracondylar line is less prominent than the lateral: it terminates at the adductor tubercle and is smooth about midway for passage of the femoral artery.

The lower extremity of the femur is somewhat cuboidal and presents anterior, medial, lateral, and posterior or popliteal surfaces. The latter is relevant to the foot because it gives origin to the two heads of the gastrocnemius muscle.

The medial and lateral condyles of the femur are separated by a notch, the intercondyloid fossa. The medial condyle runs backwards and somewhat medially and projects more distally than does the lateral when the bone is held vertically. A large tuberosity, the medial epicondyle, is apparent as the medial aspect.

The lateral condyle runs in an anteroposterior direction, and is wider and more prominent anteriorly than the medial. It demonstrates the lateral epicondyle below which is the prominent popliteal groove.

The inferior and posterior surfaces of both medial and lateral condyles are smooth for articulation with the tibia.

The femur is normally angulated about 10° laterally from the vertical as it extends upward from the knee. It ossifies from five centers: one each for the greater and lesser trochanters, the head, shaft, and lower end of the bone (1).

TIBIA

The tibia is a long bone having two extremities and a shaft. The superior surface articulates with the femur by an oval medial articular facet and an almost circular lateral articular facet. The intercondyloid em-inence is situated somewhat posteriorly relative to the two articular facets. Anterior and posterior intercondyloid fossa are rough triangular depressions that relate to the intercondyloid eminence before and behind.

The proximal extremity of the tibia is made up by two large expansive eminences that overhang the shaft posteriorly and laterally. These are the medial and lateral condyles of the tibia. These condyles are continuous one with the other anteriorly, forming a flattened triangular area, the apex of which forms the tibial tuberosity. The popliteal notch, running downward and laterally, separates the condyles posteriorly.

A rounded facet for articulation with the head of the fibula is seen on the posterior aspect of the tibia immediately below the lateral condyle. It angulates downward, backwards, and laterally.

The crest of the tibia (the shin) forms the anterior border of the bone. It is directed medially, then laterally, and again medially to terminate on the anterior border of the medial malleolus. The anterior border of the tibia gives attachment for the deep fascia of the leg.

The interosseous crest is sharp and prominent and forms the lateral border of the shaft of the tibia.

The interosseous crest diverges distally to form a roughened triangular area known as the fibular notch at the lateral extremity of the tibia. This border serves to make attachment for the interosseous membrane. The interosseous membrane is indistinct proximally and is perforated for passage of the anterior tibial vessels.

The medial border of the tibia is rounded and ill-defined except for its sharp and distinct middle half. It terminates distally at the posterior margin of the medial malleous.

The three tibial borders separate three surfaces, provide for important attachments for soft tissue structures. The medial surface is subcutaneous, smooth, and broad for most of its length. Its proximal region provides for the insertions for m. semimembranosis, m. semitendinosis, m. sartorious, and m. gracilis. Distally it is obliquely marked for passage of the great saphenous vein (1).

The lateral surface demonstrates a slight forward convexity. Its proximal two thirds gives origin to m. tibialis anterior. Distally it is smooth and is crossed from medial to lateral by the tendons of m. tibialis anterior, m. extensor hallucis longus, the anterior tibial vein, artery, and nerve, m. extensor digitorium longus, and m. peroneus tertius.

The posterior surface is broad proximally and is distinctively marked by the soleal line that runs obliquely downwards in a medial direction. A conspicuous nutrient foramen is usually present just below the soleal line. The so called vertical line also marks the posterior surface of the tibia: it runs along the longitudinal axis of the posterior surface beginning just below the soleal line to fade away about mid shaft.

The popliteus muscle inserts above the soleal line. The soleal line receives fibers of insertion of m. soleus and the fascia that covers the musculature of the deep compartment. M. flexor digitorum longus takes origin medial to the vertical line while m. tibialis posterior makes attachment lateral to it. The prominent tendon of m. tibialis posterior passes downward and medially to groove the posterior surface of the medial malleolus. M. flexor hallucis longus and the posterior tibial vessels and nerves relate to the lower end of the tibia as well.

Podiatric surgeons are becoming increasingly involved with structures in and about the ankle joint, and it is important to understand the lower end of the tibia. The three-sided shaft of the tibia becomes quadrilateral at its distal extremity: the inferior surface is smooth for articulation with the talus. The slightly convex surface extends as the articular surface of the medial malleolus.

Laterally, dense ligaments springing from the fibular notch binds the fibula to the tibia. A smooth anterior surface, a subcutaneous medial surface, and a grooved posterior surface characterize the distal end of the tibia. The medial malleolus is a short stout process that extends downward and medially. It ends at a higher level than does the fibular malleolus. It articulates with the talus by a comma-shaped lateral facet. The lower border of the medial malleolus is pointed anteriorly and depressed posteriorly. Its anterior extremity is grooved for attachment of the articular capsule of the ankle joint.

The posterior surface of the medial malleolus is grooved for passage of the tendon of m. tibialis posterior which is crossed posteriorly by m. flexor digitorum longus. Attachments of the flexor retinaculum are made by a ridge just medial to the tibialis posterior groove, and the deltoid ligament makes attachment to the anterior lower border of the medial malleolus where a rough depression can be identified.

FIBULA

The fibula is not involved in directly bearing the weight of the body as is the tibia. It presents a head, shaft, and lower end or lateral malleolus. The head of the fibula is palpable on the posterolateral aspect of the knee. It presents a circular facet that faces slightly forwards, upwards, and medially for articulation with the inferior surface of the lateral condyle of the tibia. This region provides origin for m. extensor digitorum longus, m. peroneus longus, and m. soleus. The styloid process projects from the posterolateral aspect of the head as a blunted apex of bone.

The common peroneal nerve is identifiable as it crosses the posterolateral aspect of the neck of the fibula just below the head (1). Local nerve block anesthesia can be achieved by injections at this location.

The shaft of the fibula presents three borders and three surfaces. The borders are anterior, posterior, and interosseous: the latter help to fix the fibula on the tibia by means of the interosseous membrane. The spindly shaft of the fibula is complex by virtue of twisting in response to some of the extrinsic musculature of the foot that take origin there. M. peroneus longus et brevis have fibers or origin on the proximal portion of the lateral surface of the fibula. The lateral surface twists distally so that it becomes continuous with the back of the fibular malleolus.

The medial surface is associated with the extensor muscles of the lower extremity. It is narrow above and wider below.

The posterior surface is largest and is associated with the flexor muscles of the deep compartment of the leg (1). The posterior surface presents a longitudinal ridge called the medial crest. Its medial position is in relation to the oblique and posterior orientation of the fibula relative to the tibia. It has nothing to do with the medial surface of the fibula, which tends to be placed anteriorly.

The lateral malleolus forms the lower end of the fibula. Its lateral surface is palpable and subcutaneous. The fibular malleolus lies more posteriorly and on a lower plane than the medial malleolus.

The medial surface of the fibular malleolus articulates with the talus by means of a convex triangular facet with base up, apex down. The malleolar fossa is a rough depression of bone just behind the articular facet.

The posterior surface of the fibular malleous is well grooved for passage of the tendons of the peroneus muscles.

TALUS

The talus is structurally irregular and is situated mortiselike between the tibia and fibula. It is one of two bones comprising the greater tarsus and is peculiar in that it is the only bone of the tarsus having no tendinous insertions (Fig. 1.36) The talus (astragulus) has a body described as having five sides because the anterior portion is occupied by the neck (1). The head (caput) and the medially angulated neck (collus) are described separately.

Dorsal Surface

The oblong dorsal surface is widest anteriorly. It presents a convexity from anterior to posterior and concave from side to side for articulation with the distal tibia. This suggests its pulleylike plan that gives it the descriptive designation as the trochlea of the talus. The lateral segment is wider than the medial because the groove of the "pulley" is more tibially oriented. The fibular border of the dorsal surface is triangular because of its obliquity and beveled posterior segment and is to be contrasted to the straight and softly contoured tibial border. The anterior border of the talus varies in outline from concave to convex with variations in between: it may present concave

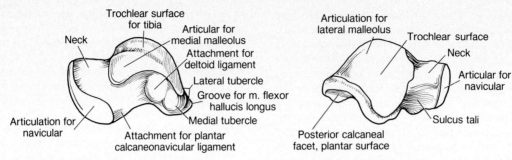

Right Talus, Medial Aspect   Right Talus, Lateral Aspect

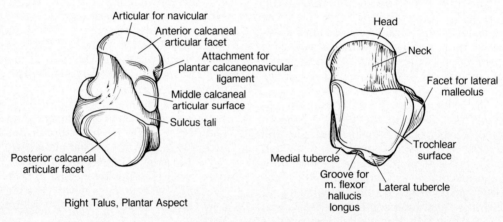

Right Talus, Plantar Aspect

Right Talus, Superior Aspect

Figure 1.36.   Talus.

medial and lateral extension facets. These are not to be confused with the so-called squatting facet that extends concave from the anterolateral trochlear surface and occurs in 30% or less of specimens (2). Because it is directed upwards and backwards it can contact the anterodistal margin of the tibia on dorsal flexion.

Medial Surface

The medial surface of the talar body presents a distinctive comma-shaped facet along its superior border that articulates with the tibial malleolus. It is the widest anteriorly and tapers posteriorly. Both anterior and posterior extremities of this articular area may be extended. When the anterior aspect is extended onto the talar neck, it is broadened and may make contact with the anteromedial margin of the tibial malleolus on strong dorsiflexion. Beneath the comma-shaped facet, the medial talar body is roughened by many vascular foramina. The deep talotibial part of the deltoid ligament makes an ovoid attachment along the posteromedial surface of the talar body.

Lateral Surface

The fibular aspect of the body of the talus is distinctive for its triangular facet for articulation with the fibular malleolus. The apex of this triangle is

directed down while its base forms the lateral border of the superior or dorsal surface of the talus. This surface is slightly convex on the transverse axis and is concave vertically. Two tubercles making attachment for the anterior talofibular ligament are seen on the anterior axis of the triangular facet. The posterior talofibular ligament makes attachment by a notched region along the posterior margin of the triangle.

Inferior Surface

The inferior surface of the body of the talus is rectangular and articulates with the posterior articular facet of the dorsal calcaneus. The long axis of the surface is concave and is angulated about 35° in an anterolateral direction. The articular surface is essentially flat from side to side. The sinus tarsi is formed in part by the convexity of the anteromedial border of the inferior surface of the talar body. Extensions of the inferior surface are occasionally seen in relation to the posterolateral and the anterolateral borders.

Posterior Surface

The posterior surface of the talar body is much reduced and irregular. It is well grooved for passage of the tendon of m. flexor hallucis longus, which passes downward and inward to curve distally into the foot. The sulcus is divided by a relatively small medial posterior tibial tubercle that gives attachment to the medial talocalcaneal ligament and to the deep and superficial components of the talotibial ligaments of the deltoid ligament.

A rare developmental anomaly, coalition of the posterior talus and calcaneous, may occur at this point. The larger posterolateral tubercle of the posterior surface of the talus may be unusually prominent: it is then referred to as the posterior process. The region provides attachment for the posterior talofibular ligament and the talofibular calcaneal ligament, as well as deep fibers of the flexor retinaculum. The os trigonum is the accessory bone associated with the lateral posterior tubercle. Its occurrence is between 3% and 8% of the population (2). The ossicle is usually deeply embedded in capsuloligamentous structures and it may groove or notch the contiguous talar surface. The trigonal process represents a fusion of the os trigonum with the lateral posterior talar tubercle.

An anterior surface of the talus is not described because the region is occupied by the neck of the talus.

Neck of the Talus

The talar neck (collum tali) is a roughened constriction of bone about 15 mm long projected downward an anteromedially. It can be described as having four surfaces: the *medial aspect* is much reduced and rounded. It orients higher than the lateral and is marked by the attachment of part of the talonavicular capsule. The *superior surface*, which is intraarticular, presents a concave cribiform fossa along its fibular aspect. The medial aspect follows the rotation of the head and is tibially angulated. It provides attachment for superficial fibers of the talotibial portion of the deltoid ligament. A cervical ridge marks the anterosuperior surface of the neck for the attachment of capsular structures. Because of the medial angulation of the head of the talus, capsular fibers of the talotibial and talonavicular joints are attached laterally on the dorsal aspect of the talar neck. An anatomical bursa is often associated with this region (3).

The *inferior surface* of the talar neck is distinctive in forming part of the sinus tarsi. The sulcus tali is a deep groove that is narrow on the tibial aspect, but wide on the fibular aspect of the inferior surface of the talar neck. The cervical tubercle is situated at the anterior margin of the sulcus tali in about one third of specimens and gives attachment for the cervical ligament. The apical part of the sulcus tali is continued medially to form the talar component of the tarsal canal. It is situated between the posterior and medial articular facets of the inferior surface of the talus. The medial facet just mentioned is the anterior articular part of the talar neck; it is smooth for articulation with the anterior calcaneal articular facet. In rare instances the tarsal canal is obliterated by coalitions. The talar portion of the tarsal canal is often ridged or roughened to give attachment to the interosseous talocalcaneal ligament and a part of the inferior extensor retinaculum.

Head of the Talus (Caput)

The head of the talus is smooth, ovoid, and convex for articulation with the navicular anteriorly, and with the medial and anterior articular facets on the superior surface of the calcaneus. The talar head glides on a fibrocartiloginous disc on the calcaneonavicular (spring) ligament and the head may demonstrate fine ridges to demarcate these three regions of articulation (4). The talar head is rotated upon the neck so that the portion articulating with the navicular is situated higher fibularward than on the tibial aspect. The head of the talus is markedly convex in all directions as it is received by the cuplike depression of the proximal navicular. Other articular surfaces, however, are essentially flat.

CALCANEUS

The calcaneus is the largest bone of the foot with an average length of 75 mm (2). It is an irregular bone, which in life demonstrates a normal upward calcaneal pitch of bone from 10° to 30°. The calcaneus or os calcis presents six surfaces (Fig. 1.37).

Superior Surface

The oblong superior surface of the calcaneus presents two roughened and two smooth articular regions. The most posterior of the four superior regions of the calcaneus is convex from side to side and rough. It is concave longitudinally from anterior to posterior. The region forms the base of a triangle in which the tendo achillis and the distal posterior aspect of the tibia provide the other two sides. The area is loosely filled with fat and connective tissue. The posterior articular facet on the dorsum of the calcaneus is sharply inclined anterior at an angle of about 65°. The area is ovoid or rectangular and is directed fibularward in addition to its forward and upward orientation for articulation with the inferior surface of the body of the talus. It is plane from side to side but concave in its longest dimension, which runs in a forward and lateral direction. Some investigators cite a screwlike behavior of the surface in one half of cases. Accessory facets may occur as anterior, posterior, and medial extensions of the posterior articular facet of the calcaneus (5).

The anterior third of the superior surface of the calcaneus is both rough and articular. The roughened surface is widest fibularly as it proceeds anteriorly in a fibularward direction and traverses the calcaneus to terminate tibially as the calcaneal part of the tarsal canal. This groove marking the superior calcaneus is known as the calcaneal sulcus. As was the case with the corresponding inferior nonarticular part of the talus, the interosseous talocalcaneal ligament and parts of the inferior extensor retinaculum make attachment to the floor of the tarsal canal or the calcaneal sulcus. A tubercle is frequently located at the lateral end of the groove. The calcaneal surface of the sinus tarsi is limited posteriorly by the posterior artic-

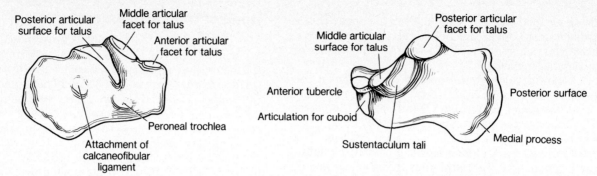

Right Calcaneus, Lateral Aspect

Right Calcaneus, Medial Aspect

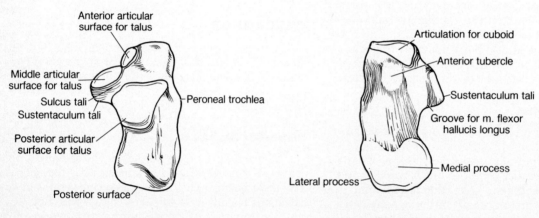

Right Calcaneus, Dorsal Aspect

Right Calcaneus, Plantar Aspect

Figure 1.37.   Calcaneus (or calus).

ular facet, laterally by the crista lateralis, and medially by the anterior articular facet and the tarsal canal. The tarsal canal is situated between the posterior and medial articular facets on the superior surface of the calcaneus. It inclines at a 45° angle confluent with the sustentaculum tali (2). The sinus tarsi is associated in part with attachments for m. extensor digitorum brevis, inferior extensor retinaculum, cervical ligament, bifurcate ligament, and the lateral calcaneocuboid ligament. It therefore has great clinical significance.

The smooth anterior articular surface is divisible into anterior and middle articular facets of variable size and shape. They may be either confluent or separated by a constriction. Both surfaces are concave longitudinally to receive the corresponding parts of the inferior talar surfaces. Their long axis is directed forward and fibularward. The anterior articular facet is associated with the calcaneal beak, while the middle articular facet occupies the superior surface of the sustentaculum tali.

Medial Surface

The medial surface of the calcaneus is somewhat quadrilateral in outline with its highest dimension posteriorly. It is an essentially smooth surface and is concave by virtue of the bulk of the medial tuberosity

behind and the sustentaculum tali that projects tibialward from the anterosuperior aspect. Important structures enter the foot from the leg in this calcaneal canal. The sustentaculum tali dominates the medial surface because it is inclined downward and forwards at a 45° angle (2). It presents a triangular appearance with the base positioned posteriorly. The superior surface is smooth and was mentioned as the middle articular facet previously. The inferior surface is usually well grooved for passage of the tendon of m. flexor hallucis longus. The tendon of m. flexor digitorum longus marks the anterior apical part of the sustentaculum tali and the recurrent bands of insertion of the tendon of m. tibialis posterior attach inferiorly. Fibers of attachment for the tibiocalcaneal part of the deltoid ligament and part of the calcaneonavicular ligaments relate to the upper medial border of the sustentaculum tali. Posteriorly on the sustentaculum tali, the medial talocalcaneal ligament makes attachment. The sustentaculum tali is about 15 mm wide and has a variable length. When its dimensions are diminutive, it is said to be "incompetent."

Lateral Surface

Like the medial surface, the lateral surface of the calcaneus is quadrilateral with its anterior dimensions more narrow than the wider posterior part. This surface, however, is convex and rough. The lateral surface is dominated by the obliquely projecting peroneal tubercle (trochlear process). Two oblique smooth grooves descend at about 45° from the posterosuperior aspect of the bone. The grooves above and below the trochlear process are for passage of the tendons of m. peroneus brevis et longus, respectively (2). A flat oval gliding cartilage may assist the gliding function of the tendon of peroneus longus, and it is situated at or near the posterior aspect of the peroneal trochlea. Occasionally an anteroinferior gliding facet is identified. Posterior to the peroneal trochlea and about midway on the lateral surface, a second prominence on the tubercle the (retrotrochlear eminence) is present. Additional tubercles may be present on the lateral surface of the calcaneus for attachments of the calcaneofibular, calcaneal part of the talocalcaneofibular, lateral talocalcaneal, and lateral calcaneocuboid ligaments. Additionally, the bone may be marked by the inferior peroneal retinaculum that binds the peroneal tendons in place. The tendon of peroneus brevis may not actually groove the lateral surface and the tendon of peroneus longus may contain an inconstant sesamoid bone.

Posterior Surface

The posterior surface of the calcaneus is ovoid with its widest dimension plantarly situated. The plantar outline is poorly defined because it curves to blend with the bone's plantar surface. The surface profile is essentially convex. Its upper third is smooth, somewhat triangular and may relate to the preachilles bursa. The insertion of the tendo achillis forms a trapezoidal striated, somewhat irregular area in the middle third of the surface. The inferior third is rough and striated because of prolongations of fibers of insertion of the tendo achillis.

Anterior Surface

The anterior surface of the calcaneus is more or less triangular and is convex transversely. Its longer medial or vertical margin presents a concave outline. It is almost wholly articular for the cuboid. The rostrum (beak) of the calcaneus is a shelf of bone overhanging the cuboid at the superior medial margin of the anterior surface. The calcaneal coronoid fossa is a posteriomedially situated groove that receives the beak of the cuboid in reciprocal fashion.

Inferior Surface

The oblong plantar surface of the calcaneus is wide posteriorly, narrow anteriorly, and is longitudinally striated. The tuber calcanei (calcaneal tuberosity) is the posterior point of weight bearing of the foot. It presents a deep longitudinal depression that separates the large medial calcaneal processes. Both are convex. A rounded eminence, the anterior calcaneal tuberosity marks the anterior aspect of the inferior surface and makes attachment for the long plantar ligament. The short plantar or calcaneocuboid ligament makes attachment anterior and deep to the long plantar ligament in relation to the anterior calcaneal tuberosity. The medial process provides for intrinsic foot muscles including m. abductor hallucis, flexor accessorious, flexor digitorum brevis, and more superficially to the plantar aponeurosis (fascia). The lateral process gives origin (along with the medial process) to m. abductor digiti minimi. The coronoid fossa represents a small depression giving attachment to the inferior calcaneonavicular ligament (6). It is situated medially between the anterior apex of the sustentaculum tali and the anterior tuberosity of the inferior surface of the calcaneus.

CUBOID

The cuboid is an irregular bone of pyramidal shape, the base of which is tibially disposed (Fig. 1.38). It constitutes part of the lateral column of the foot and is intercalated between the calcaneus proximally and the bases of the metatarsals four and five distally. It is variously described as having five or six surfaces depending on whether the lateral portion is considered to be a border or a surface (2).

Dorsal Surface

The dorsal surface is trapezoidal in outline and generally rough. It is convex transversely in continuity with the dorsal aspect of the transverse arch of the foot. The tibial aspect, which is the base of the trapezoid, marginates with both the navicular and the lateral cuneiform. A medial projection occupies the distal aspect. The lateral border is much reduced as

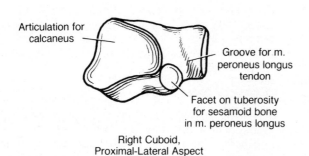

Right Cuboid, Proximal-Lateral Aspect

Right Cuboid, Medial Aspect

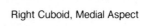

Figure 1.38. Cuboid.

the apex of the trapezoid and presents a concavity for the passage of the tendon of m. peroneus longus. The distal border is angular for approximation of the fourth metatarsal and the angular and obtuse base of metatarsal five. The proximal border is slightly convex as it approximates the calcaneus. The dorsal surface of the cuboid relates to m. extensor digitorum brevis and tendons of m. peroneus tertius and longus. Dorsomedial, dorsolateral, and lateral calcaneocuboid ligaments mark the dorsal cuboid surface, as do dorsal cubonavicular, cuneocuboid, and cubometatarsal ligaments.

Medial Surface

The thick medial cuboid surface is narrowest distally. Two articular facets may be present and the remainder of the surface is rough. The articular facet for the lateral cuneiform is variously shaped with its longest dimension oriented at the dorsal margin of the surface. A smaller variably shaped and more proximally placed facet for articulation with the navicular is present in about one half of cases. Plantar navicular and interosseous cuneocuboid ligaments make attachment at the inferior roughened portions of the surface (1).

Lateral Surface

The lateral surface is an expanded border formed by the confluence of the dorsal and plantar surfaces. It is grooved for passage of the tendon of m. peroneus longus and marks the beginning of the clinically important peroneal tunnel.

Anterior Surface

The anterior or distal surface is essentially triangular with the long axis oriented plantar and fibularward. It is nearly totally articular for the bases of metatarsals four and five, which are separated by a smooth vertical ridge. The medial articular facet for metatarsal four is oriented distally and presents a rectangular slightly concave outline. The lateral articular facet makes an angular convexity as it orients 35° in a lateroproximal direction to accommodate the base of the fifth metatarsal and its styloid process (2).

Posterior Surface

The proximal surface is variously described as triangular or saddle shaped: it is almost wholly articular with the calcaneus. The surface is smooth, convex vertically, and concave transversely. The beak of the cuboid or the coronoid process of the cuboid projects from the inferomedial angle of the posterior surface of the cuboid to undershoot the calcaneus to form a supportive bracket (2). Its direction is proximal and tibialward and limits adduction and flexion of the forefoot.

Plantar Surface

The plantar surface of the cuboid demonstrates a prolongation (the coronoid process) at the proximomedial angle. This surface, however, is otherwise similar in outline to the dorsal aspect. A small anterior and a large posterior are divided by a laterally directed prominent ridge that is the tuberosity of the cuboid. Paralleling the anterior border of the inferior surface is a deep smooth groove called the peroneal sulcus. Stieda and associates (7) challenge the opinion that the tendon of m. peroneus longus functions within the sulcus. They feel that it glides on the anterior slope of the tuberosity of the cuboid and note that a gliding facet associated with a sesamoid within the tendon of m. peroneus longus is situated on the anterolateral aspect of the tuberosity (7).

In addition, m. flexor digiti minimi, m. adductor hallucis (oblique head), and m. flexor hallucis brevis are associated with the plantar cuboid. Prolongations of fibers of insertion of m. tibialis posterior also make attachments here. Ligaments are dense in this region and include cubometatarsal, cubonavicular, and cuneocuboid, as well as elements of the long and short plantar ligaments. Two tubercles can usually be identified on the inferior surface of the cuboid. One is situated laterally on the tuberosity of the cuboid: the other is situated posteriorly on the promontory of the cuboid (1).

NAVICULAR

The navicular (scaphoid) bone is an irregular short bone intercalated between the talus proximally and the three cuneiforms distally. It has been characterized in older podiatric literature as the keystone of the medial longitudinal arch and is part of the osseous medial column of the foot. It is described as having four, five, or six surfaces depending on how the medial and/or lateral aspects are dealt with (Fig. 1.39).

Dorsal Surface

The navicular bone has a quadrilateral outline dorsally. It is concave posteriorly for reception of the head of the talus. The anterior border is generally convex but is angulated in three segments as it makes articulation with all three cuneiforms. The most lateral of these segments is situated posterolaterally. The dorsal surface is rough as attachments are given to the dorsal cubonavicular, cuneonavicular, calcaneonavicular, tibionavicular (component of the deltoid), calcaneonavicular, and talonavicular ligaments.

Medial Surface

The medial aspect is formed by the navicular tuberosity that is a principle point of insertion for expansions of the tendon of m. tibialis posterior. Both medial and plantar cuneonavicular ligaments make attachments on the tuberosity.

Lateral Surface

The lateral aspect of the navicular is quadrilateral. The plantar aspect of the surface is variably formed for articulation with the cuboid. The dorsal aspect is rough for attachment of the lateral calcaneonavicular component of the bifurcate ligament.

Posterior Surface

The proximal surface of the navicular is oval, biconcave, broadest at its fibular margin, and nearly wholly articular for reception of the head of the talus. In some cases the posterior articular facet is more plane than concave.

Anterior Surface

The general outline of the anterior surface is convex and somewhat kidney-shaped (reniform). Two soft crests divide the surface into three articular facets: the medial is convex and triangular or pear shaped; the middle is convex and triangular with its apex plantarward; the lateral facet is small and rectangular. The architecture of the anterior surfaces accommodate two phenomenona: first, it orients the distal part of the medial column of the foot in a more plantar and fibular direction. This corrects the tibial direction established by the head of the talus. Additionally, the plantar concavity of the transverse tarsal arch is established (2).

Plantar Surface

The plantar surface of the navicular, like the dorsal aspect, is quadrilateral but reduced in size. Its medial aspect blends with the navicular tuberosity. A developmental anomaly, the os tibial externum, represents a supernumerary ossicle that failed to unite with the main bone at this point (7). A bony shelf extending proximally from the mid or posterolateral aspect engages the calcaneus and is known as the beak

of the navicular or the calcaneal process of the navicular. The inferior surface is obliquely grooved for passage of tendinous slips of tendons of m. tibialis posterior that are directed anterolaterally toward the cuneiforms. The inferior surface is rough and provides attachment for the plantar cubonavicular and calcaneonavicular ligaments (8). Rarely, an articular facet for the calcaneus can be identified on the posterolateral margin of the posterior surface of the navicular (2).

FIRST CUNEIFORM

The medial or first cuneiform is the largest of the three cuneiforms and projects the farthest distally. It presents a wedge shaped outline in which the base is plantar and the apex is directed upward (Fig. 1.40). It articulates with the first and second metatarsal, the intermediate or second cuneiform and the navicular. There is no definitive superior surface because it is a crest and more like a border. The anterior third runs directly anteriorly in line with the first metatarsal, while the posterior two thirds is somewhat tibially oriented, angulating with the second cuneiform. The crest runs forward and upward overall and is rounded and smooth.

The medial surface is pentagonal or quadrilateral with a small oval face or depression at its anteroinferior angle. This is the site for part of the tendinous insertion for m. tibialis anterior. A small bursa is interposed at this location (2). This surface is generally rough except for a groove that diagonally crosses from posterosuperiorly to anteroinferiorly. Attach-

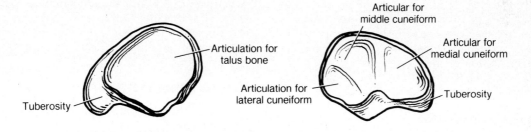

Right Navicular, Proximal Aspect   Right Navicular, Distal Aspect

Figure 1.39. Navicular.

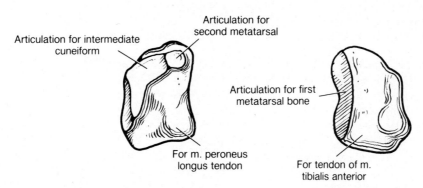

Right Medial Cuneiform, Lateral Aspect   Right Medial Cuneiform, Medial Aspect

Figure 1.40. First cuneiform.

ments for dorsal cuneonavicular, intercuneiform, cuneometatarsal (both first and second ligaments), and a medial cuneonavicular ligament are situated on this surface.

The lateral surface is also quadrilateral. It is generally concave and rough but is distinctive for its smooth articular L-shaped facets that are concave (1). The vertical arm is along the posterior border and the horizontal arm marks the superior border in part for articulation with the adjacent second cuneiform. The distal third of the larger horizontal arm is ovoid for articulation with the tibial aspect of the base of the second metatarsal. A minute bony band usually separates the two articular areas of the horizontal arm. An intercuneiform ligament makes attachment near the juncture of the vertical and horizontal articular arms. Lisfranc's ligament for attachment of the first cuneiform with the medial aspect of the base of the second metatarsal is marked by an eminence near the anteroinferior aspect of the surface. The hylum (notch) is fibularly oriented midway on the lateral border. The surface is flat and elongated on its vertical dimension, which inclines medially. The transverse axis is slightly convex. It is wholly articular for the base of the first metatarsal and is occasionally divided into two surfaces.

The *posterior surface* is concave in all directions as it articulates with the navicular. It is variously described as triangular or pear-shaped, the apex of which is up, and the base down. The *inferior surface* is quadrilateral or rectangular. It is rough and convex from side to side (1). The posterior aspect is marked by the tuberosity of the first cuneiform for attachment of the plantar cuneonavicular ligament. A rugosity at the site of insertion of the tendon of m. peroneus longus is seen fibularly and anteriorly to the tubercle. In addition, plantar intercuneiform and cuneometatarsal ligaments can be identified. These structures also mark the bones.

A case of duplication of the first cuneiform was described in the literature over 50 years ago (9).

SECOND CUNEIFORM

The second or intermediate cuneiform is the smallest of the three. This is important in fixing the base of the second metatarsal, with which it articulates, between the medial and lateral cuneiform. The bone is essentially wedge-shaped, base up, apex down (Fig. 1.41). It presents five surfaces and an inferior

crest or border (2). The rectangular dorsal surface is generally rough and convex. The somewhat longer posterior border is depressed at the medial border to form the intercuneiform fossa along with a contiguous pit in the lateral aspect of the first cuneiform. Dorsal cuneonavicular, cuneometatarsal (2-2), and medial and lateral intercuneiform ligaments (1-2) (2-3) are present.

The *medial surface* is rectangular or quadrilateral. It, like the lateral surface of the first cuneiform with which it articulates, has an L shaped articular facet. The vertical limb runs along the posterior border. The horizontal segment is wider and is situated along the superior border. The remainder of the surface is rough and presents a tubercle for attachment of the interosseous ligament.(1) The lateral surface is similar to the medial in presenting an inverted L shaped articular facet for the lateral or third cuneiform. It demonstrates posterior and superior smooth surface limbs that are sometimes modified to appear as a single pear-shaped surface, which is widest superiorly. The attachment for the interosseous cuneiform ligament (2-3) is marked by a small tubercle. The remainder of the surface is rough for attachment of cuneometatarsal ligaments (2-2) (2-3).

The *anterior surface* is triangular, base up, apex down. It is convex dorsally, as the surface as a whole on its vertical dimension for articulation with the base of the second metatarsal. The lateral border is concave. The *posterior surface* is much like the anterior. Its triangular outline demonstrates concave lateral and convex medial borders. The *inferior crest* or *border* is encroached on by the contiguous first and third cuneiforms. It is roughened for attachments of plantar cuneiform (1-2) and cuneonavicular ligaments (1). More superficially, fibrous structures giving origin to the fibular arm of m. flexor hallucis brevis and the insertion of tendinous reflections of m. tibialis posterior are identified (1).

THIRD CUNEIFORM

The lateral or third cuneiform is also triangular with its base up and apex down (Fig. 1.42). It presents five surfaces with an inferior border or crest. The *dorsal surface* is rough and is inclined upwards. It is essentially rectangular in its outline. The posterior border is inclined posterolaterally. The anterior border is concavoconvex for articulation with the third metatarsal. The medial and lateral borders provide for a

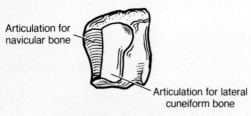

Articulation for navicular bone

Articulation for lateral cuneiform bone

Right Middle Cuneiform
Proximal-Lateral Aspect

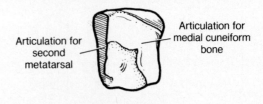

Articulation for second metatarsal

Articulation for medial cuneiform bone

Right Middle Cuneiform,
Distal-Medial Aspect

Figure 1.41.   Second cuneiform.

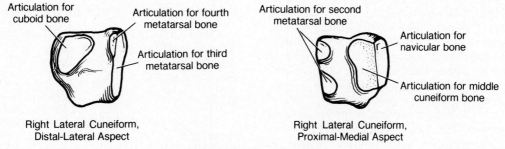

Articulation for cuboid bone
Articulation for fourth metatarsal bone
Articulation for third metatarsal bone
Right Lateral Cuneiform, Distal-Lateral Aspect

Articulation for second metatarsal bone
Articulation for navicular bone
Articulation for middle cuneiform bone
Right Lateral Cuneiform, Proximal-Medial Aspect

Figure 1.42.   Third cuneiform.

directional correction so that the third metatarsal, with which it articulates, is directed straight forward. The medial border is centrally notched and bevelled to align with the lateral aspect of the base of the second metatarsal. The lateral border is slightly angular: its posterior segment runs posteromedially while the anterior part is directed anteromedially.

The *medial surface* is quadrilateral or rectangular with two vertical articular surfaces. The anterior border is somewhat concave with a vertical facet for articulation with the base of the lateral aspect of the base of the second metatarsal. It is separated into upper and lower portions. The central constriction is for attachment of an interosseous ligament and is situated on a roughened area more posteriorly (2). A relatively large articular band is vertically placed along the posterior border for the second cuneiform. This border is extended inferiorly as a small nonarticular region and the central portion of the surface is rough.

The *lateral surface* is also quadrilateral: it presents a significant ovoid articular facet along the posterosuperior aspect for the medial surface of the cuboid. The anterosuperior angle of the surface may display a much smaller facet for articulation with the medial aspect of the base of the fourth metatarsal. The surface is otherwise generally rough for cuneometatarsal (3,4) and interosseous cuneocuboid ligaments (1). The *anterior surface* is totally articular with the base of the third metatarsal. It is triangular in outline, base up and apex down, and is essentially plane in contour.

The *posterior surface* is quadrilateral or ovoid and plane in contour for articulation with the navicular proximally. A posteromedially directed blunt shelf of rough bone may be present inferior to the articular region. The inferior border or crest of the third cuneiform is smooth and rounded. Posteriorly a tubercle is present for attachments of plantar cuneocuboid, cuneonavicular, and cuneometatarsal (3,4) ligaments that are deeply situated (1). More superficially fibers of tendinous reflections of m. tibialis posterior and parts of the origins for m. flexor hallucis brevis and adductor hallucis can be identified.

METATARSAL BONES

Five metatarsal bones articulate with the parts of the lesser tarsus, including the cuboid and all three cuneiforms. This, the tarsometatarsal joint, is fre-

quently identified as Lisfranc's joint. The metatarsal bones are numbered one through five from medial to lateral. They are morphologically and developmentally classified as long bones. The second metatarsal is longest but the first is the largest in terms of its bulk. No anatomist has recorded the first metatarsal as dominant. The accepted normal metatarsal formula is $2 > 3 > 1 > 4 > 5$.

Students of biomechanics argue about whether the foot should be described in terms of arches. However, from a purely morphological standpoint, a dome-like structure for the foot as a whole is undeniable. The metatarsal bases form a transverse arch that is highest medially and low laterally. The second metatarsal is the apex of the arcuate structure and is wedged securely between the first and third cuneiforms. Medial and lateral arches are formed by their plantar concavities and dorsal convexities as the metatarsals are plantar flexed in relation to the mid tarsus. This characteristic is far more pronounced medially than laterally. However, no transverse arch can be said to exist relative to the five metatarsal heads; they lie essentially on the same horizontal plane. Synostosis between the navicular, cuneiform, and metatarsal has been verified in comparatively recent literature (10).

First Metatarsal

There is a slight longitudinal divergence of the axis of the first metatarsal from the second. The usual range varies from 2° to 9° (2). Measurements of the various metatarsals as to length and angulation vary with development. These factors were touched on briefly in the discussion on the developmental anatomy of the foot. The first metatarsal forms the end of an obliquity of the general metatarsal alignment that orients proximally and fibularward with the second metatarsal interlocking within a depression between the first and third cuneiforms. The *base of the first metatarsal* is essentially triangular with medial, lateral, and inferior borders. The articular surface, however, is reniform and congruent with the anterior surface of the first cuneiform. The hilum of the kidney-shaped surface is situated midway along the lateral border: the surface is concave from side to side and plane on the vertical axis, and frequently upper and lower subdivisions of the articular surface are present. A tubercle at the inferomedial border makes attachment for part of the tendinous insertion of m. tibialis anterior. Parts of the tendon of insertion of m. peroneus longus make attachment at a larger posteriorly directed tubercle at the inferolateral border of the base of the second metatarsal, and it is important to remember that no interosseous ligament is present between the first and second metatarsals.

The shaft of the first metatarsal is prismatic and has three surfaces (Fig. 1.43). The *lateral surface* is plane or slightly concave, smooth, and vertical. It provides part of the origin for the first dorsal interosseous muscle that orients proximodistally. The *inferior surface* of the first metatarsal is bounded by medial and lateral borders. It is concave on its long axis and the plantar tubercles of the medial and lateral angles of the base exaggerate this feature. The *dorsomedial surface* is smooth, convex, and becomes more dorsally oriented distally. The shaft demonstrates three borders; the superior border is smooth, rounded, and separates the dorsomedial and lateral surfaces. The medial and lateral borders marginate the inferior surface and are well defined.

The *head* of the first metatarsal is quadrilateral and relatively massive. Unlike the lesser metatarsals, the first metatarsal head is wider transversely than in its vertical dimension. The anterior articular surface is expanded plantarly into two smooth sloped grooves that are prolonged posteriorly and which are separated by a longitudinal elevation of bone, which is the cristae or median eminence. The fibular groove is greater than the tibial and both relate to fibular and tibial sesamoid bones, respectively. These ossicles develop with the tendons of m. flexor hallucis brevis. The median eminence is occasionally grooved as it relates to the tendon of m. flexor hallucis longus if the sesamoids are dimunitive. The superior hallucal phalangeal articular field is convex. The dorsal articular margin terminates proximally with a posterior transverse convexity that is smooth and lips over the dorsal aspect of the metatarsal shaft. Consequently, the metatarsal head's articular surface is greater than that of the congruent base of the proximal hallucal phalanx. The superomedial and superolateral angles of the metatarsal head present a tubercle or small epicondyle for attachment of the metatarsophalangeal collateral and sesamoidal ligaments (1).

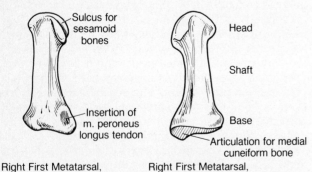

Right First Metatarsal, Lateral Aspect — Sulcus for sesamoid bones, Insertion of m. peroneus longus tendon

Right First Metatarsal, Medial Aspect — Head, Shaft, Base, Articulation for medial cuneiform bone

Figure 1.43.   First metatarsal.

Second, Third, and Fourth Metatarsals

The first and fifth metatarsals are structurally dissimilar. However, metatarsals two, three, and four demonstrate some similarities and will be discussed and compared as a group (Figs. 1.44–1.46).

Base

The second metatarsal base is cuneiform or pyramidal in outline; it has superior, medial, lateral, and posterior surfaces. The triangular posterior articular surface is slightly concave. The apex is inferior, the base is superior, and it is wholly articular with the second cuneiform. The medial surface demonstrates two articular facets: the posterosuperior angle facet is for the medial cuneiform. Usually a smaller facet for the first metatarsal is located more distally. The lateral surface bears four facets; two posteriorly are for the third cuneiform while two anteriorly are for the medial side of the base of the third metatarsal. The facets are separated by slight bony elevations. Therefore, the second metatarsal base articulates with the first and third metatarsals, and the first, second, and third cuneiforms. The superior surface is continuous with the shaft and is rough, as are the medial and lateral surfaces. Ligaments present include dorsal cuneometatarsal, dorsal and interosseous intermetatarsal, plantar cuneometatarsal, and plantar metatarsal ligaments (1). Lisfranc's ligament is represented as it firmly attaches the first cuneiform to the second metatarsal (2). The inferior crest provides insertion for tendinous slips of m. tibialis posterior and fibers of origin for the oblique head of m. adductor hallucis are identified.

The third metatarsal base, like the second, is cuneiform or pyramidal in outline with superior, medial, lateral, and posterior surfaces. The superior surface is rough and continuous with the shaft. The posterior surface is smooth and triangular, base up, apex down; it is slightly concave for articulation with the anterior articular surface of the third cuneiform. The medial surface is rough except for two articular facets, one superior, one inferior, for the base of the fibular aspect of the second metatarsal. The lateral surface is rough except for a single articular facet for the tibial aspect of the base of the fourth metatarsal. Attachments for interosseous cuneometatarsal, interosseous metatarsal, dorsal intermetatarsal, dorsal cuneometatarsal, plantar cuneometatarsal, and plantar intermetatarsal ligaments cause rugosities as they attach to their respective surface (2). Once again, reflections of the tendinous slips of insertion for m. tibialis posterior and fibers of origin of the oblique head of m. adductor hallucis relate to the rounded inferiorly situated crest.

The fourth metatarsal base is cuboidal or quadrilateral in outline (1). Like the other lesser metatarsal bones, the superior surface is rough and continuous with the shaft. The medial surface has two superiorly situated articular facets, the smaller of which marks the posterosuperior angle and is for articulation with

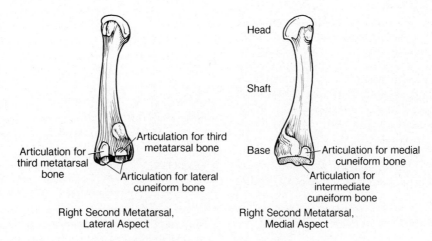

Articulation for third
metatarsal bone

Articulation for
third metatarsal
bone

Articulation for lateral
cuneiform bone

Right Second Metatarsal,
Lateral Aspect

Head

Shaft

Base

Articulation for medial
cuneiform bone

Articulation for
intermediate
cuneiform bone

Right Second Metatarsal,
Medial Aspect

Figure 1.44. Second metatarsal.

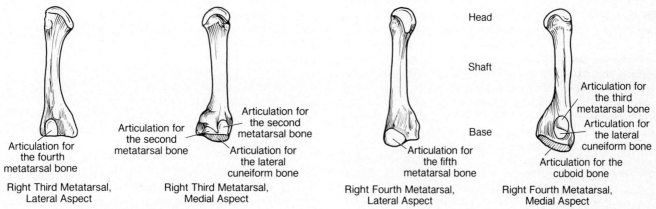

Articulation for
the fourth
metatarsal bone

Right Third Metatarsal,
Lateral Aspect

Articulation for
the second
metatarsal bone

Articulation for
the second
metatarsal bone

Articulation for
the lateral
cuneiform bone

Right Third Metatarsal,
Medial Aspect

Figure 1.45. Third metatarsal.

Head

Shaft

Base

Articulation for
the fifth
metatarsal bone

Right Fourth Metatarsal,
Lateral Aspect

Articulation for
the third
metatarsal bone

Articulation for
the lateral
cuneiform bone

Articulation for the
cuboid bone

Right Fourth Metatarsal,
Medial Aspect

Figure 1.46. Fourth metatarsal.

the third cuneiform. The larger, more anteriorly placed, facet is for the fibular aspect of the base of the third metatarsal. It is not unusual for the two facets to be confluent.

The lateral surface presents a large triangular or oval facet that is widest superiorly. It is situated at the posterosuperior angle for the tibial aspect of the base of the fifth metatarsal. A deep groove is present that parallels the anteroinferior angle of the articular facet, which is directed obliquely and somewhat vertically. It is for attachment of the intermetatarsal ligament (2). The posterior articular facet is plane or slightly concave and is congruent with the anteromedial aspect of the cuboid. Unlike the inferior aspects of the second and third metatarsal, which are merely crests, the fourth metatarsal has a plantar surface. It is small, rectangular, and often bears a tubercle for attachment of plantar intermetatarsal, plantar cuboidometatarsal, and plantar cuneometatarsal ligaments. Additionally, reflections of the tendinous fibers of insertion of m. tibialis posterior and fibers of origin for the oblique head of adductor hallucis relate to the plantar surface. Interosseous intermetatarsal, cuboidometatarsal, and cuneometatarsal ligaments are present, as are dorsal cuboideometatarsal and dorsal intermetatarsal ligaments that bind metatarsal bases three, four, and five (2).

Shafts—Metatarsals Two, Three, and Four

The shafts of metatarsals two, three, and four all have prismatic contours with dorsal, medial, and lateral surfaces. Each demonstrates an inferior smooth crest or border that is concave in its longitudinal dimension. Dorsolateral and dorsomedial borders are also present to delineate the three surfaces. The dorsal surface is flat and somewhat convex. Additionally, it is relatively large proximally and narrow distally. The medial surface tends to be convex and, with the lateral surface, converges on the inferior border or crest. The superior aspect of the lateral surfaces of the second, third, and fourth metatarsals give origin to the second, third, and fourth dorsal interosseous muscles. The medial surface of the second metatarsal shaft gives origin to the first dorsal interosseous muscle (1). The inferior aspect of the medial surfaces of the third, fourth, and fifth metatarsals give origin to the first, second, and third plantar interosseous muscles, respectively. A degree of twisting is associated with the longitudinal axis of the lesser metatarsals. For example, the second metatarsal is tapered. The superior surface of the base curves medially as it proceeds distally so that as the metatarsal head is approached, the surface is tibially disposed. Similarly, the posterolateral surfaces twist into a more dorsal position distally. The nutrient foramen is positioned midway along this surface. The surface medial at the proximal part of the second metatarsal shaft orients more inferiorly as it proceeds distally. The third metatarsal shaft is shorter than the second but demonstrates most of its morphological characteristics. The fourth metatarsal shaft does likewise so that its proximal lateral surface is oriented dorsolaterally in the narrow distal segment and the plantar crest that is centrally placed proximally is fibularly oriented distally. Nutrient foramena for the third, fourth, and fifth metatarsals are located on the medial surfaces of the shafts of these bones.

Heads—Metatarsals Two, Three, Four, and Five

The four lesser metatarsal heads demonstrate essentially quadrilateral outlines (2). Each is flattened from side to side. In profile, each forms an elliptical articular surface. This surface is classically condylar and is similar to the outline convexity of the first metatarsal head in that the plantar aspect extends more proximal than does the dorsal lip. There are two plantar condyles separated by a concave notch that relates to the passage of the respective tendons of m. flexor digitorum longus. The lateral condylar extension is invariably longer than the medial and this feature is well appreciated by podiatric surgeons dealing with related intractible plantar keratosis. Tubercles appear near the superior medial and lateral angles of the lesser metatarsal heads; these are for attachment of medial and collateral ligaments (1). A groove about the heads provides attachment of the plantar joint capsule of the metatarsophalangeal articulations.

Fifth Metatarsal

The fifth metatarsal is structurally atypical and, except for its head, needs special description (Fig. 1.47). The base of the fifth metatarsal is essentially pyramidal (2). It is distinctive for its posterolaterally directed styloid process (tubercle of the fifth metatarsal), which provides insertion for the tendon of m. peroneus brevis. This blunt projection is formed by the lateral confluence of the superior and inferior surfaces. Consequently this region can be properly characterized as an apophysis. The *posterior* surface is triangular with a medially disposed base and a lateral apex that is plane and congruent with the cuboid. This surface augments the passage of the tendon of m. peroneus longus through the cubostyloid groove by an irregular lateral field that approximates with the lateral surface of the cuboid. The *medial* surface is rough for attachment of intermetatarsal interosseous ligaments except for a large posterior oval or triangular facet for articulation with the fibular aspect of the base of the fourth metatarsal (1). The *superior* surface slopes at an angulation of about 45° in an inferolateral direction. It is generally rough and continuous with the superior surface of the shaft. It provides attachments for dorsal cubometatarsal and

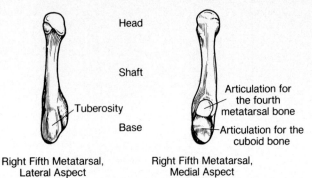

Right Fifth Metatarsal, Lateral Aspect — Head / Shaft / Tuberosity / Base

Right Fifth Metatarsal, Medial Aspect — Articulation for the fourth metatarsal bone / Articulation for the cuboid bone

Figure 1.47. Fifth metatarsal.

intermetatarsal ligaments and receives the tendinous insertion for m. peroneus tertius (peroneus brevis is inserted on the styloid process).

The *inferior* surface is rough, and in its proximal concave portion, fibers of origin for m. flexor digiti quinti brevis (flexor digiti minimi brevis) are found. The bony prominence on the inferior surface is for attachments of plantar intermetatarsal ligaments and to parts of the long and short plantar ligaments. Occasionally, some fibers of origin for m. abductor digiti minimi relate to this surface. There is no lateral surface (2). The fibular aspect of the base of the fifth metatarsal is a border formed by convergence of dorsal and plantar surfaces.

Shaft

The fifth metatarsal shaft is in continuity with the outline of the base and presents superior, inferior, and medial surfaces. Its borders are variably defined; the lateral border separates superior from inferior surfaces, but the inferior border that separates medial and inferior surfaces is poorly defined. The superior border divides medial and superior sufaces. The shaft is generally prismatic in outline with its base oriented medially and its crest in the lateral direction. The superior and inferior surfaces are convex from side to side. They are relatively broad proximally, but the shaft tapers to its neck just behind the head. The fifth metatarsal shaft demonstrates in a marked degree longitudinal rotation similar to that observed among the other lesser metatarsals. When viewed from distal to proximal, the posterior aspect of the medial surface twists clockwise into a more distal inferior position and the other surfaces follow this medial twist (2). The proximal central plantar crest becomes fibularly oriented in the distal shaft. The medial aspect of the fifth metatarsal relates to fibers of origin for the fourth dorsal and third plantar interosseous muscles. A nutrient foramen is also commonly found in the central region of the medial surface of the shaft (1).

PHALANGES

The lesser four toes are made up of four phalanges, proximal (first), middle (second), and distal (third or ungual because it relates to the toenail). The great toe has proximal and distal hallucal phalanges.

In all, there are fourteen phalangeal bones in each human foot.

The great toe is somewhat atypical and will be described first and separately. The proximal hallucal phalanx is relatively large and has a base, shaft, and head as do the lesser proximal phalanges.

Hallucal Phalanges

The *base* of the proximal hallucal phalanx presents an oval concave articular surface, which is broad from side to side (Fig. 1.48). It is smaller than the congruent articular surface of the first metatarsal head and is sometimes referred to as the glenoid cavity. The dorsal surface of the base of the proximal hallucal phalanx presents a transverse crest that overhangs the first metatarsal head to a degree. M. extensor hallucis brevis makes attachment at this point. The inferomedial and inferolateral angles also demonstrate tubercles. The larger medial one receives tendinous insertion of both m. abductor hallucis and the tibial head of m. flexor hallucis brevis. The lateral tubercle relates to tendons of the fibular head of flexor hallucis brevis and to the conjoined tendons of adductor hallucis (1). A strong plantar joint capsule invests the inferior aspect.

The *shaft* is markedly concave dorsally but slightly convex or plane inferiorly. The tendon of m. flexor hallucis longus relates to the inferior aspect of the shaft and grooves it slightly at its proximal and distal extremities. The *head* of the proximal phalanx is plane in its vertical superior aspect, but it becomes decidedly convex as the plantar aspect is approached. Small tubercles are found on the superomedial and superolateral margins of the articular cartilage for attachments of collateral ligaments. A small fossa is identified just behind the articular cartilage in the plantar aspect.

Hallucal Distal Phalanx

The ungual hallucal phalanx has a proximal articular surface that is congruent with the head of the proximal hallucal phalanx (Fig. 1.48). The bone is wide from side to side. It is concave laterally but is convex centrally. The tendon of insertion for m. extensor hallucis longus is on a broad transverse crest or tubercle immediately anterosuperior to the articular surface (11). The hallucal nail matrix is situated anterior to this point on the dorsal aspect of the bone. The collateral ligaments make attachment at the inferomedial and inferolateral angles of the base or proximal portions of the shaft of the ungual hallucal phalanx and small tubercles or rugosities may mark these locations (2). The shaft of the distal phalanx deviates laterally by an average of about 15° relative to the shaft of the proximal hallucal phalanx. This feature causes the lateral placement of the broad tendon of insertion for m. flexor hallucis longus. Consequently, the plantar aspect of the ungual hallucal phalanx presents an oblique ridge termed the "flying buttress." The *distal* aspect of the ungual hallucal phalanx is flared and tufted into a rounded structure, the ungual tuberosities.

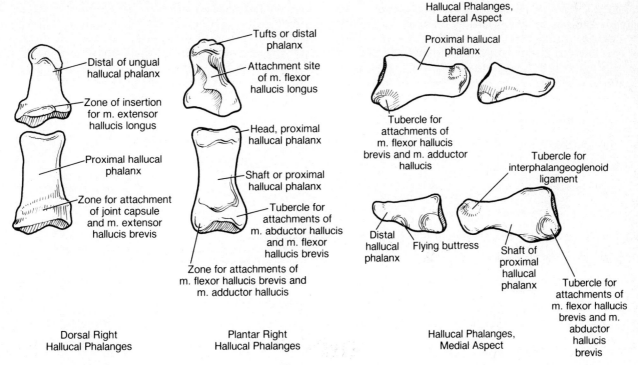

Figure 1.48.   Hallucal phalanges.

Phalanges of the Lesser Toes

The proximal phalanges of the four lesser toes are somewhat triangular or ovoid and longest on the vertical axis (Fig. 1.49). The *posterior* articular facet is smooth, concave, and congruent with the respective lesser metatarsal heads. The plantar aspect is notched and related to passage of the respective tendons of m. flexor digitorum longus. The small central concavity is surmounted by tubercles on either side that relate to the collateral ligaments. The base is slightly grooved transversely and relates to the metatarsophalangeal joint capsule and receives some fibers of insertion for dorsal and plantar interosseous muscles: the first, second, and third plantar interossei tend to adduct the respective digits and relate to the medial tubercles of the third, fourth, and fifth proximal phalanges. The dorsal interossei tend to abduct the respective lesser digits relative to a line bisecting the second ray. Some fibers of insertion for the second, third, and fourth dorsal interosseous muscles relate to the lateral tubercles of the proximal phalanges of the second, third, and fourth toes (2). The first dorsal interosseous muscle relates to the second toe.

The *shafts* of the proximal phalanges are slightly concave at the central portions of the plantar aspects both distally and proximally, and relates to the passage of the respective tendons of m. flexor digitorum longus: the inferior surface is otherwise plane or slightly concave. The shafts of the proximal phalanges are generally constricted in their central diameter but expanded at the proximal and distal extremities. The dorsal and plantar surfaces of the shaft are limited by medial and lateral borders. The *heads* of the proximal phalanges of the lesser toes are somewhat flattened dorsally where a small crescentic facet is present. The convex anterior articular surface becomes pulleylike as it proceeds plantarward. Its median groove widens as it relates to the inferior surface and the plantar articular facet is more extensive than the dorsal. Both medial and lateral sides of the respective heads are flattened and present small tubercles at their dorsal aspects that relate to the collateral ligaments (1). A depression in the bone is situated beneath each tubercle.

Middle Phalanges of the Lesser Toes

The middle phalanges of the lesser toes have bases, shafts, and heads, but these structures are much reduced in size. Their respective bases have small median vertical ridges that are expanded at the dorsal aspect to engage the crescentic lip of the dorsal distal crescentic ridge of the proximal phalanx. Two oval concave facets for articulation with the ungual phalanges are on either side of the ridge just mentioned. Tubercles are present at the inferomedial and inferolateral angles of the base that relate to the joint capsule collateral ligaments (2). The middle tendons of insertion for m. extensor digitorum longus make attachment along the dorsal aspect of the middle phalanges of the lesser toes. The shaft presents a dorsal convexity and a more or less flat plantar surface: the inferior surfaces receive the bifurcated tendons of insertion for m. flexor digitorum brevis. The heads of the middle phalanges are similar to those of the proximal row: they are convex dorsal to plantar, but broad and flattened from side to side.

Distal Phalanges of the Lesser Toes

The third, ungual or distal, phalanges appear rudimentary in that a shaft is not apparent (2). The base is congruent with the articular surface of the heads of the middle phalanges. The distal insertion of the tendon of m. extensor digitorum longus is made on the flattened superior surface. Similarly, the distal tendon of insertion for m. flexor digitorum longus is made on the flattened inferior surface. The distal end of the distal phalanges are tufted and horseshoe shaped and are termed ungual tuberosities (1). The respective nail matrixes are situated dorsally.

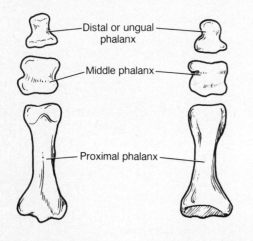

Distal or ungual phalanx

Middle phalanx

Proximal phalanx

Phalanges of Lesser Toes, Plantar Aspect

Phalanges of Lesser Toes, Dorsal Aspect

Middle phalanx

Ungual or distal phalanx

Tubercle or origin of collateral ligament of interphalangeal joint

Site of attachment of collateral ligament of interphalangeal joint

Proximal phalanx

Tubercle of attachment of interosseous muscle

Phalanges of Lesser Toes, Lateral Aspect

Figure 1.49. Phalanges of lesser toes.

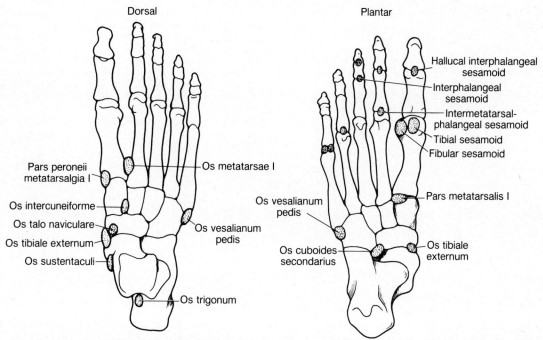

Figure 1.50. Sesamoid bones. (Modified from Warwick R, Williams PL (eds): *Gray's Anatomy*, ed 35, British. Philadelphia, WB Saunders Co, 1973.)

Synostosis or fusion of the middle and distal phalanges occur occasionally in the fourth toes, but are frequent in the fifth toe to the consternation of podiatric surgeons.

SESAMOID BONES

Sesamoid bones occur anatomically within the tibial and fibular tendinous slips of m. flexor hallucis brevis. They normally lie in smooth grooves on the plantar surface of the head of the first metatarsal and are separated by a median eminence (Fig. 1.50). These bones provide mechanical advantage through pressure absorption and a gliding mechanism. Although there are typically only two hallucal sesamoid bones, they occasionally are tripartite or, less frequently, quadripartite. The sesamoids are supported by complex ligamentous structures associated with the first metatarsophalangeal joint. These structures will be described in more depth subsequently in this chapter.

A number of inconstant sesamoid bones occur in the human foot (1,2). These include os trigonum, os sustentaculi, os tibiale externum, os talonaviculare dorsale, os intercuneiforme, os vesalianum pedis, os calcaneus secondarium, pars peroneametatarsalis I, and os cuboides secondarium. Sesamoids have also been identified on the plantar surfaces of metatarsophalangeal joints two, four, and five (the latter duplicated), the proximal interphalangeal joints of the first, second, and third toes, as well as the distal interphalangeal joint of the third toes (Fig. 1.50).

Developmentally, the bones of the foot ossify in a predictable sequence (Fig. 1.51). Failure to do so constitutes a class of disease characterized as osteochondrosis (12).

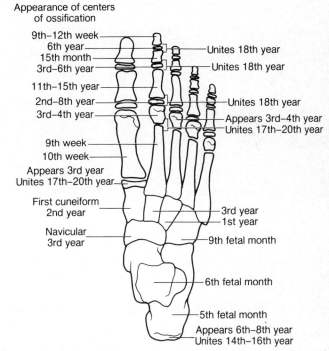

Figure 1.51. Ossification schedule of bones of foot. (Modified from Warwick R, Williams PL (eds): *Gray's Anatomy*, ed 35, British. Philadelphia, WB Saunders Co, 1973.)

References

1. Warwick R, Williams PL (eds): *Gray's Anatomy*, ed 35 British. Philadelphia, WB Saunders Co, 1973.
2. Sarrafian SK: *Anatomy of the Foot and Ankle*. Philadelphia, JB Lippincott Co, 1983.
3. Sewell RBS: A study of the astragules, part II. *J Anat Physiol* 38:243, 1904.

4. Inman VT: *The Joints of the Ankle*. Baltimore, Williams & Wilkins, 1976.
5. Laidlaw PP: The varieties of the os calcis. *J Anat Physiol* 38:133, 1904.
6. Laidlaw PP: The os calcis, part II. *J Anat Physiol* 39:168, 1905.
7. Stieda L: Der m. peroneus longus und die iuss knochen. *Anat Anz* 4:624–640, 1889.
8. Manners-Smith T: A study of the navicular in the human and anthropoid foot. *J Anat Physiol* 41:261, 1907.
9. Barclay M: A case of duplication of the internal cuneiform bone of the foot. *J Anat* 67:175, 1932.
10. Basu SS: Naviculo, cuneo-metatarsophalangeal synostosis. *Indian J Surg* 25:750, 1963.
11. Wilkinson JL: The terminal phalanx of the great toe. *J Anat* 88:537, 1954.
12. Hasselwander A: Studies on the ossification of the human foot. *Z Morphol Anthropol* 466, 1903.

Arthrology

The study of the joints of the lower extremity could easily become encyclopedic. Syndesmology or arthrology correctly includes descriptions of the mechanisms and ranges of motions that are particularly complex in the human foot. However, these parameters are best left to the chapters to follow relative to podiatric biomechanics. It will be the intent of the following comments to establish as simply as possible those morphological considerations necessary to understand the anatomy of the joints of the foot: these fundamental relationships will serve as prologue to orthopaedic considerations.

The present discussion logically begins with the ankle mortise in which the talus below is interposed between the tibia and fibula above. The distal ends of the two leg bones are closed by the extensive interosseous membrane and the anterior and posterior tibiofibular ligaments. They are characterized as strong, broad, flat connective tissue bands. The inferior aspect of the posterior tibiofibular ligament is strong and is specialized as the inferior transverse ligament that makes a deep attachment at the margin of the posterior articular surface of the talus. The fibers are directed laterally as they proceed downward from the posterior inferior aspect of the tibia.

TALOCRURAL JOINT: ANKLE JOINT

Joint Capsule

In examining the complexities of the medial and lateral ligaments of the ankle joint, it is important to remember the fibrous capsule of the ankle. It is attached to the tibial and fibular malleoli, as well as to the lower end of the tibia above and the neck of the talus below. Posterior fibers merge with those of the inferior transverse ligament (2). The capsule is thickened by collateral ligaments of either side.

The medial collateral ligament (deltoid ligament) is crossed by tendons of m. flexor digitorum longus and tibialis posterior. It has its proximal attachments on and about the notched portion of the tibial malleolus (Fig. 1.52). It is comprised of four ligamentous bands: the *anterior tibionavicular ligament* makes attachment on the navicular tuberosity. The *calcaneotibial ligament* fans out with verticle fibers about the margins of the sustentaculum tali. The *posterior tibiotalar ligament* sends fibers posterolaterally to afix on the medial tubercle of the talus. The *anterior tibiotalar ligment* makes attachment to the roughened medial surface of the talus by fibers that are the deepest of all elements of the deltoid ligament (3).

The lateral collateral ligament (lateral ligament of the ankle) is made up of three ligamentous divisions having their proximal attachments about the fibular malleolus (4). Two attach on the talus, one on the calcaneus (Fig. 1.53). *The anterior talofibular ligament* is deep and makes attachment on the lateral tubercle of the posterior process of the talus with a tibial slip passing onto the tibial malleolus. It is a strong trapezoidal band measuring about 30 × 5 mm (2). *The calcaneofibular ligament* is cordlike and rounded with its fibers directed posteriorly from the apex of the fibular malleolus above to the small tubercle on the posterolateral aspect of the calcaneus (5). *The posterior talofibular ligament* occurs with a 60% frequency. It tends to limit dorsiflexion of the foot and is often highly developed in equinus deformities. It arises from the posterolateral aspect of the fibular malleolus and makes attachments on the posterolateral tubercle of the talus and on the lateral calcaneus in a posterosuperior position (2). It characteristically has superomedial and inferolateral fibrous laminae. This ligament is extrinsically situated and relates to the sheath of the peronei and the posterior tunnel for the tendon for flexor hallucis longus. The ankle region is further markedly strengthened by fascicles that relate to the anterior colliculus. They are named the *superficial anterior tibiotalar fascicle*, the *tibionavicular fascicle*, and the *tibioligamentous fascicle* (2).

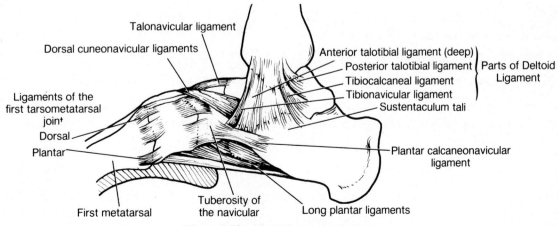

Figure 1.52. Medial ligaments of ankle.

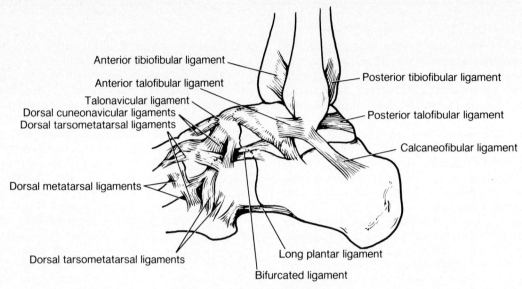

Figure 1.53.   Lateral ligaments of ankle.

GREATER TARSUS
Talocalcaneal Joint

The talocalcaneal joint is best known by podiatrists as the subtalar joint. Its patency has profound biomechanical implications. It is a modified arthrodial joint. In simple terms, the joint is comprised of the posterior articular facet of the calcaneus below and the body of the talus above. Technically, however, a portion of the anterior facet of the superior surface of the calcaneus may be cited as making up part of the articulation (2). There is a *joint capsule* surrounding the joint isolating it from all other tarsal joints and making it a simple synovial capsule. The *medial talocalcaneal ligament* makes attachment between the medial tubercle of the talus and the posterior margin of the sustentaculum tali of the calcaneus. It is closely associated with the deltoid ligament. The *lateral talocalcaneal ligament* is extended downward and posteriorly from the lateral progress of the talus to the lateral surface of the calcaneus. It is deep to the calcaneofibular ligament.

The *interosseous talocalcaneal ligament* forms the strongest bond between the talus and the calcaneus (6). It occupies most of the sinus tarsi composed of the sulcus calcanei above and the sulcus tali below and runs in an oblique transverse direction congruent with the sinus tarsi. The *cervical ligament* closes the sinus tarsi on its larger fibular portion: it extends from the superior surface of the calcaneus tibial to the origin of m. extensor digitorum brevis to a tubercle on the fibular aspect of the neck of the talus (7). The calcaneus and talus together comprise the greater tarsus. Its relationships to the lesser tarsus are significant for podiatrists.

It has been argued that the subtalar joint made by the articulation of the talus above with the calcaneus below is actually better termed a "joint and one half" (8). The designation "subtalar" is characterized as being a functional clinical term as opposed to the anatomist's view based on structure. The latter definition would include the talocalcaneal portion of the talocalcaneonavicular joint as a morphological part of the subtalar joint. It is, therefore, anatomically preferred to characterize the subtalar joint (as well as the transverse tarsal joint) as joints and one half. The subtalar joint is comprised of the talocalcaneal and portion of the talocalcaneonavicular joint whereas the transverse tarsal joint is composed of the calcaneocuboid joint plus the talonavicular portion of the talocalcaneonavicular joint. Tracy states that this one and one half concept should be borne in mind continually when the term "subtalar" or the term "transverse tarsal" is used either by the clinician or the anatomist.

Such a concept, when understood by both anatomists and clinicians, would cause considerably less confusion when the terms "subtalar" and "transverse tarsal" are to be employed (Fig. l.54).

Lesser Tarsal Joints
Talocalcaneoavicular Articulations

The head of the talus, the posterior surface of the navicular (acetabulum pedis) and the middle and anterior superior facets of the calcaneus make up this condyloid articulation (Figs. 1.55, 1.56). The primary ligamentous structure of these joints is the *joint capsule.*

The dorsal talonavicular ligament makes attachments to the superior aspect of the neck of the talus and the dorsal surface of the navicular. It is a relatively thin broad band that relates to the extensor tendons.

The lateral calcaneonavicular ligament is the tibial component of the "bifurcated ligament." It has attachment on the anterosuperior surface of the calcaneus near the angle of the sinus tarsi and fixes on the lateral aspect of the navicular. It measures about 2 × 1 cm. The fibular component of the bifurcated ligament arises lateral to the medial part and attaches to the posterodorsal aspect of the cuboid. It measures about 1.0 × 0.5 cm and is referred to as the *medial calcaneocuboid ligament* (part of the bifurcated ligament) (9).

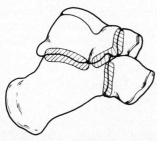

Figure 1.54. Subtalar joint (redrawn after Tracy). (Modified from Tracy EG: Definition of the subtalar and transverse tarsal joints. *J Am Podiatry Assoc* 64:56–58, 1974.)

The plantar (inferior) calcaneonavicular ligament (the "spring" ligament) makes its proximal attachment on the anterior surface of the sustentaculum tali or a bit laterally on the coronoid cavity of the calcaneus. Its fibers fan out for its distal attachment on the inferior surface of the navicular. It presents a dorsal fibrocartilaginous facet that supports the head of the talus. A thick fatty layer is found beneath the ligament.

Calcaneocuboid Articulation

The joint comprised of the anterior articular surface of the calcaneus and the posterior surface of the cuboid is enclosed by a *joint capsule* and is a saddle type joint. It has four components (Figs. 1.55, 1.56).

The *dorsal calcaneocuboid ligament* makes attachments to the dorsolateral aspect of the calcaneus proximally and to the dorsolateral aspect of the cu-

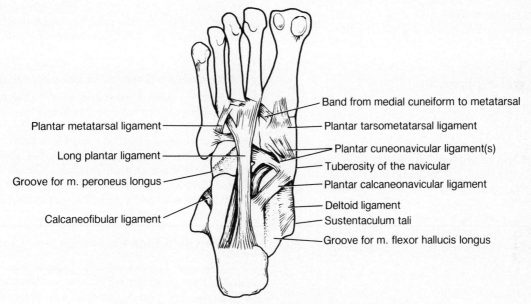

Figure 1.55. Superficial ligaments of plantar mid tarsal joint region.

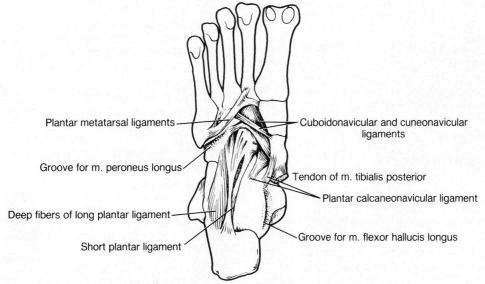

Figure 1.56. Deep ligaments of plantar mid tarsal region.

boid. It is a flat band with a separate smaller lateral segment occasionally present (2).

The *plantar calcaneocuboid ligament* makes its proximal attachment to the anterior tubercle and tuberosity of the plantar surface of the calcaneus. It fans out in an anteromedial direction to make distal attachment on the beak or promontory of the cuboid. It is called the short plantar ligament and lies deep to the long plantar ligament.

The *long plantar ligament* (long plantar calcaneocuboid ligament) makes its proximal attachment on the anterior aspect of the tuberosities of the plantar surface of the calcaneus. Its distal attachments are by deep and superficial fibers: the deep segment is thickest and is fixed on the distal aspect of the promontory of the cuboid (2). Superficial fibers form part of the tunnel for the tendon of m. peroneus longus as it cross braces the foot. It ultimately separates into four slips for attachment to the bases of metatarsals two, three, four, and sometimes five.

The *medial calcaneocuboid ligament* has been described as part of the bifurcated calcaneocubonavicular ligament.

Cuneonavicular Ligaments

The three cuneiforms articulate with the proximally situated navicular. All joints are classified as arthrodial (Figs. 1.55, 1.56).

Dorsal Cuneonavicular Ligaments. Contiguous surfaces of the medial, intermediate, and lateral cuneiforms have separate ligamentous bands attaching the posterosuperior surfaces with the anterosuperior surface of the navicular. The medial ligament extends straight forward while the intermediate and lateral elements extend obliquely forward.

Plantar Cuneonavicular Ligaments. The medial makes attachment to the plantar aspect of the navicular tuberosity. It is thick and short and is fixed on the plantar tuberosity of the medial cuneiform. Contiguous plantar surfaces of the intermediate and lateral cuneiforms make attachment to the inferior surface of the navicular by plantar ligaments. The intermediate lies deepest of the three whereas the lateral is the longest.

Medial Cuneonavicular Ligament. This makes attachment to the medial aspect of the navicular tuberosity and the medial side of the medial cuneiform. It is thick and strong. All of the plantar and medial cuneonavicular ligaments lie deep to and are masked by reflections of the tendinous expansions of m. tibialis posterior.

Cubonavicular Articulation

Dorsal Cubonavicular Ligament. Fibers of this ligament form a triangle with its base fibialward and its apex tibialward. It usually invests the third or lateral cuneiform as it makes attachments to contiguous surfaces of the cuboid and navicular dorsally (2).

Plantar Cubonavicular Ligament. Contiguous plantar surfaces of cuboid and navicular are interconnected by this rectangular band that overlaps the deep calcaneocuboid ligament. Anatomical variation of this ligament is its arrangement as two plantar triangular fascicles. In this instance, the apex is fibularly oriented on the cuboid with the base attached on the inferolateral aspect of the navicular (2).

Interosseous Cubonavicular Ligament. Strong transversely oriented fibers make interosseous attachments on the roughened bony areas below the contiguous articular facets on the fibular surface of the navicular and the tibial surface of the cuboid.

Intercuneiform Ligaments

Dorsal Intercuneiform Ligaments. The first and second and second and third cuneiforms are interconnected by relatively small rectangular bands that constitute dorsal intercuneiform ligaments.

Plantar Intercuneiform Ligaments. These make attachment between the posterolateral angle of the inferior surface of the first cuneiform and the plantar surface of the cuboid in close association with reflections of the tendinous insertions of m. tibialis posterior.

Interosseous Intercuneiform Ligaments

Strong, thick, transverse bands interconnect adjacent sides of the first and second cuneiforms. They make attachment on the posterolateral angle of the lateral surface of the first cuneiform and on the rough surface below the articular facet on the medial surface of the second cuneiform. The second and third cuneiforms have an interosseous ligament situated anterior to and between their contiguous articular facets. These ligaments are short but stout.

Cuneocuboid Ligaments

Dorsal Cuneocuboid Ligament. This is a broad, flat band that may occur as two fascicles. Its fibers orient in an anteromedially obliquity to make attachments to contiguous surfaces of the dorsal aspects of the third cuneiform and the cuboid. Along with the dorsal cubonavicular and the dorsal cuneonavicular ligaments it forms a triangle (2).

Plantar Cuneocuboid Ligament. This makes attachment between the respective crests on the plantar surfaces of the third cuneiform and the cuboid.

Interosseous Cuneocuboid Ligament. This makes interosseous attachment between the fibular surface of the third cuneiform and the tibial surface of the cuboid. It is short and thick and is placed on the roughened bone just anterior to the contiguous articular surfaces.

Tarsometatarsal (Lisfranc's Joint)

Tarsometatarsal Ligaments. The dorsal medial surfaces of the base of the first metatarsal and the first cuneiform have a single, thick, strong ligament (Fig. 1.57).

Three dorsal ligaments attach the superior aspect

of the second metatarsal with the dorsum of the first, second, and third cuneiforms by three flat bands that fan out.

The adjacent dorsal articular surfaces of the third metatarsal and the lateral cuneiform have a single flat dorsal ligament. Occasionally an accessory band that makes dorsal attachments to the base of the third metatarsal, the third cuneiform, and the cuboid can be identified (2).

The fourth metatarsal is invested dorsally with the cuboid laterally and the anterolateral angle of the third cuboid.

The fifth metatarsal base has attachment on its dorsolateral aspect to the adjacent surface of the cuboid by a single strong flat band. Normally there are eight dorsal tarsal metatarsal ligaments. Additionally, a transverse ligamentous band exists between the third cuneiform and the cuboid (2).

Plantar   Tarsometatarsal   Ligaments. These are arranged with less regularity than those on the dorsum (Fig. 1.58). Both longitudinal and oblique fibers are apparent. The first cuneometatarsal joint has the strongest of these flat bands. No plantar ligament exists between the second cuneiform and the base of the second metatarsal. Rather, the plantar aspects of the second and third metatarsal bases have oblique attachments to the first or medial cuneiform. A weaker ligamentous attachment is made plantarly to the bases of the fourth and fifth metatarsal with the contiguous border of the cuboid.

Interosseous Tarsometatarsal Ligaments. No interosseous ligaments relate to the base of the first metatarsal. There are only three such tarsometatarsal ligaments, and two relate to the second metatarsal. A constant interosseous band makes attachments between the anterolateral angle of the first cuneiform and the contiguous tibial aspect of the second metatarsal. An inconstant band makes attachments between the anteromedial angle of the third cuneiform and the adjacent base of the second metatarsal. The third makes interosseous attachments between the third cuneiform at its posterolateral angle

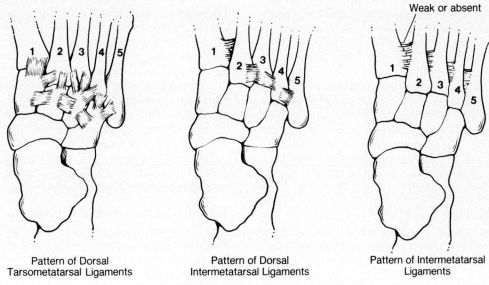

Pattern of Dorsal Tarsometatarsal Ligaments

Pattern of Dorsal Intermetatarsal Ligaments

Pattern of Intermetatarsal Ligaments

Figure 1.57.   Dorsal tarsometatarsal ligaments.

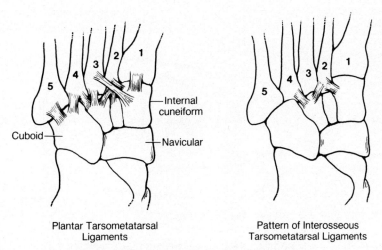

Plantar Tarsometatarsal Ligaments

Pattern of Interosseous Tarsometatarsal Ligaments

Figure 1.58.   Plantar tarsometatarsal ligaments.

and the contiguous aspect of the fourth metatarsal base. The tarsometatarsal interosseous ligaments are subject to a great degree of variation, but these are beyond the scope of this discussion (2).

Intermetatarsal Ligaments

Dorsal, plantar, and interosseous ligments make attachments between the metatarsals (Figs. 1.57, 1.58). However, the first metatarsal resembles the thumb in that no interosseous ligament exists attaching it to the second.

Dorsal Intermetatarsal Ligaments. These orient obliquely on the dorsal surfaces of the respective second and third metatarsals, the third and fourth metatarsals (the strongest) and the fourth and fifth metatarsals (2). These are thin, small, and flat fibrous bands.

Plantar Intermetatarsal Ligaments. These angle obliquely medially and slightly anteriorly as they make plantar attachments as described for the bases of the lesser metatarsals. They are, however, stronger than those on the dorsum (10).

Interosseous Intermetatarsal Ligaments. Three short but strong interosseous ligaments establish stability between the bases of the lesser metatarsals. They make attachments between adjacent surfaces of the second and third, third and fourth, and fourth and fifth metatarsals (1).

Deep Transverse Intermetatarsal Ligament. This structure, which is also called the intercapitular ligament, connects the plantar surfaces of adjacent metatarsal heads proximal to their respective heads (Fig. 1.59). The structure is a strong, flat band that stabilizes the distal intermetatarsal relationships. It will be discussed in relation to the metatarsophalangeal joints.

Metatarsophalangeal Joint(s)

The bases of the proximal phalanges and the heads of the metatarsals make articulation as spheroidal joints. There is an incomplete joint capsule plantarly, but it is absent on the dorsal aspect because of the presence of reflections of the fibrous extendor hood apparatus.

Plantar Ligaments. *The plantar capsule* is thickened by a *plantar plate* that is supported or suspended by the *collateral* and *suspensory glenoid ligaments*. The transverse metatarsal ligament invests and interconnects contiguous metatarsal plantar plates. Additionally, the plantar plate provides attachments for elements of the tendon sheath of m. flexor digitorum longus et brevis. Additionally, vertical and longitudinal(2) septae from the plantar aponeurosis, the transverse head of m. adductor hallucis, and the metatarsal adipose cushion provide support for the metatarsophalangeal joint (10).

The plantar plate makes attachments on its dorsal aspect for the metatarsoglenoid suspensory ligament: the transverse lamina of the extensor hood apparatus (aponeurosis), and the respective interossei (11).

The *phalangeal apparatus* is an anatomical unit formed by the plantar plate and structures making attachment on it (Fig. 1.60).

Metatarsophalangeal Collateral Ligaments. These make attachments on the superiorly situated lateral tubercles of the respective lesser metatarsal heads. Fibers are directed anteriorly to make a distal attachment on the inferiorly placed lateral tubercles of the bases of the respective proximal phalanges (10).

Suspensory or Metatarsoglenoid Ligament. This is a fan-shaped fibrous structure having its superior attachment on the posteroinferior aspect of the lateral tubercle of the respective metatarsal heads. The obliquely directed fibers relate to those of the collateral ligaments until they diverge to make an inferior attachment to the plantar plate of the respective plantar metatarsophalangeal joints (2) (Fig. 1.61).

Interphalangeal Joints (Lesser Toes)

The interphalangeal joints of the lesser toes are hinge or ginglymus joints. They are structurally similar to the metatarsophalangeal joints (Fig. 1.61).

Articular Capsule. The capsule incompletely

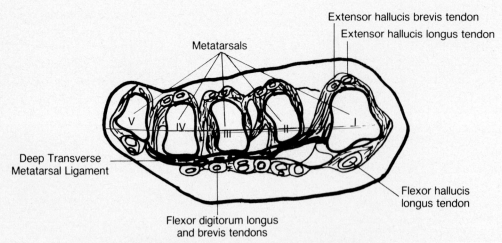

Figure 1.59. Deep transverse metatarsal ligament(s).

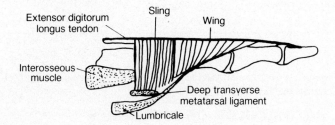

Lateral Formation of Extensor Aponeurosis

Figure 1.60. Phalangeal apparatus.

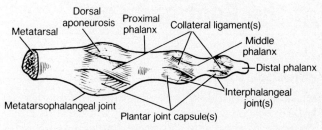

Figure 1.61. Metatarsophalangeal and interphalangeal joint organization.

invests the joint plantarly. Its deepest part is thickened to form a plantar plate or plantar ligament (1). These joints are closed dorsally by fibrous expansions of the extensor hood apparatus.

Interphalangeal Collateral Ligaments. These make proximal attachments on the superolateral aspect of the respective phalangeal heads. Fibers extend obliquely downwards to make distal attachment on the inferolateral aspect of the base of the next distal phalanx. Occasionally, interphalangeal sesamoid ossicles are present on the inferior aspect of these joints, and the collateral ligaments invest them with fibrous ligamentous extensions (2).

Hallucal Interphalangeal Joint

The interphalangeal joint of the great toe may demonstrate a sesamoid bone. Most texts relate its presence to the tendon of m. flexor hallucis longus, but the author has observed a small tendon deep to the long flexor: the author has named it m. flexor hallucis capsularis accessorious. The ossicle has several orientations. When it is distinctly intracapsular it may be marked by a transverse ridge where the joint space occurs.

Plantar Hallucal Interphalangeal Liga-

ment. This is structurally similar to those of the lesser interphalangeal joints.

Collateral Hallucal Interphalangeal Ligaments. These have proximal attachment on the superolateral aspect of the proximal hallucal phalanx. Distal attachment is made on the inferolateral aspect of the base of the ungual or distal hallucal phalanx.

References

1. Warwick R, Williams PL (eds): *Gray's Anatomy*, ed 35 British. Philadelphia,WB Saunders Co, 1973.
2. Sarrafian SK: *Anatomy of the Foot and Ankle*. Philadelphia, JB Lippincott Co, 1983.
3. Pankovitch AM, Shivaram MS: Anatomical basis of variability in injuries of the medial malleolus and the deltoid ligament: I. Anatomical studies. *Acta Orthop Scand* 50:217, 1979.
4. Prins JG: Diagnosis and treatment of injuries to the lateral ligament of the ankle. *Acta Chir Scand (Suppl)* 486:23, 1978.
5. Ruth CJ: The surgical treatment of injuries of the fibular collateral ligaments of the ankle. *J Bone Joint Surg* (A) 43:229, 1961.
6. Cahill DR: The anatomy and function of the contents of the human tarsal sinus and canal. *Anat Rec* 153:1, 1965.
7. Smith JW: The ligamentous structures of the canalis and sinus tarsi. *J Anat* 92:616, 1958.
8. Tracy EG: Definition of the subtalar and transverse tarsal joints. *J Amer Podiatry Assoc* 64:56–58, 1974.
9. Barclay-Smith E: The astragulo-calcaneo-navicular joint. *J Anat Physiol* 30:390, 1896.
10. Jones WF: *Structure and Function as Seen in the Foot*, ed 2. London, Baillier, 1949.
11. Bojsen-Moeller F, Flagstadt KE: Plantar aponeurosis and internal structure of the ball of the foot. *J Anat*, 12:599, 1976.

Aponeurosis, Retinaculae, Fascias, and Compartments of the Foot and Leg

CRURAL FASCIA

The crural fascia is the deep fascia of the leg. It invests the musculature of the leg and extends from the knee to the ankle. Along its course it sends septations between the muscles and frequently provides partial origin to the extrinsic muscles of the foot having origin on the leg. Close fibrous attachments are made to the periosteum of the medial aspect of the tibia and insertion is made to the head of the fibula. Distal attachments are made to both tibial and fibular malleoli.

Osteofascial compartmentalization of the leg divides the musculature of the leg into anterior, lateral, and posterior divisions. The posterior compartment is further divided into deep and superficial parts.

The anterior peroneal septum makes attachment to the anterolateral border of the fibula from the deep surface of the crural fascia superficially.

The posterior peroneal septum makes attachment to the posterolateral border of the fibula from the deep surface of the crural fascia.

The deep transverse intermuscular septum passes from the medial border of the tibia to the posterior peroneal septum, forming deep and superficial compartments. The muscles gastrocnemius, soleus, and plantaris are found in the superficial compartment, while m. flexor digitorum longus, m. flexor hallucis longus, and m. tibialis posterior are found in the deep compartment.

RETINACULAE OF THE ANKLE

Tough, thick connective tissue bands bind down the tendons entering the foot on its medial, lateral, and anterior aspects. Such an arrangement prevents bow-stringing and provides mechanical advantage for these strong tendons that are the extrinsic musculature of the foot.

Extensor Retinaculum (Anterior Annular Ligament)

The *extensor retinaculum* is composed of upper and lower portions (Fig. 1.62).

The *superior extensor retinaculum* or transverse crural ligament constitutes the upper limb of the extensor retinaculum. It is attached to the regions just above the tibial and fibular malleoli. Tendons of m. extensor digitorum longus, m. peroneus tertius, and m. tibialis anterior are bound down by this strong band as they approach the foot from their origins above on the leg.

The *inferior extensor retinaculum* is referred to as the anterior cruciate crural ligament because it forms a transversely oriented "Y" (or "X" in some instances). Its structure is more complex than that of the superior extensor retinaculum.

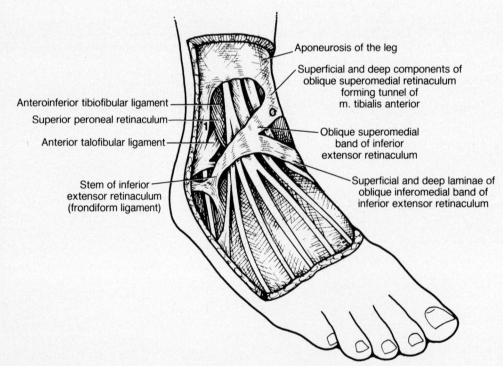

Anteroinferior tibiofibular ligament

Superior peroneal retinaculum

Anterior talofibular ligament

Stem of inferior extensor retinaculum (frondiform ligament)

Aponeurosis of the leg

Superficial and deep components of oblique superomedial retinaculum forming tunnel of m. tibialis anterior

Oblique superomedial band of inferior extensor retinaculum

Superficial and deep laminae of oblique inferomedial band of inferior extensor retinaculum

Figure 1.62. Extensor retinaculum and related structures. (Modified from Sarrafian SK: *Anatomy of the Foot and Ankle.* Philadelphia, JB Lippincott Co, 1983.)

The stem of the Y-shaped retinaculum constitutes the *frondiform ligament* and is affixed on the fibular aspect of the calcaneus near the peroneal tubercle. It has medial, intermediate, and lateral roots. The medial root forms a sling that loops around the tendons of m. peroneus tertius and m. extensor digitorum longus. A bursa is frequently demonstrated between it and the anterior talar ligaments.

The *oblique superomedial band* of the extensor retinaculum continues medially and proximally to make attachments about the tibial malleolus. This retinaculum passes over the tendon of m. extensor hallucis longus forming a recurrent loop about it. It passes under the tendon of m. tibialis anterior but bifurcates to envelop the tendon within a tunnel composed of inferior and superior retention systems.

The *oblique inferomedial band* of the extensor retinaculum forms the more distal limb of the Y-shaped retinaculum. It extends over the dorsum of the foot to attach on the medial aspect of the plantar aponeurosis (fascia) near the base of the first metatarsal. It passes over the dorsalis pedis artery, the deep peroneal nerve, and the tendon of m. extensor hallucis longus. As it proceeds in a medial direction its fibers bifurcate to invest the m. abductor hallucis and forms a distinct tunnel about the tendon of m. tibialis anterior.

In about one fourth of all specimens, an *oblique superolateral band* is present that provides the extensor retinaculum with a true cruciate or X-shaped configuration. It makes proximal attachment on the fibular malleolus.

The *peroneal retinaculum* relates to the peroneus longus et brevis musculature and is also referred to as the external retinaculum of the tarsus. It has superior and inferior components.

The *superior peroneal retinaculum* passes over the peroneal musculature with attachments on the retromalleolar groove of the fibular malleolus and passing behind to affix on the tendo achillis and the posterolateral aspect of the calcaneus. This structure is essentially quadrilateral in outline.

Distal attachment of the *inferior peroneal retinaculum* is made along the lateral rim of the sinus tarsi and is essentially continuous with the frondiform ligament. It makes attachment on the lateral surface of the calcaneus in the region of the posterolateral tubercle. The structure roofs the tendon of m. peroneus brevis above and the tendon of m. peroneus longus below within a tunnel formed in part by the peroneal tubercle that provides bony separation for the two tendons on the lateral aspect of the calcaneus. These tunnels occasionally fail to retain their respective tendons well, and surgical enhancement of these structures may be required.

The *flexor retinaculum* has been variously referred to as the medial annular ligament and the laciniate ligament (Fig. 1.63). It is a triangular structure composed of strong connective tissue fibers and is clinically important as the location of the so-called tarsal tunnel.

The apex of the flexor retinaculum is situated at the anteromedial aspect of the tibial malleolus with additional fibers extending about the contiguous parts of the tendon of m. tibialis anterior. The base of the triangle relates to the superior border of m. abductor hallucis and extends from the medial aspect of the calcaneal tuberosity and the tendo achillis behind to a line continuous with the talonavicular joint anteriorly. The more posterior margin of the flexor retinaculum relates to the deep fascias of the distal part of the leg that constitutes the *tibiotalocalcaneal canal.*

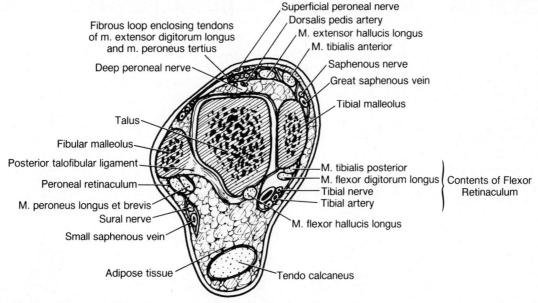

Figure 1.63. Flexor retinaculum, ankle region in cross section. (Modified from Sarrafian SK: *Anatomy of the Foot and Ankle.* Philadelphia, JB Lippincott Co, 1983.)

This structure demonstrates upper and lower canals that are the tibiotalar and the talocalcaneal tunnels, respectively.

The fascia of the proximal part of the tibiotalar canal relates to the retromedial malleolar and the posterior aspects of the distal tibia. Also included are the posterior tubercles and the posterior border and posteromedial surface of the talus. Proceeding distally, the talocalcaneal tunnel emerges to cover the medial surfaces of the talus above and the calcaneus below, as well as the sustentaculum tali.

Four canals are formed in the talocalcaneal (tarsal) tunnel. The first and most medial contains the tendon of m. tibialis posterior. It crosses the medial surface of the talus and the deltoid ligament as it proceeds to insert on the navicular and other lesser tarsal bones. The second compartment is for the tendon of flexor digitorum longus that crosses the posteromedial talar tubercle to pass over the medial surface of the sustentaculum tali.

The third compartment is for the neurovascular bundle supplying the plantar surface of the foot and includes the tibial nerve and the posterior tibial artery and vein. The nerve is situated anterior to the vessels. The fourth canal contains the tendon of flexor hallucis longus that grooves the inferior surface of the sustentaculum tali. More distally, it will cross and share a common sheath with the tendon of flexor digitorum longus. The fourth tunnel is the deepest and most laterally situated of the four canals making up the tarsal tunnel.

DEEP FASCIAS OF THE FOOT

A relatively thin membranous expansion forms the dorsal fascia of the foot. It becomes continuous with the crural fascia proximally where it becomes somewhat thicker. Distally, the dorsal aponeurosis contributes to the formation of the sheaths of the extensor tendons. It blends laterally with fibers of the plantar aponeurosis.

The sole of the foot is invested by the strong fibers of the plantar aponeurosis (Fig. 1.64). This structure has a dominant central portion with more finely structured medial and lateral componenents. The central band is structurally complex with both deep and superficial components, as well as demonstrating vertical and transverse fibers that make a variety of internal attachments including those to the dermis of the skin.

Central Component of the Plantar Aponeurosis. The major central component of the plantar aponeurosis is triangular in outline with its apex measuring about 2 cm affixed to the plantar surface of the posteromedial calcaneal tuberosity. The aponeurosis broadens as it proceeds distally with thick, glistening, gently twisted bands to the mid metatarsal shaft regions where five bands emerge. At the level of the metatarsal heads, these five bands divide into deep and superficial components.

The deep component of the plantar aponeurosis continues as five slips, each of which bifurcates to

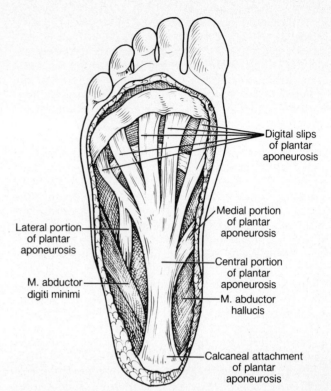

Figure 1.64. Plantar aponeurosis. (Modified from Warwich R, Williams PL (eds): *Gray's Anatomy*, ed 35 British. Philadelphia, WB Saunders Co, 1973.)

flank the tendons of m. flexor digitorum longus et brevis. This bifurcation invests the deep transverse metatarsal ligament thus forming a series of arches through which the tendons pass. The tendons of the lumbricales and the neurovascular bundles pass between these septations.

The superficial component of the plantar aponeurosis continues distally with a somewhat different orientation. The most medial slip is directed toward the great toe and the most lateral slip is similarly directed toward the fifth digit. The central three slips of the superficial component tend to be situated interdigitally. One tract is placed between the first and second toes, the second attaches either to the base of the third toe or to the interval between the third and fourth toes, and the third makes attachment either to the base of the fifth toe or to the interval between the fourth and fifth toes.

The skin of the distal forefoot has intimate attachments to the fascias of the plantar surface that orient along several planes (Fig. 1.65).

Natatory Ligament. This transversely oriented system of six to eight bands is situated deep to the longitudinal fibers of the superficial aponeurosis. It reticulates the area between the web spaces and the dermis on the ball of the foot. Longitudinal fibers of the superficial fascia contribute to the structure that covers the neurovascular bundles of the region.

Fasciculus Aponeurotica Transversum. This structure is situated superficial and proximal to the metatarsal heads. It too has transversely oriented bands, but at its medial and lateral margins fibers diverge into a more longitudinal axis. Its distal portions contribute to the formation of the natatory ligament. Adipose tissue is found liberally dispersed throughout its bands.

Sagittal Septae.   Ten (five paired) bands arise from each of the five longitudinal superficial aponeurotic bands proximal to the metatarsal heads. These septae help to flank the digital flexors and attach deeply to the fascia underlying the interossei and m. adductor hallucis (transverse head), as well as the deep transverse metatarsal ligament, the plantar plates, and the glenoid ligaments.

Vertical Fibers.   Vertical fibers make attachments to the dermis of the overlying skin with deep attachments to the adjacent superficial aponeurosis, flexor sheaths, and the deep transverse metatarsal ligaments.

Mooring Ligaments.   Mooring ligaments constitute a transverse reticular system associated deeply to the five flexor sheaths distal to the metatarsal heads that are also affixed superficially to the skin.

Encapsulated Fat Bodies.   Fat bodies are encapsulated plantar to the intermetatarsal capitular space superficial to the deep transverse metatarsal ligament. These cushions protect neurovascular bundles deep to them (Fig. 1.66).

Lateral Intermuscular Septum.   The foot contains three compartments separated by two septations. The lateral one arises from the medial calcaneal tuberosity and follows along the medial border of the fifth metatarsal (Fig. 1.67). It encloses the third plantar interosseous muscle and its tendon of insertion. Additionally, it is perforated by the long flexor tendon and the neurovascular bundle along the lateral plane.

Medial Intermuscular Septum.   This comb-like structure is frequently perforated by nerves, vessels and tendons. It is attached proximally at the margin of m. flexor accessorious and the medial surface of the calcaneus. It passes between the muscle substance of the oblique head of m. adductor hallucis and m. flexor hallucis brevis to make distal attachment to the navicular and to the lateral aspect of the first metatarsal. It provides passage for m. flexor digitorum longus and the lateral plantar neurovascular bundle.

Specialized Supportive Structures About the Metatarsophalangeal Joints

Minute structures in and about the metatarsophalangeal joints of the human foot provide for spe-

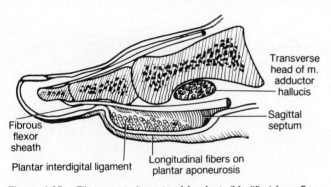

Figure 1.65.   Fibrous attachments of forefoot. (Modified from Sarrafian SK: *Anatomy of the Foot and Ankle*. Philadelphia, JB Lippincott Co, 1983.)

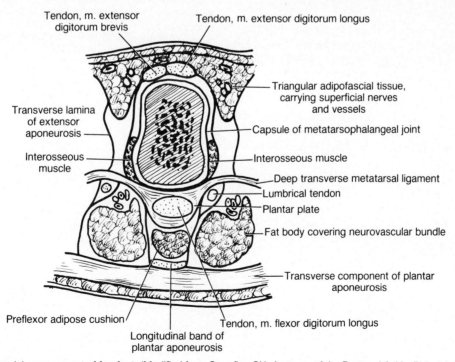

Figure 1.66.   Adipofascial arrangement of forefoot. (Modified from Sarrafian SK: *Anatomy of the Foot and Ankle*. Philadelphia, JB Lippincott Co, 1983.)

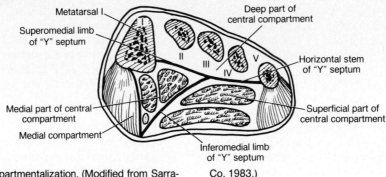

Figure 1.67. Forefoot compartmentalization. (Modified from Sarrafian SK: *Anatomy of the Foot and Ankle*. Philadelphia, JB Lippincott Co, 1983.)

cialized supportive, insulative, and shock absorbing functions. Such anatomical features are most often missed in traditional cadaver dissection, which is subject to severe dehydration and degeneration. Recent investigations have demonstrated these small structures in fresh unembalmed specimens.

Podiatrists are familiar with the so-called extensor hood apparatus. The structure stabilizes the extensor tendons of the metatarsophalangeal and interphalangeal joints. Oblique and transverse fibers fan out from either side of the centrally placed tendon to enclose the dorsal aspect of the joint. This annular structure is an aponeurosis that extends plantarly to the level of the deep transverse metatarsal ligament (Fig. 1.68). It also makes attachment to the plantar plates of the metatarsophalangeal joints along with their respective glenoid ligaments. This connective tissue reflection is the extensor sling; vertical fibers of the apparatus are referred to as the vertical lamina (Fig. 1.66).

An intertendinous segment of the common dorsal aponeurosis interconnects adjacent extensor sheaths proximal to the respective metatarsal heads. Deep to this structure is a more or less parallel dorsal interosseous aponeurosis. The two structures just named will converge in the region of the metatarsophalangeal joint as the dorsal transverse ligament.

Fascial septations pass from dorsal to plantar about the respective metatarsal heads. The vertical lamina interconnects the plantar transverse ligament with the dorsal interosseous aponeurosis.

An interaxial lamina is situated between adjacent metatarsal heads contiguous to the transverse and vertical lamina (Fig. 1.69).

The deep transverse metatarsal ligament makes attachment of adjacent metatarsal heads by a system of strong fibrous bands extending from the inferior aspects of the metatarsal heads. The structure is augmented by the plantar plate of the capsules of the metatarsophalangeal joints.

Articular cul de sacs located about the metatarsophalangeal joints are identified. Two inferolateral bodies and a single dorsal structure are present.

Adipose (fat) bodies are arranged protectively about the lesser metatarsal heads. Dorsally, an exten-

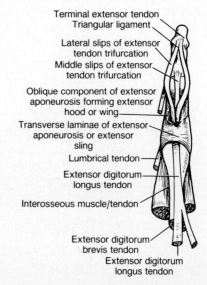

Figure 1.68. Extensor aponeurosis. (Modified from Sarrafian SK: *Anatomy of the Foot and Ankle*. Philadelphia, JB Lippincott Co, 1983.)

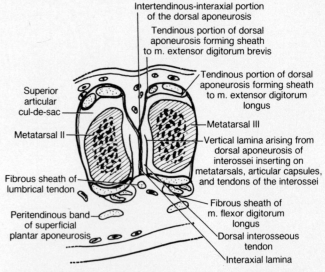

Figure 1.69. Intermetatarsal compartmentalization. (Modified from Sarrafian SK: *Anatomy of the Foot and Ankle*. Philadelphia, JB Lippincott Co, 1983.)

sive intermetatarsal capitular adipofascial complex is present. Plantarly, a single preflexor adipose cushion lies between paired lateroplantar fat bodies (Fig. 1.66).

Plantar Compartmentalization of the Foot

The plantar surface of the foot has medial, lateral, central, and interosseous compartments.

The central compartment is the largest and contains four fascial spaces. It contains the tendons and muscles flexor digitorum longus, flexor digitorum brevis, flexor accessorious, the four lumbricales, the plantar segments of tendons of insertion of tibialis posterior and peroneus longus, and both heads of adductor hallucis. It is covered dorsally by the tarsometatarsal skeleton. The medial and lateral intermuscular septum mark its medial and lateral boundaries and its superficial aspect is formed by the central part of the plantar aponeurosis.

The interosseous fascia below and metatarsals two, three, and four mark the limits of the interosseous compartment that contains the seven interosseous muscles.

The medial compartment has the plantar aponeurosis delineating its superficial and medial borders. The medial intermuscular septum forms its lateral border. The inferior surface of the first metatarsal forms the roof of the medial compartment. This compartment contains tendons of insertion of peroneus longus, tibialis posterior, and flexor hallucis longus. Additionally, m. abductor hallucis and m. flexor hallucis brevis are located here.

The lateral compartment has the lateral intermuscular septum as its medial border. The lateral segment of the plantar aponeurosis forms the lateral and superficial borders of the compartment that contains m. abductor digiti minimi, m. flexor digiti minimi brevis, and the opponens musculature.

The medial and lateral intermuscular septae are joined by a Y-shaped septum that is oriented transversely so that its two limbs form superomedially and inferomedially to attach to the inferolateral border of the first metatarsal and the plantar aponeurosis (Fig. 1.67).

Synovial Cavities of the Foot

There are six synovial cavities within the foot unless the occasional occurence of one between the cuboid and navicular is established when these bones make limited articulation. Such an instance produces a seventh small synovial cavity (Fig. 1.70).

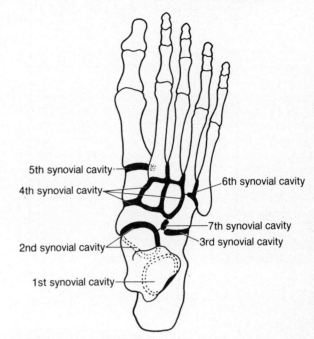

Figure 1.70. Synovial cavities of foot. (Modified from Sarrafian SK: *Anatomy of the Foot and Ankle.* Philadelphia, JB Lippincott Co, 1983.)

The first synovial cavity is situated between the posterior articular facets between the talus and calcaneus. A second synovial cavity lies between the anterior and middle facets of the calcaneus and talus extending to the talonavicular articulation. The third cavity is identified between the posterior surface of the cuboid and the anterior surface of the calcaneus (Fig. 1.70).

The fourth synovial cavity is extensive. It involves adjacent surfaces between all cuneiforms and the navicular, between the lateral cuneiform and the medial cuboid, intercuneiform articulations, and cuneometatarsal joints two and three, as well as limited areas between bases of metatarsals two, three, and four.

A fifth synovial cavity is formed between adjacent articular surfaces of the internal cuneiform and the first metatarsal. The sixth synovial cavity is situated between the articular surfaces of the bases of metatarsals four and five with the anterior articular surface of the cuboid. It extends distally for a short distance between the adjacent surfaces of the bases of metatarsals four and five as well (Fig. 1.70).

It is clinically important to keep the boundaries of these synovial cavities in mind. They provide natural barriers to the extension of infectious and inflammatory processes that might develop.

Myology

There is a sense in which valid discussions of the musculature of the lower extremity should include the myology of the low back and thigh. This is especially true whenever biomechanical principles of locomotion are to be considered. However, for purposes of the discussion of the muscles of immediate importance to the podiatric surgeon, this discussion will be contained within the parameters of the muscles operative on the foot itself. This includes, of course, the extrinsic musculature having origin on the leg. Two muscles of the triceps surae, namely, m. gastrocnemius and plantaris, involve the lower end of the femur.

MUSCLES OF THE ANTERIOR COMPARTMENT OF THE LEG

The deep peroneal nerve innervates all of the anterior crural (leg) muscles.

Tibialis Anterior

Origin

M. tibialis anterior (m. tibialis anticus, anterior tibial muscle) is a mild invertor and dorsiflexor of the foot on the leg (in the pronated foot it even becomes an evertor). Its origin involves the lateral condyle and the lateral shaft of the tibia. Soft tissue attachments also are made on the interosseous membrane, the deep surface of the crural fascia, and the intermuscular septa of the contiguous surface of m. extensor digitorum longus (Fig. 1.71).

Insertion

Insertion of the muscle is for the most part (about 90%) on the medial and plantar aspect of the first cuneiform with the remaining fibers involving the base of the first metatarsal (1). Other variations of insertion include attachment to the base of the first metatarsal and fanning out to include much of the tuberosity of the navicular (2).

Relationships

M. tibialis anterior descends vertically and is the most medial of the anterior crural muscles. It is superficial and closely related to the crest of the tibia until it passes through the most medial compartment of the superior extensor retinaculum. It then emerges from beneath the inferior extensor retinaculum to its insertion.

Extensor Digitorum Longus

M. extensor digitorum longus extends (dorsiflexes) and hyperextends the four lesser toes. It, along with m. extensor hallucis longus, acts synergistically to dorsiflex the foot on the leg. It may also assist in everting the foot.

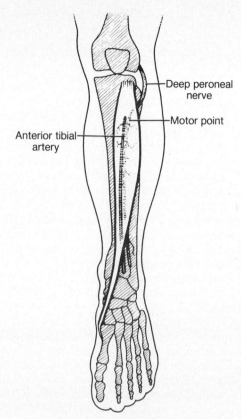

Figure 1.71. M. tibialis anterior.

Origin

The muscle origin is from the lateral condyle of the tibia and from the upper three fourths of the anterior surface of the fibula. Soft tissue attachments include the adjacent interosseous membrane and crural fascia and the intermuscular septum common to m. tibialis anterior and m. peroneus longus.

Insertion

Insertion of the muscle is made complex by the division of the tendon. Two laterally disposed tendinous slips pass alongside the middle phalanx to reunite for insertion centrally on the dorsal surface of the ungual or distal phalanx. A shorter central slip passes directly forward to insert on the base of the middle or intermediate phalanx. Each of the four lesser toes receives contributions from m. extensor digitorum longus (Fig. 1.72).

Relationships

M. extensor digitorum longus is characterized as a pennate muscle that flattens out to become tendinous in the lower one third of the leg. It passes beneath the superior and inferior extensor retinaculae where it divides into the four tendons for the four lesser toes.

As each tendon approaches the heads of the four

lesser metatarsals, each tendon gives off membranous expansions that envelop the respective metatarsophalangeal joints dorsally. This represents the so-called extensor hood apparatus and is analogous to a dorsal

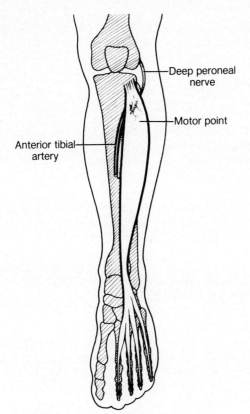

Figure 1.72. M. extensor digitorum longus.

joint capsule. This structure serves as one of the points of attachment for the dorsal and plantar interosseous muscles and the four lumbricales (Fig. 1.73).

M. extensor digitorum longus' tendons receive the tendons of m. extensor digitorum brevis on the fibular aspect of the long extensor tendon. Variations for insertion of m. extensor digitorum longus include a bifid tendon, both of which may insert on the same toe or on the toe adjacent (3).

Extensor Hallucis Longus

M. extensor hallucis longus is a powerful extrinsic foot muscle that extends the hallucal phalanges and dorsiflexes the foot on the leg. It may also aid in inverting the foot.

Origin

The muscle takes origin below or distal to those for extensor digitorum longus and tibialis anterior. Its attachments are to the anterior surface of the fibula in the middle two fourths (1). Its soft tissue attachments include the underlying interosseous membrane and the adjacent intermuscular septae (Fig. 1.74).

Insertion

Insertion of the muscle is to the dorsal aspect of the base of the distal or ungual hallucal phalanx. It may also make attachment on the proximal hallucal phalanx.

Relationships

At its point of origin, m. extensor hallucis longus is deep to and is covered by the bellies of m. extensor

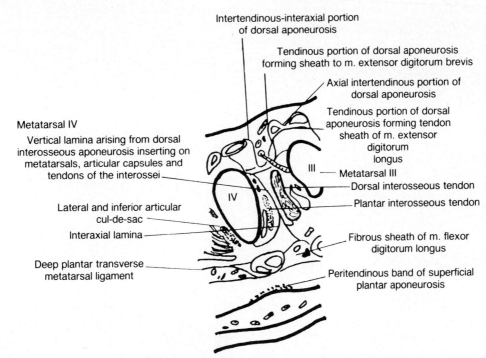

Figure 1.73. Extensor aponeurosis (hood) in relation to other metatarsophalangeal joint structures. (Modified from Sarrafian SK: *Anatomy of the Foot and Ankle.* Philadelphia, JB Lippincott Co, 1983.)

digitorum longus and m. tibialis anterior. It emerges distally to run a course between these two muscles and passes through the superior and inferior extensor retinaculae in its middle compartment. The deep peroneal nerve and the anterior tibial vessels are deep to this muscle on the lower third of the leg. As was the case with m. extensor digitorum longus, m. extensor hallucis longus gives off fibrous expansions at about the level of the head of the first metatarsal that also constitutes an extensor hood apparatus. When extensor hallucis brevis does not insert directly into the base of the proximal hallucal phalanx, it may make attachment to the inferolateral aspect of the long extensor tendon.

Muscles Accessory to M. Extensor Hallucis Longus

Extensor ossis metatarsi hallucis has insertion on the base dorsum of the first metatarsal as a tendinous slip arising from the tendon of m. extensor hallucis longus (4).

M. extensor primi internodii hallucis makes insertion as a tendinous slip on the base of the proximal hallucal phalanx after arising from the tendon of m. extensor hallucis longus itself (4).

Tate and Pachnik (5) describe an accessory tendon (extensor hallucis capsularis) arising from the tendon of m. extensor hallucis longus with a great degree of regularity that inserts into the dorsal aspect of the extensor hood apparatus. Its function appears to be to draw the joint capsule away from the joint

during dorsal flexion. Because the novice surgeon often mistakes this tendon for a nerve, it has been called the student's nerve.

Peroneus Tertius

M. peroneus tertius is not one of the muscles of the peroneal group. Rather, it belongs with the anterior crural group and is innervated by the deep peroneal nerve. It acts as a dorsiflexor and evertor of the foot on the leg.

Origin

This muscle takes origin from the lower third of the fibula on its anteromedial aspect and from the adjacent interosseous membrane.

Insertion

Insertion of the muscle is into the proximal portion of the shaft of the fifth metatarsal. Anomalous insertions include those into the base of the fourth metatarsal, into the tendon of m. extensor digitorum longus to the fifth toe, into one of the phalanges of the fifth toe, into the fifth metatarsal shaft, or on the interosseous space (Fig. 1.75).

Relationships

The muscle's course is under the superior limb of the extensor retinaculum through the lateral compartment in close association with the tendon of m. extensor digitorum longus. It emerges from beneath

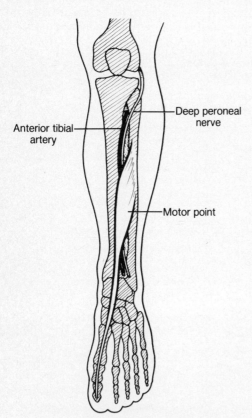

Figure 1.74. M. extensor hallucis longus.

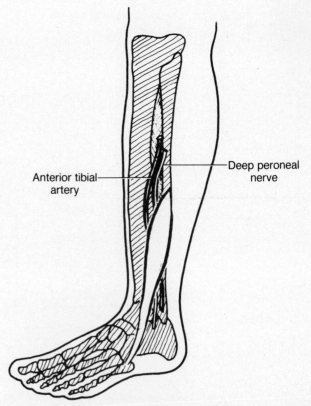

Figure 1.75. M. Peroneus tertius.

the lower limb of the extensor retinaculum and proceeds laterally towards its insertion. Peroneus tertius is not present in all subjects. It is important for surgeons to know that it is actually connected to the tendons of m. extensor digitorum longus by loose connective tissue in the compartment in which they are both contained at the level of the ankle joint.

Extensor Digitorum Et Hallucis Brevis

M. extensor digitorum brevis is an intrinsic foot muscle that will be described here because it assists the long extensor in extending the middle phalanges of the second, third, and fourth toes. The most medial tendon of the muscle acts on the proximal hallucal phalanx, however.

Origin

The muscle takes origin as a comparatively thin band of muscle associated with the tubercle at the lateral end of the calcaneal sulcus and the cervicle ligament. It, like the extrinsic extensors of the foot, is innervated by the deep peroneal nerve (Fig. 1.76).

Insertion

Insertion of the muscle is into the fibular side of the tendons of extensor digitorum longus to the second, third, and fourth toes. There is no tendon to the fifth digit. M. extensor hallucis brevis is the designation given to the muscle's most medial slip that inserts into the dorsal aspect of the proximal hallucal pha-

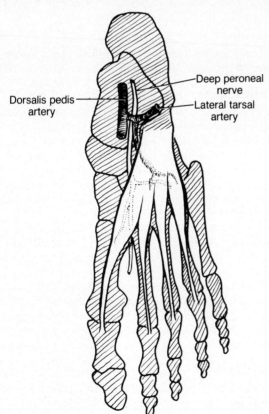

Dorsalis pedis artery

Deep peroneal nerve

Lateral tarsal artery

Figure 1.76. M. extensor digitorum brevis.

lanx. Alternatively, it may make attachment to the fibular aspect of the tendon of m. extensor hallucis longus, which is approached on the fibular side and deep to the long extensor tendon (Fig. 1.77).

Relationships

The muscle's course is from behind forward and from lateral to medial. The extensor hallucis brevis portion passes superficial to the dorsalis pedis artery. Accessory slips are common for this muscle. An accessory slip to the medial side of the head of the proximal phalanx of the second toe occurs in 34% of cases (6). Additionally, accessory slips may be found to the fourth toe or the third toe. In the latter instance, the slip comes from the fascicle to the second toe.

A *digastric muscle* may be formed from the second fascicle of extensor digitorum brevis. Such slips have attachment to the first and/or second interosseous muscle tendons.

A *trigastric muscle* attaches simultaneously to the first and second interosseous muscle tendons after originating from the second fascicle of m. extensor digitorum brevis (3).

MUSCLES OF THE LATERAL COMPARTMENT OF THE LEG
Peroneus Longus and Peroneus Brevis

M. peroneus longus and m. peroneus brevis are both evertors of the foot. *Gray's Anatomy* (1) states that m. peroneus longus is an accessory dorsiflexor of the foot. Such action occurs when the first is in eversion. M. peroneus longus, by virtue of its cross bracing of the foot, maintains the integrity of the longitudinal and transverse arch structures of the foot in tiptoeing and in takeoff in gait.

Peroneus Longus
Origin

M. peroneus longus takes its origin from the head and lateral upper half of the fibula, the anterior and posterior peroneal fascias, and the adjacent crural fascia (Fig. 1.78).

Insertion

The muscle grooves the cuboid and turns tibially beneath the long plantar ligament to make attachment to the posteroinferolateral angle of the base of the first metatarsal. About ten percent of fibers also make attachment to the contiguous surface of the first cuneiform. Other slips may relate to the bases of the third, fourth, and fifth metatarsals or to the oblique head of m. adductor hallucis.

Relationships

M. peroneus longus is a pennate muscle that runs superficially down the lateral aspect of the leg and becomes tendinous as it passes beneath the superior peroneal retinaculum. A sheath common to it and to m. peroneus brevis conduct the muscles through the

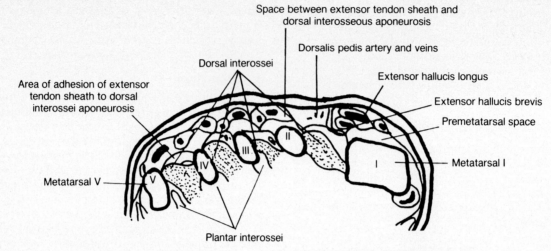

Figure 1.77.   Relationships of the extensor musculature at metatarsophalangeal joints.

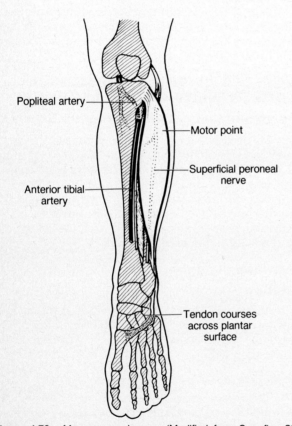

Figure 1.78.   M. peroneus longus. (Modified from Sarrafian SK: *Anatomy of the Foot and Ankle*. Philadelphia, JB Lippincott Co, 1983.)

retinaculum. Its course is then oblique along the lateral side of the calcaneus, under the peroneal trochlea and the inferior peroneal retinaculum to the groove on the lateral aspect of the cuboid bone. Here it turns tibialward in a depression inferior to the cuboid and in a tunnel formed by the long plantar ligament. A sesamoid bone may be identified in the tendon of m. peroneus longus at the level of the tubercle of the cuboid. Anterior and posterior frenular ligaments contained in a mesotendon may make attachments for

the tendon about contiguous plantar surfaces of the base of the fifth metatarsal and the cuboid tubercle (7).

Peroneus Brevis

Origin

Origin of m. peroneus brevis is anterior to that for m. peroneus longus from the lower two thirds of the lateral surface of the fibula. Soft tissue attachments relate to the anterior and posterior peroneal septa.

Insertion

Insertion of m. peroneus brevis is into the lateral aspect of the base of the fifth metatarsal (Fig. 1.79).

Relationships

Peroneus brevis is situated deep to m. peroneus longus proximally until it passes in continuity with that muscle through a sheath within the superior peroneal retinaculum. It then passes beneath the fibular malleolus above and anterior to m. peroneus longus. Its course continues along the lateral aspect of the calcaneus and above the peroneal trochlea. Considerable variation exists with respect to the peroneal musculature, especially in relation to m. peroneus brevis, which may be altogether absent. In this case it is often replaced with a muscle arising from the lateral surface of the middle one third of the fibula that has insertion by three tendinous slips. One attaches to the calcaneus, one attaches to the lateral surface of the cuboid and the ligaments contiguous thereto, and the most posterior tendon makes attachment posterior to and below the fibular malleolus.

Variations

Variations include separation of two tendinous slips from the peroneal muscle masses with attachments into the inferior extensor retinaculum and the inferolateral aspect of the calcaneus. Another variation is a cylindrical tendon measuring 2.5 × 5 cm arising from the brevis and inserting into the lateral surface of the calcaneus (3). Another variation springs from the brevis muscle by a thin tendinous slip that makes attachment to the calcaneus and the inferior part of the peroneal retinaculum. Still another variation comes off the brevis to fan out for insertions resembling a peroneal-calcaneal ligament. Attachments are made at about three locations including the tubercle on the lateral aspect of the calcaneus, an anterior slip to the distal lateral aspect of the calcaneus, and a posterior slip to the fibular malleolus.

MUSCULATURE RELATED TO THE FLEXOR RETINACULUM

The structures passing beneath the flexor retinaculum on the medial aspect of the ankle are (from behind forward), m. flexor hallucis longus, the tibial nerve and posterior tibial artery and vein, m. flexor digitorum longus, and m. tibialis posterior. All three muscles are innervated by the tibial nerve, but their actions are variable and are discussed individually.

Flexor Hallucis Longus

Origin

The origin of m. flexor hallucis longus is from the lower two thirds of the posterior aspect of the fibula. Its soft tissue attachments include the posterior portion of the peroneal septum and the deep transverse

intermuscular septum and the fascia covering m. tibialis posterior that overlaps the muscle belly (Fig. 1.80).

Insertion

Insertion of m. flexor hallucis longus is into the plantar aspect of the base of the ungual hallucal phalanx. The action of this muscle is to plantarflex the hallux in general and the distal hallucal phalanx in particular. Additionally, it assists in plantarflexion of the foot on the leg.

Relationships

The external portion of m. flexor hallucis longus is related to the deep surface of m. soleus. It is a pennate muscle that becomes tendinous just proximal to the flexor retinaculum (laciniate ligament) through which it passes in the fourth compartment. The tendon grooves the posterior distal tibia and passes between the tubercles on the posterior surface of the talus and forms a deep groove on the inferior surface of the sustentaculum tali. Its tendon crosses that of m. flexor digitorum longus in a lateral to medial direction to continue forward between the bipennate fibers of flexor hallucis brevis and between the tibial and fibular sesamoid bones invested within the tendons of the brevis muscle and on to its insertion. It sends fibers of attachment to the tendons of m. flexor digitorum longus and flexor hallucis brevis (vinculus) where the structures come into close contact.

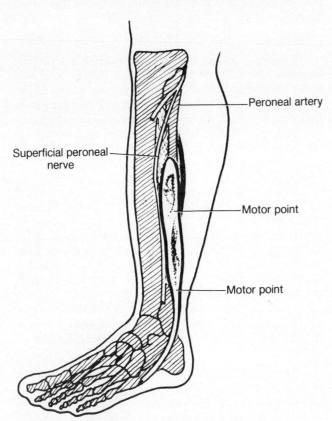

Figure 1.79.   M. peroneus brevis.

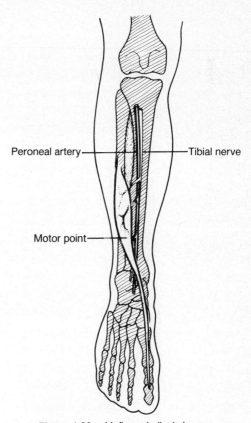

Figure 1.80.   M. flexor hallucis longus.

Flexor Digitorum Longus

M. flexor digitorum longus plantarflexes the four lateral toes at the level of the metatarsophalangeal articulations and continued action flexes the phalanges of the four lateral toes on themselves plantarward. The muscle also assists in the plantarflexion of the foot on the leg.

Origin

Origin of the muscle is from the posterior surface of the tibia in the region between the soleal line above, and an area to 7 or 8 cm proximal to the bone's distal end. Soft tissue attachments are made with the fascia of m. tibialis posterior where the two muscle bellies are associated.

Insertion

Insertion for m. flexor digitorum longus is by four tendons that make attachments to the distal or ungual phalanges on their respective plantar surfaces (Fig. 1.81).

Relationships

M. flexor digitorum longus arises first as a comparatively thin band that expands as it proceeds distally. As it becomes tendinous it crosses m. tibialis posterior superficially and enters the foot after passing through the second compartment of the flexor retinaculum. (The third compartment contains the tibial nerve and the posterior tibial artery and veins.) As

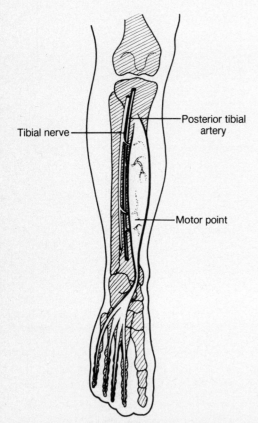

Tibial nerve
Posterior tibial artery
Motor point

Figure 1.81. Plantar aspect of foot. M. flexor digitorum longus.

the muscle's tendon enters the foot it crosses m. flexor hallucis longus in superficial relationship where it is interconnected with a vinculus. A similar situation exists where the muscle crosses m. tibialis posterior. As the four tendons destined to serve the four lateral toes, attachment is made with the intrinsic foot muscle, quadratus plantae (flexor accessorious). The four lumbricalis muscles take their origins from the tibial sides of each of the tendons of insertion of m. flexor digitorum longus.

The tendons of insertion of m. flexor digitorum brevis bifurcate to embrace the tendons of m. flexor digitorum longus as they proceed distally to their respective points of insertion.

Tibialis Posterior

M. tibialis posterior makes attachment to all tarsal bones (except the talus) on their plantar aspects and thereby cross braces and stabilizes the midfoot. This muscle is a plantarflexor of the foot on the leg and inverts the foot.

Origin

The origin of m. tibialis posterior involves both of the leg bones. It arises from the posteromedial surface of the fibula and from the posterior surface of the tibia below the popliteal line and lateral to the vertical line. Soft tissue attachments are also made on the adjacent interosseous membrane and the adjacent intermuscular septae. The muscle is overlapped by both m. flexor hallucis longus and m. flexor digitorum longus.

Insertion

The insertion for m. tibialis posterior is primarily into the tuberosity of the navicular. However, it also sends numerous fibrous bands for attachment to the plantar surfaces of all tarsal bones with the exception of the talus, which receives no muscular insertions. In addition, m. tibialis posterior makes attachment to the bases of the middle three metatarsals (Fig. 1.82).

Relationships

M. tibialis posterior is deep to the long flexors and in the lower quarter of the leg it passes deep to the flexor digitorum longus to groove the posterior aspect of the medial malleolus. It enters the foot by passing through the first (medial) compartment of the extensor retinaculum. Sarrafian (3) divides the tendon of insertion of m. tibialis posterior into anterior, middle, and posterior components.

MUSCLES OF THE SUPERFICIAL COMPARTMENT OF THE POSTERIOR LEG

The superficial compartment of the posterior aspect of the leg contains three muscles collectively referred to as the triceps surae. All three muscles insert by a common tendon in most cases into the posterior surface of the calcaneus via the tendo achillis

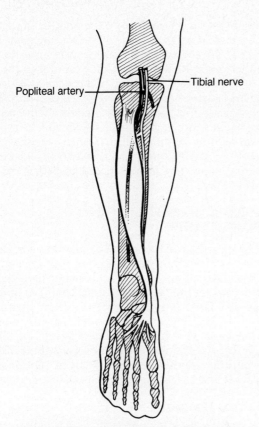

Figure 1.82. M. tibialis posterior (plantar foot).

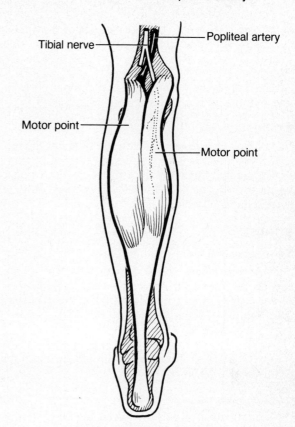

Figure 1.83. M. gastrocnemius.

or tendo calcaneus. All of these muscles are innervated by muscular branches of the tibial nerve. All act to plantarflex the foot on the leg and, in the case of m. gastrocnemius, it flexes the leg on the thigh by virtue of its origin on the posterodistal aspect of the femur to cross the knee joint.

Gastrocnemius

Origin

The origin of m. gastrocnemius is by two heads. The larger medial head is from the nonarticular region of the posterior medial condyle of the femur and the lower part of the medial supracondylar line. The smaller lateral head (which is sometimes absent) arises from the nonarticular region of the posterior part of the lateral femoral condyle and the lower part of the supracondylar line (Fig. 1.83). The medial head takes origin from the region of the depression behind the upper posterior part of the medial condyle of the femur behind the adductor tubercle.

Insertion

Insertion of m. gastrocnemius is into the middle portion of the posterior surface of the calcaneus by means of the common tendo achilles or tendo calcaneus. This tendon is the largest, thickest, and strongest tendon of the human body. It fans out as it makes attachment into the calcaneus and usually is associated at this point with m. soleus and m. plantaris (when present). An anatomical bursa is situated between the tendon and the posterior surface of the

calcaneus. An adventitious bursa is commonly present between the tendon and the overlying skin at the point where contact is made with the counter of the shoe.

Relationships

M. gastrocnemius is the most superficial muscle of the triceps surae. The two muscle masses remain separate as far as their attachment to a broad aponeurosis on the anterior surface of the muscle. Such an arrangement makes the muscle a definitely bipennate structure(1).

Some podiatric surgeons have remarked on the apparent confusion relative to the spiraling of fibers of the tendo achillis. In some living subjects, the fibers may seem to descend vertically. In anatomical specimens a rotational spiral arrangement can definitely be identified (8). Proximally, the fibers of m. gastrocnemius are posterior to those for m. soleus. Such fibers gradually rotate from medial to lateral about 12 cm proximal to the tendon's insertion (8). Soleus fibers also rotate so that fibers that were oriented anteriorly in their proximal relationships are distally seen to be more posteriorly situated. The degree of rotation is variable.

Soleus

Origin

The origin of m. soleus is from the posterior part of the head of the fibula and the upper one third of the posterior surface of the fibula. In addition, it has fibers of origin from the middle one third of the medial border of the tibia and from beneath the popliteal line.

Insertion

Insertion of m. soleus is in common with m. gastrocnemius by the tendo achillis (Fig. 1.84).

Relationships

M. soleus is a broad, flat muscle that lies deep to m. gastrocnemius. It is separated from the muscles of the deep compartment of the leg by the deep transverse fascia of the leg. Muscle fibers are oblique, bipennate, and relatively short.

Plantaris

Origin

The origin of m. plantaris is usually just medial to the lateral head of origin of m. gastrocnemius on or near the lateral supracondylar line of the posterior lateral condyle of the femur (Fig. 1.85).

Insertion

Insertion for m. plantaris is usually in common with tendo achillis.

Relationships

M. plantaris is situated between the fleshy bellies of m. gastrocnemius and m. soleus. Its course is from lateral to medial. This muscle is frequently absent and its distal attachments are subject to some variation.

In 47% of cases insertion is by a fan-shaped expansion into the medial aspect of the superior calcaneal tuberosity (3). In 36% of cases insertion is anterior and medial to the tendo achillis. It may fan out to include parts of the flexor retinaculum and the fascia covering the medial surface of the posterior calcaneus (8). In 12.5% of cases the insertion is broadly to the medial surface of the tendo achillis and 4% may make attachment as high as 16 cm proximal to the medial point of insertion of the tendo achillis to the calcaneus. Additional slips may then proceed to attach on the calcaneus itself.

INTRINSIC PLANTAR FOOT MUSCULATURE

The muscles intrinsic to the plantar surface of the foot are classically arranged into four layers. The first layer is composed of m. abductor hallucis, m. flexor digitorum brevis, and m. abductor digiti minimi. The second layer is made up of m. flexor digitorum accessorius (quadratus plantae) and the four lumbricalis muscles. The third layer consists of m. flexor hallucis brevis, m. adductor hallucis, and m. flexor digiti minimi brevis. The fourth layer contains the four dorsal and three plantar interosseous muscles.

Abductor Hallucis

M. abductor hallucis lies on the medial border of the foot. It covers over the approaches of the posterior tibial artery and vein and the tibial nerve as they enter

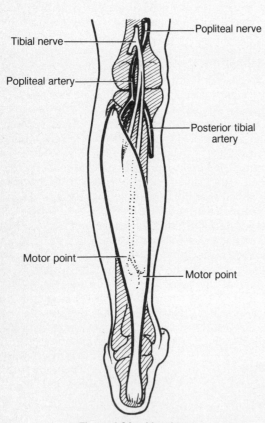

Figure 1.84. M. soleus.

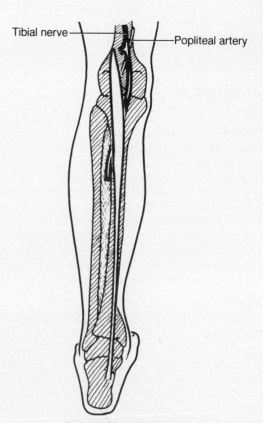

Figure 1.85. M. plantaris.

the foot to supply the plantar structures of the foot. The muscle acts to plantarflex and abduct the hallux and is innervated by the medial plantar nerve.

Origin

Origin of m. abductor hallucis is from the medial aspect of the posteromedial calcaneal tuberosity. Soft tissue attachments include the deep surface of the plantar aponeurosis, the flexor retinaculum, and the medial intermuscular septum.

Insertion

Insertion of m. abductor hallucis is on the tibial sesamoid initially by inferolateral fibers. Its tendon continues on to make attachment on the medial plantar tubercle at the base of the proximal hallucal phalanx (Fig. 1.86).

Relationships

This thick, rather flat, muscle forms the fleshy medial margin of the foot. It is adherent to the fibrous tunnel for m. tibialis posterior, m. flexor digitorum longus, and m. flexor hallucis longus.

Variations

A tendinous slip may make attachment to the tibial aspect of the base of the proximal phalanx of the second toe.

Fibers of origin may be observed from the tendon of flexor hallucis longus (9).

Flexor Digitorum Brevis

M. flexor digitorum brevis is situated deep to the central portion of the plantar aponeurosis. The muscle acts to flex the four lesser toes on the metatarsophalangeal joints and the middle phalanx on the proximal phalanges. Innervation is by the medial plantar nerve.

Origin

Bony attachment is made to the posteromedial aspect of the plantar surface of the calcaneal tuberosity. Soft tissue attachments are also made from the posterior third of the deep surface of the plantar aponeurosis and the medial and lateral intermuscular septae.

Insertion

Insertion is by four rather flat fascicles through fibro-osseous tunnels that are separated by vertical septations from the plantar aponeurosis. The belly of the muscle divides at the bases of the four lateral proximal phalanges to embrace the tendons of m. flexor digitorum longus. Final insertion is on the inferior surface of the middle phalanx where tendinous fibers reunite or decussate (Fig. 1.87).

Relationships

The muscle is wedged between m. abductor hallucis anteromedially and m. abductor digiti quinti anterolaterally and is covered superficially by the deep surface of the plantar aponeurosis.

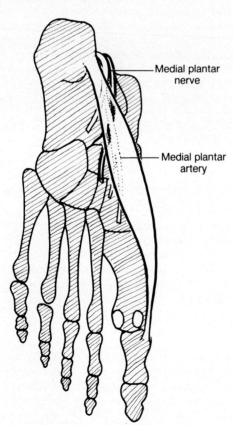

Figure 1.86. M. abductor hallucis.

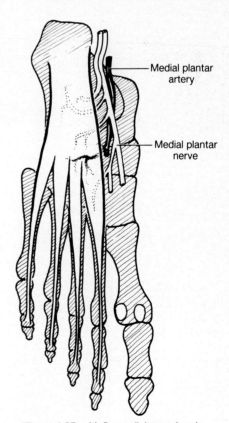

Figure 1.87. M. flexor digitorum brevis.

Variations

Variations include the presence of an additional tendinous slip of the flexor digitorum brevis to the fifth toe, which arises from the tendon of m. flexor digitorum longus.

Another variation is the presence of an additional tendinous slip of m. flexor digitorum brevis to both fourth and fifth toes, which arises from tendons of m. flexor digitorum longus.

The presence of an additional tendinous slip to the fifth toe that arises from the tendon of m. tibialis posterior can also occur.

Or, the tendon of m. flexor digitorum longus may be the sole origin of m. flexor digitorum brevis to the fourth and fifth toes.

Finally, the lateral intermuscular septum may act as the sole origin for m. flexor digitorum brevis to the fifth toe (10).

Abductor Digiti Quinti

M. abductor digiti quinti helps to marginate the lateral border of the human foot. The lateral plantar vessels and nerve are situated along its tibial border. This muscle abducts and plantarflexes the fifth toe and is innervated by the lateral plantar nerve.

Origin

Origin is from the plantar surface and the lateral process of the calcaneus. Soft tissue attachments include contiguous areas of the plantar aponeurosis and the adjacent intermuscular septa (Fig. 1.88).

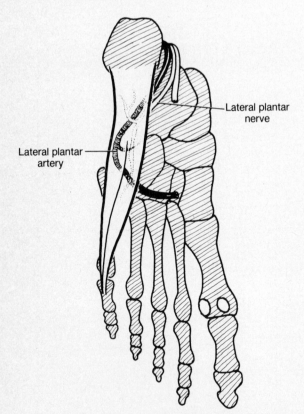

Figure 1.88. M. abductor digiti minimi.

Lateral plantar nerve

Lateral plantar artery

Insertion

The muscle makes bony insertion on the lateral aspect of the base of the proximal phalanx of the fifth digit. Soft tissue attachments include the plantar capsule of the fifth metatarsophalangeal joint with additional fibers extending to the extensor hood apparatus and the tendon itself.

Relationships

The muscle is elongated and fusiform, becoming tendinous about the level of the calcaneocuboid joint. Usually the tendon's course will relate it to the styloid process of the base of the fifth metatarsal where a bursa is usually present.

Variations

The biventral muscle, which runs deep to the main muscle belly and which takes origin from the plantar aspect of the bases of the fifth metatarsal, may be one variation.

M. abductor ossi metatarsi quinti is closely related to m. abductor digiti quinti. It takes origin from the posterolateral aspect of the lateral process of the calcaneus. Insertion is on or about the styloid process of the base of the fifth metatarsal.

M. abductor accessorius arises variously from the lateral process of the calcaneus or from the plantar and lateral aspect of the sheath of m. peroneus longus. It inserts along with m. abductor digiti minimi into the lateral aspect of the base of the proximal phalanx of the fifth toe (11).

Opponens digiti quinti arises from the sheath of m. peroneus longus as a flat triangular muscle. It follows closely to the base of the fifth metatarsal to insert on the lateral border of the shaft of the fifth metatarsal. Le Double (9) recognizes this muscle as present in 50% of specimens and believes this muscle should be regarded as a specific anatomical entity.

SECOND LAYER OF PLANTAR FOOT MUSCULATURE

Flexor Accesorius (Quadratus Plantae)

M. flexor accesorius is situated deep to m. flexor digitorum brevis. It assists in the flexion of the four lateral toes through its insertion on m. flexor digitorum longus and is innervated by the lateral plantar nerve. It has been suggested that this muscle stabilizes and corrects for the obliquity of the course of m. flexor digitorum longus as it crosses the foot from medial to lateral.

Origin

M. flexor accesorius takes origin by two heads. The medial head arises from the medial surface of the calcaneus plantarly where the bone is grooved by m. flexor hallucis longus. The lateral head takes origin from the posterolateral tuberosity of the calcaneus and the anterior aspect of the posteromedial calcaneal tuberosity. Soft tissue attachments include the calcaneocuboid ligament and the inferior surface of the intermuscular septum of the calcaneal canal (Fig. 1.89).

Insertion

Insertion of m. flexor accessorius is into the segmented portion of the tendon of m. flexor digitorum longus, mainly into the division destined for the fifth toe (3). It occasionally makes attachment to m. flexor hallucis longus where it is in close proximity with m. flexor digitorum longus.

Relationships

The two fleshy heads of this muscle come together in a comparatively narrow tendon of insertion. It tends to be sandwiched behind m. flexor hallucis brevis and its osteoligamentous frame.

Variations

Variations include fibrous attachments to the lumbricales distally or to m. flexor hallucis brevis.

Replacement for the tendon of m. flexor digitorum brevis to the fifth toe where the former is absent can also occur.

Insertion of the medial head of m. flexor accessorius into tendons of m. flexor hallucis longus where the long hallucal flexor replaces an absent m. flexor digitorum longus to the second and third toes. Insertion of the lateral head into tendons of m. flexor digitorum longus that are present only for the supply of the fourth and fifth toes is another variation (12).

The medial or lateral head of m. flexor accessorius may be absent.

Lumbricales

There are four small lumbricalis muscles that are numbered one to four from medial to lateral associated with individual tendons of m. flexor digitorum longus. These muscles act in concert to flex the four lateral toes on their respective metatarsophalangeal joints. Continued action extends their phalanges on one another. They may also tend to draw the lesser digits toward the hallux. The first lumbricalis is innervated by the medial plantar nerve. The lateral three muscles receive innervation from the deep branch of the lateral plantar nerve.

Origin

Origin of the first lumbricalis is from the tibial aspect of the medial division of the tendon of m. flexor digitorum longus.

The second lumbricalis arises from the contiguous side of the first and second divisions of the tendon of m. flexor digitorum longus.

The third lumbricalis arises from the contiguous sides of the second and third divisions of the tendon of m. flexor digitorum longus.

The fourth lumbricalis arises from the contiguous sides of the third and fourth divisions of the tendons of m. flexor digitorum longus.

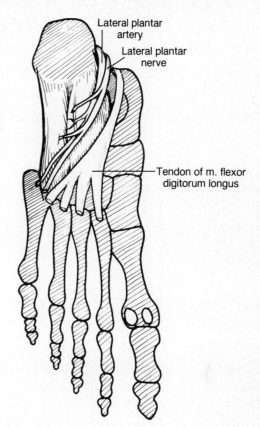

Figure 1.89. M. flexor accessorius (quadratus plantae).

Insertion

Each of the four lumbricales inserts into the tibial aspect of the membranous expansions of the respective tendons of m. extensor digitorum longus (extensor hood apparatus). Such attachments are made mainly to the middle of the proximal phalanges a bit dorsal to the midline. The first lumbricalis makes attachment to the tibial aspect of the second toe, the second to the third, the third to the fourth, and the fourth to the fifth toe (Fig. 1.90).

Relationships

Each of the four lumbricalis muscles is closely associated with the respective tendons of m. flexor digitorum longus where the lumbricalis lies fibularward of the long flexor.

Variations

Origin of the first lumbricalis may occur from the tendon of m. tibialis posterior.

Origin of the first lumbricalis may occur from the tendon of m. flexor hallucis longus.

Origin of the second, third, and/or fourth lumbricalis may occur from tendons of m. flexor digitorum brevis.

The lumbricales may be absent.

There may be duplicity or bifidity of the third and/or fourth lumbricalis (13).

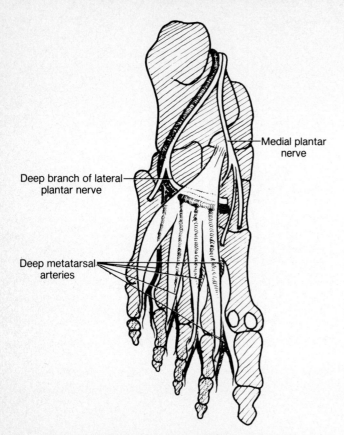

Figure 1.90.   M. lumbricales.

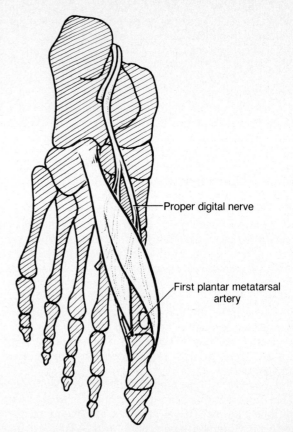

Figure 1.91.   M. flexor hallucis brevis.

THIRD LAYER OF PLANTAR FOOT MUSCULATURE

M. flexor hallucis brevis, m. adductor hallucis, and m. flexor digiti minimi brevis constitute the third layer of the plantar foot musculature. These muscles are deep and consequently shorter relative to the musculature of the second layer.

Flexor Hallucis Brevis

M. flexor hallucis brevis acts to flex the great toe (hallux) on the metatarsophalangeal joint. It is innervated by the medial plantar nerve.

Origin

Origin of m. flexor hallucis brevis is by a Y-shaped arrangement of fibers. The medial arm is from that portion of the tendons of insertion of m. tibialis posterior that are related to the metatarsal bases. The lateral arm is from the cuboid, the third cuneiform, and the sheath of m. peroneus longus along with the long and short plantar ligaments. The stem of the Y-shaped insertion of the deep part relates to the medial calcaneal tubercle (Fig. 1.91).

Insertion

Insertion of m. flexor hallucis brevis is by two tendons of insertion. The lateral head makes attachment to the lateral aspects of the plantar plate of the first metatarsophalangeal joint and the central medial aspect of the fibular sesamoid bone. Fibers of insertion continue forward to make final insertion into the lateral aspect of the base of the proximal hallucal phalanx along with m. adductor hallucis. The medial head is situated tibial to the tendon of m. flexor hallucis longus. It makes attachment to the plantar plate and to contiguous areas of the lateral portion of the central part of the tibial sesamoid bone. It continues forward to make final insertion into the medial aspect of the base of the proximal hallucal phalanx along with m. abductor hallucis.

Relationships

M. flexor hallucis brevis usually demonstrates an anatomical bursa between the proximal portions of the muscle and the first tarsometatarsal and first cuneiform joints, as well as the sheath of m. peroneus longus. M. flexor hallucis brevis divides into its medial and lateral head at the level of the neck of the first metatarsal. The muscle is crossed somewhat obliquely by the tendon of m. flexor hallucis longus.

Variations

Union of the lateral head of flexor hallucis brevis may occur with the oblique part of m. adductor hallucis.

Insertion of the medial head of m. flexor hallucis brevis into the tendon of insertion of m. abductor hallucis may occur.

Interosseous plantaris primus, which is a tendinous slip or fascicle from m. flexor hallucis brevis inserting on the first cuneiform, may be observed.

M. flexor hallucis brevis may extend a tendon to the proximal phalanx of the second toe.

Reinforcement of m. flexor hallucis brevis may occur by a tendinous extension from m. flexor digitorum longus.

Adductor Hallucis

M. adductor hallucis may be considered as two muscles sharing a common insertion. Its action is described as drawing the hallux toward the midline of the second toe and it is commonly implicated as contributing to the common foot deformity, hallux abducto valgus. However, there is some question as to whether the muscle is actually involved in producing the deformity because no increase in bulk of the muscle can be demonstrated in this condition. There can be little doubt that it fixes the position of the great toe in hallux valgus.

Origin

Origin of m. adductor hallucis is by two portions quite distinct from one another. The oblique head arises from the middle segment of the sheath of m. peroneus longus and the distal segment of the inferior calcaneal ligament. Its bony attachments include the crest of the cuboid and the bases of metatarsals two, three, and four along with the adjacent parts of the cuneiform bones. The transverse head arises from the plantar plates of the third, fourth, and fifth metatarsophalangeal joints, as well as from the transverse metatarsal ligament about the heads of metatarsals two, three, four, and five. It is composed of three fascicles of which the longest and most superficial is associated with the region of the fifth metatarsal head.

Insertion

Insertion of the two portions of m. adductor hallucis has been stated as simply to the tubercle at the inferolateral border of the proximal hallucal phalanx. Close examination of the parts involved, however, indicate somewhat greater complexity. The oblique head clearly relates to the sheath of m. flexor hallucis brevis. It also invests the lateral aspect of the fibular sesamoid with fibrous slips extending dorsally to involve the hallucal extensor hood apparatus (Fig. 1.92). The transverse head demonstrates a relatively short tendon that arises at the level of the second metatarsal head. It makes attachment to the oblique tendon of m. adductor hallucis and proceeds to the deep transverse metatarsal ligament for final attachment to the hallux.

Relationships

The oblique head of m. adductor hallucis forms an arc for passage of the lateral neurovascular bundle. It courses obliquely over the base of the fourth metatarsal in its course toward the proximal hallucal pha-

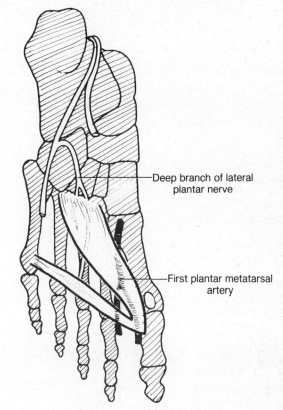

Figure 1.92.   M. adductor hallucis.

- Deep branch of lateral plantar nerve

- First plantar metatarsal artery

lanx. It is superficial to the interosseous muscles. Its medial border relates to the fibular border of m. flexor hallucis brevis.

Variations of the Oblique Adductor Hallucis

Fusion of the oblique head may occur with the lateral head of m. flexor hallucis brevis.

Insertion of the oblique head may occur on m. flexor hallucis brevis.

Tendinous slip of insertion of the oblique adductor may be observed into the lateral aspect of the base of the proximal phalanx to the second toe.

Variations of the Transverse Adductor Hallucis

Limited origin of the transverse adductor may occur, which involves only the regions of the fourth and fifth or third and fourth metatarsal heads.

Origin of the transverse adductor may be limited to the region of the fifth metatarsal only.

The transverse component of m. adductor hallucis may be totally absent or can be present merely as a slip of fibrous tissue.

The presence of an aponeurotic slip from the transverse adductor to the anterior border of the oblique adductor may be observed.

The transverse adductor tendon may receive insertion from an anomalous 1 cm triangular muscle that arises from the base and distal one third of the plantar border of the second metatarsal. This anomalous structure is interposed between the first dorsal interosseous and the oblique adductor hallucis musculature.

Flexor Digiti Minimi Brevis

The action of m. flexor digiti minimi brevis is to flex the fifth toe. Its innervation is from superficial branches of the lateral plantar nerve.

Origin

Origin of m. flexor digiti minimi brevis is from the crest of the cuboid bone and the contiguous portion

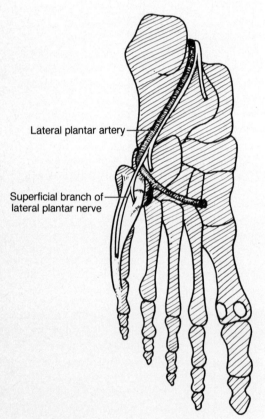

Figure 1.93. M. flexor digiti minimi brevis.

of the base of the fifth metatarsal. Soft tissue attachments include the sheath of m. peroneus longus and the contiguous parts of the plantar aponeurosis.

Insertion

Insertion of m. flexor digiti minimi brevis is into the plantar plate of the fifth metatarsophalangeal joint with final insertion on the plantar aspect of the base of the proximal phalanx of the fifth toe (Fig. 1.93).

Relationships

M. flexor digiti minimi brevis is a fusiform muscle situated fibularly to m. flexor digitorum longus. Its insertion places this muscle between m. abductor digiti minimi and m. flexor digitorum longus (Fig. 1.94).

Variations

Union may occur with m. abductor digiti minimi. Fusion may occur with m. opponens digiti quinti (14).

FOURTH LAYER OF PLANTAR FOOT MUSCULATURE

Interossei

Because the functional axis of the foot itself bisects the second metatarsal, abduction and adduction of muscles intrinsic to the foot relate to this point. Seven interossei relate to the intermetatarsal spaces along with the lumbricales already mentioned. The actions of these muscles are abduction and adduction based on the anatomical principle just defined. The dorsal interossei are abductors relative to the midline of the second metatarsal. This feature is conveniently remembered by their designation as "DAB" muscles: D meaning dorsal, AB indicating abduction. The plantar interossei are remembered as "PAD" muscles, P meaning plantar, AD indicating adduction (Fig. 1.95).

Innervation of the interossei is by deep branches of the lateral plantar nerve except in the fourth interspace, which is supplied by a superficial branch of the

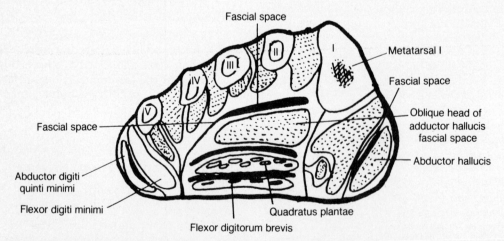

Figure 1.94. Relationships of intrinsic forefoot musculature. (Modified from Sarrafian SK: *Anatomy of the Foot and Ankle.* Philadelphia, JB Lippincott Co, 1983.)

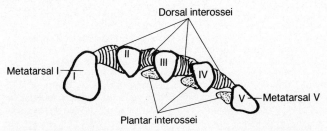

Figure 1.95. Relationships of interosseous musculature. (Modified from Sarrafian SK: *Anatomy of the Foot and Ankle.* Philadelphia, JB Lippincott Co, 1983.)

lateral plantar nerve, although some overlapping innervation exists.

Origin

Origin of the dorsal interosseous muscles is by bipennate fibers arising from adjacent sides of the metatarsal bone. The first occupies the interspace between the first and second metatarsals, the second is situated between the second and third metatarsals, the third is placed between metatarsal three and four, and the fourth is between the fourth and fifth metatarsals (Fig. 1.96).

Origin of the plantar interosseous muscles is from the tibial aspects of the third, fourth, and fifth metatarsal bones and from their respective bases. They arise from below rather than between the metatarsal bones and are named first, second, and third plantar interosseous muscles from medial to lateral (Fig. 1.97).

Insertion

Insertion of the dorsal interosseous muscles is first to the deep transverse metatarsal ligament, thence to the dorsal interosseous aponeurosis, the lateral capsule and the glenoid ligaments of the respective metatarsophalangeal joints, the respective plantar plates, and to the deep surfaces of the transverse lamina. Ultimately, they make osseous attachment to the fibular aspect of the second, third, and fourth toes and the first dorsal interosseous muscle has insertion on the tibial aspect of the second toe. They are, consequently, in position to abduct the respective digits with respect to the midline of the second toe.

Insertion of the plantar interossei is into the tibial aspects of the bases of the proximal phalanges articulated to the metatarsals from which they took origin. Because of this arrangement, these muscles adduct the third, fourth, and fifth toes relative to the midline of the second metatarsal.

Variations

Origins of the dorsal interossei may occur by single heads. The first arises from the second alone, the second from the second metatarsal, the third from the fourth metatarsal alone, and the fourth arises from a single head from either the fourth or the fifth metatarsals alone.

The first plantar interosseous muscle displaces the second dorsal interosseous muscle in the second

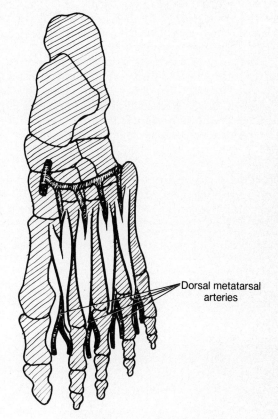

Figure 1.96. M. dorsal interossei.

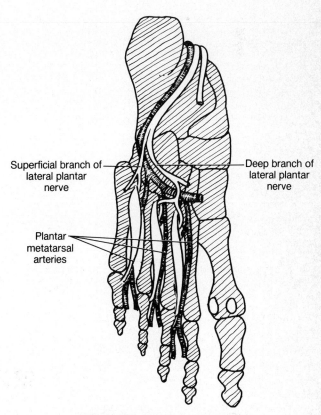

Figure 1.97. M. plantar interossei.

intermetatarsal space. In such instances it occupies the more dorsal aspect of the third metatarsal bone, as well as the plantar portion.

Plantar accessory interosseous slips may be associated with the first and second plantar interossei or the second and third dorsal interosseous muscles.

Fusions that involve the second and third dorsal interossei or the first plantar with the second dorsal interosseous muscles may be observed (15).

References

1. Warwick R, William PL: *Gray's Anatomy*, ed 35 British. Philadelphia,WB Saunders Co, 1973.
2. Seelaus HK: On certain muscle anomalies of the lower extremities. *Anat Rec* 35:187, 1927.
3. Sarrafian SK: *Anatomy of the Foot and Ankle*. Philadelphia, JB Lippincott Co, 1983.
4. Trestrit L: *Les Anomalies Musculaires Chez l'Homme Explique'es per l'Anatomie Compare' Leur Importance en Anthropologie.* Paris, Masson, 588–694, 705–732, 735–737, 741–744, 1884.
5. Tate R, Pachnik RL: The accessory tendon of extensor hallucis longus. *J Am Podiatry Asoc* 66:12, 899–907, 1976.
6. Lucien M: Les chefs accessoires du muscle court extenseur des orteils chez l'hommes. *Bibl Anat* 14:148, 1909.
7. Picou R: Insertions in ferieures du pe'ronier lateral. *Bull Soc Anat Paris* 8:7, 254–259, 1894.
8. Cummins JE, Anson JB, Carr WB, Wright rr, Hauser DWE: The structure of the calcaneal tendon (of Achilles) in relation to orthopedic surgery with additional observations on the plantaris muscle. *Surg Gynecol Obstet* 83:107, 1946.
9. Le Double AF: *Traite' des Variations du Systeme Musculaire de l'Homme et leur Signification au Point de Vue de'Anthropologie et Zoololique*, Vol II. Paris, Schleicher Freres, vol II, 1897.
10. Nathan H, Gloobe H: Flexor digitorum brevis: anatomical variations. *Anat Anz* 135:295, 1974.
11. Jones FW: *Structure and Function as Seen in the Foot*, ed 2. London, Bailliere, 1949.
12. Auvray M: Anomalies musculaires et nerveuses. *Bull Soc Anat Paris* 10:223, 1896.
13. Schmidt VR, Reissig D, Heinrichs HJ: Die mm lumbricales am Fuss des Menschen. *Anat Anz* 113:450, 1963.
14. Poirier P, Charpy A: *Traite' d'Anatomie Humaine*, ed 2, vol 2. Paris, Masson et Cie, 279, 1901.
15. Manter JT: Variations of the interosseous muscles of the human foot. *Anat Rec* 93:117, 1945.

Plan of Circulation for the Human Lower Extremities

It is axiomatic in podiatric anatomy and physiology that the ability to trace a drop of blood from the heart to the toes and back again be demonstrated. The intent of this section is to emphasize the circulation as it is observed distal to the knee as being most relevant to the podiatric surgeon. A brief review of circulation in general will, however, be included here.

Poorly oxygenated blood is returned to the right heart by way of the superior and inferior vena cavae. Blood passes from the right auricle into the right ventricle, which pumps it through the pulmonary artery for oxygenation in the lungs. Oxygenated blood is returned to the left auricle by way of four pulmonary veins. This is the only instance when venous blood is richly oxygenated. The left auricle shunts blood to the left ventricle, which expels it to the aorta from which several directions can be taken. The several orifices of the heart are valved to prevent the retrograde flow of blood. The tricuspid valve operates between the right auricle and ventricle, while the bicuspid valve is situated between the left auricle and ventricle.

The *aorta* arises from the left ventricle. It ascends and then arches posteriorly above the root of the left lung and gives off several branches to the heart itself, as well as to the head and upper and lower extremities. The *descending aorta* is about 8 inches long and extends from the arch of the aorta to the diaphragm as the *thoracic aorta*, which lies posterior to the mediastinum.

As the vessel passes through the diaphragm, it becomes the *abdominal aorta*. At the level of the fourth lumbar vertebra, the abdominal aorta bifurcates into *right* and *left common iliac arteries*. This bifurcation is a common location for the so-called saddle blockage of blood to the lower extremities. Because the aorta is situated left of the body's midline, the right common iliac artery is somewhat longer than the left. Common iliac arteries terminate as *internal* and *external iliac arteries*. The internal branch contributes to the circulation of the gluteal region, the hip, and the inner thigh.

Most of the blood destined for the lower extremities continues through the *external iliac artery*, which becomes the *femoral artery* after passing beneath the inguinal ligament. This mainstem vessel is palpable in the groin region.

The femoral artery runs downward, medially and posteriorly to pierce the m. adductor magnus where it becomes the *popliteal artery*. At this point it once again becomes palpable when pulsatory activity is patent.

ARTERIES

Popliteal Artery

The popliteal artery is the direct continuation of the femoral artery, beginning as it passes through the adductor hiatus. At the lower border of the popliteus, at the level of the soleal line, it divides into the anterior and posterior tibial arteries, its terminal branches. The popliteal artery is covered by muscles above and below, semimembranous, and the medial head of m. gastrocnemius. Its middle portion is in the popliteal fossa.

The branches of the popliteal artery are the superior muscular branch, sural arteries, cutaneous branches, medial and lateral superior genicular arteries, middle genicular artery, and medial and lateral inferior genicular arteries.

Superior Muscular Branches

The superior muscular branches, two or three in number, supply muscles above the knee, m. adductor magnus and the hamstrings, and anastomose with the terminal part of the deep femoral artery. They originate high in the popliteal fossa.

Sural Arteries

The sural arteries are two large branches arising just below the knee joint, supplying m. gastrocnemius, m. soleus, and m. plantaris. They penetrate m. gastrocnemius from its deep side.

Cutaneous Branches

The cutaneous branches arise from the popliteal artery or some of its branches, and pass between the two heads of m. gastrocnemius to be distributed to the skin on the upper part of the back of the leg.

Medial Superior Genicular Artery

The medial superior genecular artery comes off the popliteal artery very deep in the fossa, under the fat. It courses above the medial condyle of the femur, under semimembranous with the descending genicular and medial inferior genicular arteries. The other reaches across the anterior surface of the femur to anastomose with the lateral superior genicular artery.

Lateral Superior Genicular Artery

The lateral superior genicular artery branches off the popliteal artery at about the same level as its medial couterpart, also very deep in the popliteal fossa. It winds around the femur above the lateral condyle, deep to m. biceps femoris. At the front of the knee joint it divides into two branches. The lateral branch supplies m. vastus lateralis and anastomoses with the descending branch of the lateral circumflex femoral artery and the lateral inferior genicular artery. The deep branch anastomoses on the front of the femur with the descending genicular and medial superior genicular arteries.

Middle Genicular Artery

The middle genicular artery is an unpaired branch, arising from the anterior surface of the popliteal artery. It pierces the oblique popliteal ligament to supply the cruciate ligaments and the synovial membrane of the knee joint.

Medial Inferior Genicular Artery

The medial inferior genicular artery arises below the knee joint and runs medially and downwards along the upper border of m. popliteus, under the medial head of m. gastrocnemius and the tibial collateral ligament. It supplies m. popliteus. At the anterior border of the ligament it sends branches to anastomose with the descending genicular, medial superior genicular, lateral inferior genicular, and anterior recurrent tibial arteries.

Lateral Inferior Genicular Artery

The lateral inferior genicular artery arises slightly higher than its medial companion, runs laterally across m. popliteus, and then downwards under the lateral head of m. gastrocnemius and m. plantaris. It lies on the lateral condyle of the tibia. After passing beneath the fibular collateral ligament it divides into branches that anastomose with the lateral superior genicular, medial inferior genicular, anterior and posterior recurrent tibial, and circumflex fibular arteries.

Circumpatellar Anastomosis

There is an important network of arterial anastomoses on the anterior of the knee. A superficial portion surrounds the patella, and a deep portion lies on the joint capsule and adjacent condyles. Nine vessels take part in this anastomosis. Two come from above, the descending genicular artery and the descending branch of the lateral circumflex femoral artery. Four are the superior and inferior genicular arteries. Three come from below, the circumflex fibular and the anterior and posterior recurrent tibial arteries.

Anterior Tibial Artery

The anterior tibial artery begins as the popliteal artery ends at the lower border of the popliteus by dividing in two, one branch being the anterior tibial artery. It immediately passes through an opening at the superior end of the crural interosseous membrane to reach the anterior compartment of the leg. As it descends it moves slightly medially, so that it is on the anterior surface of the interosseous membrane above, but directly on the tibia below. It ends at the ankle joint by becoming the dorsal artery of the foot.

In the upper third of the leg the anterior tibial artery is between and deep to m. tibialis anterior and m. extensor digitorum longus. In the middle third it is between m. tibialis anterior and m. extensor hallucis longus. Just proximal to the talocrural joint the tendon of m. extensor hallucis longus crosses over the artery, so that in its final portion it lies between the tendons of the two long extensors; at this level it is deep to the inferior extensor retinaculum.

The branches of the anterior tibial artery are posterior recurrent tibial artery, anterior recurrent tibial artery, muscular branches, anterior medial malleolar artery, and anterior lateral malleolar artery.

Posterior Recurrent Tibial Artery

The posterior recurrent tibial artery is not always present. It is given off before the anterior tibial artery passes to the front of the crural interosseous membrane. It runs on the anterior surface of m. popliteus, which it supplies, and anastomoses with the inferior genicular artery to supply the superior tibiofibular articulation.

Anterior Recurrent Tibial Artery

The anterior recurrent tibial artery is the first branch on the front of the leg. It passes upwards and backwards in the substance of m. tibialis anterior, and takes part in the circumpatellar network by anastomosing with the circumflex fibular and inferior genicular arteries.

Muscular Branches

All the muscles in the anterior compartment of the leg are supplied by the anterior tibial artery: m. tibialis anterior, m. extensor digitorum longus, m. extensor hallucis longus, and m. peroneus tertius. Other branches pierce the interosseous membrane to reach the deep posterior muscles.

Anterior Medial Malleolar Artery

The anterior medial malleolar artery begins about 5 cm above the ankle joint and runs medially, deep to the tendons of m. extensor hallucis longus and m. tibialis anterior. There it anastomoses with branches of the posterior tibial and medial plantar arteries (Fig. 1.98).

Anterior Lateral Malleolar Artery

The anterior lateral malleolar artery arises at about the same level as its medial counterpart and goes laterally under the tendons of m. extensor digitorum longus and m. peroneus tertius. At the lateral side of the ankle it anastomoses with the perforating branch of the peroneal artery and the lateral tarsal artery (Fig. 1.99).

Dorsal Artery of the Foot

At the ankle joint the anterior tibial artery changes its name, and as the dorsal artery of the foot continues across the talus, navicular, and middle cuneiform to the first intermetatarsal space. There the artery dives deep, as the deep plantar branch, to join the plantar arch.

The artery is superficial for most of its path, being crossed only near its termination by m. extensor hallucis brevis.

There is a great deal of variation in the dorsal artery and its branches, with perhaps only 5% of all individuals conforming completely to the described pattern. It is frequently found lateral or medial to its usual site. It is commonly very small or absent and is

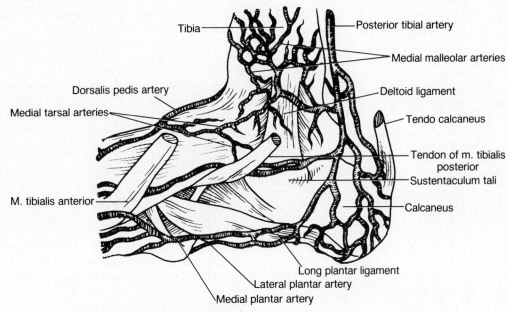

Figure 1.98. Relationships of medial blood supply of foot to contiguous structures.

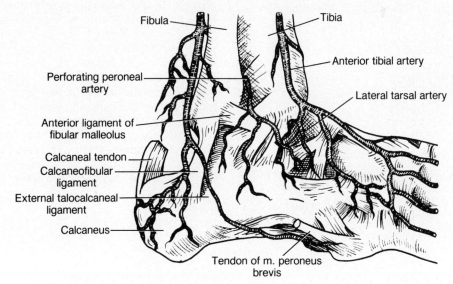

Figure 1.99. Relationships of lateral blood supply of foot to contiguous structures.

compensated for by other, mainly plantar, vessels, or it may derive from the perforating branch of the peroneal artery.

The branches of the dorsal artery of the foot are lateral tarsal artery, medial tarsal artery, arcuate artery, first dorsal metatarsal artery, and deep plantar branch.

Lateral Tarsal Artery

The lateral tarsal artery is given off as the dorsal artery crosses over the talus. It lies under m. extensor digitorum brevis and supplies it. It anastomoses with the anterior lateral malleolar, arcuate, and lateral plantar arteries and the perforating branch of the peroneal artery.

Medial Tarsal Arteries

The medial tarsal arteries are small arteries variable in number and origin, but generally two in the region of the navicular. They supply the medial border of the foot and take part in the medial malleolar anastomosis.

Arcuate Artery

The arcuate artery arises from the dorsal artery of the foot over the base of the second metatarsal, and passes laterally under the tendons of the long and short extensors. It anastomoses with the lateral tarsal artery and lateral plantar arterial branches. It gives off the second, third, and fourth dorsal metatarsal arteries.

Dorsal Metatarsal Arteries

The dorsal metatarsal arteries are numbered according to the intermetatarsal space in which they lie. They lie on the dorsal interossei, ending where the anterior perforating branches off. There they become common dorsal digital arteries, which shortly divide into proper dorsal digital arteries. Just proximal to

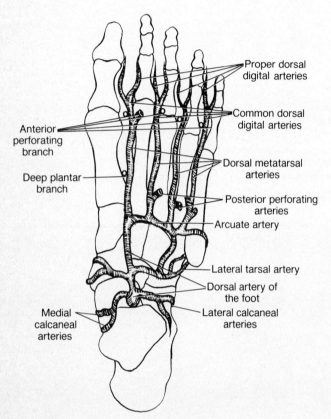

Figure 1.100. Arterial supply of the dorsum of foot.

the nail a communicating branch connects the proper dorsal digital branches of each toe.

The second, third, and fourth arteries arise from the arcuate artery. Near their bases they give off posterior perforating branches that pass between the heads of the dorsal interossei to anastomose with similar branches from the plantar arch. Anterior perforating arteries are sent off more distally, also anastomosing with plantar branches. The fourth artery usually gives off a branch for the lateral side of the fifth metatarsal and toe, but this may come directly from the arcuate artery.

The first dorsal metatarsal artery is a branch of the dorsal artery of the foot. At the base of the great toe it sends a branch under the tendon of m. extensor hallucis longus to the medial border of the toe. The first artery has only an anterior perforating branch, the posterior one being replaced by the deep plantar branch of the dorsal artery (Fig. 1.100).

Posterior Tibial Artery

The posterior tibial artery is the other terminal branch of the popliteal artery and remains on the posterior aspect of the leg. It passes downwards under m. soleus and through the deep transverse fascia of the leg, lying first on m. tibialis posterior and then m. flexor digitorum longus. In its lowest part it lies on the tibia and ankle joint (Fig. 1.101). It runs under the flexor retinaculum to end by bifurcating deep to m. abductor hallucis. Its terminal branches are the medial and lateral plantar arteries.

The branches of the posterior tibial artery are the circumflex fibular artery, the peroneal artery, a nutrient artery, muscular branches, a communicating branch, medial malleolar branches, medial calcaneal branches, the medial plantar artery, and the lateral plantar artery.

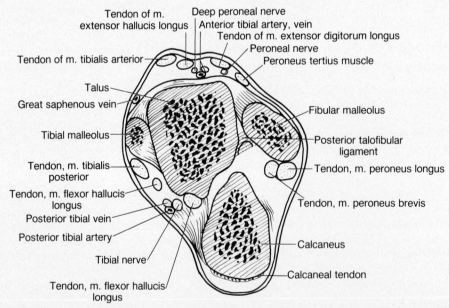

Figure 1.101. Relationships of blood supply at the ankle joint. Cross sectional representation.

Circumflex Fibular Artery

The circumflex fibular artery sometimes arises from the anterior tibial artery or popliteal artery. It passes through m. soleus, supplying it, and curves around the lateral side of the neck of the fibula. On the front of the knee it anastomoses with the inferior genicular and anterior recurrent tibial arteries.

Peroneal Artery

The peroneal artery is a large branch arising from the posterior tibial artery about 2.5 cm below the lower border of m. popliteus. It passes downwards over m. tibialis posterior toward the fibula, and then runs between m. tibialis posterior and m. flexor hallucis longus, behind the inferior tibiofibular joint, to the heel. There it breaks up into a number of lateral malleolar branches, from which calcaneal branches arise. The artery supplies muscular twigs to m. soleus, m. tibialis posterior, m. flexor hallucis longus, m. peroneus longus and m. peroneus brevis, and a nutrient branch to the fibula.

About 5 cm above the lateral malleolus a perforating branch is sent through the crural interosseous membrane to anastomose with the anterior lateral malleolar, lateral tarsal, lateral plantar, and arcuate arteries or their branches.

Slightly below the perforating branch a communicating branch runs medially, deep to m. flexor hallucis longus, and anastomoses with the communicating branch of the posterior tibial artery.

Nutrient Artery

The nutrient artery supplies the tibia and is considered to be the largest nutrient artery in the body. It arises on the medial side, about 2.5 cm below the popliteal line, and goes through m. tibialis posterior to reach the bone.

Muscular Arteries

The muscular arteries supply m. soleus and the deep posterior muscles.

Communicating Artery

The communicating artery appears about 5 cm above the lower end of the tibia and runs laterally under m. flexor hallucis longus to meet the communicating branch of the peroneal artery.

Medial Malleolar Branches

The medial malleolar branches are one or more branches from the posterior tibial artery. They join with twigs from the anterior tibial artery to form a rete over the medial malleolus.

Medial Calcaneal Branches

The medial calcaneal branches arise from the posterior tibial artery just before its terminal division. They pierce the flexor retinaculum to supply the area around the tendo calcaneus and medial side of the heel. These twigs anastomose with the posterior me-

dial malleolar branches and with the lateral calcaneal branches of the peroneal artery.

Medial Plantar Artery

The medial plantar artery is the smaller of the terminal branches of the posterior tibial artery. It enters the sole under the m. abductor hallucis, and runs forward between that muscle and m. flexor digitorum brevis, supplying them. At the base of the first metatarsal bone it usually provides a branch that joins the first plantar metatarsal artery in supplying the medial side of the great toe. Other branches run superficially to join the second, third, and fourth plantar metatarsal arteries.

It lies medial to the medial plantar nerve (Fig. 1.102).

Lateral Plantar Artery

The lateral plantar artery runs laterally and distally between m. flexor digitorum brevis and m. quadratus plantae after entering the sole under m. abductor hallucis. It lies lateral to the lateral plantar nerve. At the base of the fifth metatarsal the artery curves medially along the metatarsal bases. This part of the artery is known as the plantar arch.

The lateral plantar artery supplies all muscles of the sole except m. abductor hallucis, m. flexor digitorum brevis, and the first dorsal interosseous muscle. Superficial branches supply the skin and subcutaneous tissues in the lateral part of the sole. Deeper,

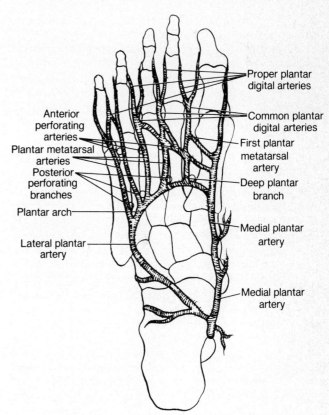

Figure 1.102. Arterial supply of plantar surface of foot.

anastomotic branches meet with branches from the lateral tarsal and arcuate arteries.

Plantar Arch

The plantar arch runs from lateral to medial, from the lateral end of the lateral plantar artery at the base of the fifth metatarsal to the first intermetatarsal space. There it anastomoses with the deep plantar branch of the dorsal artery, which often is its main source of blood. The plantar arch runs over the bases of the middle three metatarsals and the origins of the interossei, covered plantarly by the oblique head of m. adductor hallucis. Thus it is a landmark for separating the third and fourth layers of muscles.

The plantar arch gives off three perforating arteries from its deep surface that pass into the intermetatarsal spaces between the heads of the dorsal interossei. There they anastomose with the posterior perforating branches of the dorsal metatarsal arteries.

The four plantar metatarsal arteries are also branches of the plantar arch.

Plantar Metatarsal Arteries

The first plantar metatarsal artery arises at the union of the lateral plantar and deep plantar branches. The other three plantar metatarsal arteries are given off from the anterior side of the plantar arch and run distally on the ventral surface of the interossei. All give off anterior perforating arteries that meet their mates from the dorsal side, and terminate at that point by becoming the common plantar digital arteries. They end a short distance later by dividing into proper plantar digital arteries.

A branch from the first plantar metatarsal artery crosses to the medial side of the great toe to aid in its blood supply. The lateral side of the fifth toe is nourished by a branch that arises from the fourth metatarsal artery or the lateral plantar artery, and runs along the ventral surface of m. flexor digiti minimi brevis.

Malleolar Anatomoses

Under each malleolus, and extending toward the calcaneus and along the side of the foot, are networks of anastomosing arteries. On the medial side of the contributing vessels are the anterior malleolar branch of the anterior tibial artery, the medial tarsal branch of the dorsalis pedis artery, the malleolar and calcaneal branches of the posterior tibial artery, and branches from the medial plantar artery (branch of the posterior tibial artery).

The arteries taking part in the lateral malleolar network are the anterior lateral malleolar branch of the anterior tibial artery, the lateral tarsal branch of the dorsal artery, the perforating and calcaneal branch of the peroneal artery, and branches from the lateral plantar artery that anastomose with the lateral tarsal arteries.

VEINS

There are two sets of veins in the lower extremity, superficial and deep. Deep veins accompany the arteries, and there is generally a pair of veins for each of the smaller arteries. These are called venae commitantes. The superficial veins are located in the superficial fascia. Both sets have valves, although the deep veins have more.

Superficial Veins

There are two main channels among the superficial veins, the great saphenous and small saphenous veins. They have many tributaries forming an anastomosing network in the superficial fascia. Communicating branches pass from these veins to the deep veins, equipped with valves to ensure that blood does not flow back from the deeper vessels. Thus, most venous blood is carried by the deep veins.

Dorsal digital veins receive communicating branches, often called intercapitular veins, from the plantar digital veins. They then join to form the dorsal metatarsal veins, which come together in a dorsal venous arch. The arch lies over the metatarsals, and is superficial to the cutaneous nerves. Concerning the superficial veins of the foot, the dorsal venous arch is joined at one end by the medial dorsal digital vein of the great toe, thus forming the medial marginal vein that becomes the great saphenous vein, and at the other the lateral dorsal digital vein of the fifth toe joins the arch to form the lateral marginal vein, which continues as the small saphenous vein.

Superficial veins on the plantar surface of the foot drain mainly into the lateral and medial marginal veins, which run around the edges of the foot to join the saphenous veins. Some blood flows into the deep veins.

Great Saphenous Vein

The great saphenous vein is the longest vein in the body, running from the base of the great toe to the saphenous opening, where it joins the femoral vein. It enters the leg anterior to the medial malleolus, lies along its medial side, and then arches backward to cross the knee behind the condyles. In the thigh it runs somewhat anteriorly, heading toward the femoral triangle.

A part of the great saphenous vein may be duplicated. The number of valves varies, perhaps from 6 to 25, but most of them are in the leg.

Many tributaries supply the great saphenous vein, but only one is named in the thigh or leg, the accessory saphenous vein. It drains the posteromedial portion of the thigh. Another common tributary, sometimes called the lateral or anterior accessory saphenous vein, drains the anterior part of the thigh and meets the great saphenous vein high in the femoral triangle.

Just before it passes through the saphenous opening, the great saphenous vein receives the superficial epigastric, superficial external pudendal, and superficial circumflex iliac veins. The deep external pudendal vein joins it just as it enters the femoral vein.

Small Saphenous Vein

After its beginning on the dorsolateral part of the foot the small saphenous vein passes posterior to the lateral malleolus to reach the back of the leg. It lies at first lateral to the tendo calcaneus, then on it, and finally runs up the middle of the leg. Near the lower end of the popliteal fossa the vein pierces the deep fascia, passes between the two heads of m. gastrocnemius, and merges with the popliteal vein somewhat above the knee joint.

Actually, the termination of the small saphenous vein is quite variable. It may run up the back of the thigh to join the accessory saphenous vein, or it may send a branch along that route. It sometimes enters the great saphenous vein below the knee, or even ends by joining other deep veins of the leg or thigh.

Generally there are from 7 to 11 valves in the small saphenous vein, but there may be somewhat more or less.

The small saphenous vein communicates with the great saphenous and deep veins, but it has no named tributaries.

Deep Veins

Deep veins accompany the arteries and bear the same names.

Plantar digital veins unite to form four plantar metatarsal veins, after sending branches to the dorsal surface. Here, as dorsally, the metatarsal veins drain into a venous arch, the ends of which are the medial and lateral plantar veins. From this point on their paths are similar to those of the arteries, receiving tributaries comparable to arterial branches. The deep veins also receive blood from the superficial veins.

The popliteal and femoral veins are unpaired.

LYMPHATICS

Like the veins, lymphatics can be divided into deep and superficial compartments. The superficial vessels are in two sets. The medial ones, much more numerous than the lateral, follow the course of the great saphenous vein in a general way to end at the superficial inguinal lymph nodes. The lateral vessels of the leg follow the small saphenous vein and some accompany it into the popliteal fossa. The rest, along with those of the thigh, drain into the superficial inguinal nodes.

The superficial inguinal nodes, about 12 to 25 in number, receive all the superficial lymphatics of the lower extremity except those that drain to the popliteal nodes, as well as lymphatics from the genitalia and perineum. They vary considerably in arrangement but can be divided into two groups, one parallel to the inguinal ligament and one along the saphenous vein. Efferent vessels drain to the external iliac nodes.

The deep lymphatic vessels follow the arteries. Those from the foot and leg drain to the popliteal nodes, of which there are two to four, or to the small anterior tibial node on the anterosuperior part of the interosseous membrane. The efferents from these nodes, and the lymph vessels of the thigh, ultimately reach the deep inguinal nodes. There are one to three of these nodes, on the medial side of the femoral vein in the upper part of the femoral triangle. They then drain to the external iliac nodes. Part of the deep gluteal region drains to the sacral lymph nodes.

Plan of Innervation for the Human Lower Extremities

The nerve having the largest diameter supplies the human lower extremities. Its origins are from ventral divisions of the fourth and fifth lumbar vertebrae and from the first, second, and third sacral vertebrae nerves. It is known as the *sciatic nerve*. This broad nerve passes through the greater sciatic notch, passes between the greater trochanter of the femur and the ischial tuberosity. It rests on the posterior surface of m. adductor magnus, and is crossed at one point by the long head of m. biceps femoris.

In the lower third of the thigh, the sciatic nerve divides into the tibial nerve that services the posterior leg and plantar foot and the *common peroneal nerve* that will ultimately give off branches for innervation of the anterior and lateral compartments of the leg, as well as the dorsum of the foot.

COMMON PERONEAL NERVE

Lateral Sural Cutaneous Nerve (Branch of Common Peroneal)

The nerve comes off the common peroneal in the popliteal fossa proximal to where the common ceroneal nerve winds superficially about the neck of the fibula at which point the recurrent articular is given off. It supplies the upper anterior, posterior, and lateral aspects of the calf and sends a long branch distally towards the tendo achillis known variously as the peroneal anastomotic, peroneal communicating, or sural communicating nerve which unites with the

medial sural cutaneous branch of the tibial nerve to form the sural nerve. Occasionally the communicating branch to the sural nerve may arise independently from the common peroneal (Fig. 1.103).

Articular Branches

Three articular branches are distributed to the superior tibio-fibular syndesmosis and also to the knee joint. The principal branch is the recurrent articular branch.

Deep Peroneal Nerve (Anterior Tibial)

Beginning at the bifurcation of the common peroneal nerve between the fibula and the upper part of the peroneus longus, the nerve passes obliquely forward beneath m. extensor digitorum longus on the interosseous membrane where it comes in relationship with the anterior tibial vessels, just above the midline of the leg. It descends with the vessels anterior to the ankle joint where it divides into medial and lateral terminal branches.

Muscular Branches

Muscular branches supply muscles on the anterior of the leg and m. peroneus tertius.

Articular Branch to the Ankle

The deep peroneal nerve passes deep to the extensor retinaculum and terminates as medial and lateral terminal branches.

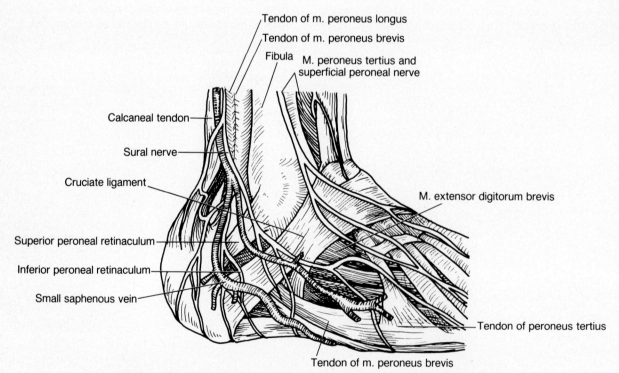

Figure 1.103.   Relationships of lateral innervation of foot to contiguous structures.

Lateral Terminal Nerve

Passing across the tarsal area beneath the extensor digitorum brevis muscle, which it innervates, the nerve becomes slightly enlarged and gives off three interosseous branches that supply the tarsometatarsal area of the second, third, and fourth interosseous muscles. This distribution is variable. The first interosseous branch sends a branch to the second dorsal interosseous muscle. It supplies the metatarsophalangeal joints of the second, third, and fourth toes.

Medial Terminal Nerve

Following the course of the dorsalis pedis artery on its lateral side, the nerve divides at the first interosseous space into two dorsal digital nerves. They supply the adjacent sides of the first and second toes (Fig. 1.104). The medial terminal branch communicates with the medial (dorsal cutaneous) nerve of the superficial peroneal. An interosseous branch given off before the division innervates the metatarsophalangeal joint of the great toe. Additionally a branch goes to the first dorsal interosseous muscle (which is also supplied by the deep branch of the lateral plantar nerve).

Superficial Peroneal Nerve (Musculocutaneous)

The superficial peroneal nerve supplies m. peroneus longus et brevis and the skin over the lower

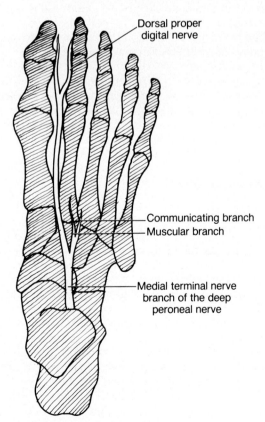

Figure 1.104.   Deep dorsal innervation of human foot.

anterior part of the leg and the dorsum of the foot. Beginning at the bifurcation of the common peroneal the nerve lies deep to m. peroneus longus and is directed distally and anteriorly. It passes between the peronei and m. extensor digitorum longus and pierces the deep fascia at the lower third of the leg. It perforates the anterolateral intermuscular septum and divides into medial and intermediate dorsal cutaneous nerves (Fig. 1.105). These relationships are important to know in such surgical procedures as transfer of the tendon of m. peroneus longus into the anterior compartment and to the dorsum of the foot.

Medial (Dorsal Cutaneous) Nerve

This branch of the superficial nerve divides in front of the ankle joint into two dorsal digital nerves. The skin of the medial side of the foot and ankle receive innervation (Fig. 1.106). The medial dorsal digital nerve supplies the medial side of the great toe and communicates with the medial terminal branch of the deep peroneal in the first interosseous space. At the level of the ankle joint it passes superficial to the extensor retinacula. The lateral dorsal digital branch of the medial dorsal cutaneous nerve supplies the adjacent sides of the second and third toes. Communicating branches anastomose with the saphenous nerve and medial terminal nerve of the deep peroneal (Fig. 1.107).

Intermediate Dorsal Cutaneous Nerve (Lateral Branch of the Superficial Peroneal Nerve)

Passing anterior and lateral to the ankle joint, this nerve is the smaller branch of the superficial peroneal nerve; it is smaller relative to the medial dorsal cutaneous nerve. It passes along the dorsal lateral aspect of the foot and divides into two dorsal digital branches. The more medial dorsal digital supplies the adjacent sides of the third and fourth toes. The lateral supplies the adjacent sides of the fourth and fifth toes. The lateral also helps to supply the dorsolateral aspect of the foot. Communicating branches anastomose with the lateral dorsal cutaneous nerve, the terminal branch of the sural nerve.

TIBIAL NERVE

The tibial nerve is the larger component of the sciatic nerve. Descending along the back of the thigh through the middle of the popliteal fossa to the lower border of the popliteus muscle, it passes with the popliteal artery beneath the soleus muscle and descends along the back of the leg with the posterior tibial vessels to the interval between the medial malleolus and the calcaneus. This relatively large nerve lies immediately beneath the transverse intermuscular septum in the deep posterior compartment of the leg. It is located between m. flexor digitorum longus medially and m. flexor hallucis longus laterally. It then divides beneath the laciniate ligament (flexor retinaculum) into medial and lateral plantar nerves to innervate the foot. In the thigh the tibial nerve is

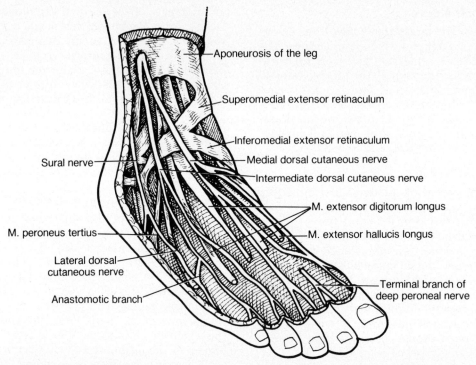

Figure 1.105.   Relationships of dorsal innervation with contiguous structures of human foot.

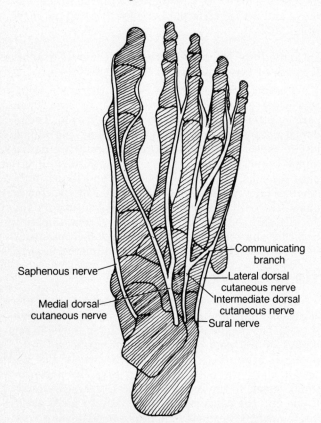

Figure 1.106.   Superficial innervation of human foot.

overlapped by the hamstring muscles. It becomes more superficial and lies lateral and some distance from the popliteal artery and vein at the popliteal fossa and the knee joint. Here the tibial nerve crosses to the medial side of the popliteal vessels. In the leg the tibial nerve

is covered by m. gastrocnemius and m. soleus. In the upper and lower parts of the leg it is covered by the fascia. In most of its lower course it lies on the lateral side of the posterior tibial artery. In the lower third of the leg it runs almost parallel to the Achilles tendon (Fig. 1.107).

The branches of the tibial nerve are the articular and the medial sural cutaneous nerve. There are usually three articulars. At the knee, a plexus is formed by anastomosing with the obturator. Distally the ankle is innervated. Medial sural cutaneous nerve passes down the back of the leg after emerging from the popliteal fossa medial or lateral to the lesser saphenous vein and unites with the sural communicating branch of the lateral sural cutaneous branch of the common peroneal nerve (peroneal anastomotic nerve) forming the sural nerve.

Sural Nerve

The sural nerve is formed by the junction of the medial sural cutaneous branch of the tibial nerve with the sural communicating (communicating ramus) branch of the lateral sural cutaneous branch of the common peroneal nerve. It passes downwards near the lateral side of the tendo calcaneus in relationship with the small saphenous vein to the interval between the lateral malleolus and the calcaneus. It then runs forward below the lateral malleolus. At this point it is continued along the lateral side of the dorsal aspect of the foot as the lateral dorsal cutaneous nerve. It communicates on the dorsum of the foot with the intermediate dorsal cutaneous nerve (branch of the superficial peroneal). In the leg it communicates with branches of the posterior femoral cutaneous nerve of

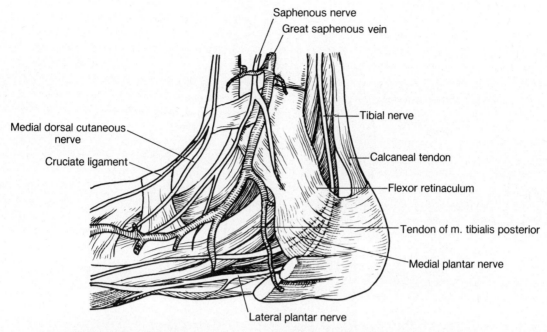

Figure 1.107.   Relationship of flexor retinaculum, tibial nerve, and contiguous structures.

the thigh. It supplies the lateral side of the fifth toe (Fig. 1.103).

The muscular branches of the tibial nerve supply m. gastrocnemius, m. plantaris, m. soleus, m. popliteus, m. tibialis posterior, m. flexor hallucis longus, and m. flexor digitorum longus.

The medial calcaneal nerve is the last branch given off by the tibial nerve before dividing into the medial and lateral plantar nerves. This branch perforates the laciniate ligament (flexor retinaculum) and supplies the skin of the heel plantarly and the medial side of the foot posteriorly.

The tibial nerve bifurcates at about the level of the flexor retinaculum (laciniate ligament) into the medial and lateral plantar nerves.

NERVES OF THE FOOT
Plantar Nerve Supply of the Foot

Medial Plantar

The medial plantar is the larger of the two terminal divisions of the tibial nerve running in the third compartment or canal of the flexor retinaculum (laciniate ligament). It accompanies the medial plantar vessels with the vessels lying along its medial side. The medial plantar nerve gives off a proper digital nerve to the medial side of great toe. Emerging from between m. abductor hallucis and m. flexor digitorum brevis it gives off three common digital nerves at the level of the metatarsal bases (Fig. 1.108).

Cutaneous Branches.   These nerves emerge from between m. abductor hallucis and m. flexor digitorum brevis to pierce the plantar aponeurosis and supply cutaneous innervation of the medial plantar aspect of the sole of the foot.

Muscular Branches.   The muscular branches for m. abductor hallucis and m. flexor digitorum brevis arise from the trunk of the medial plantar nerve before it gives off its proper digital branch. There are also branches for m. flexor hallucis brevis, by a muscular branch from the proper digital branch (medial aspect of the great toe) and the first lumbricalis muscle, from the first common digital branch plantarly.

Articular Branches.   These supply the joints of the tarsus and metatarsus.

Terminal Branches.   The proper digital or first digital nerve of the medial plantar gives a muscular branch, proximal to the first tarsometatarsal joint, which supplies m. flexor hallucis brevis. It also supplies the skin of the medial plantar aspect of the great toe (this branch penetrates through the plantar fascia at the tarsometatarsal joint level).

Three Common Digital or Second, Third, and Fourth Digital Nerves of Medial Plantar.   Each of these three nerves split into two proper digital nerves. The first supplies the adjacent sides of the great toe and the second toe. The second supplies adjacent sides of the second and third toes. The third supplies the adjacent sides of the third and fourth toes. The first common digital or second digital nerve gives off a branch to the first lumbricalis muscle. The third common digital or fourth digital branch communicates with the lateral plantar nerve. (This is the classical location of Morton's neuroma or neurofibroma.) Each proper digital nerve gives off both cutaneous and articular branches along the respective digits, terminating in the ball of each toe. At the level of the distal phalanx it sends a dorsal branch upward that is distributed to the structures around the nails, including the innervations of the nail matrix. Thus the ends and sides of the toes are supplied by the plantar nerves (Fig. 1.109).

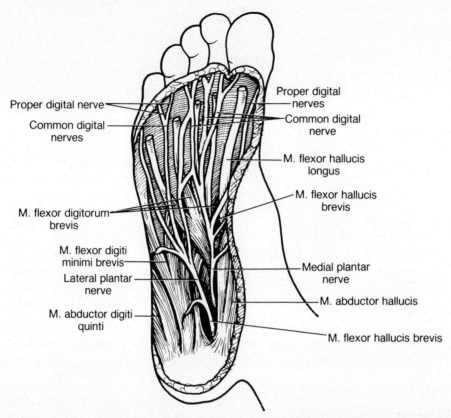

Proper digital nerve

Common digital nerves

M. flexor digitorum brevis

M. flexor digiti minimi brevis

Lateral plantar nerve

M. abductor digiti quinti

Proper digital nerves

Common digital nerve

M. flexor hallucis longus

M. flexor hallucis brevis

Medial plantar nerve

M. abductor hallucis

M. flexor hallucis brevis

Figure 1.108.   Relationships of plantar innervation with contiguous structures of human foot.

Lateral Plantar Nerve

The lateral plantar nerve is the second and smaller terminal branch of the tibial nerve. It supplies the skin of the fifth toe and the lateral half of the fourth toe, as well as most of the deep muscles of the foot.

It passes obliquely across the foot and medial to the lateral plantar vessels. From the tubercle at the base of the fifth metatarsal the nerve continues between m. flexor digitorum brevis and m. quadratus plantae. In the space between m. flexor digitorum brevis and m. abductor digiti quinti (minimi) it divides into a superficial and deep branch.

Cutaneous Branch.   It supplies the lateral aspect of the sole of the foot.

Muscular Branch.   It supplies m. quadratus plantae and m. abductor digiti minimi (flexor digitorum accessorius) from the main trunk before it divides into superficial and deep branches.

Superficial Branch.   The superficial branch divides into a proper and common digital branch. The proper digital branch supplies the lateral side of the fifth toe, m. flexor digiti minimi brevis, the third plantar interosseous, and the fourth dorsal interosseous muscles found in the fourth intermetatarsal space. It also gives off cutaneous and articular branches. The common digital branch communicates with the third common digital branch of the medial

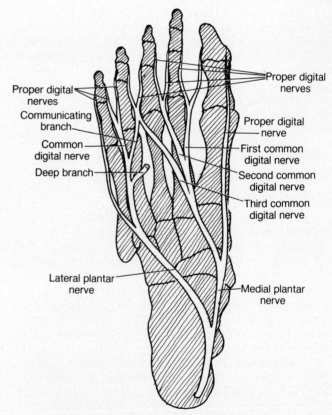

Proper digital nerves

Communicating branch

Common digital nerve

Deep branch

Proper digital nerves

Proper digital nerve

First common digital nerve

Second common digital nerve

Third common digital nerve

Lateral plantar nerve

Medial plantar nerve

Figure 1.109.   Plantar innervation of human foot.

plantar nerve. It divides into two proper digital branches that supply the adjacent sides of the fourth and fifth toes.

Deep Branch. The deep branch of the lateral plantar nerve accompanies the lateral plantar arch on the deep surface of the flexor muscles (between the third and fourth layer) and supplies all of the interosseous muscles except those in the fourth interosseous space (the third plantar and fourth dorsal interosseous muscles). It supplies all the lumbricales except the first lumbricalis. It also supplies m. adductor hallucis.

All four muscles that have origin from the plantar surface of the calcaneus are supplied by the lateral and medial plantar nerves before either divides into its branches. M. abductor hallucis and m. flexor digitorum brevis are supplied by the medial plantar nerve. M. abductor digiti minimi and the m. quadratus plantae (flexor accessorius) are supplied by the lateral plantar nerve.

Cross Sectional Anatomy - Rearfoot

GREATER AND LESSER TARSUS

Traditionally, anatomy is studied by systems. An understanding of osteology is necessary before attachments of the musculature can be understood. Arthrology explains how bones make attachment to one another. Neurology and angiology describe the innervation and vascularization of structures. However, in surgery, it is important to understand all relationships at any given point. For this reason cross sectional representations are now provided.

The muscular and tendinous attachments about the calcaneal tuberosities are best demonstrated with sections in the sagittal plane. Posteriorly, m. gastrocnemius and m. soleus make insertion into the calcaneus by means of the tendo achillis (Fig. 1.110). M. plantaris (when present) inserts into the medial aspect of the posterior two thirds of the calcaneus, but cannot be demonstrated in this example. A bursa is interposed between the upper third of the calcaneus and the tendo achillis with fat interposed superiorly between the triceps surae and the lower free portions of the tibia and fibula (1).

The tendo achillis is the strongest tendon for its length in the human body. The posterior talotibial and posterior talofibular ligaments attach to the medial and lateral tubercles of the talus, respectively, and the posterior portions of the ankle joint are closed by the joint capsule (2).

Some attachments of the first and second layers of the intrinsic foot musculature can be seen in sagittal section of the rearfoot.

M. flexor digitorum brevis of the first layer and m. flexor accessorius of the second layer, as well as the panniculus adiposus and the plantar aponeurosis are well demonstrated (Fig. 1.110).

The more posteriorly oriented sections demonstrate the orientation of the tendons of the deep posterior crural musculature into the foot. They may be organized into four compartments. M. tibialis posterior grooves the medial malleolus in the first compartment to insert by two tendinous slips, the principle of which makes attachment to the navicular tuberosity, but all tarsal bones, except the talus, receive tendinous slips of tibialis posterior. It passes superficial to the deltoid ligament, but deep to the flexor retinaculum (laciniate ligament). The tendon of m. flexor digitorum longus occupies the second compartment as it passes the medial aspect of the sustentaculum tali to cross m. flexor hallucis longus to make insertion by four tendons into the lesser digits of the foot. It receives fibers from m. flexor accessorius posteriorly and gives rise to m. lumbricalis anteriorly. The third compartment is made up of the posterior tibial nerves, arteries, and veins and the fourth compartment contains m. flexor hallucis longus. This muscle's tendon grooves the inferior surface of the sustentaculum tali and will cross the tendons of m. flexor

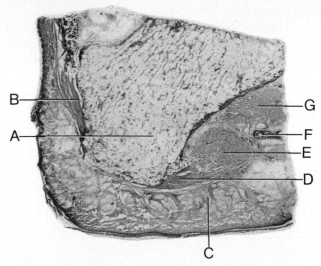

Figure 1.110. Sagittal section demonstrating insertion of triceps surae (B) into calcaneus (A). (C) Panniculus adiposis. (D) Plantar aponeurosis or fascia. (E) Flexor digitorum brevis. (F) Long plantar ligament. (G) Flexor accessorius or quadratus plantae.

digitorum longus and the lateral fibers of the belly of m. flexor hallucis brevis. These tendons are seen (in order) entering the foot proper with m. tibialis posterior most proximally oriented and m. flexor hallucis longus most deeply positioned (Fig. 1.111). These muscles relate to the deep surface of the first layer of the intrinsic foot muscles.

The intrinsic foot musculature is divisable into four layers, the first two of which relate directly to the calcaneus (2).

The first layer is constituted by three muscles described from medial to lateral. The fleshy medial border of the foot is marked by m. abductor hallucis, which takes origin in part from the medial process of the calcaneal tuberosity, but in the main from the deep fibers of the flexor retinaculum. M. flexor digitorum brevis takes origin from a small area on the medial process of the calcaneal tuberosity, but principally arises from the deep surface of the plantar aponeurosis. M. abductor digiti minimi fills out the lateral border of the foot and arises from both medial and lateral processes of the calcaneal tuberosities and contiguous soft tissue structures. All three muscles extend distally as fleshy muscle masses (3) to make insertion in the respective digits. Their deep surfaces relate to the principal blood vessel and nerve supply of the plantar surface of the foot.

The articulation between the talus and calcaneus is somewhat complex and is differentiated anatomically and clinically. Anatomically, the subtalar joint involves the posterior facets of the inferior surface of the talus and the superior surface of the calcaneus (Fig. 1.112). This constitutes the most posterior of six (sometimes seven) synovial membranes located in the human foot (2). The clinical definition of the subtalar

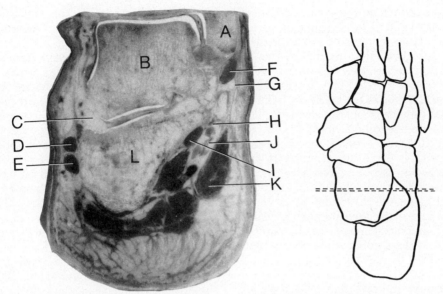

Figure 1.111. (A) (Left) Cross section of rear foot posterior to sinus tarsi, which constitutes first synovial cavity of foot. (A) Tibial malleolus. (B) Talus. (C) Lateral talocalcaneal ligament. (D) Peroneus brevis. (E) Peroneus longus. (F) Tibialis posterior. (G) Medial talocalcaneal liga-ment. (H) Flexor digitorum longus. (I) Flexor hallucis longus. (J) Posterior tibial artery, nerve, and vein. (K) Abductor hallucis. (L) Calcaneus. (Right) Cryosection intersecting talus and calcaneus (section just anterior to previous intersecting sinus tarsi).

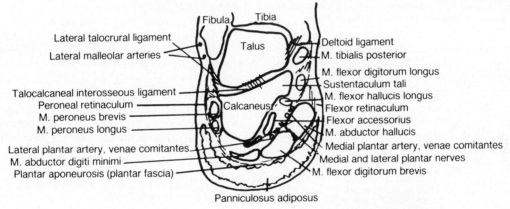

Figure 1.112. Cross section of greater tarsus in diagrammatic representation.

joint includes the middle and anterior facets of the superior surface of the calcaneus: These articulations also make connection with the talocalcaneonavicular joint. The definition of the subtalar joint therefore actually may identify one half of the joints.

The sinus tarsi occupies the middle regions interfaced by the superior surface of the calcaneus and the inferior surface of the talus. It is occupied by fat and the interosseous talocalcaneal ligament, which is the strongest ligament joining the talus and calcaneus. This area is particularly well vascularized (4). There are also anterior, medial, and lateral talocalcaneal ligaments in addition to the articular capsule closing the more anterior aspects of the joint (5).

The plantar surface of the foot is vascularized by the posterior tibial artery and its branches. The parent vessel gains entry to the foot in the third compartment of the flexor retinaculum accompanied by two venae commitantes. It lies deep to m. abductor hallucis and bifurcates into a larger lateral plantar and smaller medial plantar artery (Fig. 1.111). The medial vessel is smaller and relates to m. abductor hallucis whereas the lateral plantar artery is more extensively involved. The lateral plantar artery lies between m. flexor digitorum brevis and m. flexor accessorius in the rearfoot and it makes its medial turn in relation to m. abductor digiti minimi. Venae commitantes accompany the larger arteries of the plantar rearfoot vessels (Fig. 1.112). The dorsal vascularization will be discussed in relation to more anteriorly oriented cross sections.

The nerve supply to the plantar surface of the rearfoot is essentially planned in relation to the pattern for the blood vessels. The posterior tibial nerve enters the foot in the third compartment of the flexor retinaculum and bifurcates into a medial plantar nerve that lies fibular to the medial plantar artery and a lateral plantar nerve that lies tibial to the lateral plantar artery (6).

The second layer of foot muscles is composed of the m. flexor accessorius and m. lumbricalis, the latter of which takes origin from tendons of m. flexor digitorum longus and does not relate to the greater or lesser tarsus. M. flexor accessorius (quadratus plantae) takes origin by two heads. The larger fleshy portion arises under the groove for m. flexor hallucis longus on the medial tuberosity of the calcaneus. The fibular origin is flat and tendinous from the lateral tuberosity of the calcaneus and from the long plantar ligament that also springs from the calcaneus at this level separating the two heads of m. flexor accessorius. M. flexor accessorius extends distally to make attachment to the proximal aspect of the tendon of m. flexor digitorum longus whereas the long plantar ligament extends distally to make attachments to the plantar surface of the bases of the second, third, fourth, and fifth metatarsals and the plantar surface of the cuboid at the ridge and tuberosity.

Muscles of eversion and dorsiflexion of the foot are best demonstrated on somewhat more anteriorly oriented sections of the talus and calcaneus. M. peroneus longus becomes tendinous to run posterior to the fibular malleolus in a groove from which it emerges to run across the lateral surface of the calcaneus below the peroneal trochlea and inferior to the tendon of m. peroneus brevis and deep to the inferior peroneal retinaculum (Fig. 1.113). It grooves the plantar surface of the cuboid and passes obliquely and deep to the long plantar ligament to make insertion into the fibular aspect of the base of the first metatarsal and the medial cuneiform. Similarly, m. peroneus brevis accompanies m. peroneus longus but is anterior to it. It passes behind the fibular malleolus and crosses the lateral calcaneal surface superior to the peroneal tro-

chlea to insert into the base of the fifth metatarsal. The tendon is corklike and measures approximately 2.5 mm in diameter.

The plantar aponeurosis (fascia) of the foot is an unusually strong fibrous structure with three bands of white fibrous connective tissue. It lies deep to the panniculus adiposus (plantar fat pad) and superficial to the first layer of intrinsic musculature (Fig. 1.114). The thick central portion attaches to the medial process of the calcaneus where it separates the medial and lateral heads of origin for m. flexor accessorius (7). Its distal attachments invest numerous structures contiguous to the sulcus of the toes and consequently is beyond the scope of this study. The medial portion springs from the flexor retinaculum and thinly invests the medial dorsal aspect of the foot whereas the lateral thickened proximal portions are continuous with the dorsal fascia in the region between the lateral calcaneal process and the base of the fifth metatarsal. The panniculus adiposus is thick in the posterior foot and measures about 1 cm at the more dense locations. The region is richly vascularized by the plantar cutaneous venous network (Fig. 1.114). These veins drain into communicating vessels that connect to medial and lateral marginal veins, which in turn drain into the greater and lesser saphenous veins, respectively.

The greater and lesser tarsus make articulation at the talocalcaneonavicular and calcaneocuboid joints. A striking anatomical feature of this region is the dorsally disposed bifurcated or Y ligament that arises on the anterosuperior surface of the calcaneus and passes distally to attach to the tibial (medial) surface of the cuboid and the fibular (lateral) surface of the navicular (Fig. 1.115). Inferiorly, the short plantar ligament closes the plantar surface of the

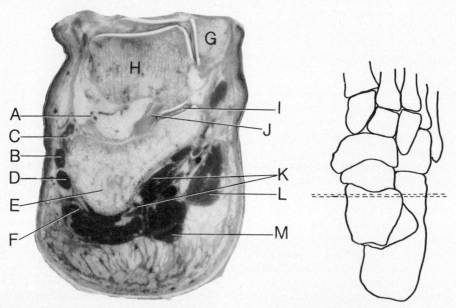

Figure 1.113. (Left) Interosseous talocalcaneal ligament (J) crosses sinus tarsi (I) obliquely. (A) Lateral talocalcaneal ligament. (B) Peroneus brevis. (C) Peroneal retinaculum. (D) Peroneus longus. (E) Lateral tuberosity of calcaneus. (F) Abductor digiti minimi. (G) Tibial malleolus. (H) Talus. (J) Interosseous talocalcaneal ligament. (K) Flexor accessorius. (L) Abductor hallucis. (M) Flexor digitorum brevis. (Right) Cryosection intersecting talus and calcaneus (section just anterior to preceding example).

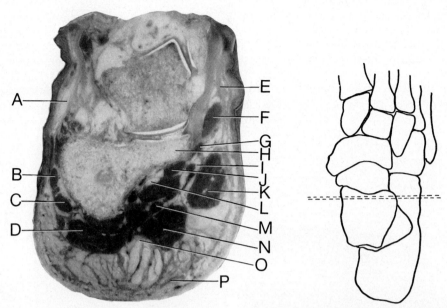

Figure 1.114. Posterior tibial artery bifurcates into medial (I) and lateral (M) plantar arteries under cover of abductor hallucis (K). (A) Peroneal retinaculum. (B) Peroneus brevis. (C) Peroneus longus. (D) Abductor digiti minimi. (E) Flexor retinaculum. (F) Tibialis posterior. (G) Flexor digitorum longus. (H) Sustentaculum tali of calcaneus. (I) Medial plantar artery. (J) Flexor hallucis longus. (K) Abductor halucis. (L) Flexor accessorius. (M) Lateral plantar artery. (N) Flexor digitorum brevis. (O) Plantar aponeurosis. (P) Panniculus adiposus. (Right) Cryosection intersecting talus and calcaneus (section just anterior to preceding example).

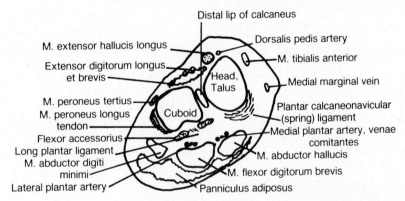

Figure 1.115. Cross sectional relationships approaching midtarsal joint diagrammatically.

calcaneocuboid joint with the dorsal calcaneocuboid closing it superiorly as it passes over the calcaneocuboid capsular ligament (2). The articulation between calcaneus and cuboid is closed with an articular capsule which constitutes the third synovial membrane of the foot (Fig. 1.115). Sections oriented in this plane usually show the fleshy 3 cm belly of m. extensor digitorum brevis that takes origin from the anterosuperior surface of the calcaneus.

The talocalcaneonavicular articulation is multiaxial and contains the plantar calcaneonavicular or spring ligament that is critical for the maintenance of the proper positioning of the head of the talus. The spring ligament is a broad, thick band situated between the anterior aspect of the sustenaculum tali of the calcaneus and the plantar surface of the navicular (Fig. 1.116). A triangular fibrocartilaginous facet is located on the dorsal surface of the ligament that articulates with a portion of the plantar aspect of the

head of the talus, thus tending to limit depression of the medial longitudinal arch. It relates medially with the deltoid ligament and is supported plantarly by the tendon of m. tibialis posterior. The lateral border of the ligament relates to m. flexor hallucis longus and m. flexor digitorum longus. The talocalcaneonavicular joint is enclosed by its articular capsule over which the dorsal talocalcaneal ligament passes (Fig. 1.116).

The cubonavicular joint is somewhat typical of the several articulations making up the lesser tarsus in that dorsal, plantar, and interosseous ligaments are usually present. If the interosseous ligament is lacking the joint will be of the plane classification and the synovial cavity and articular capsule become continuous with those of the cuneonavicular joint anteriorly. Usually there is a strong interosseous ligament with transverse fibers connecting the rough nonarticular adjacent portions of the medial cuboid and the lateral navicular. The actual articulation consists of small fibrous facets situated on the dorsal aspects of the contiguous bones (8). The dorsal ligaments of the cubonavicular joint pass forward obliquely and laterally, whereas the plantar ligament extends transversely.

The tendon of m. extensor hallucis longus, after passing deep to the superior reflection of the extensor retinaculum, enters the foot proper through the inferior portion of the extensor retinaculum. The tendon has a breadth of about 5 mm and will cross the anterior tibial vessels as it proceeds distally (Fig. 1.117). Sec-

tions through navicular and cuboid should also demonstrate most of the tendons of m. extensor digitorum longus et brevis as well as m. peroneus tertius, which is destined to insert on the dorsal aspect of the base of the fifth metatarsal (Fig. 1.117).

The lesser tarsus is characterized by interdigitations amongst the five bones constituting this region, which tends to provide for stability and motions appropriate to the location (8).

The podiatric surgeon can be deceived as to just what bone or joint surface is being exposed during

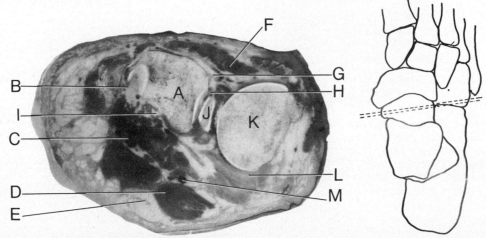

Figure 1.116.   (Left) Extensor digitorum brevis is fleshy (F) in region of talocalcaneonavicular joint. Peroneus longus (B) grooves cuboid as it changes direction to cross brace foot to make final insertion on fibular aspect of base of first metatarsal and medial cuneiform bone. (A) Cuboid. (B) Tendon of peroneus longus. (C) Lateral plantar artery. (D) Flexor digitorum brevis. (E) Panniculus adiposus. (F) Extensor digitorum brevis. (G) Dorsal calcaneocuboid ligament. (H) Bifurcated ligament. (I) Flexor accessorius. (J) Anterior tip of calcaneus. (K) Head of talus. (L) Spring ligament. (M) Medial plantar artery. (Right) Cryosection intersecting talus (head), calcaneus (distal tibial portion), and cuboid.

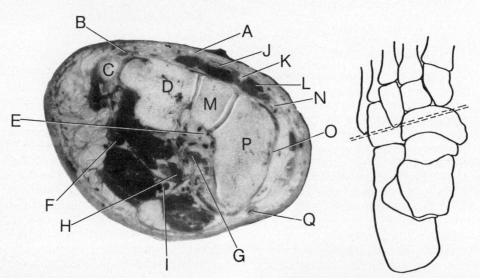

Figure 1.117.   Peroneus tertius is dorsiflexor and evertor of foot on leg and has insertion on base of fifth metatarsal. Cross sections of foot that intersect base of fifth metatarsal vary considerably depending on angle of cut because of bony recesses characteristic of articulations in region. (A) Intermediate dorsal cutaneous nerve. (B) Peroneus tertius. (C) Styloid process of fifth metatarsal base. (D) Cuboid. (E) Reflections of tendon of insertion of tibialis posterior. (F) Lateral plantar artery. (G) Tendon of flexor hallucis longus. (H) Tendon of flexor digitorum longus. (I) Medial plantar artery. (J) Extensor digitorum longus et brevis. (K) Medial dorsal cutaneous nerve. (L) Extensor hallucis longus et brevis. (M) External cuneiform. (N) Saphenous nerve. (O) Tendon of tibialis anterior. (P) Navicular. (R) Medial tarsal artery. (Right) Cryosection intersecting navicular, external cuneiform (proximal tip), and cuboid.

operative dissections directed at this particular site of the human foot. For example, an incision dorsal to the cubonavicular joint may reveal the unexpected presence of the proximal aspect of the lateral cuneiform between the navicular and cuboid (Fig. 1.117).

Vascularization to the dorsum of the foot is by branches of the anterior tibial artery that terminates at a location about mid-way between the tibial and fibular malleoli. At this point it becomes the dorsalis pedis artery (2).

The vessel crosses the articular capsule of the ankle and relates dorsally to the navicular and/or middle cuneiform. It is deep to the inferior extensor retinaculum and it lies distally between the tendons of m. extensor hallucis longus and m. extensor digitorum longus. The dorsal artery of the foot is of a caliber of about 3 mm in diameter in life, but is seen collapsed here. The vessel terminates opposite the medial cuneiform as the arcuate artery where it is deep to the tendons of m. extensor digitorum longus et brevis. The vessel crosses the bases of the metatarsals to give off dorsal metatarsal arteries.

The region just described should reveal lateral and medial anterior tarsal arteries and lateral plantar arteries. It should be noted that the dorsalis pedis artery may on occasion be anatomically absent. Venae comitantes accompany the large arteries of the ankle.

The nerve supply to the dorsum of the foot is somewhat complex. The anterior tibial nerve (deep peroneal nerve) enters the foot just lateral to the anterior tibial artery. It terminates in part as the medial terminal branch, which maintains a lateral relationship to the dorsalis pedis artery and innervates

the adjacent sides of the first and second toes (2). The lateral terminal branch lies deep to m. extensor digitorum brevis and gives off interosseous branches. The superficial peroneal nerve (musculocutaneous) terminates in medial and lateral branches. The medial branches serve the adjacent sides of the second and third toes and the medial side of the hallux. The lateral branches innervate the adjacent sides of digits three and four and four and five. The saphenous nerve usually innervates the medial side of the foot whereas the sural nerve innervates the lateral aspect. The tendon of m. peroneus longus can be seen grooving the cuboid (Fig. 1.117).

The entries of m. peroneus longus et brevis into the foot have been previously described in relation to their pulleylike mechanisms involving the fibular malleolus and the peroneal tubercle (Figs. 1.113, 1.114). Yet another pulleylike mechanism occurs as the tendon of m. peroneus longus obliquely grooves the inferior surface of the cuboid to proceed obliquely forward across the foot to make insertion at the fibular aspects of the medial cuneiform and the base of the first metatarsal. The cuneocuboid articulation, under which the tendon of m. peroneus longus passes, is characterized by dorsal, plantar, and interosseous ligaments and constitutes part of the fourth synovial membrane of the foot (Fig. 1.118). Its passage is through a canal formed by the long plantar ligament that is superficial to the tendon (Figs. 1.118, 1.119). The tendon of m. peroneus brevis can be seen making insertion into the dorsolateral aspect of the base of the fifth metatarsal (Figs. 1.118, 1.119).

One may identify tendons of m. extensor digito-

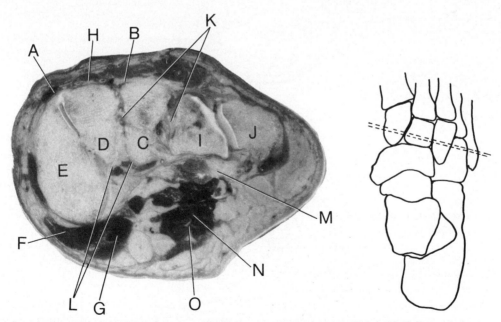

Figure 1.118. Intercuneiform and cuneocuboid joints are rigidly interconnected to provide stability for transverse arch of foot by dorsal (B) plantar (L) and interosseous (K) ligaments. (A) Tendon of extensor hallucis longus. (B) Dorsal intercuneiform ligament. (C) Lateral cuneiform. (D) Middle cuneiform. (E) Medial or first cuneiform. (F) Abductor hallucis. (G) Flexor hallucis brevis. (H) Extensor digitorum longus et brevis. (I) Cuboid. (J) Base of metatarsal five. (K) Intercuneiform interosseous ligaments. (L) Plantar intercuneiform ligament. (M) Tendon of peroneus longus. (N) Tendon(s) of flexor digitorum longus. (O) Flexor digitorum brevis. (Right) Cryosection intersecting internal cuneiform, intermediate cuneiform, external cuneiform, cuboid, and metatarsal base.

rum longus, which measures 1.5 × 3 mm, as they pass superficial to m. extensor digitorum brevis (Fig. 1.120). The tendon of m. extensor hallucis longus, measuring 1.5 × 6 mm, orients dorsal to the internal cuneiforms, and the tendon of insertion of m. tibialis anterior is also demonstrable tibially on the same bone (Fig. 1.120).

Vascularization and innervation to the plantar aspect of the foot are relatively uncomplicated. The posterior tibial artery enters the plantar foot passing midway between the medial malleolus and the medial process of the calcaneus(2). It then divides into medial and lateral branches deep to the fibers of origin of m. abductor hallucis. The medial plantar artery is the smaller of the two branches situated tibial to the medial plantar nerve. It relates to the course of m. abductor hallucis. The lateral plantar artery also begins between the tuberosities of the calcaneus (tuber calcanei) and abductor hallucis to proceed obliquely and lateralward between m. flexor digitorum brevis and m. flexor accessorius. At the base of the fifth metatarsal the vessel lies between m. flexor digitorum brevis and m. abductor digiti minimi (Fig. 1.120). Veins and venae comitantes accompany the plantar

arteries of the foot that relate to the plantar venous arch, which is well demonstrated in cryosections.

The cuneonavicular and intercuneiform joints possess dorsal and plantar ligaments, but only intercuneiform articulations have interosseous ligaments. The tendon of m. flexor hallucis longus is cordlike and measures 4 mm in this region, whereas m. flexor digitorum longus is broadening out to a dimension of 4 × 8 mm before to dividing into individual tendons to the four lesser digits (Fig. 1.120).

At the level of the bases of the metatarsals, the third layer of intrinsic foot muscles can be identified in addition to elements of the first and second layers of intrinsic foot musculature. M. flexor hallucis brevis takes origin from the medial and plantar surface of the cuboid proximal to the grooves and the contiguous surface of the external cuneiform. It frequently has fibers of origin springing from the tendons of m. peroneus longus and m. tibialis posterior. Whereas the transverse head of m. adductor hallucis takes origin distal to the limits of the present study, the oblique head of the muscle can be seen arising from the bases of the second, third, and fourth metatarsal bases, as well as from the sheath of m. peroneus longus (Fig.

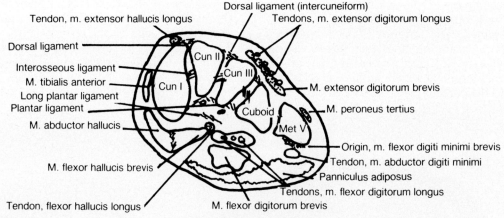

Figure 1.119. Cross sectional relationships at level of cuboid and cuneiforms diagrammatically represented.

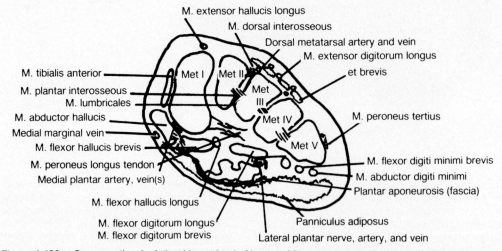

Figure 1.120. Cross sectional relationships at level of bases of five metatarsals diagrammatically represented.

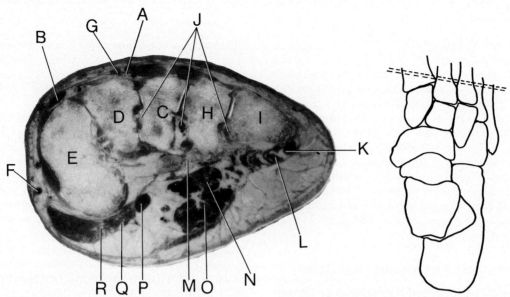

Figure 1.121. (Left) Bases of all five metatarsal bones have interosseous ligaments (J) with exception of region between first and second metatarsals. (A) Dorsal metatarsal artery. (B) Tendon of extensor hallucis longus et brevis. (C) Third metatarsal. (D) Second metatarsal. (E) First metatarsal. (F) Medial marginal vein. (G) Extensor digitorum longus et brevis. (H) Fourth metatarsal. (I) Fifth metatarsal. (J) Intermetatarsal interosseous ligaments. (K) Abductor digiti minimi. (L) Flexor digiti minimi. (M) Fibers of origin, oblique head, adductor hallucis. (N) Flexor digitorum longus. (O) Flexor digitorum brevis. (P) Flexor hallucis longus. (Q) Flexor hallucis brevis, fibular head. (R) Flexor hallucis brevis, tibial head. (Right) Cryosection intersecting metatarsal one, metatarsal two, metatarsal three, metatarsal four, and metatarsal five bases.

1.121). The two muscles just mentioned relate distally to insertions on the hallux. Finally, m. flexor digiti minimi brevis is identified arising from the medial aspect or the base of the fifth metatarsal (Fig. 1.121). The muscle is of the strap type and proceeds distally to insert at the base of the proximal phalanx of the fifth digit.

Other muscles of perhaps vestigial origin can be observed as intrinsic to the foot such as m. abductor ossis metatarsi, m. opponens hallucis, m. hallucis capsularis, and m. opponens digiti minimi (1, 2).

The first at risk structures encountered in foot surgery are the abundant venous networks that invest the foot and will be the final topic discussed relative to rearfoot cryomicrotomy studies. Deep and superficial veins drain the digits and forefoot into the medial and lateral marginal veins (Fig. 1.112). Superficial or cutaneous veins of the foot do not have corresponding arteries and they run in the superficial fascia as single vessels (2).

When arteries are deep and related to the musculature of the foot, they are accompanied by venae comitantes (double vessels). The general plan of su-

perficial venous drainage is to receive the blood of the medial marginal vein into the great saphenous vein that passes superficially in front of the medial malleolus. The lateral marginal vein drains the blood of the fibular aspect of the foot into the small saphenous vein, which proceeds up the leg behind the fibular malleolus.

References

1. Sarrafian SK: *Anatomy of the Foot and Ankle.* Philadelphia, JB Lippincott Co, 1983.
2. Warwick R, Williams PL: *Gray's Anatomy*, ed 35 British. Philadelphia, WB Saunders Co, 1973.
3. McCarthy DJ, Gorecki J: The anatomical basis of inferior calcaneal lexions. *J Am Podiatry Assoc* 69:527–536, 1979.
4. Cahill DR: The anatomy and function of the contents of the human tarsal sinus and canal. *Anat Rec* 153:1, 1965.
5. Smith JW: The ligamentous structures in the canalis and sinus tarsi. *J Anat* 92:616, 1958.
6. McCarthy DJ, Saunders MM, Herzberg AJ: The surgical anatomy of the rear foot. Part I: The greater tarsus. *J Am Podiatry Assoc* 73:607–619, 1983.
7. Laidlaw PP: The varieties of the os calcis. *J Anat* 38:133, 1904.
8. McCarthy DJ, Sanders MM, Herzberg AJ: The surgical anatomy of the rear foot. Part II: The lesser tarsus. *J Am Podiatry Assoc* 74:1–12, 1984.

Cross Sectional Anatomy of the First Ray

The first ray of the human foot begins as the first cuneiform makes articulation with the first metatarsal. It continues distally to include the proximal hallucal and ungual phalanges. This segment is vitally important to podiatric surgeons because of the frequent need operatively to correct the deformity of hallux abducto valgus. This is a complex problem requiring that different procedures be employed as a variety of variables are encountered. Surgical intervention may be directed at the cuneometatarsal joint, the base or distal shaft of the first metatarsal, or the base or shaft of the proximal hallucal phalanx, as well as the metatarsophalangeal articulation itself. All of these levels need to be considered.

FIRST CUNEOMETATARSAL REGION

The surgical distinctive of the Lapidus technique for correction of hallux abducto valgus involves a closing abductory wedge osteotomy and arthrodesis at the first cuneometatarsal joint.

The first cuneometatarsal articulation is defined as being arthroidal in type. The joint possesses its own synovial cavity and is made especially strong by dense dorsal and plantar ligaments that strengthen the capsule (Fig. 1.122). There are no interosseous ligaments between either metatarsals one and two or the medial cuneiform and metatarsal one (1). However, a well-defined interosseous ligament exists between the adjacent sides of the medial and middle cuneiforms (Fig. 1.123) (2). The medial cuneiform bone is somewhat triangular. A blunted apex orients dorsally, whereas the convex base is situated plantarly. The distal aspect of the medial cuneiform is the location of insertions of important extrinsic musculature. The inferotibial aspect is marked by the insertion of m. tibialis anterior (Fig. 1.123). The inferomedial aspect of the bone demonstrates the attachment of reflected slips of insertions of m. tibialis posterior. M. peroneus longus cross bars the foot to insert still more

inferiorly on the fibular side of the medial cuneiform (Figs. 1.122, 1.124). Two extrinsic foot muscles, m. extensor hallucis longus and m. flexor hallucis longus, cross the joint dorsally and plantarly and make for distinctive "markers."

At the level of the cuneometatarsal joint, the severity of the expression of hallux abducto valgus deformity produces minimal alteration in the position of these two tendons. A modest fibularward shift of m. extensor hallucis longus and m. flexor hallucis longus can, however, be noted in hallux abducto valgus (Fig. 1.124). Two intrinsic foot muscles operable on the first ray are observable at the level of the first cuneometatarsal joint. Tibial to and somewhat inferior to the medial cuneiform, m. abductor hallucis can be noted as a fleshy mass bordering the foot medially (Figs. 1.123, 1.124). The location of this fleshy muscle belly is in a distinctly inferior position relative to the cuneometatarsal articulation in feet with hallux abducto valgus deformity (3). Fleshy proximal parts of m. flexor hallucis brevis lie slightly deep to m. flexor hallucis longus (2). The muscle is bipennate and lies tibial and fibular to the long flexor (Figs. 1.123, 1.124). Its position is shifted fibularward in relation to m. flexor hallucis longus in the moderate and severe expressions of hallux abducto valgus.

Innervation to the area is distinctive. Dorsally the medial terminal nerve is situated fibular to the tendon of extensor hallucis longus. Tibial innervation is made by the common digital branch of the medial dorsal cutaneous nerve at the dorsotibial aspect, whereas more medially, distal elements of the saphenous nerve can be found (Fig. 1.122). Plantar innervation is supplied by two common plantar hallucal digital nerves that bifurcate proximally from the medial plantar nerve.

Vascularization of the first cuneometatarsal region is by dorsal and plantar vessels. The dorsalis pedis artery lies dorsal to and between the medial and middle cuneiforms. It lies fibular to the tendon of

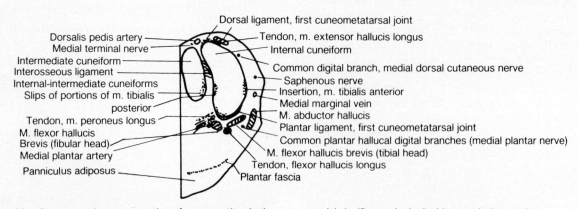

Dorsal ligament, first cuneometatarsal joint
Dorsalis pedis artery
Medial terminal nerve
Intermediate cuneiform
Interosseous ligament
Internal-intermediate cuneiforms
Slips of portions of m. tibialis
posterior
Tendon, m. peroneus longus
M. flexor hallucis
Brevis (fibular head)
Medial plantar artery
Panniculus adiposus

Tendon, m. extensor hallucis longus
Internal cuneiform
Common digital branch, medial dorsal cutaneous nerve
Saphenous nerve
Insertion, m. tibialis anterior
Medial marginal vein
M. abductor hallucis
Plantar ligament, first cuneometatarsal joint
Common plantar hallucal digital branches (medial plantar nerve)
M. flexor hallucis brevis (tibial head)
Tendon, flexor hallucis longus
Plantar fascia

Figure 1.122. Diagrammatic representation of cross sectional relationships of first cuneometatarsal joint. Structures identified have special significance in the lapidus surgical procedure.

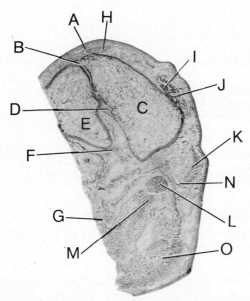

Figure 1.123. Well-defined interosseous ligament is situated between medial, middle, and lateral cuneiform bones. Tendon of m. peroneus longus makes partial insertion on the lateroplantar aspect of medial cuneiform. (A) Extensor hallucis brevis. (B) Dorsal intercuneiform ligament. (C) Medial or internal cuneiform. (D) Intercuneiform interosseous ligament. (E) Middle or internal cuneiform. (F) Plantar intercuneiform ligament. (G) Oblique head of adductor hallucis. (H) Tendon of extensor hallucis longus. (I) Medial marginal vein. (J) Insertion of tibialis anterior. (K) Abductor hallucis. (L) Tendon of flexor hallucis longus. (M) Fibular head of flexor hallucis brevis. (N) Tibial head of flexor hallucis brevis. (O) Plantar fascia. Cross section intersecting medial and middle cuneiforms.

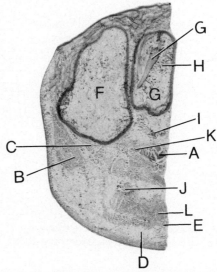

Figure 1.124. Fibularward shift of soft tissue structures relative to contiguous bone exists as hallux abducto valgus develops. This feature is especially applicable to extensor hallucis longus et brevis, flexor hallucis brevis and abductor hallucis. (A) Tendon of peroneus longus. (B) Abductor hallucis. (C) Tibial head of flexor hallucis brevis. (D) Panniculus adiposus. (E) Plantar aponeurosis (fascia). (F) Internal cuneiform. (G) Distal articular surface of intermediate cuneiform. (H) Base of second metatarsal. (I) Oblique part of adductor hallucis. (J) Tendon of flexor hallucis longus. (K) Fibular head of flexor hallucis brevis. (L) Flexor digitorum brevis. Cross section intersecting first and second cuneiforms at level of base of second metatarsal.

extensor hallucis longus. It is a dominant vessel in this region, but it is not always present and vascularization of the region may occur from other sources.

The medial plantar artery and its branches vascularize the area plantarly. Deep veins and the medial marginal vein and its superficial tributaries drain the area (Figs. 1.122–1.124).

The osseous outline is altered in proceeding distally to the base of the first metatarsal. The bone is characterized as having a reniform (kidney) shape (1). The superior surface is more concave and the inferior is more angular than that observed in relation to the medial cuneiform.

Contiguous soft tissue structures are positionally similar at this level relative to the distal medial cuneiform and the proximal portion of the base of the first metatarsal. A bursa is commonly positioned between the most proximal aspects of the first and second metatarsals.

PROXIMAL SHAFT, FIRST METATARSAL

Opening and closing abductory wedge osteotomies are applied at this location for the correction of hallux abducto valgus. The outline of the proximal portion of the shaft of the first metatarsal tends to be somewhat triangular at this point, apex up, base down (Fig. 1.125). The fibular border of the bone is straight and

normally is oriented at right angles to the ground surface. There are no ligaments attaching to this location.

The extrinsic musculature of the proximal parts of the shaft of metatarsal one demonstrate only the tendons of m. extensor hallucis longus and m. flexor hallucis longus. The former tendon is encountered relatively superficial to the dorsal crest of the metatarsal 0.3 cm below the skin and is 3 or 4 mm in diameter (4). The long flexor is about the same girth and is situated about 1 cm deep to the plantar skin surface where fleshy parts of the bipennate belly of m. flexor hallucis brevis embrace it (Figs. 1.125, 1.126).

A modest fibular shift of the tendon of m. flexor hallucis longus can be noted in specimens representative of hallux abducto valgus (3).

Intrinsic musculature involving the first ray is abundant in the region. The first dorsal interosseous muscle occupies much of the interspace between the first and second metatarsals, the adjacent sides of which provide the origins of the muscle. It lies about 1 cm beneath the free surface of the skin and is about 1 cm in both breadth and depth (Figs. 1.125, 1.126). The fleshy belly of m. abductor hallucis marks the medial border of the foot (5). It lies 2 or 3 mm beneath the free surface of the skin measuring roughly 0.3 × 0.6 cm at this location (Figs. 1.125, 1.126). This muscle adopts a distinctly inferior position relative to the first metatarsal in hallux abducto valgus deformity (3). M. flexor hallucis brevis is deep to m. flexor digitorum longus. A fibrous raphe divides the tibial and fibular

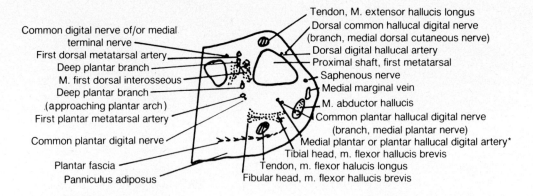

Tendon, M. extensor hallucis longus
Dorsal common hallucal digital nerve
(branch, medial dorsal cutaneous nerve)
Dorsal digital hallucal artery
Proximal shaft, first metatarsal
Saphenous nerve
Medial marginal vein
M. abductor hallucis
Common plantar hallucal digital nerve
(branch, medial plantar nerve)
Medial plantar or plantar hallucal digital artery*
Tibial head, m. flexor hallucis brevis
Tendon, m. flexor halucis longus
Fibular head, m. flexor hallucis brevis

Common digital nerve of/or medial
terminal nerve
First dorsal metatarsal artery
Deep plantar branch
M. first dorsal interosseous
Deep plantar branch
(approaching plantar arch)
First plantar metatarsal artery
Common plantar digital nerve
Plantar fascia
Panniculus adiposus

* Vessels are variable as to exact location and occurrence.

Figure 1.125. Composite diagrammatic representation of proximal shaft showing relationship to opening and closing wedge osteotomies. Diagrammatic representation of cross sectional relationships about base of first metatarsal.

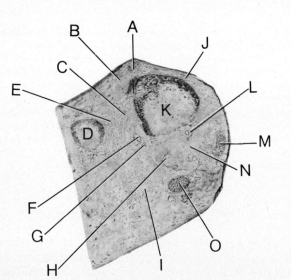

Figure 1.126. Interspace between first and second metatarsals is occupied by first dorsal interosseous muscle. This muscle assists in plantarflexion of second metatarsophalangeal joint, extends interphalangeal joints, and draws second digit towards hallux. (A) Tendon of extensor hallucis longus. (B) Tendon of extensor hallucis brevis. (C) Tibial origin of first dorsal interosseous muscle. (D) Shaft of second metatarsal. (E) Fibular origin of first dorsal interosseous muscle. (F) Artery, deep plantar branch. (G) Plantar metatarsal artery and nerve. (H) Fibular head, flexor hallucis brevis. (I) Panniculus adiposus. (J) Dorsal metatarsal artery. (K) Proximal shaft of first metatarsal. (L) Plantar metatarsal artery and nerve. (M) Abductor hallucis. (N) Tibial head of flexor hallucis brevis. (O) Tendon of flexor hallucis longus. Cross section of proximal portion of first metatarsal shaft.

bellies, each of which has a breadth of about 1 cm extending winglike to embrace the long flexor tendon (Fig. 1.126). The muscle lies about 1.5 cm deep to the plantar surface of the foot (4).

Dorsally the nerves likely to be encountered in this region may vary either because of the variability inherent in distribution or because branches vary as to the level at which they divide. The medial terminal nerve supplies the region between the first and second metatarsal by giving off a common digital branch. Either nerve may be encountered about 1.5 cm fibular

to the tendon of m. extensor hallucis longus where they have a diameter of 1 or 2 mm (6). A common digital branch from the medial dorsal cutaneous nerve is situated about 1 cm tibial to the tendon of m. extensor hallucis longus. It is relatively superficial and lies 2 or 3 mm below the free surface of the skin. The saphenous nerve frequently has a medially located representation (Fig. 1.125). The plantar nerve supply in the region of the proximal parts of the first metatarsal shaft is more deeply situated. Common plantar hallucal digital nerves originating with the medial plantar nerve are found inferior to the medial and lateral borders of the metatarsal shaft (Figs. 1.125, 1.126). Communicating nerves are also likely to be encountered at this level of the first ray.

Important arteries vascularize the region of the proximal aspect of the first metatarsal shaft.

The dorsalis pedis artery (where present) terminates proximally giving off the first dorsal metatarsal artery found midway between the first and second metatarsals about 5 mm beneath the free surface of the skin (Figs. 1.125, 1.126). In addition, the dorsalis pedis artery gives off the deep plantar branch that angles downward to "complete" the plantar arch arterial system (Figs. 1.125, 1.126). Its angle and level of bifurcation make its exact location difficult to isolate.

A medial dorsal hallucal digital branch off the first dorsal metatarsal artery is given off by the first dorsal metatarsal artery. It has a diameter of 1 or 2 mm and angles variably across the proximal part of the shaft of the first metatarsal ultimately to supply the tibial aspect of the great toe.

The lateral plantar arterial blood supply associated with the proximal portion of the base of metatarsal one is by the first plantar metatarsal artery. The vessel is about 2 mm in diameter and is a branch of the medial plantar artery. It is found in close association with the deep plantar branch that joins with the plantar arch branch of the lateral plantar artery (Figs. 1.125, 1.126). Any or all of these vessels may be encountered whenever the surgical procedure involves the proximal interspace between metatarsals one and two (7). The medial plantar artery also gives off a smaller branch, the medial plantar hallucal digital artery, which angles toward the tibial aspect of the great toe. Depending on the level of bifurcation, either the medial plantar or medial plantar hallucal digital artery may be encountered about midshaft .5 cm plantar to the first metatarsal slightly deep to and between m. abductor hallucis and the tibial belly of m. flexor hallucis brevis (3). Frequent communicating, articular, and muscular branches may be identified at this level as well. Veinous drainage of the area is by deep venae comitantes and elements of the superficial venous arch and the medial marginal vein (Figs. 1.125, 1.126).

DISTAL SHAFT, FIRST METATARSAL

Surgical corrections of hallux abducto valgus directing attention to the distal aspect of the first metatarsal shaft have been devised by Austin, Reverdin, Mitchell, and others. The outline of the metatarsal shaft at this level tends to be more oval with dorsal and plantar convex surfaces. The fibular border of the bone, however, normally remains at right angles to the weight-bearing surface (Fig. 1.127).

No ligaments are encountered at this level, although the presence of the deep transverse metatarsal ligament situated about 1 cm distally should be kept in mind (7).

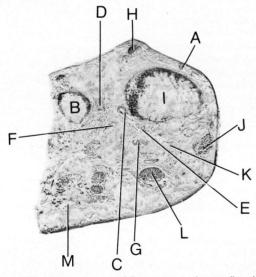

Figure 1.127. Fibular border of first metatarsal normally orients at right angles to weight-bearing surface of foot. It provides partial origin for first dorsal interosseous muscle. Dorsal and plantar surfaces of first metatarsal are essentially convex, and bone is more or less oval. (A) Dorsal digital hallucal artery. (B) Shaft of second metatarsal. (C) Anterior perforating artery. (D) First dorsal interosseous muscle. (E) First plantar metatarsal artery. (F) Oblique head of adductor halucis. (G) Fibular head of flexor hallucis brevis. (H) Extensor hallucis longus et brevis. (I) Distal shaft of first metatarsal. (J) Abductor hallucis. (K) Tibial head of flexor hallucis brevis. (L) Tendon of flexor hallucis longus. (M) Panniculus adiposus. Cross section through distal aspect of the first and second metatarsals.

Intrinsic and extrinsic muscular relationships are similar to those noted with reference to the proximal first metatarsal shaft. The more distal orientation of the first metatarsal accentuates the (apparent) fibular shift of the tendons of m. extensor hallucis longus and m. flexor hallucis longus as hallux abducto valgus deformities develop. This alteration occurs also with the intrinsic muscles associated with the first ray (3). The abductor hallucis muscle becomes more tendinous at this level and is noticeably more plantar and fibularly oriented in the hallux abducto valgus specimen than in the normal situation. The oblique head of m. adductor hallucis makes its initial appearance at this level and is in intimate association with the fibular head of m. flexor hallucis brevis. Blood vessels and nerves at this level tend to converge on the metatarsal shaft borders and are distal extensions of structures already identified.

The dorsolateral nerve supply is by a common digital hallucal nerve situated 2 or 3 mm dorsofibular relative to the metatarsal shaft (Fig. 1.128). A common dorsal hallucal nerve branching from the medial dorsal cutaneous nerve is situated on the contralateral side 2 or 3 mm dorsal and tibial to the metatarsal shaft. Common plantar hallucal digital nerves branching from the medial plantar nerve are located about 4 to 8 mm from the fibular borders of the plantar surface of the metatarsal (6). The tibial or medial common digital nerve lies deep to and between m. abductor hallucis and the tibial head of m. flexor hallucis brevis. The fibular or lateral common hallucal digital nerve lies deep to and between the fibular head of m. flexor hallucis brevis and the tibial margin of the oblique head of m. adductor hallucis. The structures are of small caliber, being about 1 or 2 mm in diameter.

The blood supply at the distal aspect of the first metatarsal shaft is variable according to levels of bifurcation and by anatomical variations occurring normally (2). Dorsally, the first dorsal metatarsal artery lies midway between the metatarsal shafts superior to the first dorsal interosseus muscle. The dorsal hallucal digital artery may be observed branching medially more closely to approximate the bone. In decidedly distal areas a portion of the anterior perforating artery may be encountered (Fig. 1.128). Other dorsal digital and plantar digital hallucal arteries are positioned at the dorsomedial, inferomedial and inferolateral borders of the metatarsal shaft at this level, 5 to 10 mm from the bone itself.

FIRST METATARSOPHALANGEAL JOINT

Surgical intervention for the correction of hallux abducto valgus invariably involves the first metatarsophalangeal joint in all techniques. McBride, Silver and others, however, limit attention to the joint area in the procedures associated with their names.

Complex ligamentous attachments characterize the first metatarsophalangeal joint where the head of the metatarsal bone tends to be quadrilateral. On the tibial aspect of the joint, tibial collateral, tibial sesamoidal, and plantar tibial sesamoidal ligaments are encountered. The contralateral side laterally demonstrates equivalent structures as identification is made of fibular collateral, fibular sesamoidal, and plantar fibular sesamoidal ligaments (7). An intersesamoidal ligament, the joint capsule proper, and the deep plantar transverse ligament are unpaired ligaments associated with the joint (Figs. 1.129, 1.130).

Resection of the medial eminence of the first metatarsal obviously involves incision and reflection of the several ligaments making up the tibial capsular structure. These structures are normally strong and compact (Figs. 1.129, 1.130). However, as the hallux abducto valgus deformity progressively worsens, these structures weaken, fray, and may appear thickened because of repeated reparative processes (Fig. 1.131). The fibular aspect of the joint capsule remains relatively intact as the condition worsens and the sesamoid bones undergo a fibular "shift" that is more apparent than real. As the head of the first metatarsal everts and arcs tibialward, the tibial sesamoid can be seen encroaching on the crista (Fig. 1.131). In severe hallux abducto valgus, the tibial sesamoid can be seen in the position originally occupied by the fibular sesamoid, while the fibular sesamoid can be seen everted into the space between metatarsals one and two. Normally, the tendon of m. extensor hallucis longus is seen dorsal and somewhat fibular to the midline of

the head of the first metatarsal. There is no joint capsule as such dorsal to the first metatarsophalangeal articulation joint. The extensor hood apparatus, however, functionally closes the joint dorsally (Fig. 1.131). The tendon of m. extensor hallucis brevis (when present) often converges on m. extensor hallucis longus near this point. The tendon of m. flexor hallucis longus normally lies immediately inferior to the crista of the plantar surface of the first metatarsal head (6). The apparent "shift" of the long flexor and extensor tendons is in direct proportion to the tibial excursion of the first metatarsal head. In hallux abducto valgus these tendons are located 0.5 to 1 cm fibular to the lateral border of the first metatarsal head (3).

The intrinsic foot musculature becomes intimately associated with the sesamoidal apparatus at this level. M. abductor hallucis is normally placed at the inferomedial angle of the first metatarsal (Fig. 1.130). As hallux abducto valgus increases, the tendon is found more inferior and fibularward relative to the first metatarsal head (3).

The tendons of m. flexor hallucis brevis are functionally attached to the tibial and fibular sesamoids, and their positions are, of course, related to these bones (6). Similarly, m. adductor hallucis, by converging its oblique and transverse heads, makes attachment to the fibular sesamoid (Fig. 1.130). In hallux abducto valgus, the muscle, by its tendon, remains essentially in situ. However, as the head of the meta-

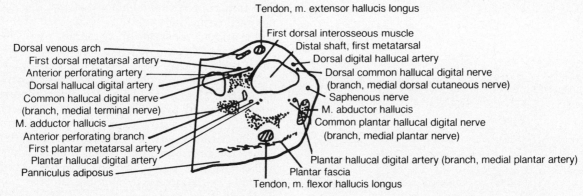

Figure 1.128. Diagrammatic representation of cross sectional relationships about distal portion of first metatarsal shaft. Composite diagrammatic representation of shaft relative to Mitchell, Austin, and Reverdin procedures.

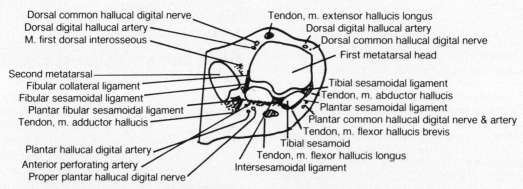

Figure 1.129. Diagrammatic representation of cross sectional relationships about head of first metatarsal. Composite diagrammatic representation of first metatarsal head relative to Silver and McBride procedures.

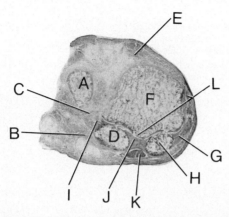

Figure 1.130. First metatarsophalangeal joint is characterized by complex ligamentous structures, most notably sesamoidal apparatus. There are tibial and fibular sesamoidal, plantar tibial, and fibular sesamoidal and intersesamoidal ligaments. Additionally, joint capsule and deep transverse metatarsal ligament relates to part. (A) Second metatarsal at surgical neck. (B) Inserting oblique head of adductor hallucis. (C) Inserting transverse head of adductor hallucis. (D) Fibular sesamoid bone. (E) Tendon of extensor hallucis longus et brevis. (F) First metatarsal head. (G) Tibial sesamoidal ligament. (H) Tibial sesamoid. (I) Fibular sesamoidal ligament. (J) Intersesamoidal ligament. (K) Tendon of flexor hallucis longus. (L) Median eminence of first metatarsal head. Cross section through head of first metatarsal.

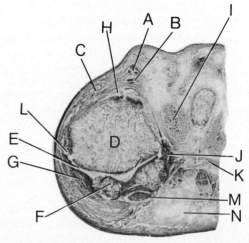

Figure 1.131. First metatarsophalangeal joint is subject to instability that may lead to deformity of hallux abducto valgus. Tendinous relationships of extensor hallucis longus et brevis, flexor hallucis longus et brevis, abductor hallucis, and adductor hallucis are altered in their course. (A) Tendon of extensor hallucis longus. (B) Tendon of extensor hallucis brevis. (C) Dorsal common hallucal artery and nerve. (D) First metatarsal head. (E) Tibial sesamoidal ligament. (F) Tibial sesamoid. (G) Tendon of abductor hallucis. (H) Hallucal extensor hood apparatus. (I) First dorsal interosseous muscle. (J) Fibular sesamoidal ligament. (K) Inserting adductor hallucis. (L) Medial plantar hallucal artery and nerve. (M) Tendon of flexor hallucis longus. (N) Panniculus adiposus. Cross section through first metatarsal head at level of second metatarsophalangeal articulation.

tarsal everts and shifts tibialward, the attachment of the hallucal adductor mirrors the position of the sesamoid and orients more dorsally (Fig. 1.131).

The blood vessels and nerves of the region are essentially the same as described for the distal part of the shaft of the first metatarsal. Dorsal digital hallucal arteries and proper dorsal digital hallucal nerves relate to the dorsomedial and lateral margins of the head of the first metatarsal about 2 or 3 mm from the bone. As with other soft tissue structures, their positions appear to shift as the metatarsal head everts and arcs tibialward. In moderate hallux abducto valgus, the medial digital hallucal artery relates more dorsofibular relative to the everted metatarsal head (Fig 1.131). Plantar digital hallucal arteries and proper plantar digital hallucal nerves relate to the inferomedial and lateral angles of the tibial and fibular sesamoid bones respectively (6). The structures are 2 or 3 mm from the ossicles. As the sesamoid bones change position with respect to the first metatarsal, these vessels just named tend to retain their position relative to the sesamoid bones, but appear to shift fibularward with reference to the metatarsal head. One important artery must be identified when discussing the region of the first metatarsophalangeal articulation. The anterior perforating artery angles downward and forward from the first dorsal metatarsal artery to join its fellow plantarly. This vessel or communicating branches from it may be encountered in the first intermetatarsal space (1). Because the inferolateral border of the first metatarsal orients more dorsally as it everts with reference to the mid sagittal plane of the body, plantar arteries and the perforating vessels are easily accessible and are at greater risk as the surgeon explores the intermetatarsal space.

The first dorsal interosseous muscle that has origin on the contiguous sides of the shafts of metatarsals one and two is well identified in several sections (Figs. 1.130, 1.131).

BASE, PROXIMAL HALLUCAL PHALANX

The base of the proximal hallucal phalanx is involved in bone resections in which hemi- or total joint replacements are involved in the surgical correction of hallux joint disorders. The base of the proximal hallucal phalanx is resected as the surgery distinctive of the Keller "bunionectomy."

The outline of the base of the proximal hallucal phalanx is triangular, apex up, base down, at this level (6).

The complex ligamentous plantar joint capsule, now structurally homogenous, envelopes the lower medial, plantar, and lateral aspects of the bone. Dorsally, the tendons of m. extensor hallucis longus et brevis can be identified along with distal elements of the extensor hood apparatus. The tendon of m. flexor hallucis longus normally bisects the inferior surface of the proximal hallucal phalanx (Fig. 1.132). These muscular relationships are altered in a fibular direction when hallux abducto valgus occurs, but not nearly to the degree observed at the level of the metatarsophalangeal joint (3).

Final attachments for fibrous elements of the intrinsic first ray musculature occur at this level. The inferolateral aspect of the proximal hallucal phalanx

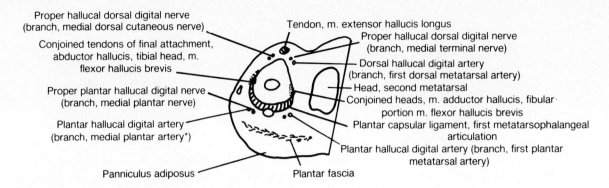

Proper hallucal dorsal digital nerve
(branch, medial dorsal cutaneous nerve)

Conjoined tendons of final attachment,
abductor hallucis, tibial head, m.
flexor hallucis brevis

Proper plantar hallucal digital nerve
(branch, medial plantar nerve)

Plantar hallucal digital artery
(branch, medial plantar artery*)

Panniculus adiposus

Tendon, m. extensor hallucis longus

Proper hallucal dorsal digital nerve
(branch, medial terminal nerve)

Dorsal hallucal digital artery
(branch, first dorsal metatarsal artery)

Head, second metatarsal

Conjoined heads, m. adductor hallucis, fibular·
portion m. flexor hallucis brevis

Plantar capsular ligament, first metatarsophalangeal
articulation

Plantar hallucal digital artery (branch, first plantar
metatarsal artery)

Plantar fascia

* Vessels are variable as to exact location and occurrence.

Figure 1.132. Diagrammatic representation of cross sectional relationships relative to base of proximal hallucal phalanx. Composite

marks the attachments for m. adductor hallucis and the fibular head of m. flexor hallucis brevis (5). On the contralateral side, the inferomedial aspect of the proximal hallucal phalanx is the location for distal attachments of m. abductor hallucis and the tibial head of m. flexor hallucis brevis (Fig. 1.133). These relationships may alter subsequent to rotational changes occurring in hallux abducto valgus (3).

Blood vessel and nerve supply to this level are similar to that occurring about the first metatarsal head. Proper dorsal neurovascular bundles occur medial and lateral to each side of the dorsal crest of the proximal phalanx (Fig. 1.133). Similarly, the plantar surface has medial and lateral proper plantar digital hallucal nerves and plantar hallucal digital arteries that are situated about 5 mm inferior to the inferomedial and inferolateral borders of the phalanx. They lie roughly in line with the dorsal structures (6).

SHAFT, PROXIMAL HALLUCAL PHALANX

Closing wedge osteotomies such as those devised by Akin are applicable to the shaft of the proximal hallucal phalanx. The surgical anatomy of this region is relatively simple.

The osseous outline remains somewhat triangular, apex up and base down as was the case for the base of the bone. The crest of the apex, however, is diminished and more rounded (Figs. 1.134, 1.135). The head of the second metatarsal usually extends well beyond the head of the first metatarsal, and this is still more accentuated when the first metatarsal is deviated medially as in hallux abducto valgus (3).

The intrinsic musculature of the first ray is no longer present at this level, having made attachments at the base of the bone. Dorsally and plantarly the now flattened tendons of m. extensor hallucis longus and m. flexor hallucis longus remain in view as they progress distally to insert on the distal hallucal phalanx (Fig. 1.135). Positional changes in relation to hallux abducto valgus are less obvious at this level (3). It should be noted, however, that the extensor hood

diagrammatic representation of base proximal hallucal phalanx relative to Keller and Akins procedures.

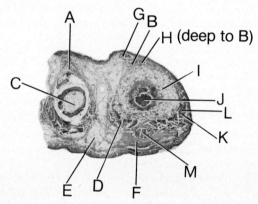

Figure 1.133. Base of proximal hallucal phalanx is important as site of attachment for intrinsic muscles of first ray including abductor hallucis and tibial head of flexor hallucis brevis on medial side and adductor hallucis and fibular head of flexor hallucis brevis on lateral aspect. (A) Tendon of extensor digitorum longus et brevis. (B) Dorsal lateral hallucal digital artery. (C) Second metatarsophalangeal joint. (D) Insertion of fibular head, flexor hallucis brevis and adductor hallucis. (E) Panniculus adiposus. (F) Plantar aponeurosis. (G) Tendon of extensor hallucis longus. (H) Insertion of extensor hallucis brevis. (I) Rim of base of proximal hallucal phalanx. (J) Central cartilage of first metatarsal head. (K) Insertion of tibial head of flexor hallucis brevis and abductor hallucis. (L) Capsule of first metatarsophalangeal joint. (M) Tendon of flexor hallucis longus. Cross section at level of first metatarsophalangeal joint.

apparatus may still be identified in this more distally situated region (Fig. 1.135). A tight plantar retinaculae binds m. flexor hallucis longus to the plantar aspect of the proximal hallucal phalanx. It is possible to sever this tendon with an oscillating saw during the course of surgery involving osteotomies of this region. The medicolegal ramifications of such complications are obvious.

Dorsal and plantar proper hallucal digital nerves occur at the medial and lateral aspects of the shaft of the proximal hallucal phalanx (1,2). Dorsal and plantar hallucal digital arteries occur similarly in close relationship to the nerves at the medial and lateral aspects of the phalanx. They are of small caliber (about 1 mm) and are positioned in the manner as

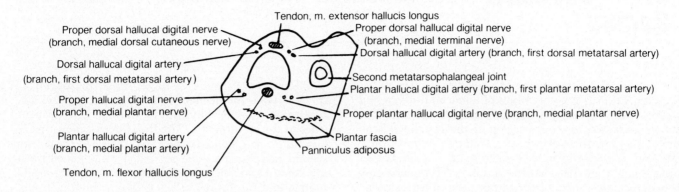

Tendon, m. extensor hallucis longus

Proper dorsal hallucal digital nerve
(branch, medial dorsal cutaneous nerve)

Proper dorsal hallucal digital nerve
(branch, medial terminal nerve)

Dorsal hallucal digital artery (branch, first dorsal metatarsal artery)

Dorsal hallucal digital artery
(branch, first dorsal metatarsal artery)

Second metatarsophalangeal joint

Plantar hallucal digital artery (branch, first plantar metatarsal artery)

Proper hallucal digital nerve
(branch, medial plantar nerve)

Proper plantar hallucal digital nerve (branch, medial plantar nerve)

Plantar hallucal digital artery
(branch, medial plantar artery)

Plantar fascia

Panniculus adiposus

Tendon, m. flexor hallucis longus

* Vessels are variable as to exact location and occurrence.

Figure 1.134. Diagrammatic representation of cross sectional relationships relative to proximal shaft of proximal hallucal phalanx.

Composite diagrammatic representation of base proximal hallucal phalanx relative to procedures of Keller and Akin.

described for the base of the proximal hallucal phalanx (Fig. 1.135).

References

1. Warwick R, Williams PL: *Gray's Anatomy*, ed 35 British. Philadelphia, WB Saunders Co, 1973.
2. Sarrafian SK: *Anatomy of the Foot and Ankle*. Philadelphia, JB Lippincott Co, 1983.
3. Grode S, McCarthy DJ: The anatomical implications of hallux abducto valgus. *J Am Podiatry Assoc* 70:539–551, 1980.
4. McCarthy DJ: The surgical anatomy of the first ray. Part II. The proximal segment. *J Am Podiatry Assoc* 73:244–255, 1983.
5. Martin BJ: Observations on the muscles and tendons of the medial aspect of the sole of the foot. *J Anat* 98:437, 1964.
6. McCarthy DJ: The surgical anatomy of the first ray. Part I. The distal segment. *J Am Podiatry Assoc* 73:111–121, 1983.
7. McCarthy DJ, Grode S: The anatomical characteristics of the first metatarsophalangeal joint. *J Am Podiatry Assoc* 70:493–504, 1980.

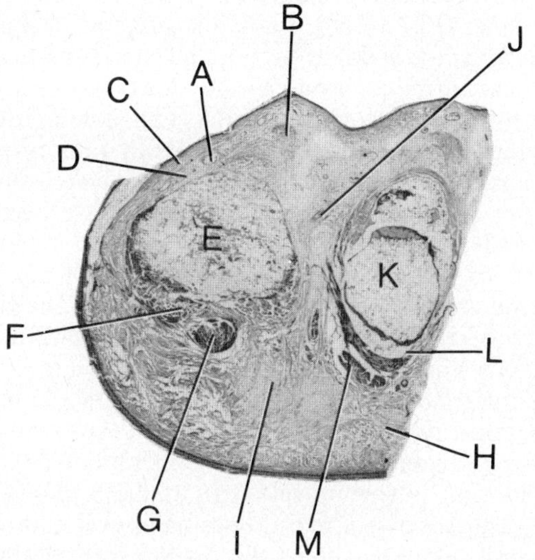

Figure 1.135. Anatomy about proximal aspect of shaft of proximal hallucal phalanx is simplified because intrinsic musculatures of first ray have already made their respective insertions. Tendons of extensor hallucis longus and elements of extensor hood apparatus and tendon of flexor hallucis longus remain in evidence. (A) Dorsal cutaneous hallucal vein. (B) Tendon of extensor hallucis longus. (C) Dorsal medial hallucal artery and vein. (D) Dorsal proper medial hallucal nerve. (E) Proximal aspect of proximal hallucal phalanx. (F) First metatarsophalangeal plantar joint capsule. (G) Tendon of flexor hallucis longus. (H) Plantar aponeurosis. (I) Panniculus adiposus. (J) Neurovascular bundle. (K) Second metatarsophalangeal joint. (L) Plantar capsule of second metatarsophalangeal joint. (M) Tendon of flexor digitorum longus et brevis. Cross section through proximal portion of proximal hallucal phalanx.

Cross Sectional Relationships of the Lesser Metatarsal Region

A significant amount of podiatric surgery is directed towards the correction of abnormalities in and about the lesser metatarsophalangeal joints. The bones and joints of this region of the foot have been discussed in some depth in a traditional way. Additional discourse would be redundant, but cross sectional anatomy as demonstrated by cryomicrotomy demonstrates a few features that need to be restated.

The apparent rotation of the lesser metatarsal shafts induces changes in the placement of their inferior crests that constitutes the apex of their triangular outlines (1). The axial rotation of the fifth metatarsal shaft is so pronounced that its apex is lateral and its base medial.

Lesser metatarsal heads are essentially quadrilateral, but they are also subject to rotational phenomenan. The present study demonstrates a tailor's bunion deformity in which the dorsal surface is inclined fibularward and the plantar surface is tilted in a tibial direction (Fig. 1.136).

The lateral condyle of the lesser metatarsals is usually much more pronounced than the medial. This frequently contributes to the formation of intractable plantar keratosis. Such a structural aberration has been demonstrated by cryomicrotomy (Fig. 1.137).

The general osseous morphology of the lesser metatarsal shafts, necks, and heads, as well as the structural features of the lesser phalanges, can be noted throughout the cryosections in several planes.

MUSCULATURE OF THE FOREFOOT

The intrinsic foot musculature most closely associated with the metatarsal bones are the four dorsal and three plantar interosseous muscles.

These seven muscles have origin on the metatarsal shafts themselves. The dorsal interossei are bipennate muscles having origin from the adjacent sides of the metatarsals. The first interosseous muscle originates in the interspace between the first and second metatarsals. The second is situated between the second and third, the third between the third and fourth, and the fourth arises between the fourth and fifth metatarsals (2).

The dorsal interosseous muscles are encountered about 1 cm beneath the dorsal surface of the foot, although this varies considerably with the amount of overlying fat and subcutaneous tissue. The muscle bellies are variable in girth, but frequently measure 1 cm or more (Fig. 1.138). Podiatric surgeons frequently encounter these reddish-brown muscles in distal metatarsal osteotomies because the muscles occupy the space between the metatarsals. The dorsal interosseous muscles become tendinous about 1 cm proximal to the metatarsal heads and are relatively small in diameter, measuring about 1 mm (Fig. 1.139). Because the dorsal interossei are abductors of the lesser toes relative to a midline through the second ray, they insert on either side of the second toe and the fibular aspects of the third and fourth toes. Additionally, tendinous slips have attachments to the plantar plate, the contiguous sides of the metatarsophalangeal joints, the glenoid ligaments, the deep transverse metatarsal ligaments, and deep portions of the transverse lamina. These muscles can assist in plantarflexion of the involved metatarsophalangeal joints and can help extend their respective interphalangeal joints. This action is because of their distal attachments to the extensor hood apparatus.

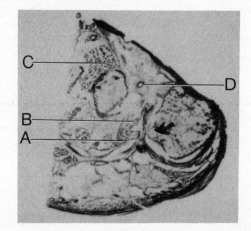
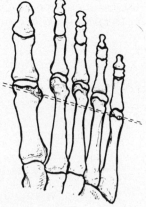

Figure 1.136. (Left) Section through fifth metatarsal head in tailor's bunion (bunionette) demonstrating inversion of fifth ray relative to everted fourth metatarsal (arrow). Note inward displacement of tendons of flexor digitorum longus (A) and fourth lumbricalis (B). Dorsal interosseous muscle (C), arising from fourth metatarsal shaft, is dorsally displaced because of inversion. (D) neurovascular bundle. (Right) Cryosection intersecting fifth metatarsal head. Details shown are tendon positioning of interossei and lumbricales.

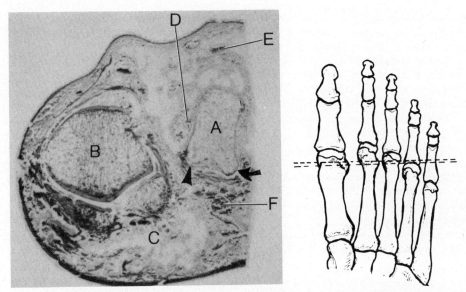

Figure 1.137. Distal portion of head of second metatarsal (A). Lateral condyle (arrow) is more prominent than medial (arrow head). Note axial rotation of this metatarsal relative to that of adjacent first metatarsal. (B) Head of first metatarsal. (C) Panniculus adiposus. (D) First dorsal interosseous muscle. (E) Extensor digitorum longus. (F) Flexor digitorum longus. (Right) Cryosection intersection of second metatarsal head region. Plantar condyle detail is shown.

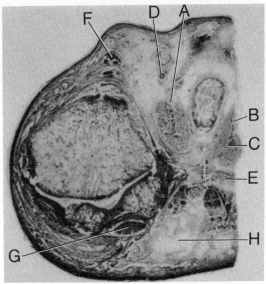

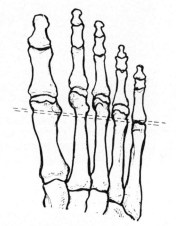

Figure 1.138. (Left) Sections through first and second dorsal interosseous muscles demonstrating their relationships to second metatarsal. (A) First dorsal interosseous muscle. (B) Second dorsal interosseous muscle. (C) First plantar interosseous muscle. (D) Neurovascular bundle. (E) Transverse head of adductor hallucis. (F) Extensor hallucis longus. (G) Flexor hallucis longus. (H) Panniculus adiposus. (Right) Cryosection intersecting shaft and second metatarsal. Detail of first plantar interosseus muscle is shown.

There are three plantar interosseous muscles. Their origins are from the inferior tibial aspects of the third, fourth, and fifth metatarsals (1,2). They have a girth of about 3 or 4 mm and insert with diminutive tendons into the tibial aspects of the bases of the third, fourth, and fifth toes. Consequently, they are adductors of the three lateral digits relative to a midline bisecting the second ray. Additionally, they have soft tissue attachments like those of the dorsal interossei. Thus they are also plantar flexors of the respective metatarsophalangeal joints and extensors of the interphalangeal joints.

Before proceeding with the myology of the forefoot, mention must be made of fibrous attachments maintaining the integrity of the metatarsophalangeal joints. These include the deep transverse metatarsal ligament and the respective metatarsophalangeal joint capsules.

The metatarsophalangeal joints consist of collateral and plantar joint capsules. In effect the proximal phalanx of each of the lesser toes is suspended from the contiguous metatarsal head by oblique cordlike collateral ligaments angled downward distally and triangularly shaped suspensory glenoid ligaments. Fibular ligaments are characteristically stronger than the medial ligaments. A dense fibrous plantar plate is identified plantarly, which is intimately associated with the deep transverse metatarsal ligament (1). The dorsum of the joints is closed by elements of the extensor hood apparatus that will be dealt with subsequently in connection with m. extensor digitorum longus et brevis. The interphalangeal joints are similar in construction to the metatarsophalangeal joint but are less densely organized. They demonstrate collateral ligaments and plantar joint capsules.

The deep transverse metatarsal ligament consists of four short but wide flattened fibrous bands that interconnect the plantar ligaments and joint capsules of the adjacent metatarsal heads.

It is a tough connective tissue structure having a thickness of about 1 mm. It traverses the forefoot just behind the metatarsal heads and is thickened on its inferior aspect by a plantarplate. It is further supported by the plantar attachments of the collateral and glenoid suspensory ligaments (Fig. 1.140). The superior surface of the deep transverse metatarsal ligament relates to the interosseous musculature. The lumbricalis muscles and the neurovascular bundle, which is of considerable significance to podiatric surgeons, lie inferior to the deep transverse metatarsal ligaments within the four intermetatarsal spaces.

M. adductor hallucis may be considered as two muscles having a more or less common insertion on and about the fibular sesamoid and the lateral aspect of the base of the proximal hallucal phalanx. The oblique head of m. adductor hallucis does not have a direct relationship to this study of the lesser metatarsal head region. However, the transverse head of

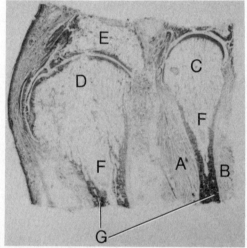
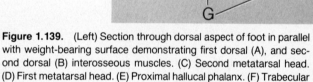
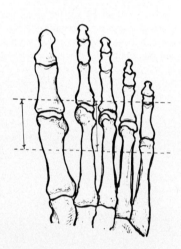

Figure 1.139.   (Left) Section through dorsal aspect of foot in parallel with weight-bearing surface demonstrating first dorsal (A), and second dorsal (B) interosseous muscles. (C) Second metatarsal head. (D) First metatarsal head. (E) Proximal hallucal phalanx. (F) Trabecular bone. (G) Cortical bone. (Right) Cryosection intersecting dorsal aspect of second metatarsal head and shaft. Detail of first and second dorsal interosseous muscles is shown.

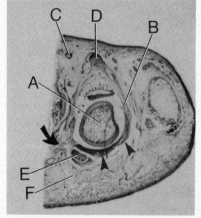
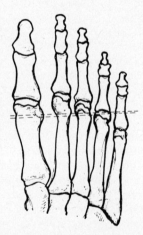

Figure 1.140.   (Left) Deep transverse metatarsal ligament between inferior surfaces of metatarsals three and four (arrow) at point of attachment of suspensory or glenoid ligament. (A) Fourth metatarsophalangeal joint. (B) Collateral ligament. Arrow heads, plantar capsule of fourth metatarsophalangeal joint. (C) Neurovascular bundle. (D) Extensor digitorum longus. (E) Flexor digitorum longus. (F) Panniculosus adiposus. (Right) Cryosection intersecting fourth metatarsophalangeal joint. Detail of fourth metatarsophalangeal joint capsule is shown.

m. adductor hallucis relates in one way or another to the third, fourth, and fifth metatarsal heads on their plantar aspects, as well as to their respective plantar-plates (3). The deep transverse metatarsal ligament gives fibers of attachment for the transverse head of m. adductor hallucis at metatarsal head two, as well as the third, fourth, and fifth metatarsophalangeal regions (Fig. 1.141). The transverse head of m. adductor hallucis constitutes part of the third layer of the foot's musculature.

The four lumbricalis muscles are the only representatives of the second layer of muscles intrinsic to the forefoot. They take fleshy origins from the tendons of m. flexor digitorum longus. The first is from the tibial side of the most medial of the four tendons that passes to the second toe. The second lumbrical arises from contiguous sides of the first and second long flexor tendons; the third is from contiguous sides of the second and third, whereas the fourth takes origin from adjacent sides of the third and fourth tendons of the long flexor muscle. Insertion of each of the four lumbricales is ultimately into the tibial aspects of the second, third, fourth, and fifth toes. These tendons are situated medial to the respective tendons of the long flexor. Initially they lie plantar to the deep transverse metatarsal ligaments. However, as they proceed distally they extend dorsally to make attachment on the extensor hood apparatus of the lesser toes. They extend the interphalangeal joints and flex the involved metatarsophalangeal joints. The individual tendons are relatively small, having a diameter of 2 mm or less.

The musculature of the forefoot is represented by at least one of the four layers constituting the foot's intrinsic composition. M. flexor digitorum brevis is of the first or most superficial of the plantar foot musculature. The muscle takes origin in the rearfoot, mainly from the medial tubercle of the calcaneus. It becomes tendinous in the distal third of the metatarsal shaft, dividing into four bands each of which has a thickness of about 1 mm. At the level of the metatarsophalangeal joints they each bifurcate to embrace the corresponding tendons of m. flexor digitorum longus. Final insertion is into the base of the middle phalanges at which point the fibers decussate or reunite (1).

The fifth metatarsophalangeal joint differs from the second, third and fourth by virtue of two intrinsic foot muscles. M. abductor digiti minimi is classified as a first layer muscle, whereas m. flexor digiti quinti brevis is representative of the third strata (Fig. 1.142).

M. abductor digiti minimi has broad origin from the rearfoot, mainly involving the lateral tuberosity of the calcaneus. Its muscle belly is fleshy and normally measures 2 cm or more as it marginates the lateral border of the foot (3). It becomes tendinous in the distal third of the shaft of the fifth metatarsal. The tendon of insertion is a broad flat band measuring 1 × 2 mm and it makes final attachment on the lateral aspect of the base of the proximal phalanx of the fifth toe. Because of the inferior placement of this tendon, it is a plantarflexor as well as abductor, of the fifth toe. It is also subject to rotational changes of the fifth metatarsophalangeal joint as seen in tailor's bunion (3).

M. flexor digiti minimi brevis is characterized as a third layer muscle intrinsic to the foot. Because it is deeply situated, its origin is more distally disposed. It

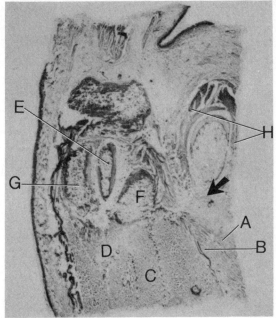
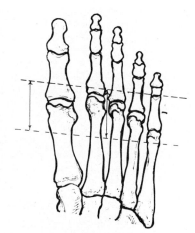

Figure 1.141. (Left) Adductor hallucis relates to plantar aspect of second metatarsal head (arrow). (A) Transverse head, adductor hallucis. (B) Oblique head, adductor hallucis. (C) Flexor hallucis brevis (fibular head). (D) Flexor hallucis brevis (tibial head). (E) Median eminence. (F) Fibular sesamoid. (G) Tibial sesamoid. (H) Capsule of second metatarsophalangeal joint. (Right) Cryosection intersecting plantar aspect of second metatarsal head and shaft (musculature). Detail of m. flexor digitorum brevis is shown.

arises from the crest of the cuboid and the base of the fifth metatarsal. The fleshy belly of m. flexor digiti minimi brevis measures about 1 cm in girth and it becomes tendinous in the distal third of the plantar surface of the fifth metatarsal. It inserts between m. abductor digiti minimi laterally and m. flexor digitorum longus medially to the plantar surface of the base of the proximal phalanx of the fifth toe. The tendon is broad and flat, measuring about 1 or 2 mm.

M. extensor digitorum brevis has origin on the superior surface of the calcaneus near the lateral end of the calcaneal sulcus adjacent to the cervicle ligament. It is a broad flat muscle that becomes tendinous by forming three slips for insertion into the fibular sides of the tendons of m. extensor digitorum longus to the second, third, and fourth toes. These tendons lie deep to the long extensor tendons and have a girth of about 2 mm.

The dorsal aponeurosis of the foot encases the foot with a stockinglike investment that sends spe-

cialized fibers and septations into the deeper recesses of the forefoot. A specialized part of the dorsal aponeurosis is the extensor hood or aponeurosis (4). It relates to both m. extensor digitorum brevis and m. extensor digitorum longus. The structure is a fibrous aponeurosis that fans out from the long extensor tendon to close the dorsal aspect of all metatarsophalangeal joints and effectively replaces a dorsal joint capsule (Fig. 1.143). Its attachments to tendons of the lumbricales and the interossei have already been mentioned. The dorsal aponeurosis demonstrates a proximal "sling" with vertically arranged fibers that relates plantarly to the plantar plate and the deep transverse metatarsal ligment. A distal "wing" of the extensor (hood) aponeurosis demonstrates proximally disposed oblique fibers that relate to the obliquity of the tendon of insertion of lumbricalis musculature (4).

M. flexor digitorum longus is an extrinsic foot muscle having origin on the posterior aspect of the tibia. It enters the foot through the second compart-

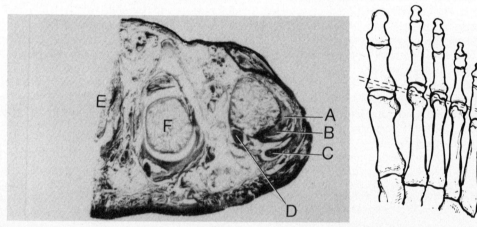

Figure 1.142.   (Left) Section intersecting base of proximal phalanx of fifth toe demonstrating insertion of tendons of abductor digiti minimi (A), and flexor digiti quinti brevis (B). Tendon of flexor digitorum longus (C), fourth lumbricalis muscle (D), metatarsal head three (E), and four (F). (Right) Cryosection intersecting base of proximal phalanx of fifth toe. Detail of tendon of m. abductor digiti minimi and tendon of flexor digiti quinti brevis is demonstrated.

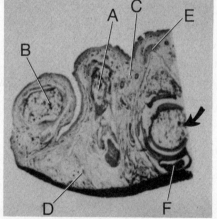
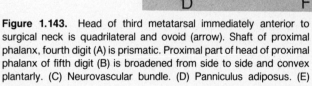
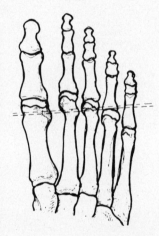

Figure 1.143.   Head of third metatarsal immediately anterior to surgical neck is quadrilateral and ovoid (arrow). Shaft of proximal phalanx, fourth digit (A) is prismatic. Proximal part of head of proximal phalanx of fifth digit (B) is broadened from side to side and convex plantarly. (C) Neurovascular bundle. (D) Panniculus adiposus. (E) Extensor digitorum longus. (F) Flexor digitorum longus. (Right) Cryosection intersecting third metatarsal head. Osseous detail of third metatarsal head base, fourth proximal phalange shaft, and proximal fifth phalanx is shown.

ment of the flexor retinaculum. It becomes tendinous in the leg well above the tibial malleolus and forms four tendons for insertion into the plantar surfaces of the distal phalanges of the four lesser toes at midfoot. The tendons are broad and somewhat flattened as they course plantar to their respective lesser metatarsophalangeal joints. They measure about 2 or 3 mm in girth. At this level, m. flexor digitorum brevis has undergone bifurcation to embrace the tendon of m. flexor digitorum longus.

The tendon of m. flexor digitorum longus normally lies in a midline position plantar to the involved metatarsals and phalanges. However, it is subject to displacement. In this respect m. flexor digitorum longus may be compared with m. flexor hallucis longus in its fibular displacement in hallux abducto valgus. The present study revealed a tibial displacement of m. flexor digitorum longus as it related to the fourth toe (Fig. 1.144). Even more severe displacements have been reported that were revealed during the course of foot surgery. This displacement may be diagnosed before surgical intervention through the use of radiopaque contrast dyes into the tendinous sheath of m. flexor digitorum longus (E. Dalton McGlamry, DPM, personal communication). Such a structural modification suggests additional displacement of contiguous structures: Certainly the lumbricalis tendons must shift and relationships to m. flexor digitorum brevis, the deep transverse metatarsal ligament, the preflexor adipose cushion, and the fat bodies must change.

The action of m. flexor digitorum longus and other plantar intrinsic foot muscles in flexing the lesser toes is antagonized in large measure by m. extensor digitorum longus. This extrinsic foot muscle has origin on the upper three fourths of the anterior surface of the fibula and the contiguous part of the lateral condyle of the tibia. It passes beneath the extensor retinaculum and expands into four somewhat

tendinous slips for insertion on each of the four lesser toes. It demonstrates a trifurcation about the level of the metatarsophalangeal joint where the extensor hood apparatus is in evidence (Fig. 1.145). A shorter middle slip inserts dorsally on the intermediate phalanx. Two lateral slips embrace the middle phalanx to insert on the superior surface of the distal phalanx (1).

The tendon of m. extensor digitorum longus usually receives tendinous attachment of m. extensor digitorum brevis on its inferolateral aspect in the region of the metatarsophalangeal joints. The extensor aponeurosis (hood) has attachment on the tendon of m. extensor digitorum longus about the metatarsophalangeal joint.

Cryomicrotomy has distinct advantages in presenting precise two-dimensional representations of cross sectional anatomy. It does not always reveal minute structures to best advantage, particularly if they are positioned tangentially. For such demonstrations, traditional dissection of fresh materials remains the best approach. The region of the lesser metatarsophalangeal joints demonstrates a great number of anomalous structures.

FIBROUS ENSHEATHMENTS OF THE FOREFOOT

Reference has been made to the fibrous annular sheath that encircles the capsule of the metatarsophalangeal joint. This extensor aponeurosis continues plantarward to make attachment to the plantar plate, as well as the deep transverse metatarsal ligament. The transverse lamina designates that proximal portion of the extensor hood along the distal part of the metatarsal shaft (5). Common intertendinous portions of the dorsal aponeurosis interconnect adjacent extensor sheaths. Deep to this fibrous sheath, a second

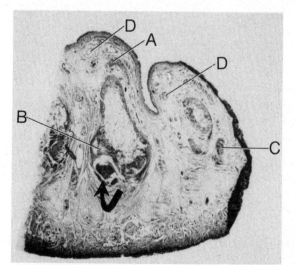
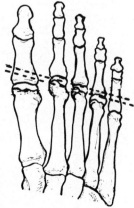

Figure 1.144. (Left) Section through base of proximal phalanx of fourth toe demonstrating tibial displacement of tendons of flexor digitorum longus and brevis (arrow). (A) Tendon of extensor digitorum longus. (B) Lumbricals tendon. (C) Tendon of abductor digiti minimi.

(D) Neurovascular bundle. (Right) Cryosection intersecting base of proximal phalanx and fourth toe. Detail of displacement of tendons of m. flexor digitorum longus et brevis is shown.

aponeurosis covers the superior surfaces of the underlying dorsal interosseous muscles. Another aponeurosis that separates dorsal from plantar interossei can also be observed. Its fibers are obliquely oriented.

In proceeding distally toward the metatarsal head, the dorsal aponeurosis forms a wedge, the apex of which extends plantarly to make attachment on the underlying dorsal interosseous aponeurosis. Vertical septations that pass between adjacent metatarsals plantarward ultimately to attach to the deep transverse metatarsal ligament now appear (1). Each interosseous tendon is therefore covered over by a "vertical lamina." Its septations pass beyond the deep transverse metatarsal ligament finally to afix on deep fibers of the plantar aponeurosis that lies beneath the metatarsophalangeal joints.

Deep fibrous septations can also be identified in association with the tendons. These thin retinaculae encircle the tendons and bind these to the underside of the joints and the respective proximal phalanges of m. flexor digitorum longus et brevis. Independent synovial sacs enclose the tendons of both the long and short tendons. They extend from the respective lesser metatarsal heads to the bases of each of the ungual phalanges of the four lesser toes. Connections between these tendons make up a vincula system (1). Vinculum morphology is variable. It may be variously likened to a tent, cord, or filament and it may orient sagittally or horizontally.

Numerous vincula complicate the relationships of the bifurcated tendon of m. flexor digitorum brevis and the intervening tendon of m. flexor digitorum longus as they insert plantar to the intermediate and distal phalanges, respectively.

M. flexor digitorum brevis has a triangular vinculus that joins the bifurcated tendinous slips. Its concave transverse free proximal border is usually located across the proximal portion of the proximal phalanx. The distal extremity of the vinculum is usually placed distally under the intermediate phalanx.

The brevis vinculum has a horizontal mesomembrane covering the bone between the two bifurcations of the tendon of m. flexor digitorum brevis. The vinculum proper of these two slips is located on their longitudinal axis. Distally, as the decussation of the short flexor insertion is about to occur, a chiasma tendineum makes its X-shaped appearance (3).

The vinculum of m. flexor digitorum longus has tent-shaped septations that join that of the brevis at its proximal border. A cordlike distal septation joins the chiasma of the brevis. The short vinculum of the long flexor tendon makes attachment to the ungual phalanx (Fig. 1.146).

ADIPOFASCIAL FOREFOOT COMPARTMENTALIZATION

A more or less constant and organized arrangement of fat bodies is situated about the metatarsal heads in a protective manner. In the intermetatarsal spaces, a triangular adipofascial complex with its base up and apex down is formed by the wedge shaped plantar disposition of the dorsal extensor intertendinous aponeurosis as it dips plantarly to meet the dorsal interosseous aponeurosis (1).

A single preflexor adipose pad is situated immediately inferior to the synovial sheath of m. flexor digitorum longus. It lies deep to the longitudinal bands of the plantar aponeurosis.

Paired fat bodies flank the head and contiguous part of the lesser metatarsal shafts. They shield the neurovascular bundles on their deep surfaces. These two fat bodies are encased on either side by thin vertical aponeurotic bands extending from the transverse fibers of the plantar aponeurosis below and the deep transverse metatarsal ligaments above.

PLANTAR APONEUROSIS

The plantar fascia (aponeurosis) of the foot is a somewhat triangular band of tough fibrous connective

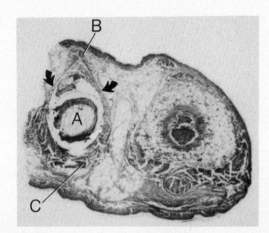
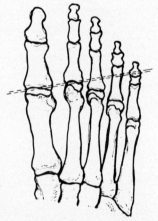

Figure 1.145. (Left) Extensor hood appartus fans outward from tendon of extensor digitorum longus to embrace dorsal aspect of metatarsophalangeal joint (arrows). (A) Second metatarsophalangeal joint. (B) Tendon of extensor digitorum longus. (C) Tendon of flexor digitorum longus. (Right) Cryosection intersecting second metatarsal head and shaft. Detail of vinculum of m. flexor digitorum longus et brevis.

tissue with proximal attachment on the inferoposteromedial aspect of the medial tuberosity of the calcaneus (2). It has deep and superficial components as it approaches the lesser metatarsophalangeal joints.

The relationships of the numerous perimetatarsal head structures can be demonstrated to good advantage by cryomicrotomy (Fig. 1.147). The superficial component of the plantar aponeurosis has transverse fibers. The lesser metatarsal region (which excludes the hallucal interphalangeal joint) usually receives distal slips to the interval between the first and second toe, the base of the third toe, and the interdigital area betwen the fourth and fifth toes (1). The most lateral slip extends to the base of the fifth toe.

The deep component of the plantar aponeurosis has longitudinal fibers also represented as separate fibrous slips that insert on and about the deep transverse metatarsal ligament at the respective metatarsophalangeal joints. They bifurcate to flank the flexor

tendons and form arches. These provide passage for the neurovascular bundles and the lumbricalis tendons as they proceed from an inferior to a more superior position in the forefoot.

The ball of the foot and the sulcus of the toes have tough fibrous interconnections between the skin and deep structures. Podiatric surgeons are familiar with the resistance encountered because of these structures in making plantar incisions. The natatory ligament consists of about eight transversely oriented bands crossing the intertriginous zones of the forefoot(1). The fasciculus aponeurotica transversum is also a system of transverse fibers, but it lies proximal to the metatarsal heads.

Mooring ligaments are found distal to the metatarsophalangeal joints (1). This is a transversely oriented reticulating system that is interposed between the flexor sheaths and the skin. Additionally, five pairs of sagittal septations flank the flexor tendons. They

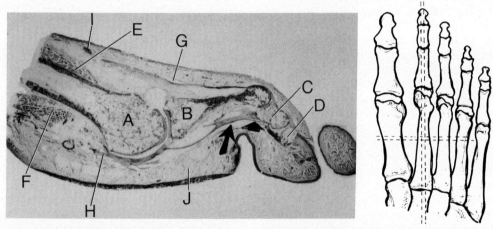

Figure 1.146. (Left) Vinculum of flexor digitorum longus tendon to lesser metatarsal. Proximal segment (arrow), distal segment (arrow head). (A) Lesser metatarsal. (B) Proximal phalanx. (C) Intermediate phalanx. (D) Ungual phalanx. (E) Dorsal interosseous muscle. (F) Plantar interosseous muscle. (G) Tendon of extensor digitorum longus. (H) Tendon of flexor digitorum longus. (I) Vein. (J) Panniculus adiposus, vertical longitudinal section. (Right) Cryosection intersecting second metatarsal head and shaft. Detail of vinculum of m. flexor digitorum longus et brevis is shown.

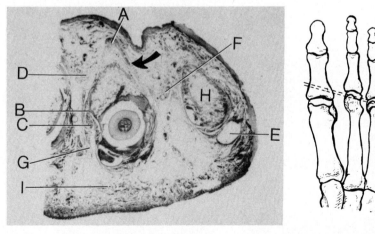

Figure 1.147. (Left) Section through fourth metatarsophalangeal joint demonstrating fine detail of extensor hood (arrow). (A) Tendon of extensor digitorum longus. (B) Transverse lamina. (C) Vertical lamina. (D) Interaxial lamina. (E) Sheath of tendon of flexor digitorum longus to fifth toe. (F) Neurovascular bundle. (G) Inferolateral fat body. (H) Fifth metatarsal head. (I) Transverse fibers of plantar aponeurosis. (Right) Cryosection intersecting fourth metatarsophalangeal joint. Detail of transverse vertical and interaxial lamina is shown.

extend from the first superficial aponeurotic bands to make deep attachments on or about the deep transverse metatarsal ligment proximal to the metatarsal heads (1).

The forefoot demonstrates a definite pattern of compartmentalization that is best demonstrated by traditional dissection techniques. The medial and lateral intermuscular septae and an intervening Y shaped septation oriented transversely form three compartments (4, 5). These are characterized as medial, central, and lateral. The medial intermuscular septum passes between the oblique head of m. adductor hallucis and m. flexor hallucis brevis. The lateral intermuscular septum follows the tibial border of the fifth metatarsal and encloses the third (most fibular) plantar interosseous muscle. The central compartment contains most of the forefoot structures and is further subdivided by a Y shaped septa with superomedial and inferomedial limbs. Its stem orients parallel with the foot's dorsal and plantar surface to make attachment laterally along the fifth metatarsal.

The vascularization and innervation of the lesser metatarsophalangeal region tends to be complex. In the forefoot small neurovascular bundles that contain the nerves, arteries, and veins are directed anteriorly through the intermetatarsal spaces where they bifurcate to serve the adjacent sides of the toes (1, 2).

The routes by which nerves and arteries enter the foot, and by which veins and lymphatics make egress, have been described earlier in this chapter. Traditional systematic methodologies are best employed to describe these relationships, but all cryosections used will demonstrate some evidences of such structures. The reader is referred to cryosections 1, 3, 5, 8, 9, and 12 for the best demonstrations of neurovascular bundles. Earlier discourses in this chapter have presented the pertinent angiology and neurology in an organized form. This information need not be repeated, but a brief review will assist in the appreciation of cryosections.

Dorsal and plantar proper digital nerves and arteries supply the adjacent sides of toes. These are derived of common digital vessels that in turn have origin from dorsal and plantar metatarsal nerves, arteries, and veins (2).

Cross sectional representations fail to recapitulate the numerous routes by which the distal parts of the foot are innervated and vascularized. The organization here is peculiar in that there is overlap and anastomosis of structures. This feature tends to preserve functional integrity in case of injury. For example, medial innervation of the hallux is accomplished by branches of the medial dorsal cutaneous nerve and the saphenous nerve.

The interspace between the first and second toes is supplied by a terminal branch of the deep peroneal nerve, whereas the intermediate dorsal cutaneous nerve from the superficial peroneal nerve supplies the second, third, and fourth interspaces. The lateral aspect of the foot is supplied by the sural nerve. This nerve is made up of anastomotic elements of the tibial nerve, which is actually related to the posterior leg.

The tibial nerve terminates as medial and lateral plantar nerves that supply the plantar surface of the foot and there is anastomosis between these structures (2).

Vascularization of the foot, like that of the hip and knee, is also protected by anastomosis and communication between vessels. Even the pulp region of the distal toes demonstrates this organization. The deep perforating and anterior perforating arteries interconnect the dorsal and plantar metatarsal arteries just posterior to the metatarsal heads. These vessels appear tangentially in some cryosections. They are best observed in traditional dissection because they change direction and orient obliquely.

The vascularization of the foot, for all practical purposes, is derived from terminal branches of the popliteal artery. Both the posterior tibial and anterior tibial arteries are derived from this parent blood vessel. The posterior tibial artery proceeds distally to supply the plantar surface of the foot. The anterior tibial artery serves the dorsum of the foot (1, 2). These divergences have been discussed earlier in traditional anatomical approaches. As is true with most human anatomy, variations are common. For example, the dorsalis pedis artery is frequently absent and blood is supplied to the dorsum of the foot by some alternative route.

References

1. Sarrafian SK: *Anatomy of the Foot and Ankle.* Philadelphia, JB Lippincott Co, 1983.
2. Warwick R, Williams PL: *Gray's Anatomy,* ed 35 British. Philadelphia, WB Saunders Co, 1973.
3. McCarthy DJ, Brandwene SM, Bartolomei FJ: The surgical anatomy of the lesser metatarsals and phalanges. *J Am Podiatry Assoc.* (in press).
4. Sarrafian SK, Topouzian LK: Anatomy and physiology of the extensor apparatus of the toes. *J Bone Joint Surg* 51:669, 1969.
5. Kamel R, Sakla BF: Anatomical compartments of the sole of the human foot. *Anat Rec* 140:57, 1961.

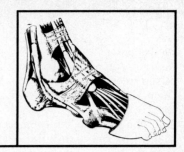

CHAPTER 2

Biomechanics

Michael J. Burns, D.P.M.

NORMAL STRUCTURAL POSITION

The positions and relationships described in this section will be considered with the individual standing in erect posture, unless otherwise specified.

Pelvis

The pelvis is level in the frontal plane. This is most easily verified by the level relationship between the anterior and posterosuperior iliac spines and the crests of the ilia. There is a normal, mild anterior tilt of the pelvis that is not readily detectable on clinical examination.

Hip

The head and neck of the femur are normally positioned in the center of its range of motion in the transverse plane. The head and neck are angulated posteriorly approximately 10°, and a normal twist in the shaft of the femur places the femoral condyles in the frontal plane. The range of motion of the adult hip in the transverse plane is approximately 45° in each direction. The hip is positioned such that the shaft of the femur is vertical in the sagittal plane. Sagittal plane range of motion of the hip is approximately 150° of flexion and 10° of hyperextension. The apparent further range of hyperextension actually consists of forward tilt of the pelvis and flexion of the opposite hip.

Knee

The knee is usually fully extended with the long axis of the shaft of the femur and the tibia being parallel to one another in the sagittal plane. There is a sagittal plane range of motion of 130° to 140° of flexion from this position. No hyperextension of the knee is normally available.

With the knee fully extended no transverse plane motion is available; however, it is available when the knee is flexed. At the beginning of flexion of the knee there is normal transverse plane motion with the "unlocking" mechanism within the knee joint. Up to 50° range of transverse plane motion of the leg relative to the femur is typically available with the knee flexed 90°.

There is usually no frontal plane movement of the leg relative to the femur available at the knee joint. A normal angulation of the femur in the frontal plane results in approximately a 170° angle laterally between the femur and the tibia. This places the knees closer together and allows the legs to remain vertical.

Ankle

The ankle is approximately 90° to the leg. Passive range of motion of approximately 10° of dorsiflexion of the foot relative to the leg with the subtalar joint neutral and knee fully extended is available in a normal individual; plantarflexion of 30° to 50° is usually available.

The ankle joint axis is deviated from both the sagittal and transverse planes by approximately 10°. The axis passes from posterior-plantar-lateral to anterior-dorsal-medial, and the motion occurring around the ankle joint axis is pronation and supination. Because of the preponderance of sagittal plane motion, plantarflexion and dorsiflexion are used to describe the motion at the ankle joint.

Subtalar Joint

The subtalar joint is in its neutral position and the posterior aspect of the heel is vertical.

The range of motion of the subtalar joint is approximately 30°. This is based on the amount of frontal plane motion of the posterior aspect of the calcaneus rather than actual rotation around the axis.

The neutral position of the subtalar joint has been described as that position at which there is congruency between the talus and calcaneus. There has also been discussion regarding this neutral position being at a point from which twice the amount of supination as pronation is available (1). The neutral position of the subtalar joint is probably closer to the end of its range of motion in the direction of pronation. The most satisfactory method of determining subtalar

111

joint neutral position is to palpate for conformity between the neck of the talus and the sinus tarsi area of the calcaneus laterally and between the neck of the talus and the tendon of m. tibialis posterior medially (2).

The subtalar joint axis is oriented from posterior plantar lateral to anterior dorsal medial. The average axis deviates approximately 42° from the transverse plane and 16° from the sagittal plane (3). As the axis becomes further angulated from a particular body plane, the amount of motion available in that plane will increase. A common example is the subtalar joint axis, which is inclined more than 42° from the transverse plane and reaches a more vertical position. This foot has a more transverse plane motion than either frontal or sagittal plane motion because of the relative position of the axis. If an axis was deviated more towards the transverse plane, then that particular subtalar joint would have more frontal plane motion and less motion available in the transverse plane (Fig. 2.1). This relative position of the axis is important in approaching the foot conservatively or surgically, because the best procedure or device to control a particular motion may be dependent on which planar motion dominates.

Midtarsal Joint

As the subtalar joint is moved through its range of motion from full supination to full pronation, the amount of motion available around the oblique midtarsal joint axis increases. When the subtalar joint is in a supinated position, there is relatively limited motion available around the oblique axis of the midtarsal joint. This is partly because of the obliquity of the axes of the talonavicular and calcaneocuboidal joints when the subtalar joint is supinated (Fig. 2.2). As the subtalar joint is moved towards the pronated position, the axes of the talonavicular and calcaneocuboidal joints become more in line with one another, thus allowing the navicular, cuboid, and the remainder of the forefoot to move together as a unit on the calcaneus and talus (4).

The oblique axis of the midtarsal joint is oriented from posterior-plantar-lateral to anterior-dorsal-medial and has been described as having an average deviation of 52° from the transverse plane and 57° from the sagittal plane (3). The position of the oblique midtarsal joint axis is quite variable among individuals; often primarily transverse or sagittal plane motion will be available, depending on the position of the axis.

As the individual pronates, the foot moves in the direction of eversion in the frontal plane. The oblique midtarsal joint axis tilts with this motion and becomes further deviated from the sagittal plane. As the axis moves in this direction, vertical loading of the forepart of the foot produces a greater moment of force around the oblique midtarsal joint axis, because the motion more closely approximates pure sagittal plane motion (Fig. 2.3).

The relative effect of the "locking mechanism" of the midtarsal joint is caused both by subtalar joint

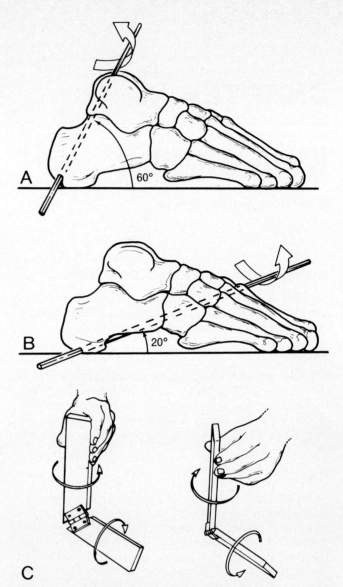

Figure 2.1.   Axis position. (A) Example of high-pitched subtalar joint axis. (B) Example of low-pitched subtalar joint axis. (C) Example of mitered hinge set at 45°.

position (relative obliquity of the talonavicular and calcaneocuboidal joints) and the relative position of the midtarsal joint axis in space.

The longitudinal axis of the midtarsal joint is also oriented from posterior-plantar-lateral to anterior-dorsal-medial and has an average deviation of approximately 9° from the sagittal plane and 15° from the transverse plane. With this position the motion around the longitudinal axis of the midtarsal joint closely approximates frontal plane motion. True motion around the longitudinal axis of the midtarsal joint does not seem to be available in all individuals. The frontal plane motion (when present) probably represents motion of several of the intertarsal and tarsometatarsal joints. As the subtalar joint is supinated, limiting motion in the midfoot, the availability of this frontal plane motion also diminishes.

Most of the surgical approaches to limit subtalar

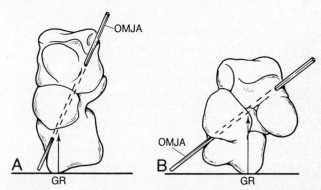

Figure 2.3. Anterior view of midtarsal joint with position of oblique midtarsal joint axis (OMJA) depicted. As subtalar joint moves from supinated (A) to pronated (B) ground reactive (GR) forces of gravity become more perpendicular to axis of motion.

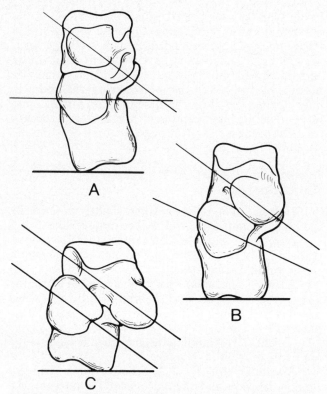

Figure 2.2. Anterior view of midtarsal joint with forefoot removed. Lines represent direction and motion available at individual facets. (A) Subtalar joint supinated. (B) Subtalar joint neutral. (C) Subtalar joint pronated. As subtalar joint moves from supinated to pronated position available range of motion of forefoot on rearfoot at midtarsal joint increases.

motion in the flatfoot (i.e. arthroereisis) depend on the secondary stabilizing effect at the midtarsal joint. If clinically supinating the subtalar joint does not reduce the mobility of the midfoot and forefoot, one must consider ancillary procedures to stabilize the midfoot.

Forefoot to Rearfoot Position

In the frontal plane the plantar aspect of the ball of the foot is aligned perpendicular to the bisection of the posterior surface of the heel. The subtalar joint is in its neutral position and the forefoot is loaded along its lateral border, pronating the forefoot relative to the rearfoot around its midtarsal joint axis. This normal arrangement does not allow the rearfoot to supinate without simultaneous motion of the forefoot in the same direction. Similarly, the forefoot cannot be pronated without rearfoot pronation. Independent motion of the forefoot or rearfoot in the other direction is available. In the transverse plane there is usually a mild amount of adduction being approximately 10° to 15°. In the sagittal plane the forefoot is plantarflexed relative to the calcaneus and the first metatarsal is approximately in line with a long axis bisecting the head and neck of the talus. The normal amount of the plantarflexion of the first metatarsal relative to the calcaneus is considerably greater than that of the fifth metatarsal, thereby producing the

more prominent "arch" at the medial aspect of the foot.

First Ray

The axis of motion of the first ray passes from posterior-dorsal-medial to anterior-plantar-lateral and is deviated from the transverse plane only slightly while deviated from the sagittal and frontal planes by approximately 45° (5). The motion that occurs around this axis is then a combination of dorsiflexion, inversion, and adduction, or plantarflexion, eversion, and abduction. Only a slight amount of transverse plane motion occurs with these motions, because the axis lies close to the transverse plane. The range of motion available around the first ray axis has not adequately been determined. Clinically, 10 to 15 mm of motion of the first metatarsal head in the sagittal plane relative to the second metatarsal head is normally available.

The relative position of the first ray and first metatarsal in the sagittal plane is important to the subsequent range of motion available at the first metatarsophalangeal joint. As will be mentioned later during the section on gait, plantarflexion of the first metatarsal is imperative to allow adequate dorsiflexion of the first metatarsophalangeal joint to occur. This is demonstrated clinically by holding the first metatarsal in a dorsiflexed position and observing the relative limitation of dorsiflexion of the hallux. In this same foot the first ray can be plantarflexed, and the amount of dorsiflexion of the hallux will be greatly increased. One can quickly see that any malfunction of the foot that necessitates the first ray functioning in a dorsiflexed position will cause jamming of the first metatarsophalangeal joint. On clinical examination the first metatarsal head seems to rest in the center of its sagittal plane range of motion and is approximately at the same level as the second, third, and fourth metatarsal heads.

Fifth Ray

The axis of motion of the fifth ray passes from posterior-plantar-lateral to anterior-dorsal-medial. The average position of the axis relative to the cardinal body planes has not been established. Clinically, the motion that occurs seems to be nearly equal in all three body planes, implying that the axis is deviated a similar amount from each plane. The position of the fifth metatarsal head, like the first, seems to rest approximately at the level of the second, third, and fourth metatarsal heads in the normal foot and approximately in the center of its range of pronatory-supinatory motion. It is difficult to evaluate the angular motion occurring at the fifth metatarsal; the position is determined by the relative position of the fifth metatarsal head to that of the third and fourth. An abnormally pronated fifth ray is abducted, everted, and dorsiflexed, making the fifth metatarsal head prominent laterally.

First Metatarsophalangeal Joint

The first metatarsophalangeal joint has two axes of motion, one oriented in the transverse plane from medial to lateral allowing primarily dorsiflexion and plantarflexion, and a second aligned in a vertical fashion from superior to inferior that allows primarily abduction and adduction. Some motion also seems to be available in the frontal plane, which would indicate the possibility of an axis passing from posterior to anterior. Some authors feel that this motion cannot occur without some subluxation of the joint (6). Range of motion in the transverse plane, pure abduction and adduction, is quite limited and is probably not significant for normal locomotion. The motion that occurs in the sagittal plane is quite important clinically.

Normally, the range of plantarflexion of the hallux relative to the first metatarsal is only slightly past parallel; however, with the normal declination angle of the first metatarsal being in excess of 20°, the hallux does not need to plantarflex significantly past a 20° dorsiflexed position for normal ambulation. The range of motion in the direction of dorsiflexion at the first metatarsophalangeal joint approximates 80° to 90°. Late in the stance phase of gait the first metatarsal will typically approach this 80° to 90° angle relative to the supporting surface while the hallux remains in contact with the ground. If this range of motion is not available, jamming will occur, and the first metatarsophalangeal joint will need to be lifted from the ground earlier during the gait cycle.

As mentioned previously, adequate plantarflexion of the first metatarsal relative to the lesser metatarsals is necessary to allow this first metatarsophalangeal joint dorsiflexion. If jamming of this joint occurs with every step, it is easy to understand the pathological changes that occur in the first metatarsophalangeal joint. In a rectus type foot (minimal metatarsus adductus) a hallux limitus or rigidus will result. In the adductus type foot, with normal digital abductus the syndrome of hallux abducto valgus occurs.

Lesser Metatarsophalangeal Joints

The axis of motion for the lesser metatarsophalangeal joints seems to be similar to that of the first, with two distinct axes noted clinically. During normal locomotion only the sagittal plane motion around the horizontal axis is significant clinically. As the heel is lifted and the metatarsal heads remain in contact with the ground, it is necessary for rotation to occur in the sagittal plane around the metatarsophalangeal joints. Motion of the lesser metatarsophalangeal joints is only slightly less than the first in the sagittal plane. Some relative tarsometatarsal plantarflexion occurs to allow adequate sagittal plane excursion in the direction of dorsiflexion.

Summary of Normal Part-To-Part Relationships

Pelvis.   The pelvis is tilted slightly anterior in the sagittal plane and level in the frontal plane.

Hip.   The hip is in the center of its transverse plane range of motion and aligned such that the femur is vertical in the sagittal plane.

Knee.   The axis is in the individual's frontal and transverse planes and the knee is fully extended. The leg is vertical in both the frontal and sagittal planes.

Ankle.   The ankle joint is aligned with the foot approximately 90° to the leg.

Subtalar Joint.   The subtalar joint is in its neutral position and the calcaneus is approximately vertical.

Midtarsal Joint.   The midtarsal joint is positioned such that the forefoot is loaded in the direction of pronation against the rearfoot and at the end of its range of motion in this direction. The forefoot rests on the supporting surface.

Forefoot to Rearfoot.   The plantar aspect of the ball of the foot is approximately perpendicular to the bisection of the heel.

First Ray.   The first metatarsal head is at the level of the second through fifth metatarsal heads and in the center of its sagittal plane range of motion.

Fifth Ray.   The fifth ray is in the center of its sagittal plane range of motion and at the level of the first through fourth metatarsal heads.

Second, Third, and Fourth Rays.   These rays are dorsiflexed, and the metatarsal heads are approximately coplanar with the first and fifth metatarsal heads.

First Metatarsophalangeal Joint.   The first metatarsophalangeal joint will be dorsiflexed 20° to 25° relative to the long axis of the first metatarsal, with the hallux resting on the supporting surface.

Lesser Metatarsophalangeal Joints.   The lesser metatarsophalangeal joints are slightly dorsiflexed in a static position, with the digit being dorsiflexed in an amount similar to that of plantar declination of the adjacent metatarsal.

NORMAL GAIT

The method by which humans move from one point to another is a complex phenomenon. The goal of normal gait is to enable the individual to move from one place to another with the least amount of energy expenditure. The body accomplishes this with a pattern of integrated joint movements and muscle functions that allow the center of gravity to be displaced minimally during locomotion.

The gait cycle can be divided into two major phases: the stance phase, during which time the foot is on the floor, and the swing phase, during which time the foot is swinging forward. The stance phase occupies approximately 62° of the total gait cycle and the swing phase the remaining 38°. Heel contact by the opposite limb is by necessity at 50° of the total gait cycle, if the individual is to walk without a limp. Stance phase of gait can be further subdivided. Contact phase occupies that portion of stance from heel contact unil 15° of the total gait cycle. Several events occur at or near 15°, making it a convenient ending point for contact phase. Midstance is from 15° of the gait cycle until the heel comes off the ground at about 40°. From heel-off until approximately heel contact of the opposite limb at 50° of the gait cycle is termed "push-off," and the remaining portion of stance phase from 50° of the gait cycle until toe-off at 62° of the gait cycle is termed "balance assist" (7). Swing phase can be subdivided by activities, the first portion (early swing phase) when the foot is being lifted and the last (late swing phase) when the limb is swung forward (Fig. 2.4).

The events occurring during the gait cycle will be discussed according to phase. Each phase will be subdivided into joint motion, center of gravity movement and energy transfer, foot-to-floor forces, muscle function, and highlight of the major events during that phase.

Contact Phase

Contact phase extends from heel contact until 15° of the total gait cycle. During this time it is necessary for the body to absorb shock, stabilize the limb for single limb support, and allow the center of gravity to move forward without interruption.

Joint Motion

At heel contact the pelvis is rotating toward the contacting limb, effectively lengthening the limb. The pelvis will continue to rotate slightly in this direction until 15° at which time pelvic rotation reverses. The hip at heel contact is flexed by approximately 30° allowing the leg to be in front of the body. From heel contact until 15° the hip is extending as the body moves forward over the supporting foot. This flexion of the thigh on the trunk is visably slowed by stance phase knee flexion. During this first portion of stance there is also internal rotation occurring at the hip joint with the femur internally rotating relative to the pelvis.

The knee joint is extended at heel contact and rapidly flexes following heel contact until 15° of the gait cycle. This rapid flexion of the knee essentially shortens the limb following heel contact, making it an important shock absorber in the sagittal plane (8).

The ankle joint at heel contact is neutral to slightly dorsiflexed. The heel hits the ground first and the ankle joint rapidly plantarflexes until the forefoot hits the ground at approximately seven percent of the gait cycle. This plantarflexion of the ankle, which is slowed by action of the pretibial muscles, is also an important sagittal plane shock-absorbing mechanism during this first portion of stance (8). Because the ankle joint axis is somewhat oblique to the three body planes, there is also a slight amount of adduction and inversion of the foot that occurs relative to the leg during this first seven percent of the gait cycle (Fig. 2.5). This motion at the ankle joint serves to increase slightly the demand on the subtalar joint for pronation during this portion of the gait cycle.

The leg is internally rotating relative to the femur during this first 15° of the gait cycle. At this time, then, the pelvis is internally rotating, the femur is internally rotating relative to the pelvis, and the tibia is internally rotating relative to the femur. The foot is also being internally rotated slightly by the adduction that occurs with ankle joint plantarflexion during the first seven percent of the gait cycle. All of this internal rotation must be absorbed by the foot as it contacts the floor and can no longer internally rotate.

The subtalar joint is that mechanism. At heel strike the subtalar joint is approximately in a neutral position, and it pronates rapidly during the first 15° of the gait cycle in response to the internal rotation of the leg. The deviation of the subtalar joint axis from vertical determines the amount of calcaneal eversion that will take place with subtalar joint prona-

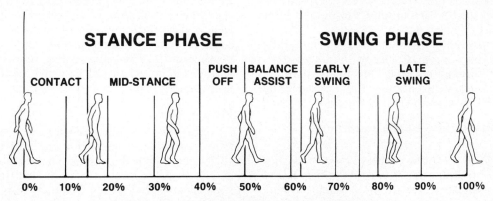

Figure 2.4.   Gait cycle divided into functional phases.

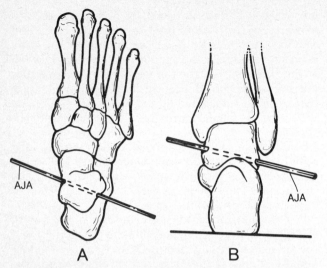

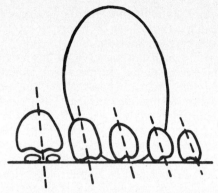

Figure 2.6. Schematic superimposition of calcaneus onto forefoot showing eversion of lesser metatarsals as similar to that of calcaneus with subtalar joint pronation. First metatarsal head is less everted because of independent axis of motion of first ray.

Figure 2.5. Axis of ankle joint (AJA) is deviated from both frontal (A) transverse (B) planes making motion that occurs around this axis pronation and supination.

tion. For example, an individual with a high-pitched subtalar joint axis might absorb this internal rotation of the leg with a minimal amount of eversion of the heel. On the other hand, an individual with a low-pitched subtalar joint axis might require a considerable amount of eversion to compensate for this leg rotation. The subtalar joint axis deviated 45° from the transverse plane would have approximately a one-to-one relationship between the amount of internal rotation of the leg and eversion of the calcaneus (Fig. 2.1).

At heel contact the midtarsal joint is supinated around both the oblique and longitudinal axes. Action of m. tibialis anterior, decelerating ankle joint plantarflexion following heel contact, has the effect of inverting the forepart of the foot, thus supinating the midtarsal joint around both the axes. As the forefoot is lowered to the ground, the lateral aspect of the forefoot hits first. When the forefoot is loaded, the midtarsal joint remains in a relatively supinated attitude because of the pronated position of the subtalar joint.

There is some dorsiflexion of the first ray at this time, with some inversion of the first metatarsal head relative to the second metatarsal head, although all the metatarsal heads are relatively everted from vertical because of the rotation around the subtalar joint axis (9) (Fig. 2.6).

The metatarsophalangeal joints have been mildly hyperextended because of activity of the long extensors following heel contact, and they should plantarflex rapidly to a neutral position as the toes reach the ground shortly following the ball of the foot.

Center of Gravity Movement and Energy Transfer

In the sagittal plane the center of gravity reaches a low point shortly following heel contact. It is raised as the body is vaulting over the now weight-bearing

limb. The sagittal plane shock-absorbing mechanisms of knee flexion and ankle plantarflexion enable this upward movement of the center of gravity to be 'minimal. Slightly less than 2 inches of total vertical displacement occurs during the gait cycle (10). At the time of heel contact the center of gravity is between the two supporting limbs and moving toward the contacting limb, so that by 15° of the gait cycle the center of gravity is over the supporting limb. The speed of advancement of the center of gravity is increasing somewhat at heel contact and continues to do so until the foot is flat on the floor, at which time the forward speed begins to slow (7) (Fig. 2.7).

As the center of gravity is elevated, the amount of potential energy present in the system will increase. Kinetic energy increases during the first half of contact phase, along with the forward speed previously discussed. From this point on through the remainder of the contact phase the kinetic energy is decreasing (Fig. 2.8).

Foot-to-Floor Forces

During contact a posterior shear develops, as momentum is trying to carry the foot forward and friction holds the foot in place on the supporting surface. This shear force continues throughout the contact phase (Fig. 2.9A). Weight is rapidly transferred to the contacting foot following heel contact; by 10% of the gait cycle approximaely 95% of the weight has been transferred, and by 15% of the gait cycle the contact limb is supporting 120% of the body weight. The raising of the center of gravity over the support limb is responsible for this increased load bearing on the foot. The peak of this vertical force is at 15% of the gait cycle, at which point it begins to decrease (Fig. 2.9B).

Muscle Function

The erector spinae are active at heel contact and help stabilize the pelvis for the anticipated weight shift that occurs during the contact phase. The hip abductors are strongly active at this time stabilizing the pelvis so that as the weight is transferred to the

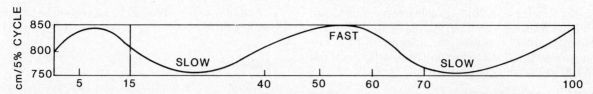

Figure 2.7. Graphic depiction of variation of forward speed during gait cycle. Energy level of body is in foot-pounds.

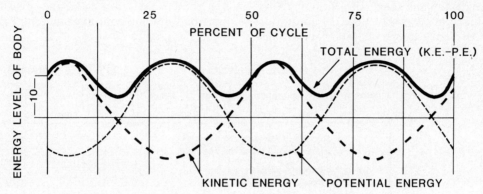

Figure 2.8. Graphic depiction of potential and kinetic changes during gait cycle.

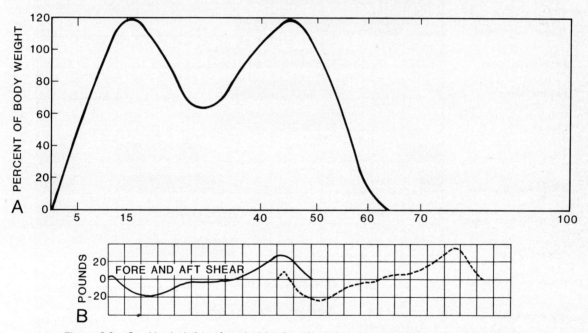

Figure 2.9. Graphic depiction of vertical loading (A) during gait cycles (B) and fore and aft shear.

contact limb, hip drop on the opposite side is minimized. The gluteus maximus is active at heel contact, and its function is related to reextending the hip during the contact phase. Action of the adductors at this time aids in stabilization of the hip and helps extend the flexed thigh. There is some internal rotation created by the adductors because of the flexed position of the hip. Hamstring activity during the contact phase is related primarily to stabilization of the knee. The quadriceps are also acting to stabilize the knee and resist knee flexion that is occurring during the contact phase. The soleus becomes active during the midportion of the contact phase just follow-

ing forefoot contact, and its activity decelerates the forward movement of the tibia helping slow knee joint flexion at this time.

The posterior tibial muscle becomes active early in the contact phase, and its function seems primarily to be one of deceleration of the subtalar joint pronation that is occurring in response to the internal rotation of the leg. M. tibialis anterior, m. extensor digitorum longus, and m. extensor hallucis longus are all active during the early portion of contact phase, decelerating the rapid ankle joint plantarflexion that occurs following heel contact. As mentioned previously, the m. tibialis anterior also inverts the forepart of the foot during this time, causing some supination around the midtarsal joint axes. M. flexor digitorum longus has some inconsistent activity during this phase, probably related to helping M. tibialis posterior decelerate subtalar joint pronation (Fig. 2.10).

Summary of Contact Phase

The important elements occurring during contact phase are: (*a*) sagittal plane shock absorption by knee flexion and ankle joint plantarflexion, (*b*) absorption of internal leg rotation through subtalar joint prona-

tion, and (*c*) smooth transfer of body weight onto the contact limb.

Midstance

This is the portion of the gait cycle from 15% until the heel comes off the ground at 40%. The opposite foot has left the floor, and it is necessary for the body to maintain its balance over the single supporting limb and continue smooth progression of the center of gravity forward.

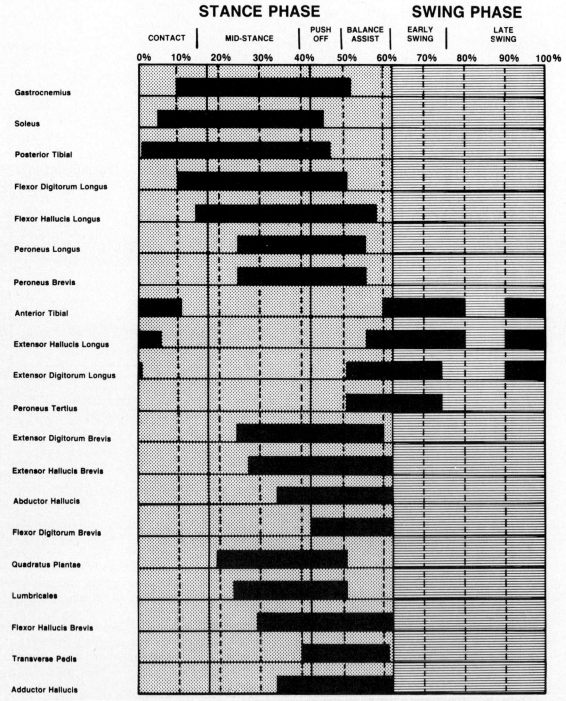

Figure 2.10. Phasic muscular activity. Graphic representation of muscular activity related to gait cycle.

Joint Function

All of the transverse plane rotations of the lower limb reverse directions at approximately 15% of the gait cycle. The pelvis begins to rotate in the opposite direction (clockwise for a supporting right limb). The hip abductors produce some frontal plane rotation, leveling the pelvis by raising the non-weight-bearing side. The hip continues to extend, reaching approximately 10° hyperextension by 40% of the gait cycle. There is external rotation of the femur relative to the pelvis occurring throughout the midstance phase.

The knee that was flexed by approximately 15° at 15% of the gait cycle is now beginning to reextend. Extension of the knee continues until the knee is fully extended at 40%, at which time the heel comes off the supporting surface. The ankle joint, which was approximately 5° plantarflexed at 15% of the gait cycle, now continues dorsiflexing until it is approximately 10° dorsiflexed at 40%. Dorsiflexion of the ankle is accompanied by some external rotation of the talus relative to the leg because of the obliquity of the ankle joint axis (Fig. 2.5). This increases the demand on the subtalar joint for supination. The subtalar joint was pronated by a few degrees when it was at 15% of the gait cycle. In response to the external rotation now occurring in the lower limb, the subtalar joint supinates converting this axial rotation into motion of the foot (Fig. 2.1).

The abrupt reversal of motion that occurs at 15% of the gait cycle is caused primarily by reversal of the rotation of both extremities and the pelvis following toe-off on the opposite limb, and secondarily by the muscles encouraging the subtalar joint to begin supinating. The subtalar joint begins to supinate from its mildly pronated position at 15% and continues to supinate throughout midstance. The subtalar joint is approximately in its neutral position at 30% and is mildly supinated at the time of heel-off at 40% of the gait cycle. This progressive supination of the subtalar joint from a mildly pronated position in turn limits the amount of motion available at the midtarsal joint and positions the rearfoot in such a way that weight bearing stress stabilizes the midtarsal joint in the direction of pronation (Figs. 2.2, 2.3).

With continued supination of the foot, relative plantarflexion of the first metatarsal is necessary to maintain firm contact between the first metatarsal head and the floor. During the midstance phase there is minimal motion occurring at the metatarsophalangeal joints.

Center of Gravity Movement and Energy Transfer

The center of gravity continues its upward movement as it passes over the supporting foot. During the midstance phase it passes from behind the supporting foot to completely ahead of the supporting foot. Forward speed reaches its low point at the middle of midstance and then accelerates as the center of gravity passes in front of the supporting foot and begins to fall (Fig. 2.7). The amount of potential energy continues to increase as the center of gravity is elevated until it reaches its maximum at approximtely 30% of the gait cycle. The amount of potential energy decreases throughout the remainder of midstance. Kinetic energy is on the decrease as the center of gravity is being elevated, and begins an increase when the center of gravity begins to fall at 30% (Fig. 2.8).

Foot-to-Floor Forces

Posterior shear decreases until the center of gravity passes over the foot, and then anterior shear takes place as the floor resists the posterior force applied on it (Fig. 2.9A). The vertical load applied to the floor is decreased to its stance phase minimum by the midportion of midstance and then begins to increase, reaching approximately 100% of body weight at heel-off (Fig. 2.9B).

Muscle Function

The hip abductors continue to be active during midstance, stabilizing the pelvis and elevating the swinging hip. M. gluteus maximus ceases activity during the early portion of midstance even though the hip continues to extend. This is because the center of gravity is moving forward, and restrained anterior movement of the tibia by the posterior leg muscles allows the hip to re-extend passively. The hamstring and quadriceps activity is ceasing during the first portion of midstance as the knee is reextending and becoming more stable.

M. gastrocnemius activity begins during midstance as the knee is reextending, possibly to put some flexion force on the knee to prevent hyperextension. M. soleus activity continues throughout midstance slowing the forward progression of the tibia, allowing the knee and hip to extend. As the subtalar joint becomes supinated, m. soleus is also able to stabilize the lateral aspect of the foot to the floor, and m. peroneus longus becomes active to hold the first metatarsal head against the floor. M. tibialis posterior continues to be active during midstance encouraging subtalar joint supination that began at 15% of the gait cycle. The m. tibialis posterior is also adding some restraining force to forward movement of the tibia aiding m. soleus in allowing the knee and hip to reextend. The anterior crural muscles are silent at this time during gait.

M. flexor digitorum longus and m. flexor hallucis longus are both active during midstance, aiding m. tibialis posterior in supinating the subtalar joint, slowing the forward motion of the leg, and also stabilizing the toes against the ground so they may begin to receive a portion of the body weight. The intrinsic foot muscles become active during the middle portion of midstance and remain active throughout midstance, helping stabilize the midtarsal joint. The intrinsic muscles attached to the base of the proximal phalanx of the hallux also aid in plantarflexion of the first metatarsal (Fig. 2.10).

Summary of Midstance Phase

The important events occurring during midstance are: (a) reversal of transverse plane motion, (b) supination of the subtalar joint with its stabilizing effect on the midtarsal joint and forefoot, (c) single limb support allowing the center of gravity to pass over the supporting foot, and (d) reextension of the knee and hip.

Push-Off Phase

Push-off phase is from heel lift at 40% of the gait cycle until heel contact of the opposite foot at 50%. During this time weight is borne only on the forepart of the supporting foot. Some upward acceleration of the leg is provided, and the body must prepare for heel strike of the opposite leg and the subsequent transfer of weight.

Joint Motion

The pelvis continues to rotate so that the hip on the supporting limb is moving posteriorly. The femur is externally rotating and the hip remains extended in the sagittal plane.

The knee begins rapidly to flex immediately following heel-off, and the tibia continues to rotate externally slightly relative to the femur. The ankle joint remains in a dorsiflexed position relative to the leg because the heel is lifted off the ground as a result of flexion of the knee rather than active plantarflexion of the ankle. During the middle portion of the push-off phase the ankle begins to plantarflex. The accompanying internal rotation of the talus relative to the leg reduces some of the supinatory demand on the subtalar joint.

The subtalar joint continues to supinate during push-off. The supination occurring around the oblique axis of the midtarsal joint, along with the subtalar joint supination, compensates for the oblique toe-break, allowing the lateral side of the ball of the foot to remain on the floor. The first metatarsal becomes more plantarflexed, enabling the first ray to continue to bear weight and increasing the available range of first metatarsophalangeal joint dorsiflexion. With the heel coming off the ground, the metatarsophalangeal joints once again begin to hyperextend and more weight is accepted by the digits.

Center of Gravity Movement and Energy Transfer

The center of gravity continues to fall during the push-off phase and moves towards the swinging limb in preparation for heel contact of the opposite side. With the fall of the center of gravity, potential energy is decreasing as kinetic energy is increasing (Fig. 2.8). Forward speed of the body increases throughout push-off (Fig. 2.7).

Foot-to-Floor Force

Anterior shear increases at this time as the heel rises off the ground. Foot-to-floor forces are increasing in a vertical direction, reaching 120% of body weight just before heel contact of the opposite limb.

Muscle Function

The erector spinae become active during the push-off phase to stabilize the pelvis in preparation for weight transfer. Hip abductor activity ceases during the midportion of push-off as the center of gravity is falling and moving toward the contacting limb. The adductors become active during the midportion of push-off in preparation for swinging the limb. M. gastrocnemius, m. soleus, and m. tibialis posterior are all active during this time supinating the subtalar joint, as well as providing for active ankle joint plantarflexion and flexion of the knee. Some of the knee flexion may directly result from activity of m. gastrocnemius; however, most of the knee flexion results from the upward push of the leg on a flexed knee.

M. peroneus brevis continues to stabilize the lateral aspect of the foot. M. peroneus longus is helping stabilize the first ray against the supporting surface. M. flexor digitorum longus and m. flexor hallucis longus are active at this time to stabilize the toes against the supporting surface, and the intrinsic foot muscles continue their activity throughout the push-off phase, helping maintain stability at the midtarsal joint and aiding in plantarflexion of the first ray. The long digital extensors show some inconsistent activity during this time, apparently in preparation for pickup (Fig. 2.10).

Summary of Push-off Phase

The important events occurring during the push-off phase are: (a) elevation of the heel from the ground, (b) active plantarflexion of the ankle providing some upward thrust of the leg, and (c) movement of the center of gravity towards the swinging limb in preparation for heel contact on the opposite side, which occurs at the end of push-off.

Balance Assist

Balance assist is that portion of the stance phase of gait from 50% until toe-off, which occurs at 62%. During this time the foot is assisting in balancing the body and completing weight transfer to the contacting limb.

Joint Motion

The pelvis continues to rotate in an outward direction, and the femur continues to rotate externally relative to the pelvis. Hip flexion is occurring as the leg begins to move forward. The tibia at this time begins to rotate externally at a relatively faster rate to the femur, corresponding to the decreasing activity of the popliteus. The rapid knee flexion occurring at this time is a passive phenomenon related to the rapid active ankle joint plantarflexion. The subtalar joint is in a supinated position at 50% and continues to supinate until shortly before toe-off, when the direction of motion reverses and the subtalar joint begins to pronate. The midtarsal joint continues to supinate, and there is plantarflexion of the forefoot on the rearfoot, along with marked plantarflexion of the first metatarsal during this phase. The digits are hyperextended at this time, and a minimum of 75° of dorsiflexion occurs at the first metatarsophalangeal joint (6).

Center of Gravity Movement and Energy Transfer

The center of gravity is moving downward and toward the opposite limb as the opposite limb is beginning to bear a greater portion of body weight. Because of the downward movement of the center of gravity, potential energy continues to decrease during the first portion of balance assist and then begins to increase as the center of gravity is elevated over the opposite (now supporting) limb. Kinetic energy increases during the first portion of balance assist, and then decreases from there until the toes leave the ground (Fig. 2.8).

Foot-to-Floor Force

Anterior shear and foot-to-floor force are rapidly decreasing as the weight is being shifted to the contacting limb (Fig. 2.9).

Muscle Function

The erector spinae continue their activity during balance assist to stabilize the pelvis as weight is transferred to the contacting limb. The adductors continue their activity flexing the thigh and preparing for swing. M. gastrocnemius, m. soleus, and m. peroneus longus et brevis all cease their activity during this phase because the limb is unweighted. M. tibialis posterior ceases its activity during the midportion of this phase, which corresponds to the beginning of subtalar joint pronation. M. tibialis anterior and long extensors to the toes begin their activity during this phase, stabilizing the toes and preparing to dorsiflex the ankle for swing. The intrinsic foot muscles remain active until the end of balance assist, stabilizing the digits and maintaining a supinatory force around the oblique midtarsal joint axis (Fig. 2.10).

Summary of Balance Assist

The important element of the balance assist phase of gait is balancing the body as weight is being transferred rapidly to the contacting limb.

Swing Phase

The swing phase of gait begins when the toes leave the ground at 62% of the gait cycle and continues to heel contact. This phase can be roughly divided into two portions: (a) when the knee is continuing to flex and the foot is being lifted off the floor, and (b) when the limb is being swung forward in preparation for the following heel contact.

Joint Function

The pelvis reverses its rotation and begins rotating so the hip on the swinging side is moving forward.

Rotation of the hip joint reverses with the femur beginning to move internally relative to the pelvis, and the hip continues to flex during the first portion of swing until approximately 75% of the gait cycle when the hip flexion stabilizes for the remainder of swing.

The knee joint flexes rapidly up to approximately 70% to 75% percent of the gait cycle, then begins to reextend in preparation for heel contact. The tibia internally rotates with the femur until heel contact. The ankle joint begins to dorsiflex following toeoff, approximating a right angle before heel contact.

The subtalar joint continues to pronate throughout the swing phase of gait, being approximately back to a neutral position by heel contact. No weight stress is passing through the forefoot and activity of m. tibialis anterior maintains the midtarsal joint in a supinated position as the subtalar joint pronates away from the forefoot.

M. tibialis anterior maintains the first ray in a dorsiflexed position. The long extensors keep the toes dorsiflexed, which aids in toe clearance as the leg swings through.

Center of Gravity Movement and Energy Transfer

The center of gravity movement during swing corresponds to the stance phase activity of the opposite limb and would be similar to that described in the stance phase. There are no foot-to-floor forces during swing phase to consider.

Muscle Function

Some activity of the erector spinae is present just before heel contact to stabilize the pelvis in preparation for heel contact. Likewise, m. gluteus maximus becomes active late in the swing phase to help stabilize the hip and to provide an extensor force around the hip joint. The adductors are active around heel contact to help extend the hip from its flexed position and to offer some stability at the hip in the frontal plane. The hamstrings become active during the reach portion of swing phase to decelerate the rapid reextension of the knee. This deceleration of knee extension tends to "pull" the body foward and is thought to imply more force to forward progression than the push that occurs following heel-off (7, 11). The quadriceps become active before heel contact to stabilize the knee in the frontal plane and in preparation for the flexion thrust that occurs following heel contact. M. tibialis anterior and the long extensors to the toes are active during swing, dorsiflexing the ankle and enabling the foot to clear the ground. It has been hypothesized that during this time the lumbricales are also active. This would reduce some of the passive flexion caused by tension on the long flexors and also help limit metatarsophalangeal hyperextension during swing (12).

Summary of Swing Phase

The important elements of swing phase are: (a) picking up of the limb in preparation for swinging it forward, (*b*) extension of the limb forward to lengthen it in preparation for heel contact, and (*c*) active restraint of knee joint extension by the hamstrings imparting a forward pull to the body, enabling continued progression.

Phasic Muscular Activity

In this section each muscle or group of muscles distal to the knee has been considered separately to clarify its function. The electrical activity within the muscles is reported as present or absent rather than being determined quantitatively. There is some question whether the strength of contraction correlates with the integrated electromyographical recordings.

In 1977 Hof and van den Berg (13) studied this problem relative to the triceps surae. They concluded that "whenever nonlinear EMG torque relations are found with other muscles the possibility that more muscles contribute to the measured torque should be taken into account." This remains somewhat controversial.

Baumann, Sutherland, and Hanggi (14) have made a preliminary report using intramuscular pressure changes during gait to delineate muscle function. It appears this method will enable measurement of "both the active and passive components of muscle function."

Bar graphs are used to present the phasic information because they are easily understood and lend themselves readily to comparison (Fig. 2.10). The gait cycle has been broken down into phases, and muscular activity is described in reference to these phases rather than exact percentages. The phasic activities recorded here are a compilation of the reports of many authors (7, 10, 15, 16–28).

Triceps Surae

The triceps surae make up the calf muscle and consist of the two heads of m. gastrocnemius and m. soleus. M. gastrocnemius arises from the posterior aspect of the femoral condyles. M. soleus originates on the posterior aspect of the head of the fibula and the upper third of the posterior aspect of the tibia. M. gastrocnemius and m. soleus have a common insertion through the tendo achillis into the middle third of the posterior surface of the calcaneus. These muscles and their tendons pass posterior to the axes of the knee and ankle and posteromedial to the axis of the subtalar joint (Fig. 2.11). Open kinetic chain function therefore consists of flexion of the knee through the two heads of m. gastrocnemius, plantarflexion of the ankle, and supination at the subtalar joint.

Because of its anatomical location m. plantaris is included with the triceps surae. M. plantaris is a muscle with a small muscle belly and a rather long slender tendon, which originates on the posterior aspect of the femur just superior to the lateral femoral condyle and inserts with the medial aspect of the tendo achillis into the posterior aspect of the calcaneus. The open kinetic chain activity of this muscle would be

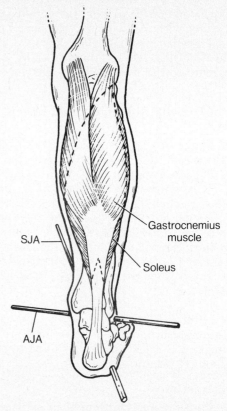

Figure 2.11. Triceps surae. Diagrammatic relationship of muscles anatomically and relative to axes of ankle and subtalar joints. (SJA) Subtalar joint axis. (AJ) Ankle joint axis.

nearly identical to that of m. gastrocnemius because of the course it follows, those being flexion of the knee, plantarflexion of the ankle, and supination around the subtalar joint axis. This muscle has not been studied with regard to phasic activity. Because of the size of the muscle belly significant functional activity of this muscle is unlikely. It has proven to be a passively powerful structure limiting dorsiflexion of the ankle joint. This is best appreciated at the time of performing tendo achillis lengthening on a patient whose m. plantaris has a separate insertion into the calcaneus; without section of this tendon it is often impossible to obtain the desired amount of dorsiflexion.

Phasic activity of the triceps surae is from shortly after heel contact until just before toe-off. The first function of the triceps during a normal gait cycle is to extend the knee. It does this through the m. soleus by slowing the forward progression of the tibia, thus allowing the femur to rotate over it extending the knee joint. The plantarflexion force transmitted by m. soleus to the foot is used for stabilization of the lateral segments of the foot to the floor. M. soleus at this time is acting as a decelerator and is actually undergoing a stretch. This physiologically economical action typifies most of the muscular activity during the gait cycle with the major exceptions of the adductors and the gastrocnemii.

The next functions of this group, those of knee flexion and ankle joint plantarflexion, occur simultaneously. The primary action at this time is plantar-flexion of the ankle, and flexion of the knee is a secondary accomplishment. The flexion force provided by m. gastrocnemius around the knee joint axis is twofold: first, the direct effect produced by the position of the muscle fibers posterior to the axis of motion, and second, the closed kinetic chain "buckling" effect derived from the limb lengthening force produced by the plantarflexion at the ankle joint.

During final propulsion when the plantarflexion of the ankle is reaching its peak the activity of m. gastrocnemius is ceasing. The ability of m. gastrocnemius to perform this task while its activity ceases is because body weight is being shifted to the other leg at this time. During midstance the triceps activity, through the supinatory force applied at the subtalar joint, assists the foot in changing from a mobile adapter to a rigid lever ensuring forefoot stability. This supinatory force at the subtalar joint also produces an external rotatory force on the leg.

Peroneus Longus

M. peroneus longus (Fig. 2.12) originates from the head and lateral aspect of the proximal two thirds of the body of the fibula. The tendon of this muscle passes posterior to the lateral malleolus and inferior to it in a groove shared with m. peroneus brevis. It continues out along the calcaneus to the lateral side of the cuboid. The tendon then runs plantar to the

cuboid in the peroneal groove and continues obliquely across the foot to insert into the lateral plantar aspect of the base of the first metatarsal and the medial cuneiform. To review the position of the tendon in relation to the axes of the joints, it crosses posterior to the ankle joint having a potential weak plantarflexion force. The tendon passes dorsolateral to the subtalar joint axis becoming a potential open kinetic chain pronator at this joint. The tendon passes dorsolateral to the oblique midtarsal joint axis and plantar to the longitudinal axis of that joint, making it a potential pronator at the oblique axis and evertor at the longitudinal axis in an open kinetic chain situation. The insertion of this tendon into the base of the first metatarsal is nearly perpendicular to the axis of motion of the first ray. Activity of m. peroneus longus produces simultaneous plantarflexion and eversion around the first ray axis when weight stress is not passing through the foot.

The motion produced at various levels by this muscle in a closed kinetic chain is somewhat different than its action in an open kinetic chain. The motion we see in a closed kinetic chain is caused by the action around the first ray axis and the ground resists any actual plantarflexion.

The motion becomes relative to the rest of the foot producing inversion of the remainder of the forefoot to the floor, being translated into supination at the subtalar joint. This mechanism helps one understand the cavus type foot that is seen in the individual

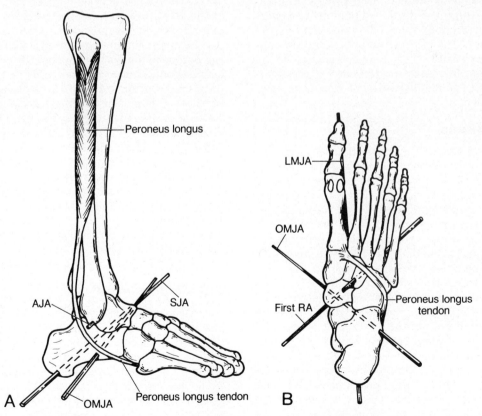

Figure 2.12. Peroneus longus. Position of muscle and tendon relative to axes crossed. (A) lateral view, (B) plantar view. (LMTJA) longitudinal mid tarsal joint axis and first ray axis.

with isolated spasticity of m. peroneus longus or weakness of m. tibialis anterior.

In gait this muscle is active during the last half of midstance and push-off. It is at this time during the gait cycle that the medial metatarsals need to be stable to allow the weight stress to be transferred medially within the forefoot. This stabilization of the medial aspect of the forefoot by m. peroneus longus takes place primarily around two joint axes, the first ray and the longitudinal axis of the midtarsal joint.

Rather than producing an actual movement at the joints crossed, this muscle's function is primarily one of stabilization. There are certain circumstances that must be met before effective stabilization can be produced. The primary prerequisite is stability of the cuboid, so it will act as a fulcrum instead of moving when m. peroneus longus becomes active. For the cuboid to be stable, the subtalar joint must be near neutral or supinated, the midtarsal joint fully pronated around the oblique axis, and m. peroneus brevis and the triceps actively stabilizing the lateral border of the foot to the supporting surface. With a stable fulcrum m. peroneus longus stabilizes the medial aspect of the forefoot.

Assisting m. peroneus longus with this stabilization of the medial border of the forefoot are m. tibialis posterior, the long plantar musculature, the plantar fascia, and the osseous locking mechanism of the midtarsal joint. The latter three continue this stabilization through the balance assist phase. Isolated loss of m. peroneus longus muscle power results in metatarsus primus elevatus and a dorsal bunion. The overall integrity of midfoot function is apparently preserved because of the other structures acting in concert with this muscle. This makes sacrifice of m. peroneus longus for transfer attractive if the overpowering of first ray dorsiflexion by m. tibialis anterior can be controlled.

Peroneus Brevis

M. peroneus brevis (Fig. 2.13) originates from the lateral aspect of the distal two thirds of the body of the fibula, deep to m. peroneus longus. The tendon of this muscle passes posterior and distal to the lateral malleolus in a common groove with m. peroneus longus. It then continues anteriorly to its insertion into the lateral aspect of the styloid process on the base of the fifth metatarsal. Looking at the relation of the tendon of m. peroneus brevis to the joints it transverses, to determine the potential open kinetic chain movements, one notes the following: the tendon passes posterior to the ankle joint axis where it exerts a weak plantarflexion force when the ankle joint is approximately at a right angle; it passes dorsolateral to the subtalar joint and oblique midtarsal joint axes providing a pronatory moment around these axes. M. peroneus brevis has a slightly better mechanical advantage at these two axes than the peroneus longus. The relation of the tendon of m. peroneus brevis to the axis of the fifth ray enables production of a slight pronatory movement at this level. Most of its action

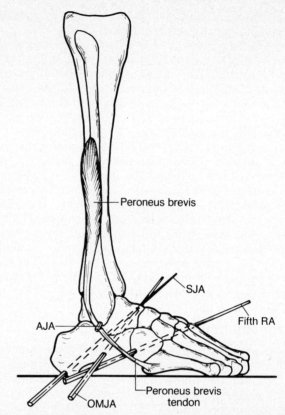

Figure 2.13. Peroneus brevis. Position of muscle and tendon relative to axes crossed.

at this level, however, is being directed across the fifth metatarsocuboidal and calcaneocuboidal articulations.

M. peroneus brevis is active slightly longer than the peroneus longus during the gait cycle. It becomes active about midway through midstance and continues until before prior to toe-off. In a closed kinetic chain situation this muscle is able to accomplish very little movement. Its chief purpose seems to be stabilization of the lateral segment of the foot, particularly the calcaneocuboidal articulation. As was discussed earlier, this is an important prerequisite for effective function of M. peroneus longus.

The use of the tendon of m. peroneus brevis in whole or part is common for lateral ankle stabilization. In an otherwise normally functioning foot, loss of this muscle has minimal consequences. Increased forefoot adductus by unopposed m. tibialis posterior activity is possible, but seldom significant clinically.

Tibialis Posterior

M. tibialis posterior (Fig. 2.14) originates from the lateral posterior aspect of the body of the tibia, the medial aspect of the body of the fibula, and the interosseous membrane in the proximal two thirds of the leg. The tendon passes posteromedial to the medial malleolus, and then, passing over the deltoid ligament, inserts into the tuberosity of the navicular. It gives off a number of fibrous expansions: one passing backwards to the sustentaculum tali, and others continuing beneath the plantar calcaneonavicular ligament, dis-

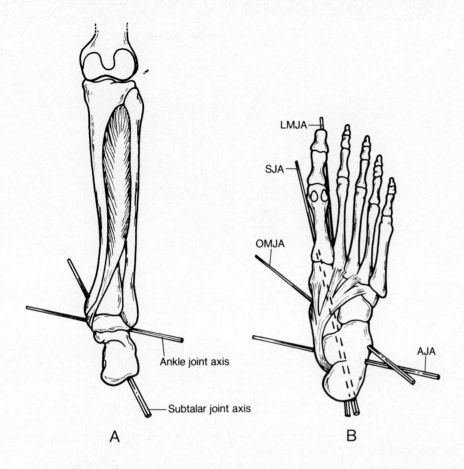

LMJA

SJA

OMJA

AJA

Ankle joint axis

Subtalar joint axis

A

B

Figure 2.14. Tibialis posterior tendon. Position of muscle and tendon relative to axes crossed.

tally and laterally to the cuneiforms, the bases of the second, third, and fourth metatarsals, and the cuboid.

Looking at the course of this muscle with respect to the joint axes it crosses, one can determine the open kinetic chain motion it is able to produce. The tendon passes just posterior to the ankle joint axis, being a weak plantarflexor. The tendon passes medial plantar to the subtalar joint axis giving it a potential supinatory movement at this level. At its insertion into the navicular m. tibialis posterior has the potential to create an inversion force around the longitudinal axis of the midtarsal joint. The sum of its insertions makes its line of force nearly perpendicular to the oblique axis of the midtarsal joint and plantar to it.

Phasically, this muscle becomes active shortly after heel contact and remains active through the push-off phase of the gait cycle. M. tibialis posterior assists in decelerating the pronation that is taking place in the subtalar joint until 15% of the gait cycle. It then stabilizes the midtarsal joint and helps reverse the leg rotation through subtalar joint supination. This muscle's stabilization of the midtarsal joint is in the direction of supination primarily around the oblique axis. This action by m. tibialis posterior helps counteract the pronatory force created by ground reaction at the metatarsal heads. The importance of m. tibialis posterior to normal foot function is readily appreciated by the clinician who has seen the patient with a loss of this muscle. The architecture of this

patient's foot literally collapses despite apparent patency of all other supporting structures.

When contemplating transfer of m. tibialis posterior, one must consider the potential for pronatory collapse of the foot. With a transfer through the interosseous membrane to the dorsum even a medial placement of the insertion will not be adequate protection. Successful phasic conversion to assist with dorsiflexion eliminates any potential stabilizing effect during stance.

The triceps surae, the peroneals, m. tibialis posterior, and the long plantar musculature are all active to assist the osseous and ligamentous elements in stabilization of the foot to the floor during the first half of the gait cycle.

Pretibial Group

The pretibial group includes m. tibialis anterior, m. extensor digitorum longus, m. extensor hallucis longus, and m. peroneus tertius (Fig. 2.15). These muscles are grouped together because their activity is similar and it would be redundant to discuss them all separately. In gait they become active before toe-off, continue activity throughout the swing phase, and cease activity midway through the contact phase. These muscles are classically considered swing phase muscles; however, by definition they are biphasic. The stance phase activity of these muscles takes place when there is limited weight stress passing through

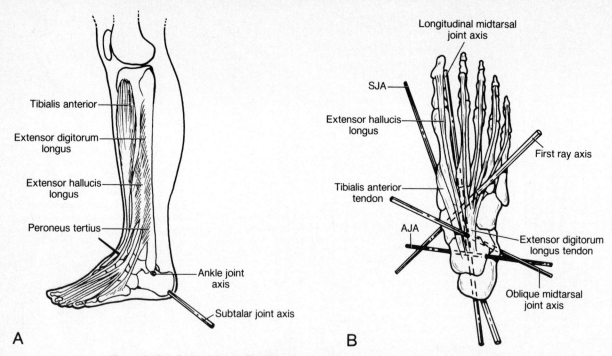

Figure 2.15. Pretibial group. Position of muscles and tendons relative to axes crossed.

the foot. Therefore functional potential is evaluated in an open kinetic chain situation.

M. tibialis anterior originates from the lateral condyle and the proximal one half to two thirds of the lateral surface of the body of the tibia. After passing through the medial compartment of the extensor retinacula, its tendon inserts into the medial and plantar surfaces of the medial cuneiform and the base of the first metatarsal. The tendon of m. tibialis anterior passes anterior to the ankle joint giving it dorsiflexion capability at this level. The tendon then passes through the subtalar joint axis when the subtalar joint is in its neutral position. It becomes a supinator when the subtalar joint is supinated and a pronator when it is pronated. The tendon of m. tibialis anterior passes plantar medial to the oblique axis of the midtarsal joint with a slight supinatory capability around this axis. The tendon's effect at the longitudinal axis of the midtarsal joint is strong inversion.

M. extensor digitorum longus arises from the lateral condyle of the tibia and the proximal three fourths of the anterior surface of the body of the fibula. Its tendon passes under the lateral portion of the extensor retinacula, splits into four tendons, and courses distally to insert into the extensor expansion of the four lesser toes. It passes anterior to the ankle joint where it has a dorsiflexion moment of force. As it continues anteriorly it passes dorsolateral to the subtalar joint axis and has a long pronatory force arm at this joint (Fig. 2.15).

The tendon also passes dorsolateral to the oblique axis of the midtarsal joint and produces a pronatory force at this level. Other than translatory stabilization of the talonavicular joint, m. extensor digitorum longus has little effect at the longitudinal axis of the

midtarsal joint. By its insertion through the extensor expansion this muscle produces dorsiflexion at the metatarsophalangeal and extension of the interphalangeal joints.

M. peroneus tertius can be thought of as part of m. extensor digitorum longus. Its origin is on the distal third of the anterior surface of the fibula, and the tendon passes under the extensor retinacula with m. extensor digitorum longus and inserts into the dorsal surface of the base of the fifth metatarsal. Its action at the ankle, subtalar, and oblique midtarsal axes is similar to m. extensor digitorum longus. M. peroneus tertius possesses a potential pronatory force at the fifth ray axis because of its dorsolateral relationship to this axis.

M. extensor hallucis longus arises from the middle half of the anterior surface of the fibula, and its tendon courses distally under the extensor retinacula between m. tibialis anterior and m. extensor digitorum longus. It continues distally to be inserted into the dorsal aspect of the base of the distal phalanx of the hallux. This tendon passes anterior to the ankle and dorsolateral to the oblique midtarsal joint axis, being able to produce dorsiflexion at the former and pronation around the latter. The tendon lies slightly dorsolateral to the subtalar joint axis and its function around this axis is dependent on subtalar joint position. It produces extension of the interphalangeal joint of the hallux and dorsiflexion of the first metatarsophalangeal joint through the extensor expansion.

These muscles, which are active simultaneously during gait cycle, are antagonistic at the subtalar and midtarsal joints and synergistic at the ankle joint, where physiological function is exerted during normal walking. The primary activities of this muscle group are decelerating the plantarflexion of the ankle joint immediately following heel contact to avoid a "foot slap" and dorsiflexion of the foot and toes to clear the ground during the swing phase of gait.

Sacrifice of the long extensor function at the metatarsophalangeal and interphalangeal level does not seem to cause difficulty clinically if the remaining structures acting on the digits are intact. This makes transfer of the insertion of these muscles attractive. The primary procedure is elimination of digital function to enhance ankle joint dorsiflixion or to remove a deforming force from the digits (i.e. Hibbs' suspension). Attempts to effect sagittal plane position of the metatarsals (i.e. Jones' suspension) probably is effective by removing the deforming force on the digit.

M. peroneus tertius (when present) does not have enough independent strength to be useful for transfer. The tendon is frequently useful for anchoring tendon transfers (i.e. split tibialis anterior transfer).

Because of the approximation of m. tibialis anterior to the subtalar joint axis, two types of transfer are frequently considered. First, with a significant cavus deformity m. tibialis anterior becomes a strong supinator during swing, which can result in fixed deformity in this direction. Transfer of the insertion laterally eliminates this effect. Transfer too far laterally may result in a pes valgus foot deformity. In a mildly supinated foot the effect is to require more activity of the long extensors to balance ankle dorsiflexion. This results in "extensor substitution" and contracture of the digits. A split tibialis anterior transfer is useful for this situation. Second, a severely pronated foot causes m. tibialis anterior to lose its

effect of positioning the foot in a neutral to slightly supinated attitude at contact. This can be counteracted by the transfer of the tendon posteriorly. The Young procedure adds to this the effect of creating an additional ligament along the plantar aspect of the medial arch. This is seldom adequate as an isolated procedure in a significant pes valgus foot deformity.

Long Flexor Group

M. flexor digitorum longus and m. flexor hallucis longus (Fig. 2.16) will be considered together because their action is very similar and occurs nearly simultaneously.

M. flexor digitorum longus originates from the middle half of the posterior aspect of the tibia below the popliteal line. This muscle's tendon inserts into the base of the distal phalanx of the four lesser toes. As it courses distally it passes posterior to the ankle joint axis where it is a weak potential open kinetic chain plantarflexor. The tendon then passes plantar medial to both the subtalar and oblique midtarsal joint axes where the muscles can produce open kinetic chain supination with moderate force. The tendon also passes plantar medial to the longitudinal axis of the midtarsal joint where muscular activity would produce an inversion moment, along with translatory stabilization at the talonavicular joint. The action of m. flexor digitorum longus on the digit is one of plantarflexion of the interphalangeal and metatarsophalangeal joints in an open kinetic chain situation. In a closed kinetic chain situation, with a stable digit, the effects of activity of m. flexor digitorum longus are

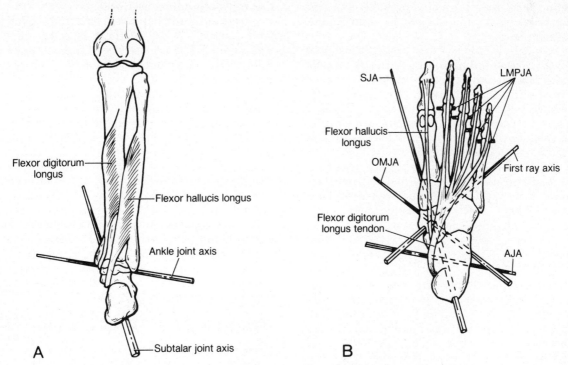

Figure 2.16.   Long flexor group. Position of muscles and tendons relative to axes crossed.

translatory stabilization and production of the plantarflexion moment of force at the metatarsophalangeal and interphalangeal joints.

M. flexor hallucis longus originates from the distal two thirds of the posterior surface of the fibula and inserts into the plantar aspect of the base of the distal phalanx of the hallux. The tendon of this muscle follows much the same course as m. flexor digitorum longus, passing posterior to the ankle joint and plantar medial to both the subtalar and oblique midtarsal joint axes. Its effect around these axes is similar, except at the ankle joint where it has a longer plantarflexion lever arm. Its tendon may or may not cross the longitudinal axis of the midtarsal joint, depending on the location of this axis in each foot. When the tendon does cross the axis, its action would be similar to that of m. flexor digitorum longus. M. flexor hallucis longus' effect on the hallux is similar to the effect of m. flexor digitorum longus on the lesser digits.

M. flexor digitorum longus becomes active about 10% earlier in the gait cycle than m. flexor hallucis longus, both becoming active in early midstance and terminating during the balance assist phase. Knowledge that m. flexor hallucis longus ceases being active before toe-off and that foot-to-floor force is decreasing during the last half of the propulsive phase of gait leads one to the conclusion that toe-off is a lifting of the foot off the ground rather than an active push.

With their activity occurring during stance phase, one is interested in the closed kinetic chain effect produced by these muscles. When the proximal joints are stable, activity of these muscles stabilizes the digits against the reactive force of the ground. They also add stability to the metatarsophalangeal joint because of their translatory vector of force at that level. Their most useful function during gait is probably assisting m. tibialis posterior around the subtalar and oblique midtarsal joint axes.

Two typical situations arise where transfer of these muscles is useful. With contracted digits transfer of the long flexor to the proximal phalanx removes the buckling effect that is present at both the metatarsophalangeal and interphalangeal joints. This same stabilization is more typically accomplished through fusion of the interphalangeal joints, which effectively transfers the muscle function.

The muscles are also useful to replace or supplement m. tibialis posterior when inserted at the midfoot level. Sacrifice of the original insertion causes minimal dysfunction if other structures affecting the metatarsophalangeal joints are intact.

Intrinsic Muscles of the Foot

For the sake of discussion, these muscles are divided into two groups: (a) those that have some potential effect at the midtarsal joint, and (b) those with their effect limited to the metatarsophalangeal joints and digits.

The first group includes m. abductor hallucis, m. flexor digitorum brevis, m. abductor digiti minimi, and m. quadratus plantae (all on the plantar aspect), and m. extensor digitorum brevis and m. extensor hallucis brevis on the dorsum. These muscles originate from the body of the calcaneus and insert into the proximal phalanx of the appropriate toe(s), with the exception of m. quadratus plantae and m. flexor digitorum brevis. M. quadratus plantae insert into the tendons of m. flexor digitorum longus, which continue to the distal phalanx of the four lesser toes, and m. flexor digitorum brevis sends its tendons to the intermediate phalanx of the second, third, and fourth toes. All of these muscles can produce a posterior translatory force at the oblique and longitudinal midtarsal joint axes, and thus can be considered stabilizers of these joints during gait. The four of these muscles on the plantar aspect would, when active, produce a supinatory force around the oblique midtarsal joint axis. The two on the dorsum of the foot would have a moment of pronatory force around the oblique midtarsal joint axis, but their primary effect would be one of translatory stabilization.

The second group of intrinsic muscles originates distal to the midtarsal joint and inserts into the proximal phalanx of the toe on which it acts. The muscles in this group are m. adductor hallucis, m. flexor hallucis brevis, m. flexor digiti minimi brevis, the dorsal and plantar interossei, and the lumbricales. These, along with the abductors hallucis and digiti minimi, produce a posterior translatory force, as well as a plantar rotatory force, at the metatarsophalangeal joints. M. flexor digitorum brevis has a posterior translatory force at both the metatarsophalangeal and proximal interphalangeal joints in the stable toe, as well as its flexor capabilities. M. extensor digitorum and hallucis brevis provide a dorsiflexion moment at the metatarsophalangeal joint, along with the posterior translatory force at this level.

This author is not aware of a study involving the phasic activity of all of these muscles individually. The combined phasic activity of these muscles is considered, as one would tend to agree with Mann and Inman's (27) conclusion, "The intrinsic muscles of the foot act as a functional unit." As such, they can be considered active from early midstance until just before toe-off. The plantar muscles crossing the midtarsal joint become important supinators around the oblique midtarsal joint axis once the heel is raised. Mann and Inman (27) also offered evidence that the intrinsic musculature in a pronated foot becomes active earlier and remains active a longer time during each cycle. This is probably an attempt to reduce the amount of hypermobility around the oblique midtarsal and subtalar joint axes. Jarrett, Manzi, and Green (12) have proposed that the lumbricales fire with the long extensors during swing phase. This would relieve the passive pull of the long flexor and reinforce interphalangeal extension (Fig. 2.17).

COMMON STRUCTURAL VARIATIONS

Forefoot Varus

Forefoot varus is a structural variation in which the plantar aspect of the forefoot is inverted relative

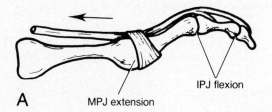

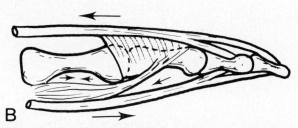

Figure 2.17. (A) Diagram depicting action of extensor digitorum longus around metatarsophalangeal joint and interphalangeal joint. Note dorsiflexion of metatarsophalangeal joint and plantarflexion of interphalangeal joint in non-weight-bearing situation. (B) Diagram depicting normal physiological contraction of a lumbricale tendon and a distally directed pull on the long flexor tendon. This force both reduces and counteracts the deforming force of the flexor tendons with long extensor contraction.

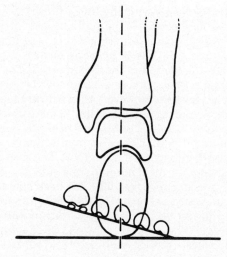

Figure 2.18. Diagrammatic depiction of forefoot varus.

to the bisection of the posterior surface of the calcaneus when the subtalar joint is in its neutral position and the midtarsal joint is maximally pronated against the rearfoot (Fig. 2.18). In evaluating the position of the forefoot relative to the rearfoot, it is important that the bisection of the heel be accurate. Because of the difficulty in palpating the medial border of the posterior surface of the calcaneus, often the mistake is made of making the bisection parallel to the lateral border that is in fact everted to an actual bisection of the calcaneus. If one is using such a line, the amount of forefoot varus apparently found during examination will be exaggerated.

A second problem increasing the amount of apparent forefoot varus is caused by examining with the subtalar joint supinated from its neutral position. The neutral position of the subtalar joint is one at which the subtalar joint is congruent, and not necessarily a position from which there is a two-to-one relationship in the amount of inversion to eversion. When evaluating the position of the forefoot relative to the rearfoot care should be taken not to supinate the midtarsal joint around its longitudinal axis, which inverts the medial aspect of the forefoot. This can be prevented by being sure that the loading of the midtarsal joint is done laterally around the head of the fifth metatarsal or the fifth metatarsal shaft, and that no dorsiflexory force is placed against the medial aspect of the forefoot.

The first ray is in its neutral position when evaluating the forefoot position relative to the rearfoot. This can be checked by grasping the lesser metatarsal heads and moving the first metatarsal head through its dorsal and plantar excursion. The neutral position

of the first ray is approximately at the center of its range of motion. Normally, when loading the lateral aspect of the forefoot the first ray will rest in the center of its range of motion; therefore it does not require positioning before the measurement is made.

An individual can have a forefoot varus with a plantarflexed first ray. This is the case if the lesser metatarsals are inverted, the first ray is plantarflexed, and the plantar plane of the first and fifth metatarsal heads remains inverted relative to the posterior bisection of the heel. This is not a common situation, and this foot functions as a forefoot varus during gait.

The forefoot varus foot type compensates through subtalar joint pronation. The eversion of the foot gained through subtalar joint pronation allows the forefoot to reach the supporting surface. If subtalar joint pronation is not adequate to allow full compensation, a partially compensated forefoot varus is present.

The individual with forefoot varus frequently complains of postural fatigue (i.e. vague foot, leg, and back fatigue). He or she may experience rather sharp discomfort around the subtalar and/or midtarsal joints. M. tibialis posterior or tendon strain is frequently associated with forefoot varus. Plantar fasciitis or heel spur syndrome is commonly present. Midtarsal joint movement on weight bearing is probably more responsible for this type of heel pain than subtalar joint motion. Forefoot symptomatology is related to the unstable position of the midtarsal joint resulting from subtalar joint pronation. The strain on the common digital nerves caused by midfoot and forefoot movement on loading may result in neuroma symptoms. Midtarsal joint instability causes first ray instability, which results in pressure concentration beneath the second metatarsal head and frequent tyloma formation in this area. First ray instability also leads to hallux abducto valgus formation in the adductus foot and hallux limitus in the rectus type foot. The pronated foot also develops varus rotation and contracture of the lesser digits.

During gait the individual with compensated forefoot varus functions with the knee internally rotated at heel contact because of the subtalar joint pronation that is present. The external rotation of the knee that occurs later in the stance phase is decreased. There may be some reduction in the amount of flexion of the knee during stance phase because of the pronated position of the foot; however, this will probably not be detectable during gait analysis. The knee would be fully extended at heel contact and heel-off. Following heel contact normal ankle joint plantarflexion occurs with smooth contact of the forefoot. The heel should leave the ground at a normal time just before heel contact of the opposite limb. At heel contact the calcaneus is everted usually to the end of its range of motion, and the heel stays everted during the stance phase of gait. The subtalar joint will be in a pronated position at heel contact, and very little subtalar joint motion will be noted during the stance phase of gait. Occasionally in a mild forefoot varus there is a less pronated position at heel contact with subtalar joint pronation occurring late in the contact phase of gait.

The midtarsal joint is unstable, and if subluxation occurs there will be a dorsiflexory break with the heel leaving the floor followed by "peeling off" of the remainder of the foot (Fig. 2.19). Motion around the metatarsophalangeal joints will be normal at heel contact with no hyperextension of the digits. The function of the metatarsophalangeal joints during the propulsive phase is somewhat altered in that the first metatarsal may not plantarflex normally as a result of midtarsal joint instability. This decreases the available dorsiflexion of the first metatarsophalangeal joint, but will probably not be noticeable during gait unless a clinically significant deformity has resulted.

Forefoot Valgus

Forefoot valgus is a structural abnormality in which the plantar aspect of the forefoot is everted relative to the posterior bisection of the calcaneus, when the subtalar joint is in its neutral position and the midtarsal joint is maximally pronated against this position (Fig. 2.20). Difficulties with evaluation of forefoot valgus are essentially the same as those enumerated under forefoot varus.

The most common problem with evaluating the forefoot valgus type foot probably relates to the position of the subtalar joint during the measurement. As the subtalar joint is supinated, the forefoot inverts faster than the rearfoot because of the limitation of motion created at the midtarsal joint. The reverse of this is also true; as one pronates the subtalar joint, the forefoot everts more rapidly than the rearfoot (Fig. 2.21). If the forefoot variation is measured with the subtalar joint supinated from its neutral (congruent) position, the amount of forefoot valgus measured will be reduced.

The position of the first metatarsal head relative to the lesser metatarsal heads is important in evaluating the forefoot valgus type foot. Frequently, with a forefoot valgus type foot the first metatarsal head will be located somewhat plantar to the second metatarsal

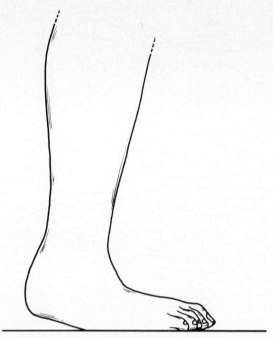

Figure 2.19.   Sagittal plane break at the midtarsal joint.

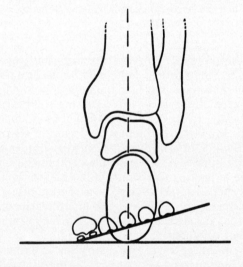

Figure 2.20.   Diagrammatic depiction of forefoot valgus (total type).

head when the first ray is in its neutral position. This relative plantarflexion increases the amount of forefoot valgus. It is important during evaluation to note the total amount of eversion of the forefoot relative to the rearfoot because the foot functions in response to its first-to-fifth metatarsal head position. Using this definition approximately 70% of individuals with frontal plane forefoot variation have forefoot valgus (29).

Forefoot valgus can be divided into two broad functional categories: one being rigid type forefoot valgus that compensates for the everted position of the forefoot relative to the rearfoot through subtalar joint supination, and the second being nonrigid forefoot valgus that does not compensate through subtalar joint supination. Some supination around the midtar-

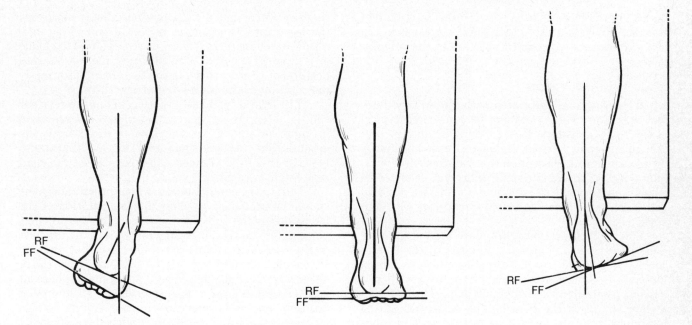

Figure 2.21. Diagrammatic illustration of effect of subtalar joint on position of plantar surface of forefoot. (A) Subtalar joint supinated. Forefoot slightly inverted relative to rearfoot. (B) Subtalar joint neutral. Forefoot perpendicular to rearfoot. (C) Subtalar joint pronated. Forefoot everted relative to rearfoot.

sal joint axes occurs in nonrigid forefoot valgus, as well as dorsal excursion of the first ray. Two subcategories can be delineated under both of these broad categories: (*a*) total type forefoot valgus, and (*b*) plantarflexed first ray type. From a functional standpoint the difference is between rigid and nonrigid, and from a structural standpoint it is between the total type and the plantarflexed first ray type of forefoot valgus.

Nonrigid Forefoot Valgus

During stance the patient with a nonrigid type of forefoot valgus will present with the subtalar joint in a neutral or pronated position. Occasionally there is an additional contributing pronatory force when this type of foot functions in a pronated position. However, nonrigid forefoot valgus alone will usually present with pronated subtalar joint function. This pronation of the subtalar joint seems to be caused by the lack of stability in the midtarsal joint. Approximately 70% of the individuals with forefoot valgus function in a nonrigid fashion (29).

Symptoms associated with nonrigid forefoot valgus would include postural symptoms and those associated with midtarsal joint hypermobility. Plantar fasciitis or heel spur syndrome is frequently seen in this foot type. Hallux abducto valgus in the adductus type foot and hallux limitus in the rectus type foot are common. Trauma plantar to the second metatarsal head results from first ray instability and reduced subtalar supination following heel lift. One would also expect to see varus rotation and contracture of the lesser digits and neuroma symptoms in the nonrigid forefoot valgus type foot that functions in a pronated attitude.

With nonrigid type forefoot valgus the knee will function either normally or internally rotated from its normal position, depending on whether the subtalar joint functions pronated. With pronation of the subtalar joint the knee would be internally rotated at heel contact, and there would be a reduced amount of external rotation during the remainder of stance phase. The knee would be fully extended at heel contact and heel-off, and it would have a nearly normal amount of flexion during the stance phase. Normal plantarflexion at the ankle joint would be expected following heel contact in this type foot with the forefoot being gently lowered to the floor. Heel-off would be at its normal time, approximately 40% of the total gait cycle. The position of the calcaneus at heel contact would be either vertical or everted. There are three possibilities for subtalar joint function in this type of foot: (*a*) near neutral at heel contact with normal subtalar joint pronation occurring during the first portion of stance with minimal resupination during the latter portions of stance phase, (*b*) pronated from heel contact through the stance phase, and (*c*) either position at heel contact and a quick resupination immediately following heel lift.

Commonly, an individual will exhibit different types of subtalar function on various strides. Normally a midtarsal joint break is not present following heel-off unless there is some additional pronatory force. In the foot with nonrigid forefoot valgus the first ray usually dorsiflexes when loaded, decreasing the available range of motion of the first metatarsophalangeal joint. Resultant first metatarsophalangeal joint symptoms and deformities are a frequent occurrence. Lesser metatarsophalangeal joint function should be normal following heel contact with no hyperextension of the digits. The toes remain in contact with the floor until the ball of the foot has been lifted. Varus rotation and contracture of the lesser digits may be present in the foot with primarily pronated function at the subtalar joint.

Rigid Forefoot Valgus

The symptoms associated with a rigid type forefoot valgus are varied and can be considered typical of the rigid cavus type foot. Postural symptoms that accompany rigid forefoot valgus are caused primarily by a lack of shock absorption that can cause low back, lateral hip, or lateral knee pain. This pain seems to be a compression induced pain, and an active individual will often relate maximum symptomatology with foot strike.

The supination that takes place around the subtalar joint axis to enable the forepart of the foot to come down to the ground often results in a lateral instability of the rearfoot. This lateral instability is present primarily at the subtalar joint. Through secondary injury to the ligamentous structures of the lateral aspect of the ankle, true lateral ankle instability is a frequent consequence.

Heel pain when seen in an individual with a rigid forefoot valgus seems to be the result of a lack of shock absorption, and often the individual will complain of a "bruise" type pain rather than the plantar fascial type pain experienced with the pronated foot. The high arch type foot that often results from a rigid type forefoot valgus may have a plantar fascia that is somewhat tight, and pain may be present in the central portion rather than the proximal insertion, which is more frequently inflamed in the flatfoot.

Tyloma formation beneath the first metatarsal head (specifically the tibial sesamoid) and the fifth metatarsal head is pathognomonic of rigid forefoot valgus. The cause of these lesions, with the rigidly plantarflexed first ray type forefoot valgus, is obvious. However, the lesion pattern is present frequently with the total type rigid forefoot valgus as well. As the subtalar joint supinates to compensate for the rigid forefoot valgus, available motion is limited around the oblique midtarsal joint axis causing the forefoot to become relatively inverted to the rearfoot. This supination at the midtarsal joint causes plantarflexion of the first ray leaving the first metatarsal in a slightly plantarly located position relative to the second.

The hammertoes seen with the rigid type forefoot valgus are typically direct dorsal contracture type deformities. The increase in metatarsal declination that is seen in the supinatory compensation for rigid forefoot valgus undoubtedly leads to some muscular imbalance around the metatarsophalangeal joints, and a combination of these two factors produces the dorsal contracture.

During gait the rigid type forefoot valgus causes some significant alterations. The sagittal plane motion that occurs at the knee can be limited with rigid type forefoot valgus. The internal rotation of the leg relative to the thigh, which is necessary during the first portion of knee flexion, can be blocked by the external rotatory force that a rigid forefoot valgus places on the leg during the contact period of gait. This may result in a decrease in stance phase flexion of the knee, or occasional function with the knee in a more flexed position at contact to avoid the requirement for internal rotation of the leg relative to the thigh.

The lateral instability that occurs in the rearfoot can be noted during the contact phase, but seems to be more prominent as the heel is lifted from the ground. The normal supinatory motion that takes place at this time is accentuated because of the rigid type forefoot valgus.

During the contact phase, when the subtalar joint should be pronating to allow internal rotation of the leg to occur, the subtalar joint is supinating to compensate for the rigidly everted position of the forepart of the foot. This supination causes external rotation of the leg, eliminating one of the important shock absorbing mechanisms during the contact phase of gait. The subtalar joint maintains itself in a supinated position, and following heel lift this supination increases as the leg continues to rotate externally.

Because of the supinated position of the subtalar joint throughout the entire stance phase of gait, the midtarsal joint remains "locked," and the ability to accommodate for terrain variation is limited. With the relatively plantarflexed position of the first ray, the first metatarsophalangeal joint motion is usually not limited, and a deformity resulting from jamming of the first metatarsophalangeal joint is unusual in the rigid type forefoot valgus.

The lesser metatarsophalangeal joints remain in a dorsiflexed position throughout the entire gait cycle once the typical dorsal hammertoe formation has occurred. This also has a tendency to displace the fat pad beneath the metatarsal heads anteriorly, enhancing the likelihood of the formation of lesions beneath the lesser metatarsal heads during propulsion.

Rearfoot Varus

Rearfoot varus is defined as a structural variation in which the posterior bisection of the calcaneus is inverted relative to vertical when the subtalar joint is in its neutral position and the individual is in the base and angle of gait (Fig. 2.22). Rearfoot varus by definition can include tibial varum, genu varum, subtalar varum, and a varus twist within the calcaneus, and is typically a combination of two or more of these. The most reliable method to determine the total amount of rearfoot varus is through a stance measurement in which the person is placed in the base and angle of gait, both feet are placed with the subtalar joint in its neutral position, a posterior bisection of the calcaneus is made, and the amount of inversion of the posterior aspect of the calcaneus relative to vertical is measured. It is useful to think of rear foot varus as "whole foot varus" because the forefoot will also be in an inverted position relative to the ground if no forefoot variation is present.

Compensation for rearfoot varus takes place through the eversion component of subtalar joint pronation. If adequate subtalar joint range of motion is available, the foot will evert until the heel is perpendicular to the supporting surface. This is a fully compensated rearfoot varus. If adequate subtalar jont eversion is not present and the heel remains inverted relative to the supporting surface when the subtalar joint is maximally pronated, then this is a partially compensated rearfoot varus. The individual with a rearfoot varus may experience postural symptoms in the form of foot, leg, and back fatigue. He or she may also present with knee joint complaints, particularly if the rearfoot varus is not fully compensated. Forefoot symptoms associated with rearfoot varus are minimal. There may be some callous formation under the fourth and fifth metatarsal heads. This would be accentuated with an uncompensated type rearfoot varus. There are no typical digital deformities associated with rearfoot varus.

During gait this individual would function with the knee joint fully extended both at heel contact and heel-off. The leg may be somewhat internally rotated at heel contact, and some internal rotation would occur if subtalar joint motion were available from this point. During the latter half of stance phase of gait normal external rotation of the leg occurs. Plantarflexion at the ankle joint following heel contact would be normal in this individual with a normal forefoot contact. Time of heel-off would be essentially normal. Position of the heel at contact would normally be vertical; however, if the rearfoot varus is not fully compensated, the heel remains in an inverted position.

The subtalar joint is normally pronated at heel contact, and some further subtalar joint pronation may occur during the first portion of stance. During the push-off phase subtalar joint supination should occur with inversion of the heel. A midtarsal joint break is usually not seen in an individual with rearfoot varus, because the midtarsal joint remains quite stable unless the calcaneus is everted. There would not be extensor substitution following heel contact, and the toes should contact the ground in the normal fashion. At toe-off the digits remain in contact with the ground until the adjacent portion of the ball of the foot has left the ground.

Equinus

Equinus will be defined as a condition in which less than 10° of ankle joint dorsiflexion is available when the subtalar joint is in its neutral position and the knee joint is fully extended (Fig. 2.23). This requirement for dorsiflexion will be used because of the normal 10° of hyperextension present at the hip at heel-off. When measuring ankle joint dorsiflexion it is important that the subtalar joint be in a neutral position, because pronation of the subtalar joint dorsiflexes the foot giving a false measurement. It is also important that the knee joint be fully extended, because flexion of the knee joint relaxes m. gastrocnemius, which may be the structure limiting ankle joint dorsiflexion.

Normally ankle joint dorsiflexion is measured using the lateral border of the foot from the most plantar aspect of the calcaneus to the fifth metatarsal head as the reference line; if a midtarsal joint break is present, a line from the most plantar aspect of the

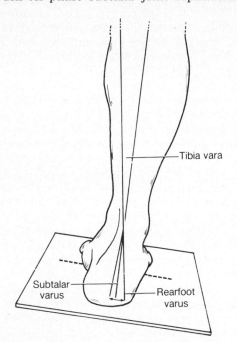

Figure 2.22. Diagrammatic depiction of rearfoot varus. When rearfoot varus exists as single structural variation entire foot is in inverted position.

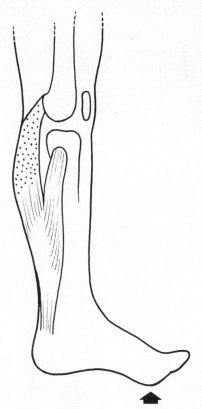

Figure 2.23. Equinus. Less than 10° of dorsiflexion of foot to leg available with knee extended and subtalar joint neutral.

calcaneus to the fifth metatarsal base should be used. Compensation for an equinus condition can occur in several ways. (A) Early heel-off with or without knee joint flexion. This is the most straightforward method of compensation for an equinus: if adequate ankle joint dorsiflexion is not available the heel may come off the ground before the hip becomes hyperextended 10°. (B) Short steppage. An individual shortens the stride so there is less hyperextension of the hip, reducing the requirement for ankle joint dorsiflexion. (C) External rotation at the hip. The individual who walks with a widely abducted gait has less of a requirement for ankle joint dorsiflexion. An individual walking with the feet abducted 90° to the line of progression will require no ankle joint dorsiflexion. (D) Abnormal subtalar and midtarsal joint pronation. This type of foot gains the amount of necessary dorsiflexion during the stance phase of gait through dorsiflexory motion at the midtarsal joint. For the midtarsal joint to be able to dorsiflex, the subtalar joint must be in a pronated position to increase the range of motion. A considerable portion of this dorsiflexion occurring at the midtarsal joint is the result of subluxation of this joint.

In March 1978 at Doctors Hospital Surgical Symposium in Atlanta, Smith presented an interesting idea regarding this type of compensation for equinus that essentially was as follows: Subtalar joint pronation occurs during the swing phase to enable the foot to get into a dorsiflexed position so that the shock absorption obtained by allowing the heel to strike first and slowly plantarflexing the foot can be used. If the ankle cannot become dorsiflexed adequately to allow the heel to contact first, one of the important shock absorption mechanisms at heel contact is lost. The requirement for dorsiflexion during the stance phase is then made up through motion at the midtarsal joint (S.D. Smith, unpublished observation). The swing phase requirement for subtalar joint pronation, to allow the heel to contact first, certainly seems to be a reasonable explanation for the function seen with this type of compensation.

An individual with an equinus frequently has symptoms of postural fatigue in the legs and back. Postural fatigue in the foot will be present if subtalar and midtarsal joint pronation is a method of compensation. Plantar fasciitis and heel spur syndrome might be present more commonly in the pronated foot. Forefoot abnormalities seen in an individual with equinus likewise depend on the midtarsal joint stability. If the midtarsal joint is unstable, then the individual will have pressure beneath the second metatarsal head, along with varus rotation and contracture of the digits. Neuroma symptoms are frequently encountered in this foot type as well. Hallux abducto valgus formation is common when there is adduction of the forefoot. With a rectus type forefoot, hallux limitus would be a common finding. In a less pronated foot, plantar lesions across the entire ball of the foot might be present. Extensor substitution frequently causes dorsal contracture of all of the digits.

The gait variations seen with short steppage or external rotation for compensation are quite straightforward.

The individual who compensates for the equinus with an early heel-off will frequently function with the knee slightly flexed throughout the stance phase of gait. The knee will be somewhat flexed at heel contact; the flexion might increase during midstance for normal contact phase flexion, but it will never fully extend at heel-off. This individual when standing erect may demonstrate a mild genu recurvatum that is not evidenced during gait. A variation that occurs with this type of function is a mild hyperextension of the knee just before heel contact. As the leg swings forward, it actually becomes hyperextended relative to the femur and then begins to flex, and is flexed by the time the heel contacts the ground. Rather than being an actual compensatory mechanism for equinus, this seems to protect the knee from abnormal stress in a fully extended position. In a severe equinus a "backknee" function may be present. This is seen when the lack of ankle joint dorsiflexion forces the knee into hyperextension during the stance phase of gait.

The ankle will be approximately at a 90° angle at heel contact unless the equinus is severe, at which time it is possible that contact will be foot flat rather than heel first, or possibly ball first contact. The important shock absorbing mechanism of ankle joint plantarflexion following heel contact will be hindered in either of these latter situations. Following foot flat the ankle will then dorsiflex to the limit of its range of motion, at which time heel-off will occur. In the individual who is functioning with an early heel-off this will be substantially before heel contact of the opposite limb. Timing of this early heel-off is quite variable and can be from immediately following contact until just before the normal time. The earlier the heel is off the ground the sooner excessive load is placed on the ball of the foot, and the more likely stress induced symptomatology of the ball of the foot will occur.

The subtalar joint will typically be neutral to slightly supinated at contact, and although a mild amount of subtalar joint pronation might occur during the early portion of stance, it is foreshortened, and the subtalar joint is in a supinated position before the time the heel comes off the ground. This relatively supinated position of the subtalar joint serves to protect the midtarsal joint both by limiting the amount of motion available at the midtarsal joint and by inverting the oblique midtarsal joint axis so that the moment arm creating pronation is shortened.

The individual compensating through subtalar and midtarsal joint pronation would have the knee internally rotated at heel contact, and there would be a lack of normal internal rotation following heel contact. Less external rotation than normal would occur during the latter portion of stance phase. The knee generally is extended at heel contact; however, it may be flexed somewhat as with the individual who compensates with an early heel-off. At heel-off the knee should be fully extended again; however, frequently slight flexion will persist. Ankle joint motion at contact will be normal in appearance. Heel-off will usually be early with a midtarsal joint break (Fig. 2.19). At heel contact the calcaneus will be everted, and there will be minimal subtalar joint motion present during the stance phase of gait with the heel remaining everted.

Midtarsal joint hypermobility results in first ray instability. The subsequent limitation of first metatarsophalangeal joint dorsiflexion may be noticeable if a clinically significant hallux abducto valgus or hallux limitus has developed. The metatarsophalangeal joints will be hyperextended at heel contact because of the substitution phenomenon of the long extensors to the toes. At toe-off the toes will not maintain their contact with the ground after the ball of the foot has left the ground, because the extensors become active early to assist in dorsiflexion at the ankle.

This overview should serve as a reminder that most pedal symptoms and deformities amenable to surgical intervention are the direct result of abnormal function.

References

1. Sgarlato T: *A Compendium of Podiatric Biomechanics.* San Francisco, California College of Podiatric Medicine, 1971, p 60.
2. Burns LT, Burns MJ, Burns GA: A clinical application of biomechanics: Part 1. *J Am Podiatry Assoc* 69:24, 1979.
3. Manter JT: Movements of the subtalar and transverse tarsal joints. *Anat Rec* 80:397, 1944.
4. Elftman H: The transverse tarsal joint and its control. *Clin Orthop* 16:41, 1960.
5. Hicks JH: The mechanics of the foot. 1. The joints. *J Anat* 87:345, 1953.
6. Root ML, Orien WP, Weed JH: *Normal and Abnormal Function of the Foot.* Los Angeles, Clinical Biomechanics Corp, 1977.
7. Perry J: The mechanics of walking. A clinical interpretation. *Phys Ther* 47:778, 1967.
8. Whitney AK: Podokinetics. *J Am Podiatry Assoc* 47:383, 1957.
9. Oldenbrook L, Smith C: Metatarsal head motion secondary to rearfoot supination and pronation. *J Am Podiatry Assoc* 69:24, 1979.
10. Saunders JB, Inman VT, Eberhart HD: The major determinants in normal and pathological gait. *J Bone Joint Surg* 35A:543, 1953.
11. Inman VT: Human locomotion. *Can Med Assoc J* 9:1047, 1966.
12. Jarrett BA, Manzi JA, Green DR: Interossei and lumbricales muscles of the foot. *J Am Podiatry Assoc* 70:1, 1980.
13. Hof AL, van den Berg JW: Linearity between the weighted sum of the EMGs of the human triceps surae and the total torque. *J Biomech* 10:529, 1977.
14. Baumann JU, Sutherland DH, Hanggi A: Intramuscular pressure during walking: an experimental study using the wick catheter technique. *Clin Orthop* 145:292, 1979.
15. Eberhart HD, Inman VT, Bresler B: *The Principal Elements in Human Locomotion. Human Limbs and Their Substitutes.* New York, McGraw-Hill, 1959, p 437.
16. Battye CK, Joseph J: An investigation by telemetering of the activity of some muscles in walking. *Med Biol Eng Comput* 4:125, 1966.
17. Basmajian JV, Lovejoy JF, Jr: Functions of the popliteus muscle in man: a multifactorial electromyographic study. *J Bone Joint Surg* 53A:556, 1971.
18. Sutherland DH: An electromyographic study of the plantar flexors of the ankle in normal walking on the level. *J Bone Joint Surg* 48A:66, 1966.
19. Murray MP, Drought AB, Kory RC: Walking patterns of normal men. *J Bone Joint Surg* 46A:335, 1964.
20. Houtz SJ, Walsh FP: Electromyographic analysis of the function of the muscles acting on the ankle during weightbearing with special reference to the triceps surae. *J Bone Joint Surg* 41A:1469, 1959.
21. Suzuki R: Electromyographic kinesiology of the lower limb. *J Japan Orthop Assoc* 46:139, 1972.
22. Mann RA, Hagy JL: The popliteus muscle. *J Bone Joint Surg* 59A:924, 1977.
23. Simon SR, Mann RA, Hagy JL, Larsen LJ: Role of the posterior calf muscles in normal gait. *J Bone Joint Surg* 60A:465, 1978.
24. Gray EG, Basmajian JV: Electromyography and cinematography of leg and foot ("normal" and flat) during walking. *Anat Rec* 161:1, 1968.
25. Shefield FJ, Gersten JW, Mastellone AF: Electromyographic study of the muscles of the foot in normal walking. *Am J Phys Med* 35:223, 1956.
26. Advisory Committee on Artifical Limbs National Research Council: The pattern of muscle activity in the lower extremity during walking. Series 11, Issue 25, Berkeley, Institute of Engineering Research, University of California, 1953.
27. Mann R, Inman VT: Phasic activity of intrinsic muscles of the foot. *J Bone Joint Surg* 46A:469, 1964.
28. Elftman H: The function of muscles in locomotion. *Am J Physiol* 125:357–366, 1939.
29. Burns MJ: Orthotic control following surgical correction of hallux abducto valgus. *J Foot Surg* 18:89–95, 1979.

Additional References

Bogdan RJ: *Range of Motion of the Subtalar Joint and Ankle Dorsiflexion of the Developing Child. Decision Making in Foot Surgery.* New York, Symposia Specialists, 1976, p 73.
Bresler B, Brankel JP: The forces and moments in the leg during level walking. *American Society of Mechanical Engineers, Trans.* 72:27, 1950.
Close JR, Inman VT: The action of the ankle joint. *Advisory Committee on Artificial Limbs National Research Council* Series 11, Issue 22, April 1952.
Close JR, Inman VT, Porr PM, Todd FN: The function of the subtalar joint. *Clin Orthop* 50:159, 1967.
Close JR: *Motor Function in the Lower Extremity.* Springfield, Ill, Charles C. Thomas, 1964.
Elftman H: Biomechanics of muscle. *J Bone Joint Surg* 48A:363, 1966.
Goss CY: *Gray's Anatomy,* ed 28. Philadelphia, Lea & Febiger, 1966.
Inman VT: *DuVries' Surgery of the Foot,* ed 3. St Louis, The C.V. Mosby Co., 1973.
Inman VT: The influence of the foot-ankle complex on the proximal skeletal structures. *Artif Limbs* 13:59, 1969.
Isman RE, Inman VT: Anthropometric studies of the human foot and ankle. *Bull Prost Res* Spring 1968, Technical Report 58, p 97.
Karpovich PV, Wilklow LB: A goniometric study of the human foot in standing and walking. *US Armed Forces Med J* 10:885, 1959.
Levens AS, Inman VT, Blosser JA: Transverse rotation of the segments of the lower extremity in locomotion. *J Bone Joint Surg* 30A:859, 1948.
Morris JM: Biomechanics of the foot and ankle. *Clin Orthop* 122:10, 1977.
Parlasca R, Shoji H, D'Ambrosia RD: Effects of ligamentous injury on ankle and subtalar joints: A kinematic study. *Clin Orthop* 140:266, 1979.
Perry J: Kinesiology of lower extremity bracing. *Clin Orthop* 102:18, 1974.
Ralston HJ, Lukin L: Energy levels of human body segments during level walking. *Ergonomics* 12:39, 1969.
Schoenhaus H, Gold M, Hylinski J, Keating J: A preliminary report of computerized analysis of gait. *J Am Podiatry Assoc* 69:2, 1979.
Schwartz PR, Heath AL: The definition of human locomotion on the basis of measurement: with description of oscillographic method. *J Bone Joint Surg* 29:203, 1947.
Steindler A: *Kinesiology of the Human Body.* Springfield, Ill, Charles C Thomas, 1964.
Sutherland DH, Hagy JL: Measurement of gait movements from motion picture film. *J Bone Joint Surg* 54A:787, 1972.
Wright DG, Desai SM, Henderson WH: Action of the subtalar and ankle joint complex during the stance phase of walking. *J Bone Joint Surg* 46A:361, 1964.

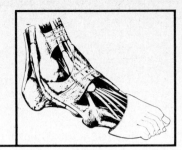

CHAPTER 3

Radiology

Barbara S. Schlefman, D.P.M.

This chapter covers the basic techniques used in podiatric radiology of the foot and ankle, as well as some of the new, sophisticated procedures coming into vogue. It is our job as practitioners constantly to improve on our radiographic quality and eliminate unnecessary exposure. Proper use of intrinsic x-ray factors (mAs, kVp) and extrinsic factors (focal spot size, object film distance, focal film distance), as well as an understanding of proper collimation, filtration, and x-ray development procedures will improve the radiographic quality. Reducing retakes reduces unnecessary radiation exposure.

STANDARD RADIOGRAPHIC PROJECTIONS OF THE FOOT

Dorsoplantar Projection

Dorsoplantar (DP) projection is actually an anteroposterior (AP) projection of the foot; only the terminology is appropriately altered. Where possible the DP projection should be taken on weight-bearing. An orthoposer or podium will facilitate weight-bearing views. The film should be placed flat on the orthoposer and the patient should stand on the film. Where angle and base of gait x-ray films are desirable, one foot should be exposed at a time, using a lead shield to protect the other half of the plate. The x-ray head is angled 15° from the vertical posteriorly toward the calcaneus (Fig. 3.1). The central ray is directed at the navicular (Fig. 3.2). When both feet are filmed simultaneously, the central ray is directed equally between the feet (1–4).

In cases where weight-bearing views are not possible (i.e. trauma, postoperatively, the elderly), a non-weight-bearing DP projection is advisable. It is best to place the patient supine with the knee bent and the sole of the foot resting flat on the plate. The tube is angled 15° from the vertical (Fig. 3.3).

The DP projection allows an accurate representation of the phalanges, metatarsals, navicular, cuboid, medial cuneiform, and to a lesser extent the middle

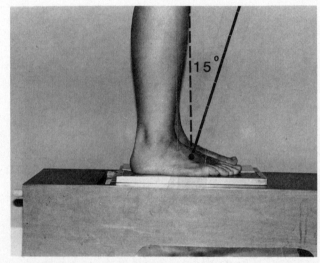

Figure 3.1. Weight-bearing dorsoplantar projection.

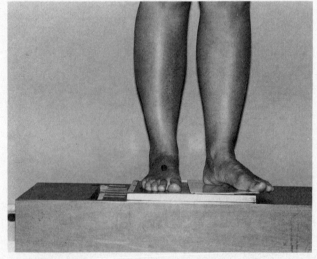

Figure 3.2. Weight-bearing dorsoplantar projection.

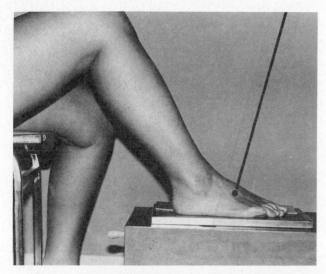

Figure 3.3. Non-weight-bearing dorsoplantar projection.

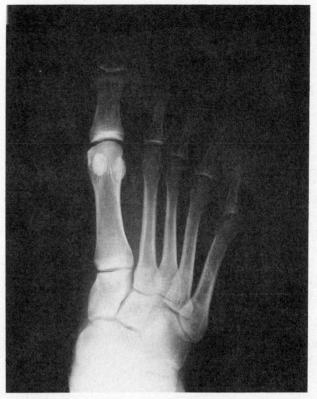

Figure 3.4. Dorsoplantar view.

and lateral cuneiforms. The distal portion of the talus and calcaneus, as well as the midtarsal joint, Lisfranc's joint, the metatarsophalangeal joints and interphalangeal joints may be observed (1–3) (Fig. 3.4).

Often a DP projection is taken with lesion markers, a small circular lead or soft wire fixed to the plantar of the foot with tape, to locate precisely the position of a questionable lesion in relation to underlying bone (Fig. 3.5).

Lateral Projection

The x-ray cassette is placed vertically in the lead-lined well of the orthoposer. The patient places one foot on each side of the film with the medial aspect of the foot in question touching the film. Angle and base of gait x-ray films are easy to obtain with proper positioning. The tube is angled 90° from the vertical

and the central ray is aimed at the first cuneiform (Fig. 3.6). This view adequately depicts the talus, calcaneus, cuboid, and to a lesser extent the navicular and medial cuneiform. The metatarsals and phalanges overlap to varying degrees (Fig. 3.7). Any digit may be elevated to a plane above the others by a radiolucent object so that the digits may be individually evaluated. This is commonly done with the hallux (Fig. 3.8).

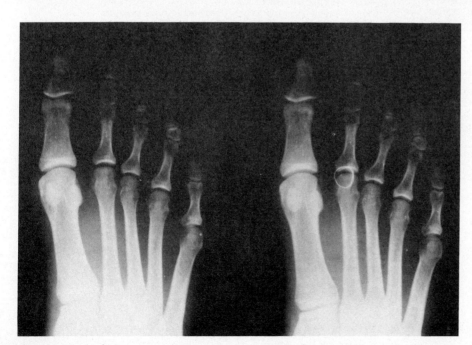

Figure 3.5. Dorsoplantar view with lesion marker beneath second metatarsal head.

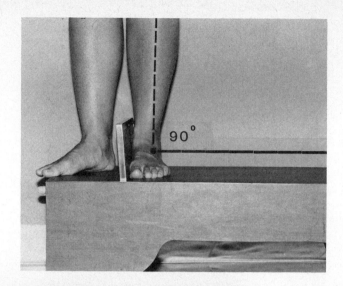

Figure 3.6.   Weight-bearing lateral projection.

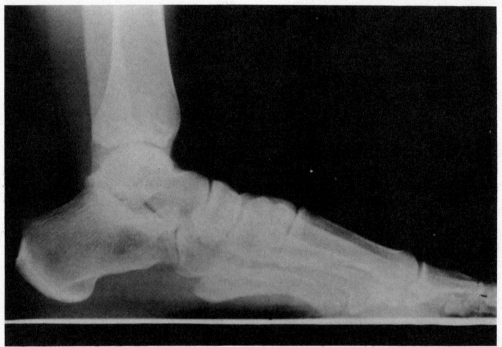

Figure 3.7.   Weight-bearing lateral view.

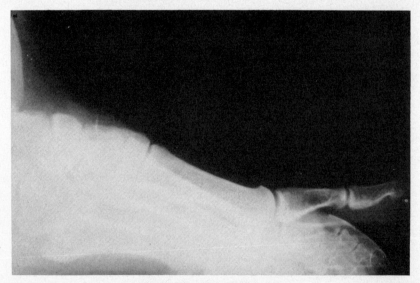

Figure 3.8.   Raised hallux view.

In taking a non-weight-bearing lateral, one places the patient supine on the unaffected side with the medial malleolus in contact with the film. The central ray is directed perpendicularly to the midpoint of the foot (Fig. 3.9).

Medial Oblique Projection

There is much disagreement about terminology when discussing medial oblique (MO) and lateral oblique projections of the foot. By definition, a projection is defined as the direction the central ray passes through the part. Hence, in an MO, the central ray should enter the foot from an MO position. This is in fact not how most people define an MO. In the weight bearing projection, the patient stands on the x-ray cassette with the most lateral border of the foot against the edge of the cassette. The tube is angled 45° from the vertical and is aimed at the cuboid bone (Fig. 3.10). This is the most common oblique in podiatric usage. It gives a magnified and distorted pres-

entation of the bones of the foot (Fig. 3.11). Variations from the 45° angle may be more useful for observing one bone over another bone. A 15° oblique projection shows the medial cuneiform, a 30° oblique projection shows the lateral cuneiform, and a 60° oblique projection shows the cuboid and anterior facet of the talocalcaneal joint.

The non-weight-bearing projection is similar to a DP projection. With the foot resting on the x-ray plate, the patient adducts the knee until the sole of the foot makes an angle of 30° to 45° with the plane of the film. The central ray is then aimed perpendicularly to the film directed to the third cuneiform (Fig. 3.12).

Lateral Oblique Projection

For a lateral oblique (LO) projection the foot is placed on the cassette that is flat on the orthoposer with the medial aspect of the foot against the edge of the film. The central ray is directed 45° from the verticle to the navicular (Fig. 3.13). This view is only beneficial for evaluating the most medial structures of the foot including the first and second metatarsals, the first and second cuneiforms, and the tibial and fibular sesamoids (Fig. 3.14). An alternative non-weight bearing projection involves flexing the knee

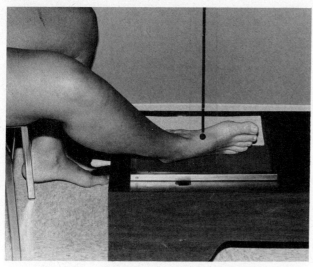
Figure 3.9. Non-weight-bearing lateral projection.

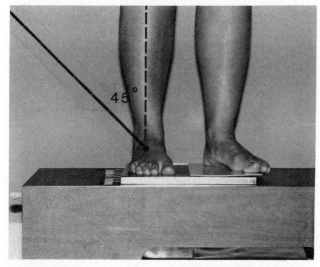
Figure 3.10. Weight-bearing medial oblique projection.

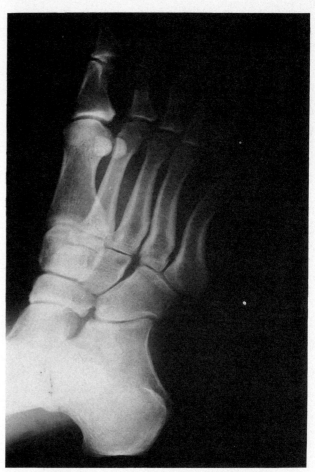
Figure 3.11. Weight-bearing medial oblique view.

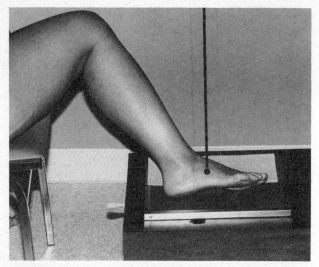

Figure 3.12.   Non-weight-bearing medial oblique projection.

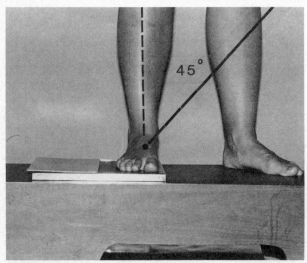

Figure 3.13.   Weight-bearing lateral oblique projection.

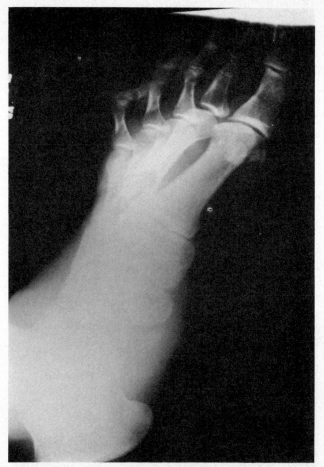

Figure 3.14.   Weight-bearing lateral oblique view.

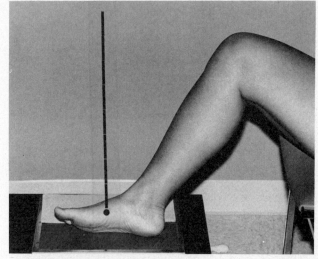

Figure 3.15.   Non-weight-bearing lateral oblique projection.

and abducting it until the plantar aspect of the foot makes a 15°, 30°, 45°, or 60° angle with the film. The central ray is directed perpendicular to the film to the first cuneiform (1–3) (Fig. 3.15).

Axial Sesamoid Projection

For an axial sesamoid projection the film is placed vertically in the slot in the orthoposer and the patient faces the film with the toes dorsiflexed against the film. The patient then raises up on the heels. The central ray is directed perpendicular to the center of the foot (or center of the film if both feet are done simultaneously) (Fig. 3.16). Many positioning devices have been designed to aid the axial sesamoid projection. An alternative positioning involves placing the patient prone or on hands and knees with the film flat on the x-ray table and the toes dorsiflexed, placing the ball of the foot perpendicular to the horizontal. The central ray is directed vertically to the metatarsophalangeal joints (Fig. 3.17).

This view is used to evaluate the sesamoid bones and their relationship with the first metatarsal head. It has questionable value in evaluating the relative declination of the metatarsal heads in relation to each other (1–7) (Fig. 3.18).

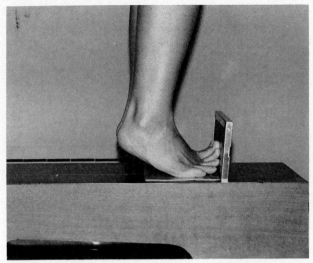

Figure 3.16. Axial sesamoid projection.

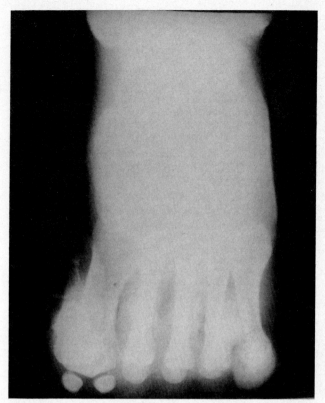

Figure 3.18. Axial sesamoid view.

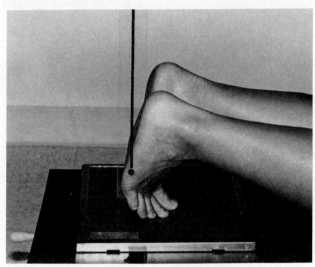

Figure 3.17. Axial sesamoid projection.

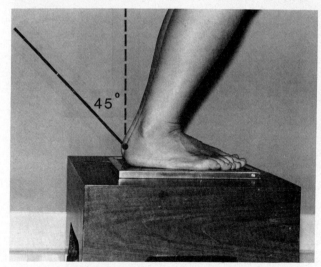

Figure 3.19. Axial calcaneal projection.

Axial Calcaneal Projections

For axial calcaneal projections, the film is placed flat on the orthoposer and the patient stands with the heel at the most posterior edge of the film. The central ray is directed at a 45° angle to the posterior aspect of the calcaneus (Fig. 3.19). An alternative method involves the patient sitting with the leg stretched out over the cassette. The ankle joint is dorsiflexed to 90°, a long piece of gauze looped around the forefoot may be used to aid dorsiflexion. The central ray is directed to the distal plantar aspect of the calcaneus at a 45° angle from the vertical (Fig. 3.20). This projection is used to examine the calcaneus for fractures or possible abnormalities in shape (1–3). It is also used to evaluate the position of internal fixation devices used in triple arthrodesis (Fig. 3.21).

Harris and Beath Projection (Coalition View)

The Harris and Beath projection is taken similar to the weight-bearing axial calcaneal projection. The main difference is that multiple angles are required to allow visualization of the subtalar joint. A scout lateral x-ray will allow one to approximate the declination of the posterior facet of the subtalar joint in reference to the weight bearing plane. Three projections are recommended. One is taken 10° above, 10° below, and at the measured angle (i.e. 30°, 40°, and 50° if the measured declination is 40°). The patient should flex the knees and ankles slightly before the film is shot. This projection gives an axial view of the calcaneus, the inferior aspect of the talus, as well as the middle and posterior facets of the talocalcaneal articulation (1–3) (Fig. 3.22).

Isherwood Projections

The Isherwood projections consist of three positions to fully visualize the joints of the subtalar joint. The oblique dorsoplantar or oblique lateral demonstrates the anterior joint (Fig. 3.23), the medial oblique axial demonstrates the middle and posterior joints (Fig. 3.24), and the lateral oblique axial demonstrates the posterior joint in profile (Fig. 3.25). A 30° and 45° wedge of wood, plaster, or any radiolucent material is

needed for positioning. The patient is seated in a chair with the leg extended over the orthoposer or lies supine on a table top.

Oblique Dorsoplantar or Oblique Lateral. The foot is positioned on the 45° wedge with the medial aspect of the foot resting on the x-ray cassette. The knee is flexed to obtain a 90° relationship of the foot to the leg. The central ray is directed vertically

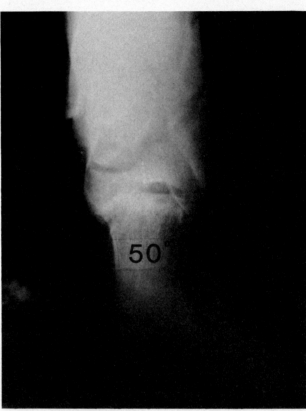

Figure 3.22. Harris and Beath view at 50°s.

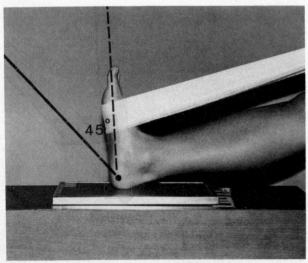

Figure 3.20. Axial calcaneal projection.

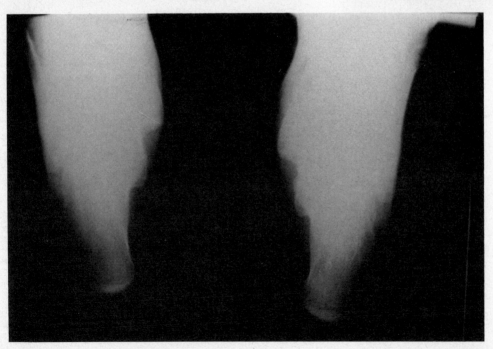

Figure 3.21. Axial calcaneal view.

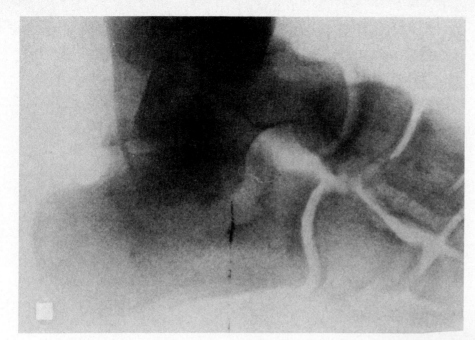

Figure 3.23. Oblique dorsoplantar or oblique lateral view.

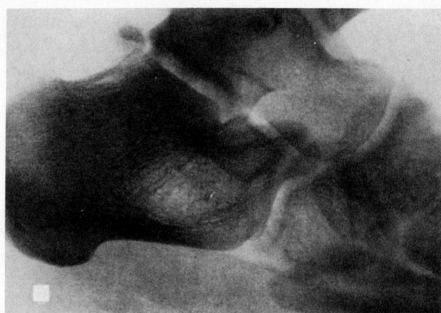

Figure 3.24. Medial oblique axial view.

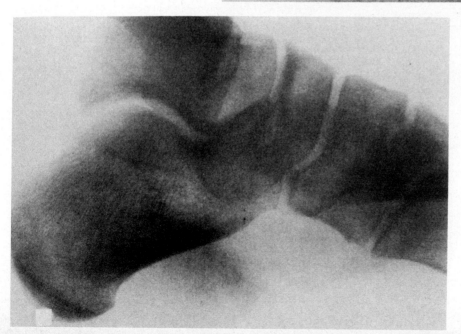

Figure 3.25. Lateral oblique axial view.

to a point 1 inch below and 1 inch anterior to the lateral malleolus (1–3, 8, 9) (Fig. 3.26).

Medial Oblique Axial.   The foot is positioned on a 30° wedge with the medial aspect of the foot resting on the x-ray cassette. The foot is held in maximum dorsiflexion and inversion with the help of a sling. The central ray is directed to a point 1 inch distal and 1 inch anterior to the lateral malleolus at an angle of 10° cephalad from the vertical (Fig. 3.27).

Lateral Oblique Axial.   The foot is positioned on a 30° wedge with the lateral aspect of the foot resting on the x-ray cassette. The foot is held in maximum dorsiflexion and eversion with the help of a sling. The central ray is directed to a point 1 inch distal to the medial malleolus at an angle of 10° cephalad from the vertical (1–3) (Fig. 3.28).

As one can readily see, positioning is very difficult with the Isherwood projections. The author believes that the benefits derived from these projections are minimal. It is probably better first to take standard radiographic projections (DP, oblique, lateral) and if

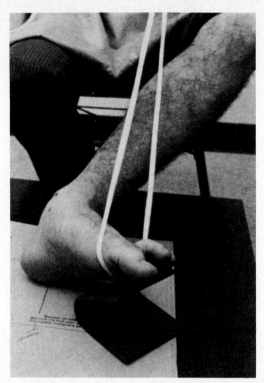

Figure 3.28.   Lateral oblique axial projection.

these do not suffice, then advanced techniques such as tomograms and computerized tomography should be used.

STANDARD RADIOGRAPHIC PROJECTIONS OF THE ANKLE

Anteroposterior Projection

For an AP projection, ankle x-ray films should be taken weight bearing where practical. The x-ray cassette is held vertically in the orthoposer. The patient stands with the posterior aspect of the heel against the film and the foot pointed straight ahead. The central ray is directed perpendicular to the film, entering midway between the malleoli (Fig. 3.29). In the non-weight-bearing projection, the patient is placed supine with the leg extended over the cassette, which is placed flat on the table. The central ray is directed vertically. This projection gives an adequate presentation of the ankle joint, including the distal ends of the tibia and the fibular and trochlear surface of the talus (1–3) (Fig. 3.30).

Mortise Projection

The mortise projection is similar to an AP projection with the exception of a 15° internal rotation of the leg placing the malleoli on a plane parallel to the film (Fig. 3.31). This projection shows a better representation of the lower tibiofibular articulation (1–3) (Fig. 3.32).

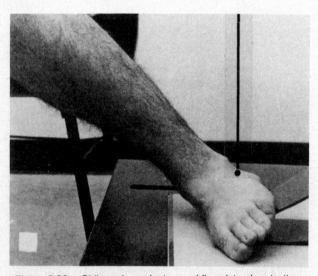

Figure 3.26.   Oblique dorsoplantar or oblique lateral projection.

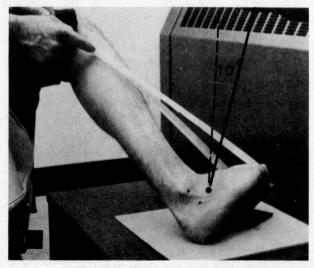

Figure 3.27.   Medial oblique axial projection.

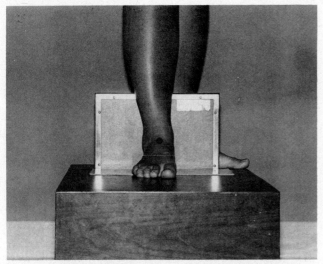

Figure 3.29. Weight-bearing anteroposterior projection.

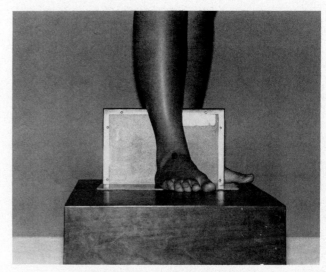

Figure 3.31. Mortise projection.

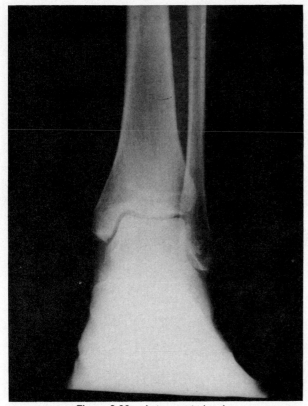

Figure 3.30. Anteroposterior view.

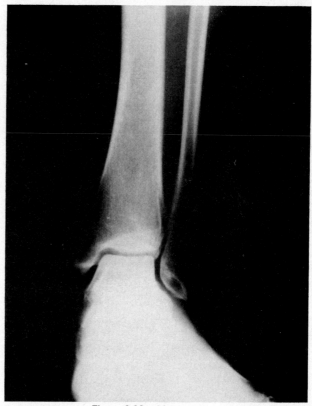

Figure 3.32. Mortise view.

Medial Oblique Projection

The MO projection is again similar to the AP and mortise projections. The leg is internally rotated 45° (Fig. 3.33). This further opens up the tibiofibular syndesmosis (1–3).

Lateral Oblique Projection

In the LO projection the leg is externally rotated approximately 45° (Fig. 3.34). Any variation in degrees

of internal or external rotation may be used when examining an ankle for trauma (1–3).

Lateral Projection

Like the lateral projection of the foot, the medial aspect of the foot is placed in contact with the x-ray cassette and the central ray is directed perpendicular to the film. The film is positioned vertically so that more of the ankle and leg is shown at the expense of the toes and forefoot (Fig. 3.35). The trochlear surface

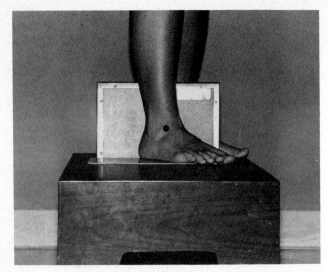

Figure 3.33.   Medial oblique projection.

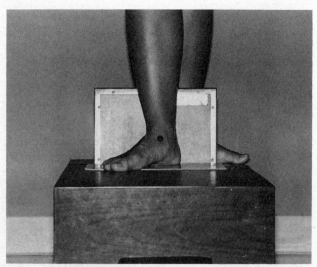

Figure 3.34.   Lateral oblique projection.

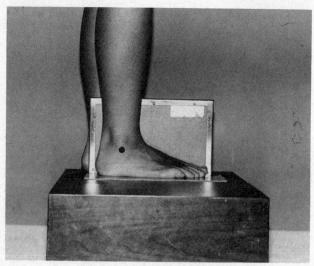

Figure 3.35.   Lateral projection.

of the talus and its articulation with the tibia and fibula are visualized well in this view (1–3) (Fig. 3.36).

Stress Dorsiflexion Projection

The stress dorsiflexion projection is similar to the lateral weight bearing projection of the ankle. The opposite leg is placed forward of the one being exposed. The patient forcefully flexes the knee and ankle of the affected side to obtain as much dorsiflexion of the foot on the leg as possible (Fig. 3.37). This projection is used to demonstrate any anterior ankle impingement as in ankle equinus (1–3) (Fig. 3.38).

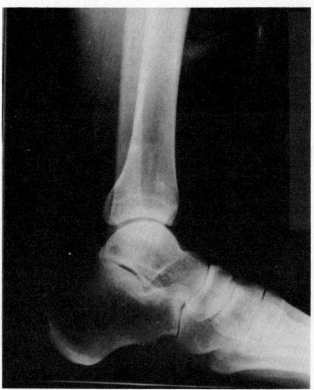

Figure 3.36.   Lateral view.

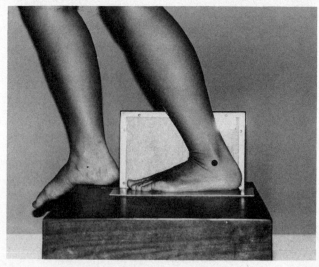

Figure 3.37.   Stress dorsiflexion projection.

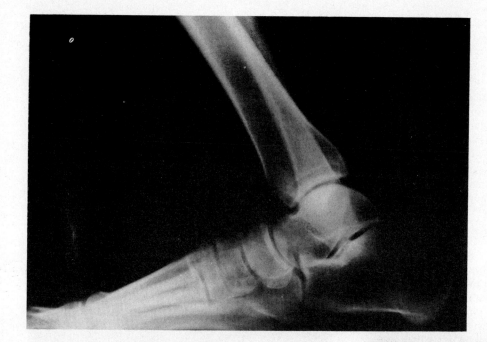

Figure 3.38.   Stress dorsiflexion view.

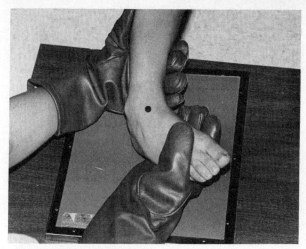

Figure 3.39.   Inversion stress projection.

Inversion Stress Projection

Inversion stress radiographs are usually performed following ankle inversion sprains when no bony pathology is noted on standard ankle radiographs. The patient lies supine on the x-ray table with the leg extended and the foot positioned over the cassette. The examiner stabilizes the lower leg with one hand while forcefully inverting (supinating) the foot with the other hand. The central ray is directed vertically to the central portion of the ankle joint and the x-ray is made at the time when the ankle is held in the most extreme inversion (Fig. 3.39).

The examiner's hands should be protected with lead gloves and a lead apron should be worn. Often the injured area must be anesthetized before examination. This may involve either local infiltration of a local anesthetic or the use of a high common peroneal nerve block. The uninjured side should be examined

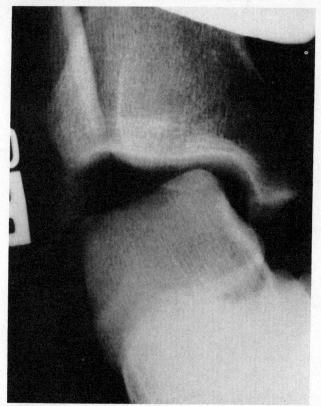

Figure 3.40.   Inversion stress view showing significant talar tilt.

in a similar fashion for comparison. The tilting of the talus in the ankle mortise is compared (1–3) (Fig. 3.40).

Bonnin (11) felt that 15° of talar tilt indicated rupture of the anterior talofibular ligament, 15° to 30° of talar tilt indicated rupture of the anterior talofibular and calcaneofibular ligaments, and over 30° of talar tilt indicated rupture of all three lateral ligaments. Other findings fail to support these statistics (10–12).

It is difficult to define what values are normal or abnormal because there is much variability. Tilting of less than 5° is probably normal, whereas tilting from 5° to 25° can be normal or abnormal. Over 25° of talar tilting is definitely abnormal. A positive stress test is helpful in identifying pathological but a negative stress test does not necessarily exclude ligamentous damage unless the patient is under general or spinal anesthesia and all reflex muscle splinting has been eliminated.

Forced eversion may also be performed to evaluate pathological conditions of the deltoid ligaments. Talar tilting over 10° seems to be pathological (10).

Anterior Drawer Projection (Push-Pull Stress)

Like the inversion stress projection, an anterior drawer projection is taken following ankle trauma where disruption of the soft tissue structures are suspected. The patient is placed supine with the leg extended and the lateral aspect of the foot placed against the underlying cassette. The examiner places one hand against the anterior aspect of the leg and the other hand placed behind the heel. Opposite forces are then applied attempting to pull the talus forward out of the ankle mortise. The central ray is directed perpendicular to the film entering at the medial malleolus (Fig. 3.41). Again, the examiner should be

shielded and bilateral views should be taken for comparison.

It is difficult to report on normal or abnormal values. If the talus can be forcefully dislocated anterior to the ankle mortise, then it would appear that some type of ligamentous disruption must have taken place (Fig. 3.42A, B).

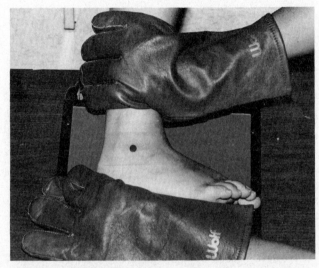

Figure 3.41.   Anterior drawer projection.

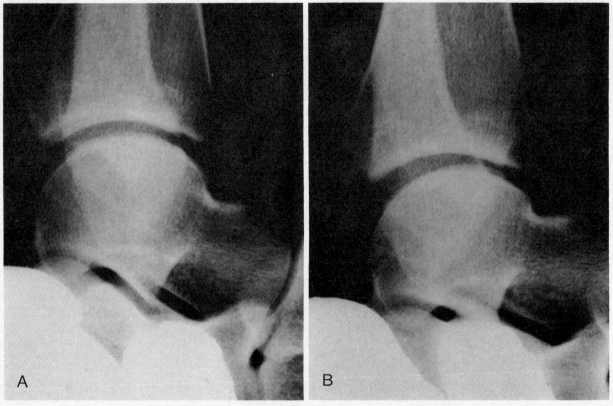

Figure 3.42.   Anterior drawer view showing comparison of normal foot (A) and abnormal foot (B).

NUCLEAR MEDICINE (BONE SCANNING)*

(Much information used in the following section was taken from Shuer ML, Hartshorne MF, Peters VG: Nuclear medicine: implications for podiatry. J Am Podiatry Assoc 75:90–98, 1985, and used with the authors' permission.)

The term "radioactive" was coined in 1898 by Marie Curie with her discovery and isolation of radium. A radioactive element or isotope is one that can spontaneously change into a different element with the emission of alpha, beta, or gamma radiation. Alpha and beta emitting isotopes do not produce a penetrating ray and thus only expose the patient to radiation but do not produce useful images. Gamma-emitting radionuclides are incorporated into radiopharmaceuticals and are used as tracers in patient examinations. The physical half-life of the element is the time for one half of the radioactive material to undergo transformation. The biological half-life is the time required for the patient to eliminate one half of the substance through normal processes such as urine, feces, exhalation, or perspiration (13).

Bone scanning developed during the 1940s and early 1950s, and its continued sophistication is seen today. In nuclear medicine, all radioactive compounds, called radiopharmaceuticals, are artificially produced. Following slow intravenous injection, the radiopharmaceutical localizes in a specified organ. A scintillation probe or detector is positioned over the organ and the emitted gamma photons are converted into visible light and counted. A photomultiplier tube converts the light into an electronic pulse. The information is then transferred to an electronic analyzer that differentiates among various gamma ray energies. A two-dimensional photodisplay unit records the image on film. The number of counts recorded reflects the amount of radiopharmaceutical concentration. In some scans normal areas are demonstrated by an increase in the number of dots and abnormal areas as "cold" areas with no dots. In other scans normal areas contain no dots, and an increased number of dots represents an abnormality (13, 14).

An ideal radionuclide should have a minimum of particulate emission (alpha and beta rays), a primary photon energy between 50 and 500 KeV, a physical half-life greater than the time needed to prepare the material for injection, a biological half-life longer than the examination time, low toxicity, stability, and a suitable chemical form and reactivity to study the part in question. The procedure is considered safe, although radioactive isotopes should not be given to pregnant women (3, Podiatry News 2:1, 1983).

The first practical bone imaging agents were strontium-85 and strontium-87m, which were able to localize in the skeleton by exchanging with calcium in the bone matrix. However, skeletal detail was not well shown because of the low count rate from these isotopes (14–17). Fluorine-18 has now been widely replaced by technetium-99m (Tc-99m) which is a derivative of molybdenum and is probably the agent of choice today because of its lower toxicity, decreased cost, and increased availability. It is combined with an appropriate bone imaging agent.

Tc-99m methylene diphosphate (MDP) has a physical half-life of six hours, a useful 140 Kev gamma photon, and rapid osteoblastic mediated chemabsorption onto the surface of hydroxyapatite crystals. Because 50% of the injected dose is excreted by the kidney, it is important to have the patient well hydrated with frequent voiding to reduce the radiation dose to the bladder wall. The patient is imaged two to four hours following intravenous injection. Normal radionuclide uptake is seen at areas of tendon insertion, constant stresses and osseous remodeling, and the epiphyseal plates in children (17, 18).

Three-phase bone scintigraphy is composed of a radionuclide angiogram, an immediate postinjection blood pool image, and a three to four hour delayed image. Tc-99 MDP is injected into a peripheral vein removed from the area of interest. Dynamic visualization of the blood flow is achieved by rapid sequence pictures taken one to three seconds apart as the blood approaches the extremity. This radionuclide angiogram is complemented by an immediate static blood pool image that quantifies the relative hyperemia or ischemia of the extremity. The delayed image follows these preliminary steps three to four hours later. Thus information is first obtained about the relative arterial supply of the area examined, then about the relative arterial blood present in the capillary and venous system, and finally about the regional rates of bone metabolism (19–24).

Tc-99m pyrophosphate (Pyp) is an older bone scanning agent that has been discarded for skeletal imaging because of its relatively poor image quality, which results from soft tissue activity. However, because it accumulates well in muscle tissue undergoing necrosis, it has become useful in the evaluation of myocardial infarction. The same ability to locate damaged, nonviable muscle has application in the lower extremities in thermal, electrical, and other injuries (25–27).

Gallium-67 (Ga-67) citrate is a diagnostic tracer used for neoplasms and inflammatory disorder localization. It is known that Ga-67 binds to white blood cells, plasma proteins, transferrin, ferritin, lactoferrin, and siderophores and travels to areas of inflammation. It is not as dependent on blood flow as Tc-99m MDP. Imaging is performed 6 to 24 hours following injection for infections and 24 to 72 hours for tumor evaluation. The half-life is quite long (78 hours) and excretion is by the kidneys (28–31).

Indium-111 (In-111) oxine white blood cells is another inflammatory imaging radiopharmaceutical. It binds to the cytoplasmic components of the white blood cell membrane. High radiation exposure is seen in the spleen and liver because of white blood cell destruction at these locations. In-111 may be more accurate in detecting acute infections, while Ga-67 may be more sensitive in assessing subacute and chronic infections. In-111 does not localize in neoplasms. Because of their high affinity for platelets, they may be used in the detection of thrombotic disease. In-111 oxine white blood cells has many advantages over Ga-67 for inflammatory imaging. Ga-67 imaging may be delayed because of slow blood flow and slow tissue clearance of the radionuclide. Ga-67 has poor physical imaging characteristics, emitting many low energy photons with a relatively large radiation dose (28, 32–38).

Tc-99m macroaggregated albumin (MAA) is an important tool in assessing capillary bed perfusion in diabetics, patients with atherosclerotic disease, and others with dysvascular feet. Its primary medical application has been in imaging pulmonary microcirculation but use in the lower extremities has led to valuable diagnostic information regarding the healing potential of ischemic ulcers (39).

Thallium-201 (TI-201) has also been used to assess foot perfusion. It is commonly used as an agent to study myocardial perfusion under stress and rest conditions. TI-201 has the advantage of intravenous administration with the resultant ability to image both extremities at the same time. To obtain bilateral imaging with Tc-99m MAA, a translumbar aortic catheter must be used for the intra-arterial infusion of the MAA, an invasive procedure. TI-201 may be used for both stress and rest imaging of the lower extremities. Tl-201 injected immediately at the end of exercise will reflect muscular perfusion under conditions of maximum metabolic demand. With time, gradual redistribution of the isotope will occur and muscular perfusion at rest can be determined. In contrast, MAA particles can only be administered during the resting state. TI-201 offers great promise as a tool to quantify capillary perfusion in the lower extremities before and after revascularization surgery or therapeutical manipulations (40–42).

Indications for bone imaging include detection and staging metastatic disease, diagnosing benign and malignant disease, differentiating monostatic versus polyostotic disease, differentiating between osteomyelitis and cellulitis, determining bone viability, infarction, or aseptic necrosis evaluation or radiographically difficult to see fractures and prosthetic joints (for infection or loosening), evaluating osseous healing following either bone grafting or osteotomy procedures, selecting biopsy sites, evaluating pain that is not clearly nonskeletal in origin particularly where the pain is ill-defined or diffuse, and skeletal survey searching for the cause of a significantly elevated alkaline phosphatase such as in Paget's disease.

Increased blood flow to an extremity will result in greater nuclide uptake. Vascular insufficiency results in poor delineation of bone in that extremity. Infarction (sickle cell infarct), aseptic necrosis, or congestive heart failure result in decreased uptake. Areas of decreased uptake are referred to as photopenic or photon-deficient. Osteoporosis shows a generalized decrease in tracer uptake. Metabolic bone disorders may also be apparent on bone scans by virtue of an unusually low, unusually high, or spotty bone accretion (28).

Increased uptake is seen following loss of sympathetic control (sympathectomy) in stoke and certain cases of neuropathy. Focal abnormalities of bone such as fractures, osteomyelitis, infarction, or new growths may interrupt the interosseous sympathetics and produce this hyperemic effect. Tracer uptake may be seen in cases of plantar fasciitis, Reiter's syndrome, and reflex sympathetic dystrophy (28,43).

Technetium phosphate compounds have a proposed two-phase mechanism for deposition in bone. The vascular phase is dependent on increased blood flow to bone. The bone phase is dependent upon the radionuclide interaction. Therefore it is vital that there be an adequate amount of viable bone for radionuclide exchange because sending an increased amount of tracer to an area is not enough to demonstrate an increased uptake on bone scans. Conversely, an increase in vascular supply is needed to bring the radionuclide to that area, if increased uptake is to be evident (17, 28, 44).

Technetium phosphate compounds have been used predominently in the diagnosis of hematogenous osteomyelitis. A well defined focus of increased radioactivity in the bone image with an identical area on the blood pool image is seen. In chronic osteomyelitis, the extent of a nonviable bone sequestrum (photon deficient) is accurately defined, as well as a viable bone involucrum, shown as an increased uptake caused by new bone formation. Increased uptake in the involved area is noted for as long as six months following clinical recovery from osteomyelitis due to the long period of osteogenesis occurring in the involved area. Technetium bone scans cannot be used to assess the progression of antibiotic therapy (19, 20, 28). Cellulitis produces a diffuse increase in radioactivity involving the soft tissue and the bone in both the blood pool and bone images. Septic arthritis has a similar appearance because of the hyperemia involving the joint (19) (Fig. 3.43, 3.44).

Because technetium is a bone imaging radionuclide and gallium is an inflammatory imaging nuclide, combined scans may give more information than either scan alone. If both gallium and technetium are used, technetium should be given first, followed in 24 to 48 hours with gallium (17). A positive technetium scan and negative gallium scan is indicative of chronic osteomyelitis. A negative technetium scan and a positive gallium scan represents cellulitis. A positive technetium scan and a positive gallium scan reveals active acute osteomyelitis or septic arthritis. A normal scan is one in which both the technetium and gallium scans are negative. Lisbona and Rosenthall (45) believe that cellulitis is generally defined more clearly by gallium than by technetium blood pool images and that gallium was more accurate in the pediatric group because of the increased concentration of technetium normally seen at the epiphyseal plates (28, 44–46).

Occasionally the pathological area is cold on scanning and this false negative may result in a misdi-

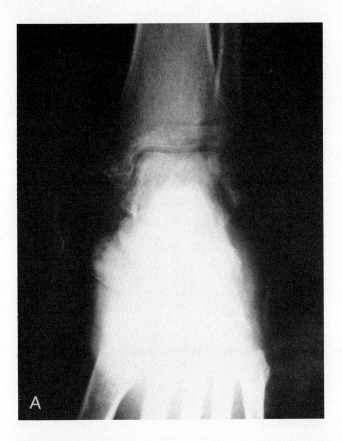

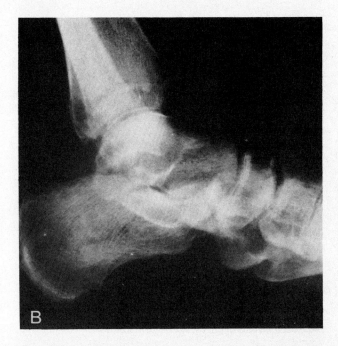

Figure 3.43. (A) Anteroposterior and (B) lateral views of right ankle six weeks following ankle arthroplasty and ankle stabilization procedure. Postoperative infection was diagnosed and treated five days following surgery. Note erosive changes present in midfoot, rearfoot, and ankle.

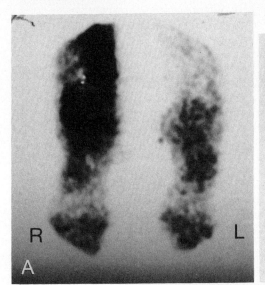

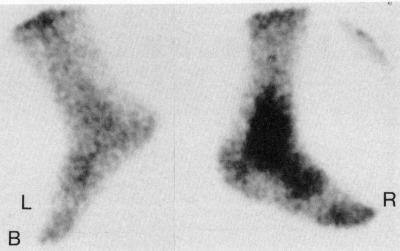

Figure 3.44. (A) Anteroposterior and (B) lateral scintigraphic scans of both ankles following injection with Technetium-99m MDP. Note "hot spots" in area of midfoot, rearfoot, and ankle of right side. Osteomyelitis was confirmed following surgery.

agnosis. The cold phase is hypothesized to be the result of vessel thrombosis and ischemia. Following surgical or spontaneous relief of pressure by decompression of the intraosseous or subperiosteal pus, hyperemia results with the subsequent deposition of increased amounts of radionuclide. The gallium scan is sometimes more effective in demonstrating acute osteomyelitis. Therefore a gallium scan is recom-

mended if a routine technetium bone scan is nondiagnostic (44, 45, 47, 48) (Fig. 3.45).

Bone scanning in the neurotrophic foot for the detection of osteomyelitis offers few advantages. An increased uptake may be the result of a true infection but it is difficult to differentiate this from a repair process secondary to a previous neurotrophic destructive process. Constant bony remodeling will frequently

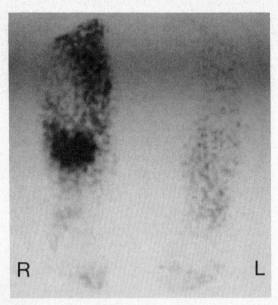

Figure 3.45. Positive 24-hour gallium scan supports diagnosis of acute osteomyelitis of patient in Figs. 3.43 and 3.44.

present with a positive technetium scan. Bone biopsy and bone culture are more reliable in diagnosis (28, 44).

A radiographic skeletal survey is fairly expensive, quite specific, and imposes a large radiographic exposure to the patient. The bone scan is currently the procedure of choice in the search for osseous metastatic disease. Bone scanning is very sensitive but even more expensive and nonspecific. It may predict occult metastatic lesions. The major downfall is its nonspecificity with a considerable number of false positive readings. Therefore all positive findings should be correlated with clinical data and additional radiographic evaluation to represent true positive (metastatic) from false positive (benign) results (45).

Differentiation between benign and malignant lesions is readily seen with bone scanning. Most tumors, unless a purely lytic process, are represented by an increase in tracer concentration on bone scans (Figs. 3.46, 3.47). Malignant lesions tend to be more hyperemic than benign lesions in the blood pool images. Technetium presents with diffusely increased activity in the adjacent epiphysis and metaphysis in malignant lesions but not in benign lesions. Therefore if increased activity in contiguous bone is present in the scan, the lesion is more likely to be malignant (28, 50, 51).

Ga-67 is a more reliable tracer for differentiating between benign and malignant lesions. It is also more accurate in delineating the local extent of primary bone tumors. Gallium scans generally show a marked increase in scintigraphic intensity in patients with malignant disease (except chondrosarcomas). The lesion is usually benign if a gallium scan shows no increase in activity. A mild increase in activity is usually attributed to benign lesions (50).

Unlike technetium scans, gallium scans do not demonstrate the diffuse increase activity in the con-

tiguous bone with malignant lesions. Thus gallium scans demonstrate the amount of local extension of a tumor better than a technetium scan. In both gallium and technetium scans the local extent of a malignant lesion was not underestimated (50).

Bone fracture is evident on a technetium scan by evidence of tracer uptake. Fractures can be revealed within seven hours following injury. Failure to reveal focal uptake excludes the diagnosis of fracture. The use of imaging to detect multiple injuries in the battered child syndrome will minimize radiation doses (28, 38, 52).

Bone scanning has been found to be especially important in the early diagnosis of stress fractures (Figs. 3.48, 3.49). Stress fractures or fatigue fractures occur primarily in the lower extremity because of unaccustomed strenuous activities. Previously most commonly found in military recruits, today stress fractures predominate in sports enthusiasts such as ballet dancers, long-distance runners, joggers, and weekend athletes. The metatarsals, calcaneus, tibia, femur and pelvis are most commonly involved. Radiographic confirmation is made by evidence of the healing phase, either medullary sclerosis in metaphyseal areas or periosteal new bone formation in diaphyseal areas. Confirmation of a stress fracture by routine radiographs ranges from three weeks to three months and without the proper diagnosis and treatment continued activity may proceed to a complete fracture. Therefore early diagnosis is imperative (53–55).

Bone scans may be used to differentiate between shin splints or periostitis and stress fractures. If periosteal irritation is present the bone scan shows a focal increase in tracer along the cortical surface of the bone. In stress fractures increased tracer uptake is noted across 50% or more of the cortex (38).

Bone scintigraphy for fractures changes over a period of time with three rather distinct stages being evident. In the acute stage (phase one) a diffuse area of increased tracer concentration about the fracture site persists two to four weeks following injury. In the subacute stage (phase two) a well-defined linear abnormality at the site of the fracture is noted. This phase persists 8 to 12 weeks and shows the most intense uptake at the fracture site. The healing stage (phase three) is characterized by a gradual decrease in the intensity of tracer uptake until it returns to normal. This time extends well beyond the time of clinical or radiographic healing because of the increased metabolic activity occurring during the remodeling process. Patterns may be accelerated in younger patients. When healing results in malalignment, scans remain positive for a much longer time (38, 56).

Atrophic nonunion appears as an area of diminution in radioactivity at the fracture site and reactive nonunion appears as an area of expected or increased tracer. Atrophic nonunion may be seen as a decrease in radionuclide because of the inability of the bone ends to respond properly in the healing process or as an area of essentially absent radioactivity often caused by a pseudarthrosis with an actual synovial-lined cav-

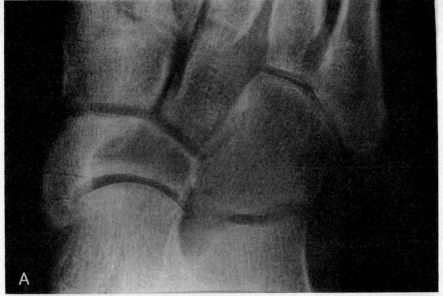

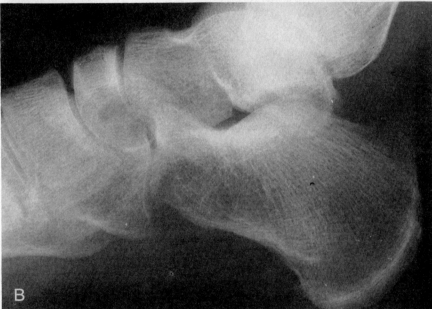

Figure 3.46. (A) Dorsoplantar and (B) lateral radiographs of osteolytic bone tumor of navicular bone, right foot.

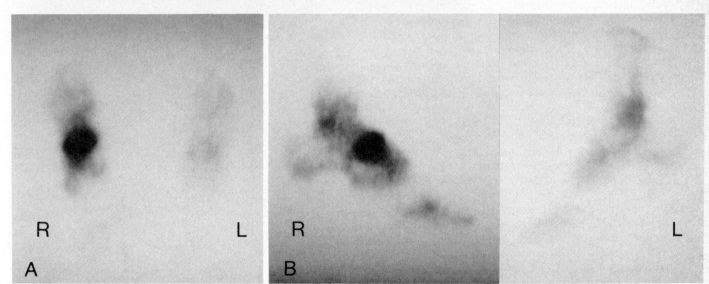

Figure 3.47. (A) Dorsoplantar and (B) lateral technetium scintigraphic scans demonstrating increased uptake in region of tarsal navicular bone. Chondroblastoma was confirmed following surgical excision of tumor.

153

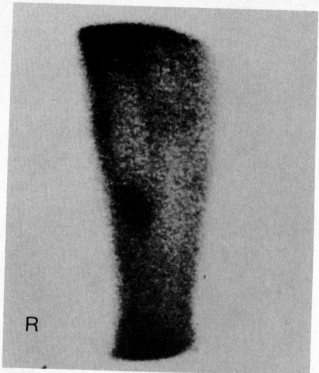

Figure 3.48. Technetium-99 mdp bone scan showing abnormal increased uptake at junction of mid and lower thirds of right leg near tibia. This sharply marginated oval or fusiform area of increased radioactivity is characteristic of stress fracture. Patient had continued symptoms for six weeks. (Reproduced by permission from *J Am Podiatry Assoc* 71:578, Figure 1, 1981.)

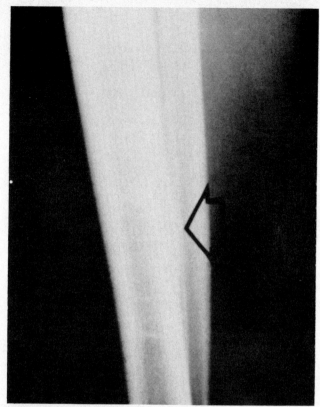

Figure 3.49. Cone down radiographs taken at same time revealed slight irregularity in cortex in one view, indicative of reactive bone. (Reproduced by permission from *J Am Podiatry Assoc* 71:578, Figure 2, 1981.)

ity and synovial fluid, the interposition of soft tissue, the location of an infectious process, or a region of interrupted blood supply (38) (Figs. 3.50, 3.51).

A delayed union does not have a specific radiographic sign differentiating it from nonunion. A study to determine standardized time sequences of radionuclide uptake of osteotomies in humans is needed (38, 56).

Bone scanning before insertion of an electrical stimulating device may enhance the percentage of success. Only the reactive nonunion group has shown significant improvement following percutaneous electrical stimulation (38).

Bone scanning has some merit in evaluating graft viability or nonviability. Increased concentration of radiopharmaceuticals is associated with a viable graft, whereas a nonviable graft does not show this increase (38).

Bone scans aid in the evaluation of postoperative implant arthroplasty. Focal uptake at the stem tip and at the implant collar where implant seats on the bone may be noted with loose implants. Infected joint implants are characterized by a diffuse and marked uptake of tracer. Comparison of a technetium and gallium scan has merit. A positive technetium scan and negative gallium scan usually indicates implant loosening, ectopic bone, heterotropic bone, or normal bone reaction. When both scans are positive and are con-

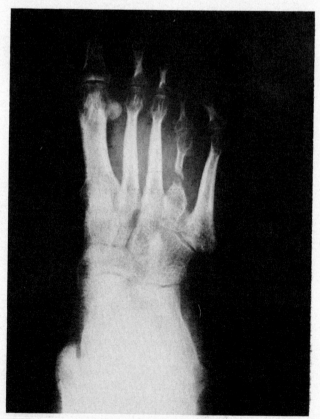

Figure 3.50. Atrophic nonunion following bone grafting for brachymetatarsia is noted.

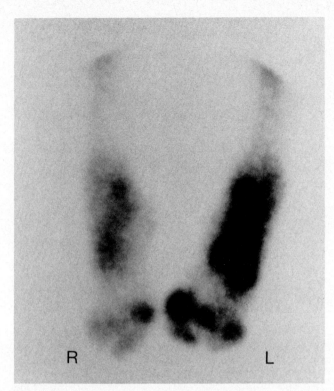

Figure 3.51. Technetium bone scan shows decreased uptake in region of fourth metatarsal right foot corresponding to lack of bone healing.

gruent (of similar size and shape) again, only implant loosening, ectopic bone, heterotropic bone, or normal bone reaction is suggested. Infection is a possibility where an intensely positive gallium scan is noted. Infection is very likely in incongruent scans where the technetium scan is larger than the gallium scan. Bursitis, cellulitis, or some other nonbony problem should be considered when the gallium scan is larger than the technetium scan (56).

COMPUTERIZED TOMOGRAPHY

Hounsfield first demonstrated the usefulness of computerized tomography (CT) in England in 1967. CT, first introduced in the United States in 1973 at the Mayo Clinic and Massachusetts General Hospital, was initially used to evaluate the brain. Ledley in 1974 introduced the whole body scanner at the Georgetown University Medical Center. The technique is safe, noninvasive and essentially without complications (57–59)

CT is synonymous with computerized transverse axial tomography (CTAT), computer-assisted tomography or computerized axial tomography (CAT), computerized tomography (CT), reconstructive tomography (RT), and computerized transaxial transmission reconstructive tomography (CTT)(60). CT reconstructs a complete cross-sectional plane of the body with minimal superimposition of body structures. In conventional radiography, low density soft tissue

structures are often obscured by more dense (i.e. bone) structure because of extensive superimposition of the various body structures. Conventional tomography minimizes superimposition at the expense of image blurring and decreased contrast due to increased scatter radiation. Both radiography and tomography fail to demonstrate slight differences in contrast of soft tissue body structures. CT can resolve differences in adjacent tissue densities as low as 0.5% (58). It cannot differentiate a homogeneous object of nonuniform thickness from a uniformly thick object of varying composition (60).

By visualizing cross sectional anatomy in CT scanning, unwanted planes or layers of the body's anatomy are eliminated. The specific location of pathological areas can be determined with extreme accuracy (58).

CT uses a scanning gantry that houses an x-ray generator and detector system, a data processing system (computer), a viewing console (cathode ray tube), and a storage system (computer). Cost varies from several hundred thousand to 1 million dollars (61–62).

At present there have been four generations of scanners. First and second generation scanners work on the rotate/translate principle. In first generation scanners a single x-ray beam and one or two detectors rotate in 1° increments a total of 180° around the patient's head taking 4.5 to 5.5 minutes per scan. Multiple cross sections tremendously increase examination time. Second generation scanners use a fan beam scanning technique and multiple detectors, thus increasing the angular increments and decreasing scanning time to .5 to 3.5 minutes. Spatial resolution is also improved. Third generation scanners use a continuously rotating pulsed fan belt with an array of detectors decreasing scanning time to 5 to 10 seconds. Multiple fixed detectors forming a ring around the object, as well as a moving x-ray source around the object, through 360° further minimizes the time to 2 to 10 seconds in fourth generation scanners (Fig. 3.52).

Fifth generation scanners are presently in production at the Mayo Clinic (58, 60, 61, Syllabus for the categorical course on computed body tomography. Presented at the annual meeting of the American Ray Society, New Orleans, May 9–14, 1982, pp 1–17). This combination of multiple detectors with a moving x-ray tube around the part results in several thousand measurements of x-ray intensity. The varying x-ray attenuation values are converted to electrical signals and rapidly collected by a computer and displayed as a matrix composed of picture elements (pixels) displayed on a cathode ray screen. Each voxel (volume element) represents the area of the pixel multiplied by the thickness of the slice (58–60, 63, 64) (Fig. 3.53).

The various attenuation values can be displayed as a digital readout expressed as computed tomography numbers (or Hounsfield numbers) ranging from −1000 for air, 0 for water, and +1000 for dense bone. These readings can be translated into a gray scale where higher densities appear white, lower densities

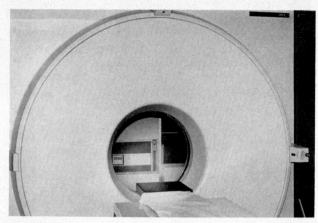

Figure 3.52. Gantry of fourth generation scanner. Multiple fixed detectors form ring around object and x-ray source moves 360° around object.

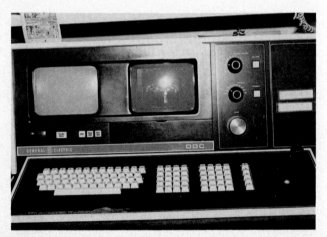

Figure 3.53. Data processing system (computer), viewing console (cathode ray tube), and storage system (computer).

appear black, with varying shades of gray for densities in between. A color image may also be produced. A magnetic tape or disc stores the data (58–60, 63, 64).

With the information stored in a computer, the printed readout may be altered in many ways. Density and contrast changes, as well as magnification of the image, may be produced. Sagittal and coronal sections may be produced without the need for additional radiation exposure to the patient (58).

The radiation dose of each slice is approximately equivalent to a single conventional x-ray. With the need for several slices, the exposure increases and is more comparable to that received in barium studies of the gastrointestinal tract, angiography, or polytomography. To compensate for a shortened scanning time of the newer units, the dose of irradiation must be increased somewhat and the average radiation absorbed dose (rad) at the skin surface in some of the new machines ranges between 0.5 and 3.0 (62).

Very thin slices for optimum detail range from 1.5 mm to 5 mm. The thickness of the part to be examined should be considered to determine the thickness of each slice. Although thinner slices provide

more accurate resolution, more slices would be required, increasing radiation exposure to the patient. Slices of bone are usually 0.5 cm thick and soft tissue lesions are 1.0 cm thick. The charge for an examination varies with the number of slices needed and ranges from $150 to $400 per study (58, 61, 62).

Most examinations require 15 to 30 minutes or longer, thus limiting the use of the scanner to 15 to 30 examinations per eight-hour day. Where adequate contrast in detail is available, the resolving power of conventional radiography is better than that of CT (58).

The podiatric uses of CT are increasing. CT can establish the presence and nature of tumors. The exact location will aid in accurate percutaneous aspirational biopsy of deep lesions and may negate the need for open surgery. CT has enhanced the success of en bloc resection surgery for malignant tumors. The precise knowledge of tumor location, size, margination, and involvement of vital nervous, vascular, and osseous structures may be determined. Muscle and soft tissue involvement may also be delineated. The extent of the neoplasm in cross section is accurately delineated; its longitudinal extent may also be delineated. At least one scan above and below the mass should be normal. If a tumor has close proximity to neighboring blood vessels, a contrast medium is needed to enhance its identification. A scan of the opposite, normal, extremity should be done for comparison (57, 64, 65). The density and invasive characteristics are noted. Tissue density differences of approximately 25% may be detected (66).

Elevation of the attentuation values in the marrow space of long bones is an early sign of acute osteomyelitis. The progression and/or recession of disease may be closely monitored (59) (Figs. 3.54, 3.55).

Fine structures of internal bone architecture and trabecular bone mineralization changes within an accuracy of plus or minus 2% may be detected by high resolution CT scanners. Thus noninvasive clinical investigations of aseptic necrosis, osteoporosis, osteomalacia, and other metabolic bone diseases may be obtained (57, 59, 67). Changes in mineralization during any regimen of therapy may be serially assessed (61). Muscular atrophy and hypertrophy may also be evaluated (64). Use of CT for diagnosis of a rare plantar ganglion cyst in a child has been reported (68). CT has been used to evaluate unilateral extremity swelling (69).

CT has use in evaluating trauma. Metatarsal stress fractures may be evaluated. Calcaneal or talar fractures with involvement of the subtalar joint and fractures otherwise invisible by conventional radiography may be evaluated (Figs. 3.56, 3.57). Fractures and dislocation of the midtarsus will be more readily detected (59).

CT is most promising for the diagnosis of tarsal coalition and degenerative changes of the tarsus or lesser tarsus where superimposition during conventional techniques has always presented a problem.

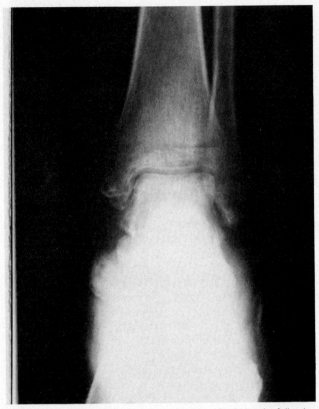

Figure 3.54. Anteroposterior view of right ankle six weeks following postoperative infection.

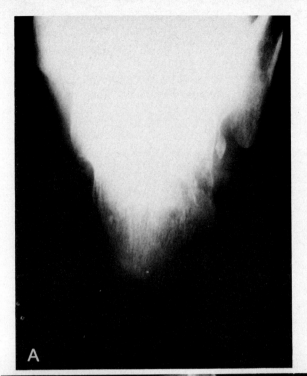

A

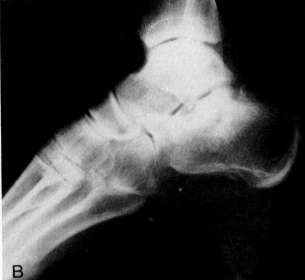

B

Figure 3.56. (A) Axial calcaneal and (B) lateral projection of foot reveals calcaneal fracture that is difficult to visualize.

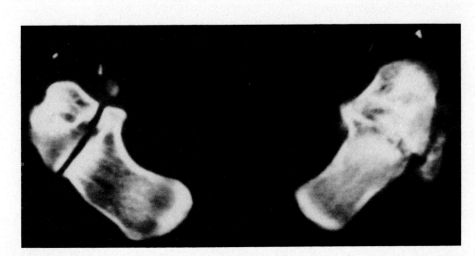

Figure 3.55. Computerized tomography in frontal plane of ankle and rearfoot showing severe degenerative changes characteristic of osteomyelitis in right foot and normal left foot.

Accessibility to the small joints of the feet are provided with high resolution CT (64).

A scout film should always be taken before the computerized tomographic study. This indicates the level that is being scanned. Figure 3.58 demonstrates

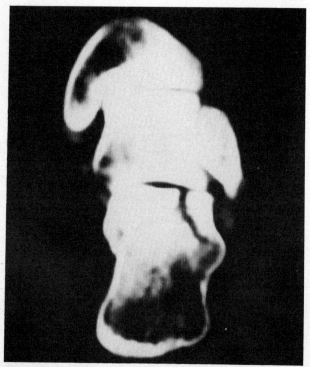

Figure 3.57. Frontal plane computerized tomogram clearly shows the intra-articular nature of this difficult to manage calcaneal fracture.

a scout film of the rearfoot (subtalar joint) and ankle joint. Vertical lines demonstrate each section that is going to be taken. Figure 3.59 demonstrates the first slice in this series. At this level the ankle joint and subtalar joint are visualized. The epiphyseal plates of the tibia and fibular are still open. The calcaneal apophysis is also noted. Figure 3.60 represents a slice more anterior (distal) to the previous slice. Here the subtalar joint is shown. The posterior and middle facets are clearly open. The sustentaculum tali is evident. Figure 3.61 represents a similar section demonstrating a middle facet subtalar joint coalition. There is osseous fusion of the talus and calcaneus at this level.

Figure 3.62 demonstrates a scout film of the midfoot (midtarsal joint). Again the vertical lines demonstrate each section that is going to be taken. Figure 3.63 shows a clear appearance of the navicular and cuboid. Figure 3.64 is more anterior than Figure 3.63 and demonstrates the cuboid and three cuneiform bones. Figure 3.65 is more anterior to Figure 3.64 and demonstrates the five metatarsal bones.

The use of CT in research is limited only by one's imagination. Bone growth and development, the nature of clubfoot and other congenital foot deformities, the anatomical distortions secondary to paralytic foot disorders, and metabolic disorders may all be more easily understood.

Optimally all foot examinations should be done with the patient weight bearing. This is impossible in CT scanning because most gantry diameters are less than 60 cm. With a movable extension table raised to about 10% and with knee and hip flexion with the patient supine, an accurate talocalcaneal relationship

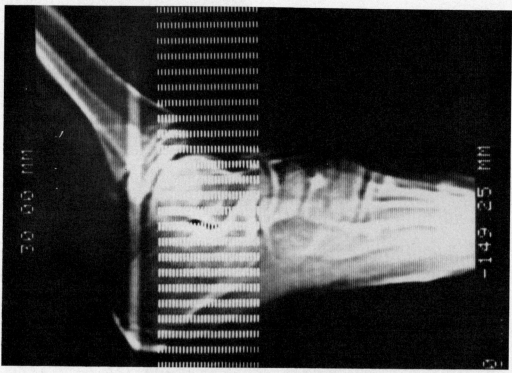

Figure 3.58.   Scout film of ankle and rearfoot.

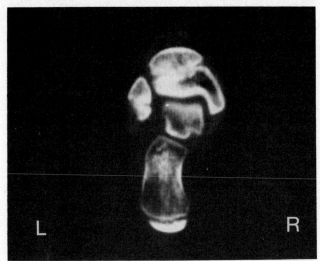

Figure 3.59. Frontal plane section through normal ankle and rear-foot.

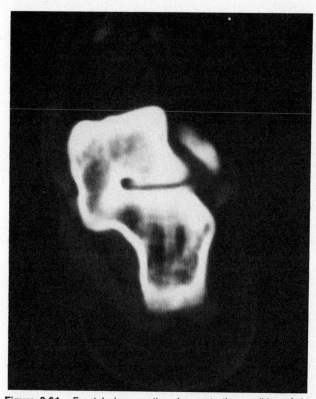

Figure 3.61. Frontal plane section demonstrating coalition of the middle facet of subtalar joint.

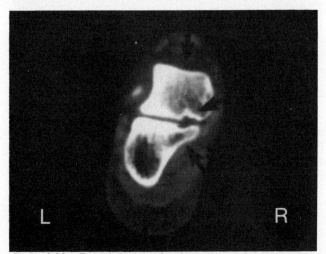

Figure 3.60. Frontal plane section through normal subtalar joint.

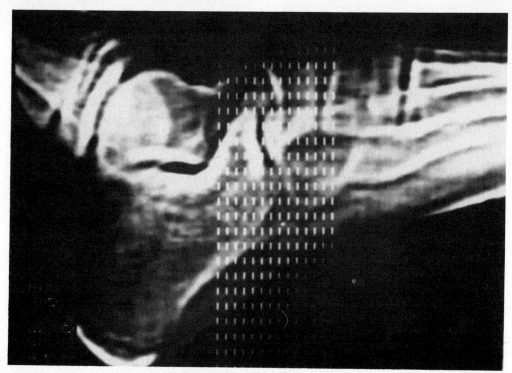

Figure 3.62. Scout film of midfoot.

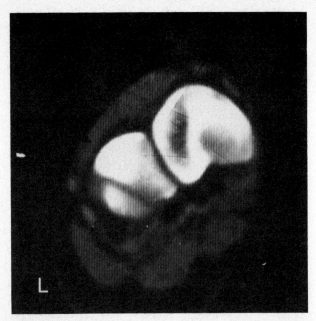

Figure 3.63.   Frontal plane section through normal navicular and cuboid bones.

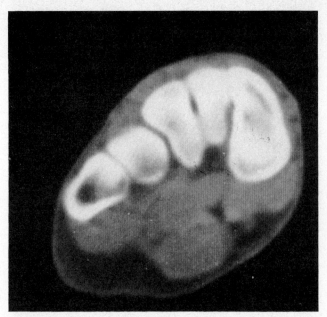

Figure 3.65.   Frontal plane section through normal metatarsals.

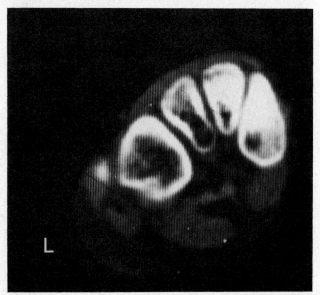

Figure 3.64.   Frontal plane section through normal cuboid and cuneiforms.

may be assessed. The gantry and the x-ray beam may be tilted to accommodate various needed changes (70).

CT scanners today cost $550,000 to $750,000 or more. The estimated annual operating cost is $250,000 to $400,000. Thus it is obvious that a unit must be fully used to make it cost effective. Increasing the mean operating time each week is one consideration. Use of a mobile unit, shared by several hospitals, is also cost effective. The American College of Radiology has adopted CT guidelines to justify purchase of a unit. These are (a) an unserved population of 150,000 people, (b) a hospital with 250 acute beds, and (c) current performance of 30,000 general imaging procedures per year (71).

MAGNETIC RESONANCE IMAGING

Magnetic resonance imaging (MRI) is a fairly new technique and its present clinical uses are still very limited and very costly. At present systems range from $600,000 to $1.6 million. It is expected that the future potential uses may surpass the benefits obtained from computerized tomography. Nuclear magnetic resonance (NMR) spectroscopy has played an important role in organic chemistry. The concept was first introduced in 1946 and imaging has been used since 1973. In 1980 the first clinically useful images were produced in various research centers. This noninvasive technique is harmless to the patient. There is no exposure to ionizing radiation or to radioactive isotopes. The system is very similar to CT scanners except that it uses a magnetic gantry in lieu of the moving x-ray tube and detectors. It is hoped that with the continued marketing of the scanners, the cost will decline (72–75).

MRI uses a strong uniform magnetic field in the range of 1000 to 3000 gauss, approximately 7000 times stronger than the earth's magnetic field. Three pairs of coils produce two-dimensional localization. One pair of coils produces excitation in the longitudinal plane. The other two coils are superimposed to form a gradient passing transversely through the body. These two gradients may then be used to localize a given point in the body. The current in the gradient coils and electromagnetic coils is provided by a power supply. No moving parts or physical movement of the patient is required. Electrical conductivity controls the direction of the second magnetic field gradient in MRI scanning. At the beginning of a procedure the patient is aligned to the anatomical reference point of three laser beams, localizing the specific region to be examined. The magnets and coils are housed in a structure resembling a CT scanner gantry that is operated by a control panel. A computer and image handling unit (cathode ray screen) completes the equipment (72).

Only nuclei with an odd number of nucleons (protons or neutrons) produce a net spin and therefore lend themselves to MRI spectroscopy or tomography (75). MRI measures the reaction of hydrogen atoms (photons) when exposed to a powerful magnetic field. The nucleus of the hydrogen atom spins and generates a small magnetic field. Water has a high content of photons and thus MRI discreetly measures the water content of various body tissues. CT only measures the specific gravity. Because tumors differ from the surrounding tissues primarily in water content rather than specific gravity, MRI would be a more useful diagnostic tool over CT. The main potential use of MRI is in the evaluation of myocardial ischemia, cerebral vascular accidents, and cerebral edema (73). The brain or any body part can be imaged by MRI in any desired cross sectional plane: transverse, coronal, or sagittal (Fig. 3.66).

The use of MRI in musculoskeletal evaluation in the lower extremities is quite different from that of CT. Bone is invisible in MRI, making the soft tissue structures even more so detectable. Therefore we may see an upswing in the use of MRI for detecting tumors, angiography, and the effects of radiation therapy and chemotherapy (72). MRI may be particularly good at detecting necrotic tissue and degenerative diseases of various kinds. At this time the full potential of MRI is still not unveiled. The Food and Drug Administration (FDA) presently limits the use of MRI tomography to research geared toward determining clinical efficacy. Much research is still needed but it is expected that MRI will have a tremendous impact on clinical usefulness.

TOMOGRAPHY*

(* This section is taken in part from Schlefman BS, Katz FN: Tomographic interpretation of the subtalar joint. J Am Podiatry Assoc 73:65–69, 1983.)

The radiographic technique of tomography was pioneered in 1922 by Bocage, who called it moving film roentgenograms. Since that time it has been described as stratigraphy by Vallebona (76), planigraphy by Ziedses des Plantes (77), and laminography by Andrews (78) and Kieffer (79). Grossman (80) first called it tomography, and that is the appropriate term used today.

Tomography minimizes the problem of superimposition that occurs when a three-dimensional object is projected onto a two-dimensional film. One plane or section, known as the focal plane, remains in focus while objects either above or below it will be blurred. Like conventional radiography, tomography requires a source of radiation, an object, and radiographic film. In addition tomography requires that the x-ray source and film move synchronously in opposite directions during exposure. A power source and linkage mechanism are required to provide vibration-free movement (81).

Figure 3.67 demonstrates the tomographic principle. The x-ray source begins at point A and travels along a path to point B during exposure. The film cassette moves in the opposite direction of the x-ray beam from point (a) to point (b). Any object that lies on the focal plane, such as the black dot, will remain in focus on the film. Any object that lies off the focal plane, such as the white dot, will be blurred.

The length of the arc of the radiation source, known as the exposure angle, determines the thickness of the plane of tissue that remains in focus. As the arc

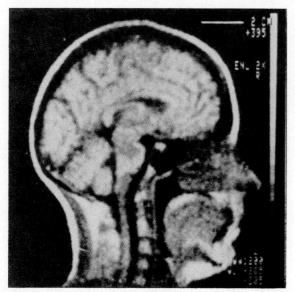

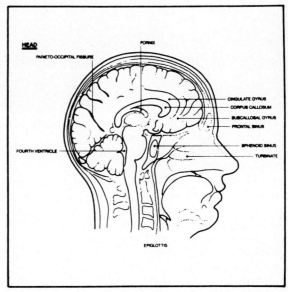

Figure 3.66. MRI of the brain. (Reproduced with permission from Wenstrup BR: Diagnostic imaging with NMR. *The First Ray* 10:21, 1984.)

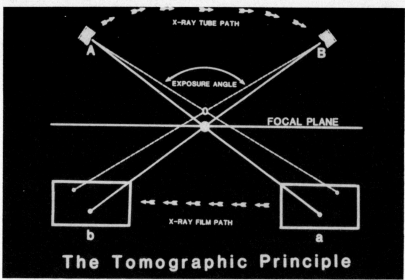

Figure 3.67.   Tomographic principle.

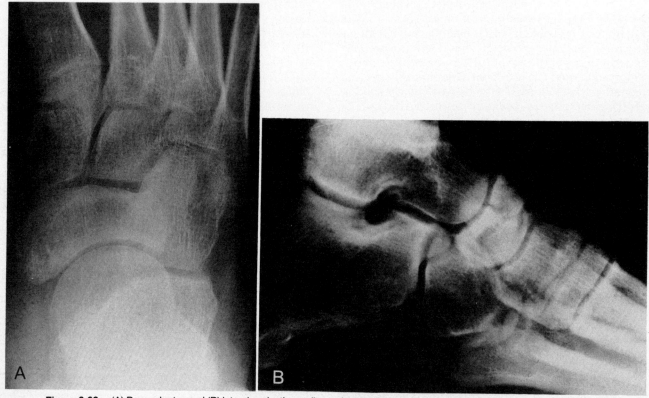

Figure 3.68.   (A) Dorsoplantar and (B) lateral projection radiographs of young man who complained of pain for over one year.

increases (wide-angle tomography) the section thickness decreases (1 to 5 mm) and objects both near to and far from the focal plane will be blurred. In narrow-angle tomography (zonography) the section thickness in focus is increased (1 cm to 2.5 cm). Objects far from the focal plane will be blurred but those near the focal plane will remain in focus. The thickness of the structure or structures to be examined and their proximity to other structures outside the focal plane determines whether a wide or narrow exposure angle should be used. Different sections through the tissue are ob-

tained by changing the focal plane either by adjusting the height of the table top (grossman principle) or by adjusting the height of the fulcrum (planigraphic principle) (81). In the foot, where structures are small and optimum detail with a decrease in overlap is desired, wide angle tomography at multiple focal planes is recommended (82).

Tomography is presently used to aid in the diagnosis of suspected fractures that are not seen on conventional radiographs, especially when complex bone structures are involved (Figs. 3.68A, B, 3.69,

3.70). Brantigan and associates (83) have used stress tomography to diagnose abnormal subtalar joint inversion in association with ankle joint inversion following trauma. DeLee and Curtis (84) used polytomography to identify osteochondral fractures of the subtalar and talonavicular joint following subtalar dislocation.

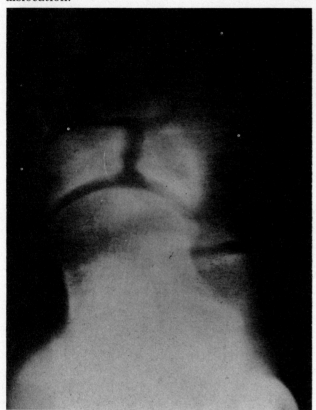

Figure 3.69. Tomogram in dorsoplantar projection revealed unhealed intra-articular fracture of navicular bone.

Beckly and associates (85) report that lateral tomograms of the subtalar joint may help distinguish between a rare anterior talocalcaneal coalition and an anomalous articulation, which is often viewed. Superimposition of the lateral talar articular surface and the posterior margin of the sustentaculum tali on the medial side of the calcaneus may result in this misleading appearance (11). Tomography may also be used in the diagnosis of soft tissue pathological conditions, differentiation between benign and malignant lesions in the lungs, abdominal radiography, intravenous pyelograms, and intravenous cholangiograms (81).

Tomograms disclose exquisite detail of joints, revealing marginal osteophytes and subchrondral cysts that may be obscured in conventional radiographs by the concomitant reactive sclerosis. Therefore tomography has proven to be of value in inflammatory conditions including rheumatoid arthritis.

Tomograms are helpful in the evaluation of adequate placement of internal fixation devices. Followup evaluation of osteotomy or arthrodesis sites may be more critically examined with the aid of tomograms.

Tumor evaluation is enhanced by tomography. Tomograms may be used to see if a soft tissue lesion has penetrated into bone and to evaluate bone lesions more thoroughly. The extent of bone destruction, the status of the cortex of bone, the presence of any periosteal reaction to the lesion, changes in the bone matrix, new bone formation, and the status of the zone of the bone between the disease and normal bone is more readily seen with tomography. Critical calcification permitting the recognition of a cartilaginous tumor, the nidus of an osteoid osteoma, or evidence of a very small tumor may sometimes be seen only with tomography (Figs. 3.71, 3.72).

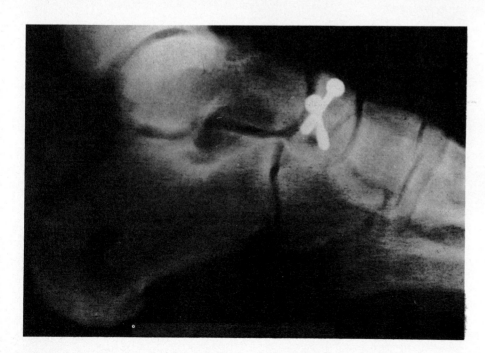

Figure 3.70. Open reduction with ASIF screw fixation remedied patient's problem.

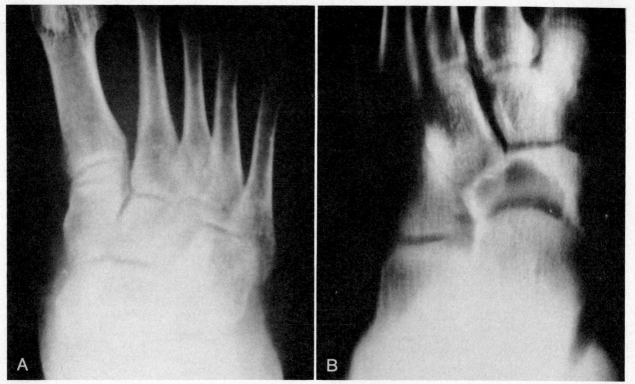

Figure 3.71. (A) Mild radiolucency is noted in body of navicular but extent of any space occupying lesion is not evident. (B) Dorsoplantar tomogram reveals full extent of this lytic tumor. Pathological diagnosis was chondroblastoma following surgical resection and packing with homologous bone graft.

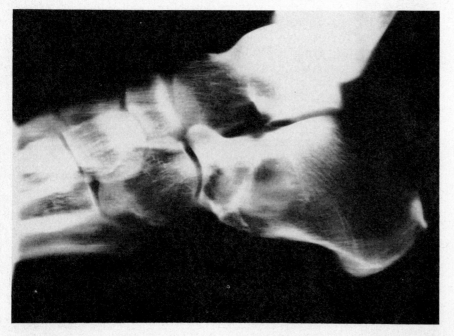

Figure 3.72. Lytic lesion of calcaneus.

XERORADIOGRAPHY

Xeroradiography was invented by Chester F. Carlson, a physicist and patent attorney, in 1937. Medical usage was begun in 1952 by John F. Roach at the Albany Medical College and its use for mammography was implemented in 1966 by J.N. Wolfe. Xerography does not use a photochemical process as is used in conventional roentgenography. It is a dry, photoelectric process using metal plates coated with selenium, a semiconductor, instead of conventional silver bromide coated film (90, 91).

Xerographic plates contain an aluminum base with a thin layer of vitreous selenium, a photoconductor. The plate is stored in a cassette that protects it from surface damage and exposure to ambient light.

The plate is inserted into a charging unit where a voltage potential is established placing a positive electrostatic charge on the free surface of the selenium layer. The plate is now charged and may be exposed to an x-ray beam as is done in conventional roentgenography. The photoconductor is discharged in amounts proportional to the densities through which the radiation passes producing an electrostatic charge pattern of the part examined. The plate is placed into a developing unit containing the toner, a blue, negatively charged plastic powder. The toner is attached to the plate in amounts proportional to the remaining positive charge. The powder image is then transferred from the plate to a plastic coated paper. Pressure and heat are required during this process to produce the final product (90, 92–95).

A small residue of toner usually remains on the plate after use, so the plate must be prepared for reuse. A relaxing unit is used to clean and neutralize the plate. Heat (135° C.) for 30 seconds will clear any remaining electrical memory and prevent a faint "ghost" image appearing along with a new image (90).

Positive and negative mode xerography are available. In the positive mode, areas of the subject that would be white on conventional films are rendered as a deep blue and other densities appear as varying shades between white and blue. A negative xerograph has the same tonal relationships as x-ray film; exposed areas are dark blue and unexposed areas are white (90, 91, 93).

Because of the phenomenon of edge enhancement, fine definition and contrast gradation are appreciated on the xeroradiogram. There is a slight increase of powder on one side and a slight decrease on the other side of a boundary of the electrostatic charge. Therefore the edges are accentuated so that normal structures and pathological lesions are clearly demarcated. On the other hand, differences in object density over a broad area are recorded with greater contrast on the conventional roentgenographic film system (90–92).

The kVp used in foot xerography is 120 kVp and the mAs varies from 10 to 40 mAs. Therefore the amount of radiation exposure is greater per film than conventional screen x-ray film. However, fewer xerograms are required to achieve superior diagnosis, and therefore the total radiation exposure is less than with conventional x-ray film. The radiation exposure is less per film compared to nonscreen film radiography (90, 94).

Xerography is less useful for trunk examinations because of the thickness of the part and therefore the increase of radiation needed. The thickness of the photoconductive layer determines the speed of the xerograph. It is increased with thicker selenium layers because there is more change from interaction with the x-rays (94).

The materials used for xeroradiography are insensitive to radiation and therefore cannot be destroyed by accidental exposure. The image can be viewed by ordinary room light because the image is opaque (94).

Xeroradiographs record the sharp differences in densities, as in fractures, better than do conventional films. Visualization of trabecular patterns, hairline fractures, subtle trauma of cortical margins, soft tissue damage, joint effusion, ligament trauma, the arthritides, and casted extremity evaluation is improved with xeroradiography. Subcutaneous swelling, tears of the gastrocnemius and Achilles tendon and hematomas are also better visualized. Metabolic bone disease such as periosteal bone resorption of hyperthyroidism may be demonstrated by xerograms. Intermetatarsal neuromas appear as an asteroid (star shaped) shadow as compared to the surrounding globular looking fatty tissue (90, 96).

Griffiths and D'Orsi (97) demonstrated the use of xerography with double-contrast arthrography to demonstrate damage to soft tissue, the cruciate ligaments, and bone with one lateral exposure of the knee.

The use of xeroradiography in the detection of foreign bodies in soft tissue has been reviewed. Metallic foreign bodies are imaged equally well on both xerograms and conventional radiograms. Glass, chicken bone, fish bone, and gravel are imaged slightly better on xerograms. Wood, rubber, graphite (lead pencil), and a plastic pick show much better visualization on xerograms (98).

Routine extremity studies for the detection of metallic foreign bodies should be performed with negative imaging. Positive images are especially useful for visualization of silicone joint replacement prostheses and other nonmetallic foreign objects such as graphite, wood, and plaster. Glass is equally well visualized in both imaging modes (90, 98).

FLUOROSCOPY

Today computerized fluoroscopy and image intensification are being used more widely, replacing traditional film studies. The images formed have low electrical interference, moderate resolution, and a satisfactory diagnostic quality.

The x-ray beam, having passed through the patient, is absorbed by a layer of cesium iodide (CsI) phosphor in the image intensifier. This produces light that is detected by electronics within this glass enclosed vacuum. The light is then electronically amplified and is emitted by the image intensifier by another light-emitting phosphor. A television camera converts the light intensity into an electric current with formation of a video image that is displayed on a television monitor. The scanning rate is very fast and the observer only sees a two-dimensional image on the television screen. The image may be further processed by the computer and stored on tapes or discs for later visualization. Thus with the aid of computerized fluoroscopy one can obtain a visual two-dimensional video picture (99).

The initial use of computerized fluoroscopy has been in the area of intravenous angiography. Podiatric uses include localization of foreign bodies to aid surgical removal, aid in closed reduction of fractures, and proper evaluation of internal fixation devices used in fracture repair, arthrodesis, and osteotomy procedures.

The C-arm machine is a portable fluoroscopic unit that is commonly used in the operating room. X-rays are produced continuously on demand to give a real-time, dynamic x-ray image that is displayed on a television screen (Figs. 3.73 and 3.74). The operator depresses the foot pedal to yield the fluoroscopic image. The longer the fluoroscope is producing x-rays, the greater the radiation dose absorbed. The amount of radiation dose must always be kept in mind and kept to a minimum. All personnel and the patient in the operating room should be shielded with a lead apron (100).

The lixiscope is a portable, hand-held fluoroscope where an x-ray image is first converted to a visible light image by a scintillator or phosphor converter and then into an electron image by a photocathode. The image may be recorded on fast instant processing films or other image recording and processing devices. The radiation exposure is far lower than with conventional radiography. Other benefits appear to be in the evaluation of joint structure and function because the part can be viewed through a range of motion. The action of joint implants may be observed. Magnification of the bony architecture is noted. Some of the drawbacks presently include its poor resolution, considerable expertise is needed before use, and it has insufficient penetrating power thoroughly to examine thicker structures such as the rearfoot (101).

ARTHROGRAPHY

Arthrography is the radiology of a joint to evaluate its soft tissue structures. It uses an injection of a contrast material, usually a water-soluble iodinated medium. Plain films should always be taken first to rule out bony pathology and to establish correct exposure factors. The skin is prepped using an antiseptic solution and draped with sterile towels. Arthrography can be performed on any joint but its use is limited in the small joints of the foot. This discussion will be limited to ankle and subtalar joint arthrography (102, 103).

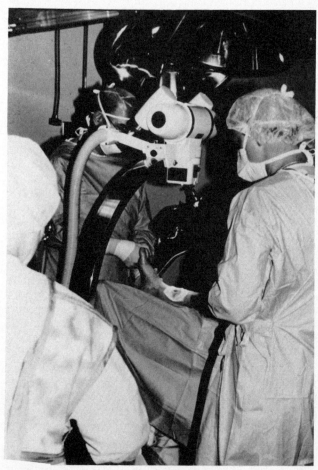

Figure 3.73. C-arm is noted. Part would be placed within "C" before imaging. Sterile field can be easily maintained.

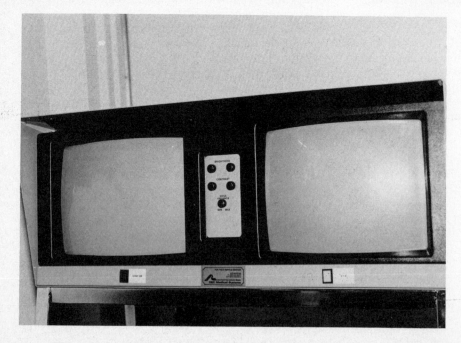

Figure 3.74. Image is noted on television screen.

The ankle joint is entered anteromedially between the tendons of m. tibialis anterior and m. extensor hallucis longus with a 1½ inch, 20 or 22 gauge needle (Fig. 3.75). Where medial damage is suspected, the injection is made further lateralward. Fluoroscopic control is advantageous but not mandatory. Following puncture into the joint space a local anesthetic is infiltrated and any joint effusion is aspirated. The syringe is then changed to one containing the contrast material. A 30% to 50% solution of contrast medium is used. Approximately 5 to 10 cc of contrast material may be injected into a normal joint, depending on pain or resistance as a limiting factor. In excess of 10 cc and up to 20 cc may be injected easily if the capsule or ligaments are torn (103, 104).

The needle is then removed and the ankle is put through a range of motion to spread the injected material throughout the joint and through any tears in the capsule or ligaments, if present. Anteroposterior, oblique, and lateral projections are then taken. Stress films may also be taken. Arthrography should be employed as soon following injury as possible because delays may result in false negative results if organized clots or adhesions seal tears in the capsule or ligaments. After two to four days when the capsule has sealed arthrography is of questionable value (104).

In the normal arthrogram the ankle joint capsule is intact (Figs. 3.76, 3.77). The anterior and posterior capsular recesses are well defined, as are the lateral and medial recesses. A recess between the tibia and fibula at the syndesmosis may also be noted.

Capsule tears are defined as either small or large. In small tears there is some resistance to injection and the normal recesses do fill with dye. Contrast material is seen to escape through the small capsular defects. There is very little resistance to injection with large capsular tears. Contrast material escapes so rapidly that the capsular recesses are poorly filled and difficult to visualize (103).

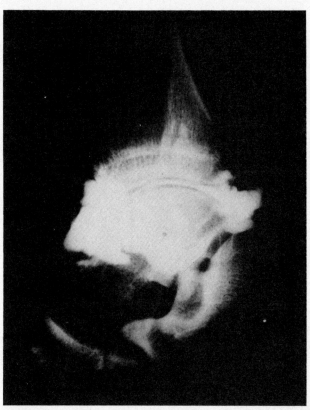

Figure 3.76. Lateral arthrogram of normal ankle reveals well-defined anterior and posterior recesses and talotibial joint space.

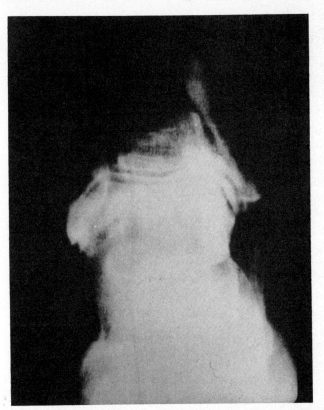

Figure 3.77. Anteroposterior arthrogram of normal ankle reveals medial and lateral recesses and talotibial joint space.

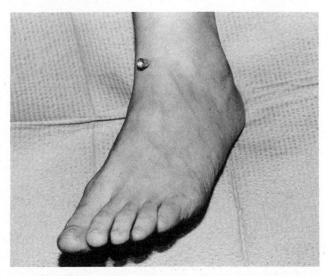

Figure 3.75. Needle placement for ankle arthrography.

Ligamentous tears are diagnosed by the pattern of contrast material as it leaks out of the joint. Bronstrom (105–108) discusses all aspects of ankle sprains and the radiographic evaluation of these injuries in his four articles. Extravasation of the contrast material anterior to the lateral malleolus and laterally alongside the lateral malleolus is seen with rupture of the anterior talofibular ligament (Fig. 3.78). The medium may be seen spreading medially over the syndesmosis anterior to the ankle joint when viewing an anteroposterior projection. The inner aspect of the tendon sheath of m. peroneus longus tears along with the calcaneofibular ligament allowing contrast material to fill along its sheath because it is now in communication with the ankle joint. Where damage to the posterior talofibular ligament occurs in conjunction with the anterior talofibular and calcaneofibular ligaments, the pattern is similar but gross instability of the ankle with minimal strain should be noted on inversion stress radiographs (104, 109).

The site of a deltoid ligament tear is usually localized by the site of extravasation of contrast material in relation to the medial malleolus. With a complete tear, massive extravasation is noted. Escape of contrast medium anterior to the normal tibiofibular syndesmosis with disruption of the normal recess is indicative of a tear of the anterior tibiofibular ligament (104).

Subtalar joint arthrography requires two separate injections adequately to visualize the entire joint. The subtalar joint contains two compartments. The posterior compartment contains the posterior facet and is enclosed by the posterior capsule. The anterior compartment contains the anterior and middle facets and is enclosed by a capsule that is contiguous with the talonavicular joint capsule. Thus the anterior compartment is actually the talocalcaneonavicular joint. Subtalar joint arthrography should be performed to evaluate for the presence of tarsal coalitions and in the evaluation of the joint for degenerative arthritis (87, 110).

Following antiseptic and anesthetic preparation of the area, a 22 gauge 1½ inch needle is first inserted dorsomedially to the talonavicular joint (Fig. 3.79). The injection should be made approximately 1 cm medial to the pulsation of the dorsalis pedis artery. Fluoroscopic control is required for proper needle placement. Approximately 2 to 3 cc of contrast material are injected. Routine radiographs are then taken. On the lateral projection the dye can be seen extending from the talonavicular joint across the plantar calcaneonavicular (spring) ligament to the sustentaculum tali (Fig. 3.80). There is no communication with the posterior subtalar joint. The presence of positive contrast material within the sustentaculartalar joint excludes the presence of a middle facet coalition. On a Harris and Beath projection a thin horizontal joint space may be visualized on the medial side of the foot (111–113).

The injection of the posterior subtalar joint compartment is more difficult and can be done from a medial or lateral approach. Medially the needle is introduced beneath the medial malleolus, 1 cm posterior and inferior to the pulsation of the posterior tibial artery, and is directed anterosuperiorly into the posterior joint space (Fig. 3.81). Laterally the needle is

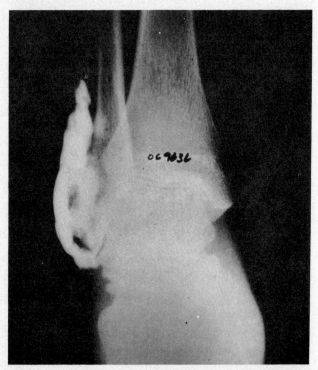

Figure 3.78. Anteroposterior arthrogram shows extravasation of dye anterior to lateral malleolus and laterally alongside lateral malleolus caused by rupture of anterior talofibular ligament.

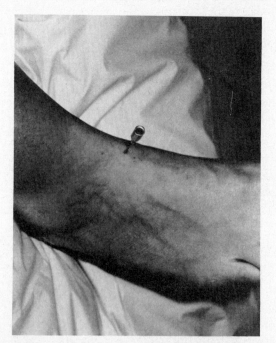

Figure 3.79. Needle placement for talocalcaneonavicular joint arthrography.

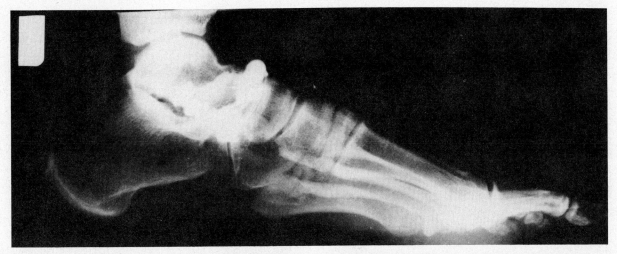

Figure 3.80. Normal arthrogram of talocalcaneonavicular joint. Dye fills entire joint space.

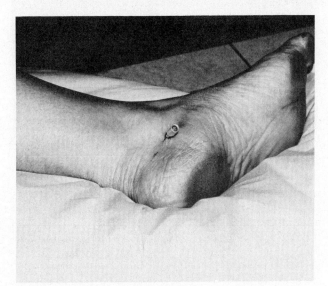

Figure 3.81. Needle placement for posterior talocalcaneal joint arthrography.

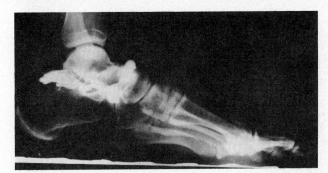

Figure 3.82. Normal arthrogram of posterior talocalcaneal joint demonstrating joint space, as well as recess at posterior aspect of joint.

introduced into the sinus tarsi with the foot supinated and is directed posteriorly to penetrate the posterior compartment. Again, fluoroscopic control is required. On a lateral radiograph contrast material fills the posterior compartment as a thin linear density between the talus and calcaneus (Fig. 3.82). A recess is noted at the posterior aspect of the joint. In approximately 20% of the cases there is communication between the subtalar and ankle joints (Fig. 3.83). Again, there is no communication with the anterior talocalcaneonavicular joint space. A thin horizontal joint space should be visualized on the lateral side of the foot on a Harris and Beath projection. Failure to fill the joint space is evidence in favor of a posterior facet coalition (112).

Dye may be injected into a sinus tract to see how far it penetrates and if it has any communication with any deeper structures (sinogram). Dye may also be injected into a tendon sheath (tenogram) to evaluate any stenosis or constriction. Figure 3.84 demonstrates

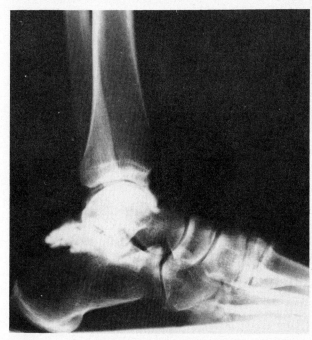

Figure 3.83. Communication between ankle and subtalar joint.

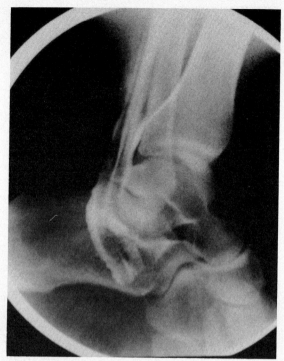

Figure 3.84. Normal peroneal tenogram.

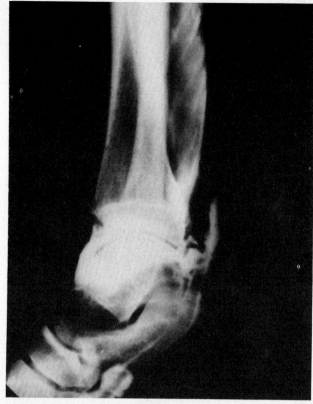

Figure 3.85. Peroneal tenogram demonstrating rupture of ankle joint capsule and lateral collateral ligaments.

a normal tenogram of the peroneal tendons. An opaque medium is injected into the synovial sheaths of the peroneal tendons above the lateral malleolus. The sheaths part as they cross the calcaneus with the m. peroneus brevis being above the trochlear process, and m. peroneus longus being above the trochlear process. The ankle joint is never connected with the synovial sheaths of the peroneal tendons, except where there has been rupture of the articular capsule in association with disruption of the lateral collateral ligaments of the ankle (Fig. 3.85).

THERMOGRAPHY

Galileo in 1595 was the first to attempt to measure body temperature by instrumental means. The early use of medical thermography dates back to the early 1950s. An excellent historical summary is provided by Gershon-Cohen (114), and a description of the instrumentation is provided by Curcio and Haberman (115).

The body's skin constantly emits infrared radiation. Wave lengths of the rays extend just beyond the red end of the visible spectrum. Infrared thermography involves the detection, measurement, and imaging of the body's naturally emitted radiation. A heat detector converts the measured heat into electrical signals that are amplified to operate a gas-discharge tube, which emits visible light in various intensities according to the amount of heat being detected. The light is then reflected onto photographic film to produce the thermogram, or thermal display (116, 117).

In a typical thermogram temperature is represented by varying shades of gray. Most frequently the

warmer temperatures appear as lighter shades of gray (whiter areas) and cooler areas as darker shades. Most apparatus may demonstrate both types of polarity and it is the option of the user to decide which is preferable. Normally the foot is approximately 4° cooler than the groin. A normal thermogram would show even consistency. A mottled pattern may be a normal variant where dark and light tones are randomly dispersed throughout a limb. Optimally satisfactory brightness is reached when the warmest temperature of the subject approaches but does not reach saturated white. The current thermographs afford temperature discrimination of about 0.2° to 0.5° C. (116–118).

Liquid crystal thermography is somewhat different from infrared thermography. Polarized light is selectively reflected in a narrow band of wave lengths as the liquid crystal material is pressed against the desired surface. The readout is a color scheme ranging from dark brown for the lowest temperatures to dark blue for the highest temperatures. Shades of light brown, red-brown, yellow, green, and light blue represent intermediate surface temperatures with each color representing a relative temperature differential of 0.2° C. (119).

Before thermographic recording thermal equilibrium between the lower extremities and the surrounding ambient temperature should be obtained. The patient should lie supine, with the lower extremities exposed up to the umbilicus for 15 minutes. The legs are externally rotated at the ankles and separated 10 to 15 cm and supported by rubber pads. Mild elevation will avoid venous pooling in the lower extremity. Tight panties may raise the temperature of the upper thigh and should not be worn. Loose fitting briefs are satisfactory (118).

The heat generated by tissue metabolism, the conduction of heat by vessels, and the heat of underlying tissues and organs produces the skin's temperature. External conditions, such as the temperature of the immediate surroundings, humidity, and evaporation also affect skin temperature. Physiological and pathological processes that affect body tissue temperatures produce surface temperature changes that may be recorded. Skin that is inflamed, swollen, or situated directly over blood supplies such as veins will appear hotter than normal. Conversely, skin over areas of decreased blood supply, which is characteristic of arteriosclerosis and thrombosis, will appear cooler (116, 117).

The uses of thermography include detection of breast cancer and other tumor masses, fetal and placenta evaluation, rheumatic disease, orthopedic diseases, vascular and cerebrovascular disease, and opthalmological and dermatological disease. Thermographic patterns are noted for malignant tumors (both localized and widespread), by fractures, abrasions, contusions, dislocation, burns, frostbite, localized infections, arthritis, and disturbances of the peripheral vascular system. Most recently thermograms have been used to identify an organic basis for pain (116, 117).

Thermograms are considered positive for breast cancer if an abnormal overall breast pattern is coupled with a significant temperature elevation in a localized area or the entire breast. Many studies support the high correlation of metastatic disease and abnormal thermography (120, 121). Unlike conventional roentgenography, thermography employs no ionizing radiation and can be used with complete safety to the fetus. The placenta is warm and therefore appears white (116).

Thermographic patterns above the sites of fractures reveal residual heat long after the bone fragments have united. This is attributed to the slow healing of the injured soft tissues and blood vessels. Devitalized tissue from frostbite or burns can be precisely mapped for removal by the surgeon. Skin graft viability may be portrayed by thermography (117).

Deep venous thrombosis is represented by a diffuse area of raised temperature in the calf or thigh and the absence of an area of tibial and/or patellar coolness. When thrombosis is in the soleal or posterior tibial veins the area of increased temperature occupies the whole or greater part of the calf. Bilateral involvement is easily identifiable. The increased temperature is caused by inflammation, as well as an increased skin blood flow caused by the release of vasoactive substances. Thermography in the diagnosis of deep venous thrombosis is rapid, noninvasive and shows a high diagnostic agreement with phlebography (118, 122).

Thermography may be used in the diagnosis of arterial obstruction. Arterial occlusions in the lower limbs produce abnormal skin temperature. Distal to the obstruction the skin is generally colder but the skin proximal to the obstruction is often warmer because of increased flow through collateral vessels, most of which are superficial. Because thermography studies the skin, a region remote from the site of major arterial pathology is not adequately represented and it is unlikely to replace arteriography as a method of localizing obstruction (123). Thermograms may be useful following a course of vasodilators or thrombolytic agents, as well as in evaluation following a sympathetic block (119).

Characteristic thermographic patterns may be found to be associated with the various types of rheumatic diseases. Temperature increase is marked and limited to the involved joints in rheumatoid arthritis. The thermographic pattern of degenerative joint disease resembles that of normal subjects. Progressive systemic sclerosis usually shows a decrease in temperature in the distal extremities, especially when it is associated with Raynaud's phenomenon (124).

It appears that the use of thermography as a diagnostic adjunct has a bright future. One obstacle may be the rapid rise in cost of the apparatus, now about $25,000.

References

1. Kinsman S, Kroeker R: *Leg-Podiatric Radiology*. Sacramento, California State Department of Health, 1973, pp 89–121.
2. Gamble FO, Yale I: *Clinical Foot Roentgenology*, ed 2. Huntington NY, Robert E Krieger Publishing Co, Inc, 1975, pp 324–360.
3. Weissman SD: *Radiology of the Foot*. Baltimore, Williams & Wilkins, 1983, pp 13–37.
4. Estersohn HS, Wolf KL, Day JC: The podium. *J Am Podiatry Assoc* 71:222–223, 1981.
5. Kehr LE: Radiology: A simplified axial view. *J Am Podiatry Assoc* 68:130–131, 1978.
6. Throckmorton JK, Gudas CJ: Radiographic axial sesamoid projection in the diagnosis of sesamoid fractures. *J Am Podiatry Assoc* 68:96–100, 1978.
7. Crystal L, Orminski D: Axial views and angle and base of gait. *J Am Podiatry Assoc* 71:331–332, 1981.
8. Pinsky MJ: The Isherwood views: a roentgenologic approach to the aubtalar joint. *J Am Podiatry Assoc* 69:200–206, 1979.
9. Isherwood I: A radiologic approach to the subtalar joint. *J Bone Joint Surg* 43B:566–574, 1961.
10. Olson RW: Arthrography of the ankle: its use in the evaluation of ankle sprains. *Radiology* 92:1439–1446, 1969.
11. Bonnin JD: Radiological diagnosis of recent lesions of the lateral ligaments of the ankle (discussion). *J Bone Joint Surg* 31B:478, 1949.
12. Fordyce AJW, Horn CV. Arthrography in recent injuries of the ligaments of the ankle. *J Bone Joint Surg* 54B:116–121, 1972.
13. Hamilton HD, Rosenfeld S: Nuclear medicine. In Ballinger PW: *Radiographic Positions and Radiologic Procedures*, ed 5. St Louis, The CV Mosby Co, 1982, pp 877–890.
14. Clark WD, Fann TR, McCrea JD, Venson JN: Use of bone scanning in podiatric medicine. *J Am Podiatry Assoc* 68:621–630, 1978.
15. Mettler FA, Guiberteau MJ: *Essentials of Nuclear Medicine*. New York, Grune & Stratton, 1983.
16. Papier MJ: An introduction to bone scanning. *J Am Podiatry Assoc* 68:101–103, 1978.

17. Hughes S: Radionuclides in orthopaedic surgery. *J Bone Joint Surg* 62B:141–150, 1980.

18. Kirchner PT, Eckelman WC, Goldsmith SJ: *Nuclear Medicine Review Syllabus*. New York, The Society of Nuclear Medicine, 1980.

19. Gilday DL, Eng B, Paul DJ, Paterson J: Diagnosis of osteomyelitis in children by combined blood pool and imaging. *Radiology* 117:331–335, 1975.

20. Duszynski DO, Kuhn JP, Afshani E, Riddlesberger MM: Early radionuclide diagnosis of acute osteomyelitis. *Radiology* 117:337–340, 1975.

21. Kozin F, Soin JS, Ryan LM, Carrera GF, Wortmann RL: Bone scintigraphy in the reflex sympathetic dystrophy syndrome. *Radiology* 138:437–443, 1981.

22. Maurer AH, Chen DCP, Camargo EE, Wong DF, Wagner HN, Alderson PO: Utility of three-phase skeletal scintigraphy in suspected osteomyelitis: concise communications. *J Nucl Med* 22:941–949, 1981.

23. Park HM, Wheat LJ, Siddiqui AR, Burt RW, Robb JA, Ransburg RC: Scintigraphic evaluation of diabetic osteomyelitis: concise communication. *J Nucl Med* 23:569–573, 1982.

24. Greene G, Maurer AH, Malmud LS, Charles ND: "Cold spot" imaging with gas gangrene in three phase skeletal scintigraphy. *Clin Nucl Med* 8:410–411, 1983.

25. Izquierdo C, Devous MD, Nicod P, Buja LM, Parkey RW, Bante FJ, Willweaon JT, Lewis SE: A comparison of infarct identification with technetium-99m pyrophosphate and staining with triphenyl tetrazolium chloride. *J Nucl Med* 24:492–497, 1983.

26. Siegel BA, Engel WK, Derrer EC: Localization of technetium-99m diphosphonate in acutely injured muscle. *Neurology* 27:230–238, 1977.

27. Bruback RA: Muscle accumulation of Tc-99m diphosphonate in myophosphorylase deficiency and other disorders of muscle glycogenolysis/glycolysis. *Clin Nucl Med* 8:165–166, 1983.

28. Hetherington VJ: Special studies: bone scans and computerized axial tomography. In Weissman SD: *Radiology of the Foot*. Baltimore, Williams & Wilkins, 1983, pp 442–456.

29. Deysine M, Rafkin H, Teicher I, Silver L, Robinson R, Manly J, Aufses AH: Diagnosis of chronic and postoperative osteomyelitis with gallium 67 citrate scans. *Am J Surg* 129:632–635, 1975.

30. Thakur ML: Gallium-67 and indium-111 radiopharmaceuticals. *Int J Appl Radiat Isot* 28:183–201, 1977.

31. Hoffer P: Gallium: mechanisms. *J Nucl Med* 21:282–285, 1980.

32. Raptopoulos V, Doherty PW, Goss TP, King MA, Johnson K, Gantz NM: Acute osteomyelitis: advantgage of white cell scans in early detection. *AJR* 139:1077–1082, 1982.

33. Thakur ML, Coleman RE, Welch MJ: Indium-111 labeled leukocytes for the localization of abscesses: preparation analysis, tissue distribution, and comparison with gallium-67 citrate in dogs. *J Lab Clin Med* 89:217–228, 1977.

34. McAfee JG, Thakur ML: Survey of radioactive agents for in vitro labeling of phagocytic leukocytes. 1. Soluble agents. *J Nucl Med* 17:480–487, 1976.

35. Zakhireh B, Thakur ML, Malech HL: Indium-111 labeled human polymorphonuclear leukocytes: viability, random migration, chemotaxis, bactericidal capacity, and ultrastructure. *J Nucl Med* 20:741–747, 1979.

36. Dutcher JP, Schiffer CA, Johnston GS: Rapid migration of Indium-111 labeled granulocytes to sites of infection. *N Engl J Med* 304:586–588, 1981.

37. Coleman RE: Radiolabeled leukocytes. *Nuclear Medicine Annual*, New York, Raven Press, 1982.

38. Matin P: *Clinical Nuclear Medicine*. Garden City, NY, Medical Examination Publishing Co, 1981.

39. Siegel ME, Williams GM, Giargiana RA, Wagner HN: A useful, objective criterion for determining the healing potential of an ischemic ulcer. *Diag Nucl Med* 16:993–995, 1975.

40. Siegel ME, Stewart CA: Thallium-201 peripheral perfusion scans: feasibility of single-dose, single-day, rest and stress study. *Am J Radiol* 136:1179–1183, 1983.

41. Siegel ME, Stewart CA, Kwong P, Sakimura I: TI-201 perfusion study of "ischemic" ulcers of the leg: prognostic ability with doppler ultrasound. *Radiology* 143:233–235, 1982.

42. *ACR Nuclear Radiology III Syllabus*. Chicago, American College of Radiology, 1983.

43. Khalkhali I, Stadalnik RC, Wisner KS, Shapiro RF: Bone imaging of the heel in Reiter's syndrome. *Am J Radiol* 132:110–112, 1979.

44. Hetherington VJ: Technetium and combined gallium and technetium scans in the neurotrophic foot. *J Am Podiatry Assoc* 72:458–463, 1982.

45. Lisbona RM, Rosenthall L: Observations on the sequential use of 99m-Tc phosphate complex and Ga-67 imaging in osteomyelitis, cellulitis, and septic arthritis. *Radiology* 123:123–129, 1977.

46. Heden RI, Lemont H: Early diagnosis of osteomyelitis with technetium bone scan. *J Am Podiatry Assoc* 67:733–736, 1977.

47. Jones DC, Cady RB: "Cold" bone scans in acute osteomyelitis. *J Bone Joint Surg* 63B:376–378, 1981.

48. Teates CD, Williamson BR: "Hot and cold" bone lesions in acute osteomyelitis. *Am J Roentgen* 129:517–518, 1977.

49. Freundlich IM, O'Mara R, Pitt MJ: Thermographic, radionuclide and radiographic detection of bone metastases. *Radiology* 122:665–668, 1977.

50. Simon MA, Kirchner PT: Scintigraphic evaluation of primary bone tumors. *J Bone Joint Surg* 62A:758–764, 1980.

51. Thrall JH, Geslien GE, Corcoron RJ, Johnson MC: Abnormal radionuclide deposition patterns adjacent to focal skeletal lesions. *Radiology* 115:659–663, 1975.

52. O'Reilly RJ, Cook DJ, Gaffney RD, Angel KR, Paterson DC: Can serial scintigraphic studies detect delayed fracture union in man? *Clin Orthop* 160:227–232, 1981.

53. Geslien GE, Thrall JH, Espiosa JL, Older RA: Early detection of stress fractures using 99m-Tc-polyphosphate. *Radiology* 121:683–687, 1976.

54. Norfray JF, Schlachter L, Kernaham WT, Arenson DJ, Smith SD, Roth IE, Schlefman BS: Early confirmation of stress fractures in joggers. *JAMA* 243:1647–1649, 1980.

55. Schlefman BS, Arenson DJ: Recurrent tibial stress fracture in a jogger. *J Am Podiatry Assoc* 71:577–579, 1981.

56. Jacobs AM, Klein, S, Oloff L, Tuccio MJ, Radionuclide evaluation of complications after metatarsal osteotomy and implant arthroplasty of the foot. *J Foot Surg* 23;86–96, 1984.

57. Paul DF, Morrey BF, Helms CA: Computerized tomography in orthopaedic surgery. *Clin Orthop* 139:142–149, 1979.

58. Johnson KC: Computed tomography. In Ballinger PW: *Radiographic Positions and Radiologic Procedures*, ed 5. St Louis, The CV Mosby Co, 1982, pp 827–838.

59. Melincoff RH: Computerized tomography—the CT scanner. *J Am Podiatry Assoc* 70:161–171, 1980.

60. Seeram E: *Computed tomography technology*. Philadelphia, WB Saunders Co, 1982, pp 12–46.

61. Genant HK, Wilson JS, Boville EG, Brunelle FO, Murray WR, Rodrigo JJ: Computed tomography of the musculoskeletal system. *J Bone Joint Surg* 62A:1088–1101, 1980.

62. O'Connor JF, Cohen J: Computerized tomography (CAT scan, CT scan) in orthopaedic surgery. *J Bone Joint Surg* 60A:1096–1098, 1978.

63. Schumacher TM, Genant HK, Korobkin M, Movill EG: Computed tomography. *J Bone Joint Surg* 60A:600–607, 1978.

64. Hetherington VJ: Special studies: bone scans and computerized axial tomography. In Weissman SD: *Radiology of the Foot*. Baltimore, Williams & Wilkins, 1983, pp 442–455.

65. Heelan RT, Watson RC, Smith J: Computed tomography of lower extremity tumors. *Am J Radiol* 132:933–937, 1979.

66. Phelps ME, Hoffman EJ, Ter-Pogossian MM: Attenuation coefficients of various body tissues, fluids and lesions at photon energies of 19 to 136 kev. *Radiology* 117:573, 1975.

67. Reis ND, Zinman C, Besser MIB, Shifrin LZ, Folman Y, Torem S, Forindlick D, Zaklad H: High resolution computerized tomography in clinical orthopaedics. *J Bone Joint Surg* 64B:20–24, 1982.

68. Engdahl DE, Kaufman RA, Hopson CN: Computed tomography in the diagnosis of a rare plantar glanglion cyst in a child. *J Bone Joint Surg* 65A:1348–1349, 1983.

69. Levinsohn EM, Vryan PJ: Computed tomography in unilateral extremity swelling of unusual cause. *J Comput Assit Tomogr* 3:67, 1979.

70. Smith RW, Staple TW: Computerized tomography (CT) scanning technique for the hindfoot. *Clin Orthop* 177:34–38, 1983.

71. Abrams HL, McNeil BJ: Computed tomography: cost and efficacy implications. *Am J Roentgenol* 131:81–87, 1978.

72. Ross RJ: Nuclear magnetic resonance. In Ballinger PW: *Radiographic Positions and Radiologic Procedures*, ed 5. St Louis, The CV Mosby Co, 1982, p 871–876.

73. Oldendorf WH: NMR imaging: its potential clinical impact. *Hosp Pract* 17:114–128, 1982.

74. Bradley WG: NMR—how does it work. *Pod Sports Med* 1:36–37, 1983.

75. Pykett IL: NMR imaging in medicine. *Sci Am* 246:78–88, 1982.

76. Vallebona A: Radiography with great enlargement (microdiography) and a technical method for the radiographic dissociation of the shadow. *Radiology* 17:340–341, 1931.

77. Ziedes des Plantes BG: Eine neue methode zur differenzierung des roentgengraphie. *Acta Radiol* 13:182–191, 1932.

78. Andrews JR: Planigraphy I. Introduction and history. *AJR* 36:575–587, 1936.

79. Kieffer J: The laminagraph and its variations: applications and implications of the planigraphic principle. *AJR* 39:497–513, 1938.

80. Grossman G: Practical considerations of tomography. *Fortschr Geb Rongenstr* 52:44, 1935.

81. Ballinger PW: *Merrill's Atlas of Radiographic Position and Radiologic Procedures*, ed 5. St Louis, The CV Mosby Co, 1982, 257–280.

82. Norman A: The use of tomography in the diagnosis of skeletal disorders. *Clin Orthop* 107:139–145, 1975.

83. Brantigan JW, Pedegana IR, Lippert FG: Instability of the subtalar joint. *J Bone Joint Surg* 59A:321–324, 1977.

84. DeLee JC, Curtis R: Subtalar dislocation of the foot. *J Bone Joint Surg* 64A:433–437, 1982.

85. Beckly DS, Anderson PW, Pedegana LR: The radiology of the subtalar joint with special reference to talo-calcaneal coalition. *Clin Radiol* 26:333–341, 1975.

86. Shaffer HA, Harrison RB: Tarsal pseudo-coalition: a positional artifact. *J Can Assoc Radiol* 31:236–237, 1980.

87. Schlefman BS, Ruch JR: Diagnosis of subtalar joint coalition. *J Am Podiatry Assoc* 72:166–170, 1982.

88. Schlefman BS, Katz FN: Tomographic interpretation of the subtalar joint. *J Am Podiatry Assoc* 73:65–69, 1983.

89. Harris RI, Beath T: Etiology of peroneal spastic flatfoot. *J Bone Joint Surg* 30B:624–634, 1948.

90. Winiecki DG, Biggs EW: Xeroradiography and its application in podiatry. *J Am Podiatry Assoc* 67:393–400, 1977.

91. Wolfe JN: Xeroradiography: image content and comparison with film roentgenograms. *Am J Roentgen, Rad Ther, Nucl Med* 117:690–695, 1973.

92. Campbell CJ, Roach JF, Jabbur M: Xeroroentgenography: an evaluation of its use in diseases of the bone and joint of the extremities. *J Bone Joint Surg* 41A:271–277, 1959.

93. Chesney DN: Xeroradiography: system 125. *Radiology* 39:21–24, 1973.

94. Wolfe JN: Xeroradiography of the bones, joints, and soft tissues. *Radiology* 93:583–587, 1969.

95. Xeroradiography. *Lancet* 2:1186, 1972.

96. Pagliano JD, Wexler CE: Xeroradiography for detection of neuromas in podiatry. *J Am Podiatry Assoc* 68:38–40, 1978.

97. Griffiths HJ, D'Orsi CJ: Use of Xeroradiography in cruciate ligament injuries. *Am J Roentgen, Rad Ther Nucl Med* 121:94–96, 1974.

98. Woesner ME, Sanders I: Xerogradiography: a significant modality in the detection of nonmetallic foreign bodies in soft tissue. *Am J Roentgen, Rad Ther Nucl Med* 115:636–640, 1972.

99. Kruger RA: Digital radiography. In Ballinger PW: *Merrill's Atlas of Radiographic Position and Radiologic Procedures*, ed 5. St Louis, The CV Mosby Co, 1982, pp 819–826.

100. Puhl RW, Altman MI, Seto JE, Nelson GA: The use of fluoroscopy in the detection and excision of foreign bodies in the foot. *J Am Podiatry Assoc* 73:514–517, 1983.

101. Gorecki GA, Weissman S, Kidawa AS: Lixiscope: a podiatric evaluation. *J Am Podiatry Assoc* 72:304–309, 1982.

102. Ballinger PW: *Merrill's Atlas of Radiographic Position and Radiologic Procedures*, ed 5. St Louis, The CV Mosby Co, 1982, p 87–90.

103. Callaghan JE, Percy EC, Hill RO: The ankle arthrogram. *J Can Assoc Radiol* 21:74–84, 1970.

104. Olson RW: Arthrography of the ankle: its use in the evaluation of ankle sprains. *Radiology* 92:1439–1446, 1969.

105. Bronstrom L: Sprained ankles: I. Anatomic lesions in recent sprains. *Acta Chir Scand* 128:483–495, 1964.

106. Bronstrom L, Liljedahl SO, Lindvall N: Sprained ankles: II. Arthrographic diagnosis of recent ligament ruptures. *Acta Chir Scand* 129:485–499, 1965.

107. Bronstrom L: Sprained ankles: III. Clinical observations in recent ligament ruptures. *Acta Chir Scand* 130:560–569, 1965.

108. Bronstrom L, Sundelin P: Sprained ankles: IV. Histologic changes in recent and "chronic" ligament ruptures. *Acta Chir Scand* 132:248–253, 1966.

109. Lindholmer E, Roged N, Jensen JT: Arthrography of the ankle. *Acta Radiol* 19:585–598, 1978.

110. Reinherz RP: Contrast media in the foot. *J Am Podiatry Assoc* 72:569–571, 1982.

111. Pavlov H: Talo-calcaneonavicular arthrography. In Freiberger RH(ed): *Arthrography*, New York, Appleton-Century-Crofts, 1979, pp 257–260.

112. Resnick D: Radiology of the talocalcaneal articulations. *Radiology* 111:581–586, 1974.

113. Kaye JJ, Ghelman B, Schneider R: Talocalcaneonavicular joint arthrography for sustentacular-talar tarsal coalitions. *Radiology* 115:730–731, 1975.

114. Gershon-Cohen J: A short history of medical thermometry. *Ann NY Acad Sci* 121:4–11, 1964.

115. Curcio B, Haberman J. Infrared thermography: a review of current medical application, instrumentation and technique. *Radiol Technol* 42:233–247, 1971.

116. Freimanis AK: Thermography. In Ballinger PW: *Merrill's Atlas of Radiographic Position and Radiologic Procedures*, ed 5. St Louis, The CV Mosby Co, 1982, p 865–870.

117. Gerson-Cohen J: Medical thermography. *Sci Am* 216:94–102, 1967.

118. Cooke ED, Pikcher MF: Deep vein thrombosis: preclinical diagnosis by thermography. *Br J Surg* 61:971–978, 1974.

119. Dribbon BS: Application and value of liquid crystal thermography. *J Am Podiatry Assoc* 73:400–404, 1983.

120. Wallace JD: Thermography in bone disease. *JAMA* 230:447–449, 1974.

121. Farrell CB, Wallace JD, Mansfield CM: The use of thermography in detection of metastatic breast cancer. *Am J Roentgen Rad Ther Nucl Med* 111:148–152, 1971.

122. Bergqvist D, Ofsing HO, Hallboo T: Thermography: a noninvasive method for diagnosis of deep venous thrombosis. *Arch Surg* 112:600–604, 1977.

123. Evans AL, James WB, Forrest H. Thermography in lower limb arterial disease. *Clin Radiol* 27:383–388, 1976.

124. Haberman JD, Ehrlich GE, Levenson C: Thermography in rheumatic disease. *Arch Phys Med Rehabil* 49:187–192, 1968.

Additional References

Ambrose J: Computerized transverse axial scanning (tomography), part 2. Clinical application. *Br J Radiol* 46:1023–1047, 1973.

Harris EG, Galinski AW: The evaluation of ankle pathology with arthrography. *J Am Podiatry Assoc* 64:202–215, 1974.

Hounsfield GN: Computerized transverse axial scanning (tomography), part 1. Description of system. *Br J Radiol* 46:1016–1022, 1973.

Ross JA, Lepow GM: The use of computerized tomography in the foot. *J Foot Surg* 21:111–113, 1982.

Seltzer SE, Weissman BN, Braunstein EM, Adams DF, Thomas WH: Computed tomography of the hindfoot. *J Comput Assist Tomogr* 8:488–497, 1984.

Solicito V, Jacobs AM, Oloff LM, Soave R, Bernstein A: The use of radionuclide bone and joint imaging in arthritic and related diseases. *J Foot Surg.* 23:173–182, 1984.

Visser HJ, Jacobs AM, Oloff L, Drago JJ: The use of differential scintigraphy in the clinical diagnosis of osseous and soft tissue changes affecting the diabetic foot. *J Foot Surg.* 23:74–85, 1984.

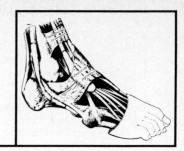

CHAPTER 4

Surgical Principles

Stephen J. Miller, D.P.M.

Reconstructive foot surgery is a strict discipline not unlike the surgical subspecialty that isolates the hand and its controlling structures. Where the hand surgeon is especially concerned with the preservation or restoration of dexterity and function, the foot surgeon must do the same not only with regards to function but with the added burden of dependency and weight bearing as mitigating factors. All planning, technique, and management revolves around these considerations, leaving little room for error.

For foot surgery to achieve its highest objectives requires that the surgeon scrupulously follow several surgical principles (Table 4.1). Careful planning, anatomical dissection, atraumatic technique, and a thorough knowledge of healing are the foundation for optimal results and minimal complications. Close adherence to such principles will reduce tissue trauma, hemorrhage, edema, fibrosis, and disability, as well as decrease convalescence time.

Successful surgery has three prerequisites: (a) adequate disciplined diagnosis (includes planning), (b) meticulous operative technique (anatomical dissection), and (c) responsible postoperative management (follow-up). This section is concerned with those principles and fundamentals directly related to the surgery itself.

PREOPERATIVE PLANNING
The Whole Patient

Francis Moore (1) put preoperative planning in perspective when he quoted a skilled senior surgeon of the older generation with the phrase "The most important thing before an operation . . . is what I think about the night before." Creating a plan is an all-encompassing task that should become a systematic routine tailored to the individual needs of each patient.

The first thing to do is to establish a preoperative checklist, actually printing such a form and attaching it to the patient's chart. In this manner the surgeon can relieve his or her mind of many details with the assurance that no important factor will be overlooked.

The next step is to stand back and view the patient as a whole. One reviews the medical history and notes any background details that might affect the anesthesia or surgery itself. Diabetes, hypertension, thrombophlebitis, rheumatic fever, heart disease, pulmonary disorders, and peptic ulcers, for example, should alert the surgeon to further preparation and workup. Are there any other systemic diseases or conditions that might result in complications? The

Table 4.1
Surgical Principles

Principle	Application
Planning	Relating to patient as a whole, setting realistic goals.
Conceptualization	Visualization. Thinking in physical and abstract dimensions.
Antisepsis	Site preparation and maintenance.
Wound Healing	Detailed understanding of tissue healing; skin, fascia, ligament, bone, tendon.
Surgical Approach	Plotting the incision and relating to local anatomy.
Anatomical Dissection	Using anatomical reference points as guides to minimal tissue disruption.
Atraumatic Technique	Gentle tissue manipulation minimizing cell death.
Hemostasis	Controlling vessel disruption and fluid extravasation.
Instrumentation	Appropriate application to minimize damage and optimize results.
Wound Protection	Liberal irrigation to remove debris and avoid cell death by dessication.
Drainage	Removal of extraneous fluids and cellular debris.
Implants	Towards tolerating foreign bodies and avoiding infection.
Fixation	Internal immobilization.
Intraoperative Analysis	Examine for alignment (radiograph), function, and surgical achievement.
Dressings/bandages	Protection and immobilization.
Immobilization	A protective environment for healing.
Postoperative Management	Wound care, immobilization, rehabilitation.

surgeon makes sure all the preoperative blood work and laboratory studies appropriate to that individual patient have been ordered. Then the surgeon critically reviews them before initiating surgery. One watches for "red flags" and is prepared to cancel or postpone the surgery if further workup or treatment is warranted or if contraindications arise. The surgeon must resist the temptation to push on.

One must be aware that in obese patients one can expect an increase in the rate of wound infection, as well as the incidence of pulmonary complication. In fact one study found severe obesity to be associated with an increased postoperative infection rate of 18.1% (2).

One reviews the patient's current medications, and has the patient take them as usual right up to and, if possible, including the day of surgery. Some anesthesiologists even allow patients to take their regular medications with a sip of water the morning of surgery. This helps maintain the equilibrium already established.

Preoperative apprehension should be anticipated. Prescribing a mild tranquilizer or sedative for one or two days before the operation, especially the night before, will help the patient maintain a positive attitude uncluttered with fear and confusion in anticipation.

If there are any doubts about or questions regarding the medical status, the surgeon consults with the patient's family physician or internist.

A paramount consideration is the circulatory status of the patient. The surgeon reviews the initial findings and doublechecks if there is any uncertainty. Backup doppler or plethysmographic examinations should be conducted if necessary. One should beware of the "Raynaudian" type patients. They tend to have cold feet "all the time" and are usually somewhat anxious the majority of the time. Their peripheral vascular system is quite sensitive, if not over-reactive, to cold, trauma, and epinephrine, all three of which may be inflicted simultaneously in the operating room. Intense and prolonged vasoconstriction can threaten the surgical results with ischemia, so much so that gangrene could be the result. Appropriate precautions should be integrated into the preoperative plan. The surgeon considers the use of peripheral vasodilators and asks for warm irrigating solutions and warm blankets for the patient.

Finally, one listens to the patient. Most people know themselves very well from years of personal experience. Statements such as "I heal slowly" or "I bruise easily" should not go unheeded. One investigates a little deeper and plans accordingly. Supplemental diets and vitamins can enhance the patient's healing capacity. It also gives the patient a sense of participation.

Conceptualization

Understanding the pathological condition is the key to achieving a successful outcome. It must be mentally animated in three dimensions and should be reviewed before the surgery. In fact a good clinician may reexamine the patient and laboratory studies on several occasions only to discover new data to complete the composite picture.

Once the pathological condition is well grasped then the goals of the surgery should be set. One determines a percentage restoration to normal or improved function, and mentally visualizes the desired result. What will the foot look like postoperatively? How will it function? Will there be any restricted joint motion?

Radiographs can be extremely valuable diagnostic tools. They are simply extensions of the eyes. Special views should be used to help in the visualization process. Mentally, they should be converted into three dimensions when viewing them. Tracing cutouts off x-ray films is another method of helping to visualize the results, especially where osteotomies are part of the surgery to be performed (3).

If any doubts linger, the surgeon seeks the advice of a consultant, whether a podiatrist or another subspecialist. It does not blemish a surgeon's reputation to request a consultation. Both the patient and the medical community will respect the doctor more because of the willingness to do so.

Alternative Planning

Anticipating potential problems will save time and avoid frustration, even if they do not occur. They should be included in the plan by establishing backup procedures should the initial procedure be inadequate. A rule of thumb is to have two backup procedures ready for every procedure already planned.

The critical consideration, then, is when to change course. This should also be anticipated in advance. Pilots are trained to establish some point on the runway before which they can abort a take-off. After that point, the plane's momentum will be too great to halt the take-off before reaching the end of the runway. A surgeon should not let himself or herself reach the end of the runway before having to change course. Some point in the surgery should be selected that might be termed the "critical point." At or before that point an alternate course can be undertaken.

Communication

Once the surgical plan is well established in the surgeon's mind, the essentials should be communicated clearly to the family, as well as to the hospital and operating room staff. Preparing the patient and family will avoid unpleasant surprises and help reinforce and preserve that "chemistry of confidence" (1). A good habit is to have the patient and family come routinely to the office for a "preoperative consultation" within the week before elective surgery. The majority are happy to pay for such an enlightening session. The surgeon should then review the proposed surgery, its goals, the procedures, the time involved, the possible complications (including "unforeseen" complications), and the usual convalescence and rehabilitation required. Radiographs, illustrations, and models will greatly augment the discussion. The patient and family should be encouraged freely to ask questions.

Finally, the surgeon should make sure the operating room staff, whether office or hospital, understand the surgical plan. Special irrigation, perioperative antibiotics, or equipment should be requested in advance.

If the surgery is to be performed in the hospital and the patient has no limiting medical condition requiring close monitoring or workup, a strong argument can be made in favor of early pre-admission. In other words, the patient comes to the hospital during the week before the operation date and completes the necessary paperwork, blood analysis, and other laboratory studies. In this manner the preoperative in-hospital stay begins only on the morning of surgery. This is advantageous because a direct correlation between the preoperative hospital stay and the rate of postoperative wound infection has been demonstrated (2).

Site Preparation

Positioning

Although the supine position is most frequently used for foot surgery a variety of procedures require special positioning of the patient. When doing so, the objective is threefold: patient comfort, surgeon comfort, and wound access.

The patient's respiration should not be mechanically compromised and there should be no points where prolonged pressure can result in ecchymosis or ischemia. The surgeon should decide whether to sit or stand and position the patient accordingly. The surgeon should not have to stand stooped over or in an awkward stance because this will cause rapid fatigue and compromise surgical skills. The extremity should be positioned for unrestricted access to the wound. If there is to be more than one wound, allowances should be made to rotate the extremity as necessary throughout the case, and to turn the patient completely if necessary. It is important that the operating room staff be notified of such intentions in advance.

For example, the prone position is appropriate for surgery on the tendo achillis or posterior heel. Ankle work is best done in the lateral position (Fig. 4.1). When an incision is to be made on the lateral aspect of the foot, and other work is best done with the patient supine, then supporting devices should be placed under the hip and leg to help rotate the extremity medially. Before draping, the limbs can be taped or strapped into the desired alignment. Sometimes a commercial positioning device can be used, such as a special "bean bag" that hardens when evacuated of air.

Antisepsis

Paramount to appropriate site preparation is antiseptic cleansing of the skin. It is impossible completely to sterilize the skin without destroying or damaging it (4). However, the total number of bacteria present can be drastically reduced by disinfecting the skin, keeping in mind that these bacteria can be divided into "transient" and "resident" flora (5). The important practical distinction, though, is between superficial organisms that can be almost completely removed either by washing with soap and water or by disinfection, and the more adherent organisms that are removed much more effectively by disinfection than by washing (6).

It is not necessary to shave the site until just before scrubbing it. Also, presurgical preps the night

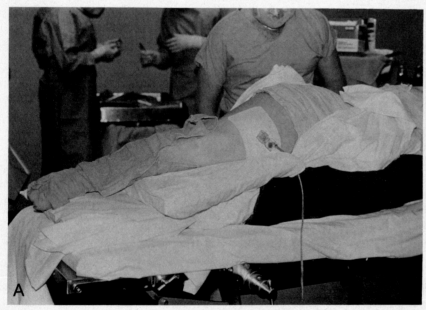
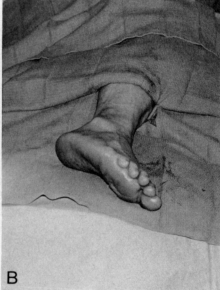

Figure 4.1.   (A, B) Positioning for lateral ankle stabilization procedure.

before surgery have been shown to be of no more value than those first done in the operating room (2). In fact they might even alter the skin flora by suppressing some species and allowing others to proliferate, especially from sweat gland ducts and hair follicles. Also, multiple superficial abrasions result in the exudation of tissue fluids that favor bacterial growth. If removal of hair is necessary the night before, it is best done with a depilatory. A simple shower with an antiseptic soap, usually hexachlorophene, the night before surgery will help initially to remove unwanted and excess bacteria.

An appropriate antiseptic for presurgical prep should be selected by the surgeon and used regularly as the agent of choice. The ideal antiseptic is one that is rapidly lethal to all forms of bacteria and their spores, capable of bactericidal activity for a prolonged period, has no injurious effects on wound tissues or skin, identifies the operative site, and is easily applied and removed (7). Backup agents should be available if there are known hypersensitivities present (Table 4.2).

The preparation of the operative site should be done by a trained person with sterile gloves, with or without sponge forceps, using sterile supplies from a "prep table." The leg should be isolated above the operating table, preferably held by an assistant, and towels used to catch excess liquids. These are to be removed before draping. Neither the foot nor the leg should touch the table until sterile foundation drapes are laid in place.

The scrub technique established should be adhered to meticulously. First, the area should be gently "scrubbed" for a specified period of time, not less than five minutes, with an antiseptic and detergent combination. Beginning at the surgical site single direction linear strokes are preferred to circular motions on an extremity. Careful attention should be paid to the intertriginous areas between the toes. The goal here is to remove surface debris and dirt and to desquamate the skin and its attendant bacteria. Sponges should be changed frequently and care taken to scrub all areas evenly. Three separate cleansing passes should be performed, starting each time at the surgical site and progressing away from it or at the toes and progressing proximally. If there is any break in antisepsis, then the scrub should be started over again. To complete this step the skin is liberally rinsed with alcohol. A final antiseptic tincture or solution should be painted on the skin with two separate passes to dry as a film.

Selection of effective antiseptic agents is difficult because of the large amount of literature that yields many conflicting findings (8, 9). Although povidone-iodine preparations are in wide use, chlorhexidene gluconate is emerging as a superior agent, especially with regard to quantified bacterial reduction (10–12). Suggested preparations are: (a) povidone-iodine detergent scrub followed by alcohol rinse; (b) chlorhexidene gluconate detergent scrub followed by alcohol rinse; (c) either scrub followed by tincture of iodine paint or iodophor solution, allowed to dry; or (d) either scrub followed by tincture of chlorhexidene. One of the most effective combinations for surgical prep was proven by Cruse and Foord (2). A povidone iodine detergent scrub followed immediately by a preoperative paint

Table 4.2
Common Antiseptic Agents Used for Skin Preparation

Agent	Preparation	Properties
Alcohol	70% or 100%	Bactericidal but ineffective against spores. Effects immediately lost with rapid evaporation. Increases the efficacy of other antiseptics when used in combination.
Iodine Tincture	Weak solution of 1%–2.5% (weight in volume) in alcohol	Low solubility in water. Caustic to skin and mucous membranes at higher concentration. Frequent skin sensitivity reactions. High levels of free iodine result in rapid bacterial action. Stains skin and garments.
Quarternary Ammonium Compounds	0.133% benzalkonium chloride 0.1% cetylpyridinium chloride	Surface-active agents with ability to precipitate or denature protein. More bacteriostatic than bacteriocidal. May be inactivated by anionic soaps. Relatively slow action.
Hexachlorophene	3% detergent	More effective against gram-positive than gram-negative bacteria. Will accumulate in the skin with repeated use. Leaves an active film. Inactive against spores. Suspected teratogenicity.
Povidone-iodine (Iodophor)	2% surgical scrub 10% solution	Available iodine is only one-tenth complex concentration with little free iodine. Bactericidal activity is only moderate compared with iodine solutions. Better activity against gram-negative bacteria. Protective film for prolonged effect is easily washed off with water. Blood on hands moderately decreases efficacy. Does not irritate open tissues in solution form. Frequent skin reactions.
Chlorohexidine	4% aqueous emulsion 1% aqueous solution 0.5% tincture in 70% alcohol	The agent disrupts the plasma membrane of the bacterial cell. Active against gram-positive and gram-negative bacteria although rare gram-negative bacteria may be resistant. Leaves a film for a persistent effect. Activity remains in the presence of blood. No known contact sensitivity.

with chlorhexidene tincture produced a significant reduction in the infection rate to 1.2% for 1,810 patients.

Draping

There are a myriad of draping techniques. Whichever one is selected, several principles should be observed. The objective of this procedure is to isolate the extremity into its own sterile field. It is performed by gowned members of the surgical team, although gloved hands should not contact the prepped skin before the first incision. Double gloving while prepping will help prevent such contact.

When the prep is completed, a double layer of impervious foundation drapes is placed on the table. A smaller drape or towel is then wrapped around the leg or thigh and double clamped in place to isolate the distal extremity. A sterile stockinette from the toes proximally provides further isolation and the limb is placed on the cleanly draped table. It is then covered with one or two top drapes that are clamped on either side of the leg. The uppermost drape should be full length. This completes the preparation of the sterile field.

If both extremities are involved in the surgery, then a split drape or extremity drape can be used for a top cover. Otherwise each limb is draped individually with plenty of working room in between them for bilateral cases.

If the drapes become wet during the surgery, they should promptly be covered by another layer of sterile draping material. Adhesive drapes can provide further local wound isolation but they do not necessarily decrease the wound infection rate (2). Although especially useful for covering toenails, they do tend to come loose when exposed to fluids along the edges.

OPERATING ROOM CONDUCT

Once the draping is complete, the surgeon is responsible for verbally positioning each member of the surgical team. He or she should carefully survey the set-up before initiating the operation. It is the responsibility of the first assistant to position the operating table and the light so that the field will be properly illuminated (9).

There should be no talking unless initiated by the operating surgeon. Besides the distraction, it has been shown that bacterial contamination of the operating room atmosphere increases with the amount of talking. Similarly, there should be a limited amount of movement about the surgical suite. The door should be closed and movement through it restricted to absolute necessity only.

An effort should be made to pass instruments properly and keep the surgical field clean and neat. The scrub nurse is responsible for passing the instruments. This requires cooperation from the operating surgeon and assistants. All participants must avoid leaning on the patient. Finally, Nealon (13) describes the duties of the individual assistants:

The primary function of the first assistant is to anticipate the needs and moves of the surgeon, and to help him proceed quickly, surely, and without interruption or irritation. The first assistant is allowed considerable opportunity to act as he thinks necessary, unless advised otherwise by the surgeon. The good first assistant anticipates the moves of the surgeon and tries to facilitate them. He attempts to create maximum exposure of the operative site with proper retraction and keeps the field clear of obstruction, removing blood and clots. He keeps the operative field from being cluttered with instruments. He prevents drying of the exposed tissues by covering them with moist packs or periodically wetting them. He makes suggestions with discretion when indicated.

The second assistant carries out the wishes of the surgeon or the first assistant. He should restrict his activities to holding instruments and retractors as instructed by either the first assistant or the surgeon; he should make suggestions only when sure of his ground and of the temperament of the operating surgeon.

Local Injections

Local anesthetic agents with or without epinephrine can be used to the surgeon's advantage. Besides providing anesthesia for the surgical site, local or regional infiltration when using general anesthesia allows the patient to be carried on a lighter and safer plane.

A word of caution is advised when using proximal nerve trunk blocks without the use of a tourniquet. The sympatholytic effect will cause considerable vasodilation distally. This is usually more powerful than the vasoconstrictive ability of epinephrine locally and can therefore result in much small vessel seepage during surgery, a problem difficult to control.

Local infiltration, particularly of the subcutaneous tissues, with an epinephrine solution can provide valuable hemostasis throughout the surgery besides retarding the absorption of the local anesthetic (14). However, it must be used judiciously. Although quite safe when used locally (15), one must be aware that the myocardium has an increased sensitivity to epinephrine when halothane is present. Contraindications to large doses of epinephrine include coronary artery disease, arrhythmia, severe hypertension, peripheral arterial disease, diabetes, and patients taking monoamine oxidase inhibitors or beta blocking agents. Otherwise, it has been shown to be quite safe in toes (16–20) (Fig. 4.2).

Epinephrine is effective only against bleeding from arterioles and capillaries and does not control venous oozing or hemorrhage from larger vessels. The duration of its local effects is determined by its rate of absorption into the surrounding vessels, as well as by the unique physiology of the individual patient. Usually subcutaneous infiltration will maintain vasoconstriction for two to four hours in the average person.

The suggested safe concentration for tissue hemostasis including digits is 1:100,000. However, a dilution to 1:200,000 has been shown to carry less risk in terms of potential tissue damage (20).

It should not be used in the vascularly compromised patient nor in the "Raynaudian" type of patient.

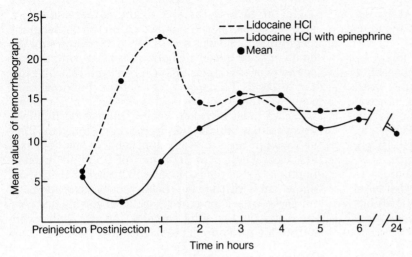

Figure 4.2. Comparison of mean values of hemorheograph readings on toes receiving plain 1% lidocaine versus toes receiving 1% lidocaine with epinephrine 1:100,000. (From Scarlet JJ, Walter HH, Bachman RJ: Digital blood perfusion following injections of plain lidocaine and lidocaine with epinephrine—a comparison. *J Am Podiatry Assoc* 5:339–346, 1978.)

Surgical Approaches

Aside from applying skin mechanics, the key principle here is that surgical approach selection should be based on sound knowledge of the anatomy plus assessment of the pathological condition in the area of surgery. Incisions must be planned and tailored to the individual patient's needs. Incisional names have little value when there is a failure to study the local anatomy.

Several other principles are involved in the planning and executing of surgical approaches: (*a*) anatomical landmarks including vital structures should be identified and marked or noted before initiating the incision; (*b*) tension on the healing incision must be avoided; (*c*) there should be adequate easy access to all the structures involved; (*d*) the incision should be long enough to avoid excess traction on the wound margins, recalling that skin heals from side-to-side and not end-to-end (21); (*e*) vital nerves and blood vessels should be identified and preserved or protected if possible to avoid vascular disruption and nerve damage; (*f*) excess manipulation and damage to the deeper tissues must be avoided by following the lines of cleavage and planes of fascia; and (*g*) scars over bony prominences or weight-bearing surface points should be avoided.

Skin Mechanics

The planning of elective skin incisions requires an understanding of the relationship between normal lines of skin tension and the resultant collagen production (22).

Favorable lines of surgical incision in relation to subsequent wound healing were first described as lines of cleavage by Langer in 1861 (23), and reinvestigated by Cox in 1941 (24). (Fig. 4.3A–C) In general these cleavage lines conform to the flexion creases at joints, except in the sole where there are at least four different rows of these lines and along the extensor surface of the ankle. When practical, skin incisions should parallel or at least closely parallel the natural creases

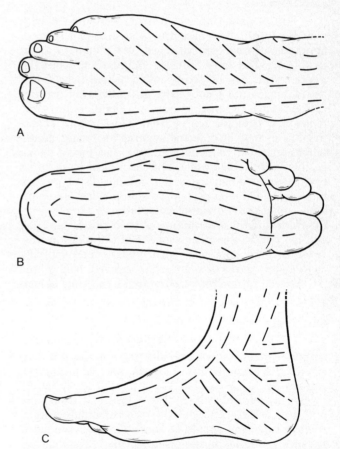

Figure 4.3. (A, B, C) Cleavage lines on skin of foot. Although incisions within skin lines are thought to leave fine scars, use of creases and dermatoglyphic lines is also important. Incisions across lines of tension tend to leave wide scars. (Adapted from Cox HT: The cleavage lines of the skin. *Br J Surg* 29:234, 1941.)

of the skin to avoid unsightly scar formation. Locating the incision in relation to these "relaxed skin tension lines" (RSTL) is a critical factor in determining the degree of fibroplasia and quality of the scar (25). Otherwise, incisions, especially longitudinal ones, should be located in areas where there is relatively little skin movement, such as the dorsum of the midfoot.

As Cox (24) discovered, the reason for following the flexion creases is because elastic and collagenous connective tissue fibers are arranged parallel with these lines, because tension across them is minimal (26). Skin expands and contracts along the direction of muscle pull, so that if an incision is made parallel to this direction, then the body responds by depositing increased amounts of collagen to strengthen the scar. Thus longitudinal incisions that cross flexion or extension surfaces of joints should be avoided or at least made in a curvilinear fashion to allow for flexibility and scar contracture. When taut skin is already present a Z-plasty approach will help lengthen the tissue at the same time.

Landmarks

Skillful palpation can provide the surgeon with valuable information essential to creating the surgical approach. Bony prominences, particularly about joints, are the most obvious landmarks. However, nerve trunks can be gently rolled beneath the finger tips for accurate localization and pulsating arteries can be traced. For smaller vessels, a Doppler ultrasonic blood flow detector can be used. More subtly, superficial veins may be detected by observation and gentle palpation, with tendons and their movement being easily recognizable by feel. The exact location of joints can be ascertained using a combination of passive movement while palpating the subtle ridges and condyles about the individual articulations.

Marking these structures with a special skin pen will help avoid the misplacement of the incision line. If one or more curves are incorporated then applying cross-hatch marks or even suture tags will help to line up the wound margins accurately at the time of closure.

Old Scars

The method of using a healed cicatrix from a past surgery depends on its age, plus the volume and density of the tissue within it. If the scar is young and thick, still within its maturation phase then it should be sharply excised at both of its edges. If it is very old and its color blends well with the surrounding skin, then the incision should be made directly through it because a parallel incision is unjustified (27). Peacock and Van Winkle (28) recommend excising old scars as well. A Z-plasty works very effectively to lengthen a contracted scar or to provide a bend in the new one if necessary and may be used in conjunction with removing the old scar.

Anatomical Approaches

Toes

The toes are the end appendages of the lower extremities. As in the fingers, their blood supply comes uniquely from four vascular complexes situated roughly at each of the four digital corners and they end in an anastomatic complex within the digital pulp. Longitudinal incisions across dorsal or plantar creases should only be made with plans for their contracture. Lateral or medial incisions will heal well allowing the scar to bend. Transverse and oblique incisions heal nicely whether they are double elliptical or not; however, care must be taken not to transect both dorsal neurovascular bundles within the digit. Long curvilinear incisions are especially applicable to the first and fifth toes. These will be described in detail in later chapters. Dorsal toe incisions will interrupt the dorsal venous circle of the superficial venous network (29), and these vessels should be occluded for hemostasis. The distal pulp is quite vascular and may be incised to the bone for approaches in this area (Fig. 4.4).

First Metatarsophalangeal Joint

Only the dorsal and medial surfaces are available for approaches to the first metatarsophalangeal joint. Rarely is the plantar surface violated. Most approaches are dorsal, dorsomedial, or medial running longitudinally across the joint. Curves should be incorporated when possible and an incision at the junction of the plantar and dorsal skin will yield a very fine scar. Care should be taken to avoid severence or entrapment of the neurovascular structures, especially dorsomedially and plantomedially. For hallux valgus correction the incision can be made to curve along the dorsomedial lines of the deformity. No incision should be made directly over the tendon of m. extensor hallucis longus (Fig. 4.5).

Lesser Metatarsophalangeal Joints

The pliability of the dorsal skin can usually accommodate longitudinal incisions in the lesser metatarsophalangeal joints. A lazy-S incision will help allow for scar contracture. However, when there are severe digital dorsal contractures, or previous scars, Z-plasties may be necessary to lengthen the skin when straightening the toes. For entering the intermetatarsal spaces, the incisions should be somewhat curvilinear, especially when entering more than one through the same incision. All three lateral intermetatarsal spaces can be entered through one well-planned, lazy-C or lazy-S incision (Fig. 4.6). If individual longitudinal incisions are used, they should be no closer than 1 cm from each other to respect blood supply to the intervening skin. A single transverse dorsal incision can only be used when there is no evidence of vascular disease, as long as the underlying longitudinal structures are respected.

Dorsal Midfoot

Longitudinal incisions are also well tolerated in the dorsal midfoot because of limited skin movement and tension (Fig. 4.7). However, transverse incisions across the foot can be used when necessary, provided that once through the dermis the nerves and larger blood vessels are identified, retracted, and protected

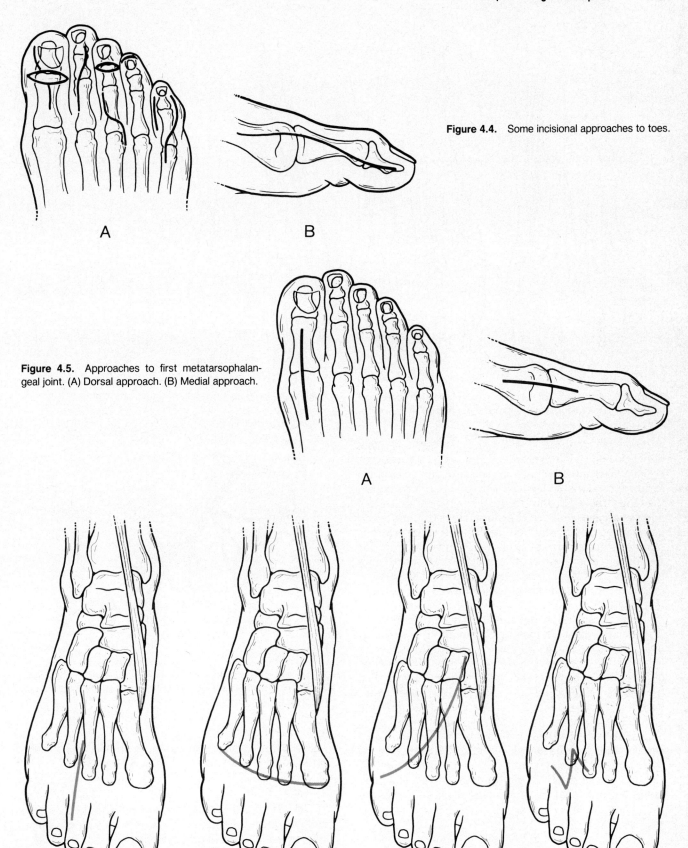

Figure 4.4. Some incisional approaches to toes.

Figure 4.5. Approaches to first metatarsophalangeal joint. (A) Dorsal approach. (B) Medial approach.

Figure 4.6. Some dorsal approaches to the forefoot. (A) Neurectomy— McKeever, 1952; Kitting and McGlamry, 1973. (B) MP joint resection— Clayton, 1963. (C) Hibbs' tendosuspension. (D) Z-plasty for MP joint release.

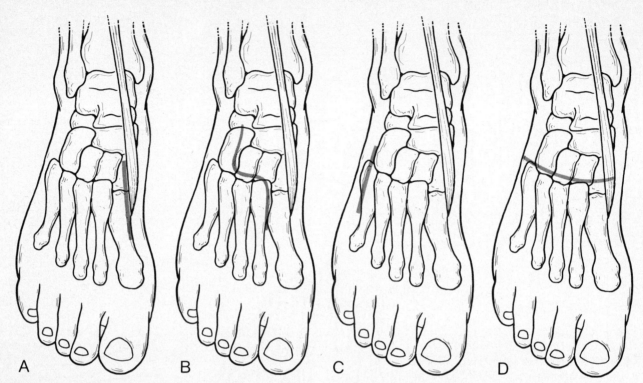

Figure 4.7. Some midfoot incisions. (A) First metatarsocuneiform articulation. (B) Midfoot lazy-S approach. (C) Access to fifth meta- tarsal base. (D) Midfoot capsular release.

as much as possible. The superficial dorsal venous network imposes a generous supply of vessels to negotiate. Care must be taken in this area not to damage extensor tendons, superficial peroneal nerve branches, the marginal veins, and the dorsal venous arch (unless necessary), as well as the dorsalis pedis and deep peroneal neurovascular bundle. Other arteries encountered on the dorsum of the foot include the anterior peroneal (when present), the arcuate with its branches, and the lateral tarsal arteries. The inferior extensor retinaculum should be respected and repaired if severed.

The dorsal osteoaponeurotic space of the foot, as it is termed and described by Sarrafian (29), is subdivided into four fascial gliding spaces and three layers of tissue. The first layer is formed by the tendon slips of m. tibialis anterior and the long extensor. The peritendinous coverings are connected with each other with loose connective tissue. The second layer, being muscular, is formed by m. extensor digitorum brevis and its investing fascia. It protects the dorsalis pedis vessels and deep peroneal nerve that together make up the third tissue layer united by an adipose-connective tissue network. These anatomical relationships are important to appreciate during surgical dissection.

Medial Foot

Vital structures in the medial foot include the medial marginal vein, the dorsalis pedis artery, and the posterior tibial neurovascular plexus, as well as the anterior and posterior tibial tendons. The venous network is quite intricate, requiring a working knowledge of its design (Fig. 4.8). The inferomedial band of

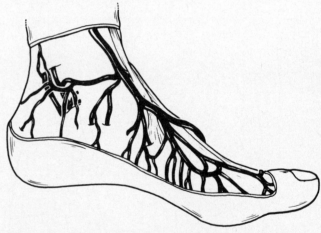

Figure 4.8. Venous network medial foot. (Redrawn from Sarrafian SK: *Anatomy of the Foot and Ankle*. Philadelphia, JB Lippincott Co, 1983.)

the inferior extensor retinaculum should be identified and repaired when severed (Fig. 4.9).

Lateral Foot

Approaches in the lateral foot should avoid the intermediate and lateral (sural) dorsal cutaneous nerves and preserve the lateral marginal vein when possible (Fig. 4.10). The perforating or anterior peroneal artery and lateral tarsal arteries are quite anomalous in this area and are frequently encountered, as are the tendons of the peroneal and m. extensor digitorum longus. As in the medial side of the foot there

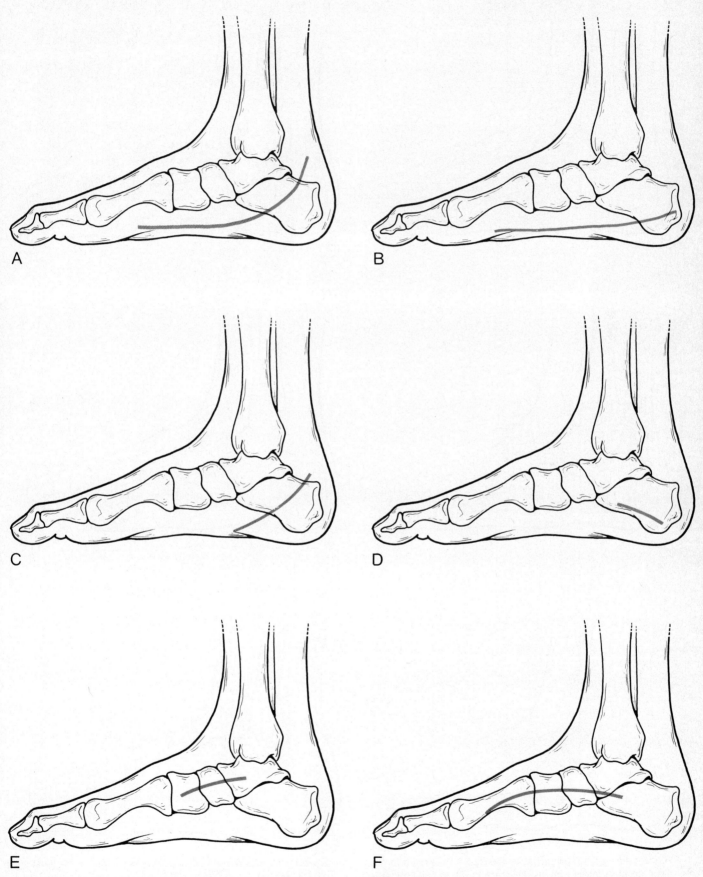

Figure 4.9. Some approaches to medial foot. (A) Ober, 1920; Brockman, 1930. (B) Henry, 1957. (C) Dwyer, 1959. (D) DuVries, 1965. (E) Access to talonavicular joint. (F) Access for medial arch reconstruction.

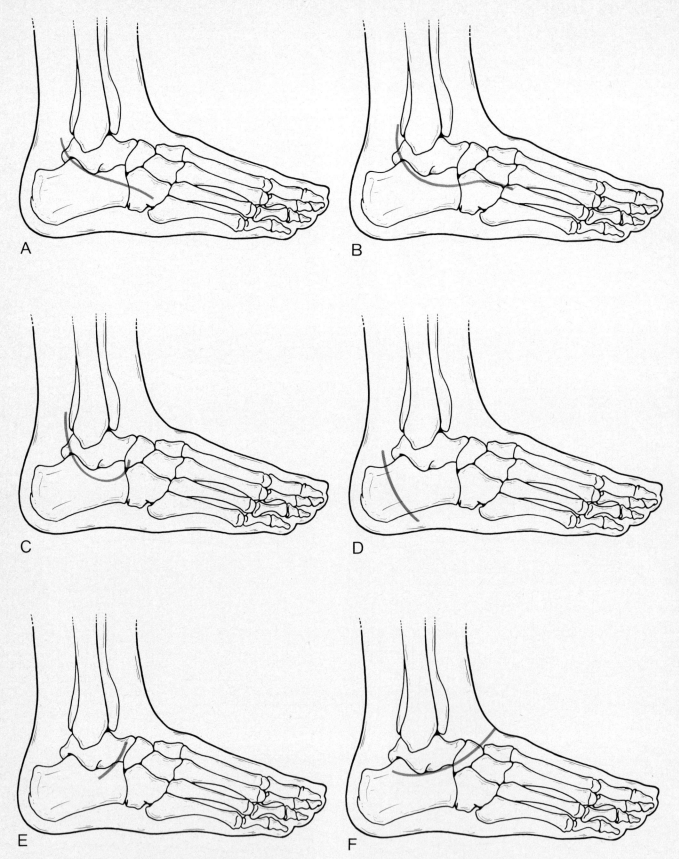

Figure 4.10.   Some approaches to lateral foot. (A) Access to posterior facet of subtalar joint. (B) Approach to subtalar and calcaneocuboid joint. (C) Kocher's approach, 1911. (D) Dwyer, 1959; Banks and Laufman, 1953. (E) Approach to sinus tarsi. Grice, 1952; Westin and Hall, 1957. (F) Ollier incision, 1891.

is a generous plexus of veins carrying blood plantarly to dorsally (Fig. 4.ll).

Medial and Lateral Heel

More arteries supply the skin of the medial heel than the lateral heel (29). The medial calcaneal arterial branches arise mostly from the lateral calcaneal artery, although one may arise from the posterior tibial artery. Care must be taken when cutting along the medial rearfoot (as in heel spur surgery) so as not to initiate a tarsal tunnel syndrome. Also, when using this approach it is almost impossible to do so without severing the medial calcaneal and muscular branches of the lateral plantar nerve (30). Although they should be preserved, their severence can lead to stump neuromas and painful scar formation. When the laciniate ligament is violated in this area, the contents of each compartment of the tibiotalocalcaneal tunnel must be clearly identified and protected.

The arteries supplying the skin of the lateral surface of the heel arise from the posterior peroneal artery above and the lateral tarsal artery below. Vital structures coursing in the area include the short saphenous vein, the sural nerve, and the peroneal tendons, the latter two of which can be palpated. The calcaneofibular ligament must be identified when encountered and repaired if cut.

Plantar Approaches

Incisions directly over the weight-bearing metatarsal heads and plantar heel are generally contraindicated in foot surgery. However, painful plantar metatarsal head lesions have been excised without leaving a painful scar by careful closure and three weeks non-weight-bearing (31, 32). A transverse incision distal to the metatarsal heads can be used for neurectomies (33, 34) (Fig. 4.12) but is difficult for access to panmetatarsal head resection (Fig. 4.13). Although dorsal approaches for the latter make the osteotomies less awkward, a double elliptical transverse plantar incision at the level of the metatarsal heads has three advantages: immediate access to the bones with minimal dissection, drawing the anteriorly

displaced fat pad proximally into a weight-bearing position, and locating the scar where there are no weight-bearing bony prominences (35). Incisions meticulously placed between the metatarsal heads have been successfully used for removal of Morton's neuroma (33). With careful surgical technique, many disorders can be approached safely via plantar incisions (36, 37) because the plantar skin is as well vascularized as the skin of the scalp (38).

Adequate incisions for entering the non-weight-bearing longitudinal arch area especially with reference to access to the plantar fascia for resection of plantar fibromatosis were reviewed by Curtin (37) and by Burns and Harvey (38). Using infrared photography Curtin demonstrated that the standard longitudinal arch incision violates most of the arterial supply to the skin beneath this area. All three authors used curvilinear incisions as shown in Figure 4.14. These yield good access to the majority of the plantar fascia that need to be resected without endangering local circulation.

Incisions to access plantar structures should otherwise be along the dorsal plantar margins of the foot, when possible, where scars form very nicely. A longitudinal plantar heel approach is a tempting but precarious alternative for approaches to plantar fascia and heel spurs. This method has been reported as not producing a painful scar but follow-up time was less than 16 months (39). It is not a recommended incision at this time.

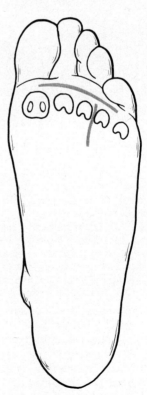

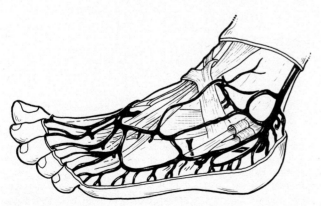

Figure 4.11. Venous network lateral foot. (Redrawn from Sarrafian SK: *Anatomy of the Foot and Ankle*. Philadelphia, JB Lippincott Co. 1983.)

Figure 4.12. Plantar approaches for neurectomy. Transverse incision— Hoffman, 1911; Nissen, 1948; Burns & Stewart, 1982. Longitudinal incision —Hoadley, 1893; Betts, 1940; Mulder, 1951.

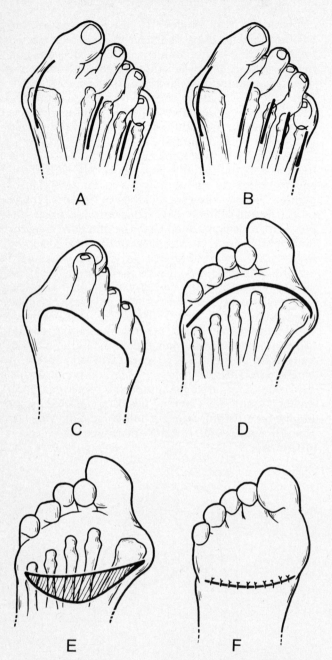

Figure 4.13. Approaches for panmetatarsal head resection. (A) Three incisional dorsal longitudinal approach. (B) Five incisional dorsal longitudinal approach. (C) Dorsal transverse approach. (D) Plantar transverse approach. (E) Plantar elliptical approach. (F) Closure of plantar ellipse draws fat pad proximally. (Redrawn from Hodor L, Dobbs BM: Pan-metatarsal head resection, a review and new approach. *J Am Podiatry Assoc* 73:287–292, 1983.)

Deep to the plantar aponeurosis, the intermuscular septa divide the planta pedis into three compartments: central, lateral, and medial. Guidelines have been devised for access to these septa (Fig. 4.15). The medial intermuscular septum separates m. abductor hallucis from m. flexor digitorum brevis whereas on the other side the lateral intermuscular septum separates m. abductor digiti minimi.

The central compartment contains three layers

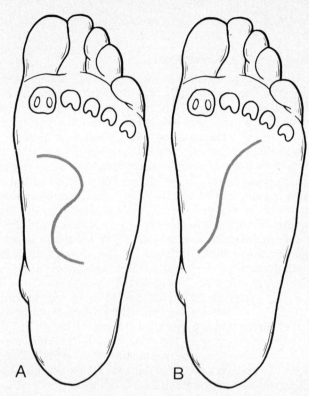

Figure 4.14. Approaches for plantar fibromatosis. (A) Curtin, 1965. (B) Burns and Harvey, 1983.

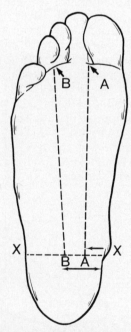

Figure 4.15. Guidelines for plantar access to intermuscular septa. XX' is plantar continuation of line drawn tangentially to posterior of tibia. B is midpoint of xx' and A is midpoint of BX. AA' is line drawn from A to first web space and indicates location of medial intermuscular septum. BB' is line drawn from B to third web space and indicates location of lateral intermuscular septum. (Adapted and redrawn from Sarrafian SK: *Anatomy of the Foot and Ankle.* Philadelphia, JB Lippincott Co., 1983.)

of muscles that are separated by four fascial spaces (29). A fifth plantar fascial space has been described as a subcutaneous space located superficial to the calcaneus and plantar aponeurosis (40). An incision for access to these plantar fascial spaces to drain diabetic foot abscesses and to explore puncture wounds was created by the same authors (Fig. 4.16).

Posterior Heel

Access to the posterior calcaneus and Achilles tendon insertion should be made, with the patient prone, through either a longitudinal or transverse incision. Central incisions across the most prominent posterior heel are best avoided to prevent future shoe irritation from the counter area. Even though a transverse incision will more correctly follow the creases of

relaxation, this incision should only be made above the level of the heel counter with the following exception: When deep access to plantar structures is necessary then a low transverse incision will allow the heel pad to be flapped inferiorly. The split heel incision advocated by Gaenslen (41) is discouraged. The medial or lateral surface of the calcaneus can be adequately exposed through curved incisions close to the posterior heel (Fig. 4.17).

Anterior Ankle

The two basic approaches to the anterior ankle are anteromedial, between the tendons of m. extensor hallucis longus and m. extensor digitorum longus or anterolateral, immediately in front of the anterior edge of the fibula (Fig. 4.18). Either incision should be

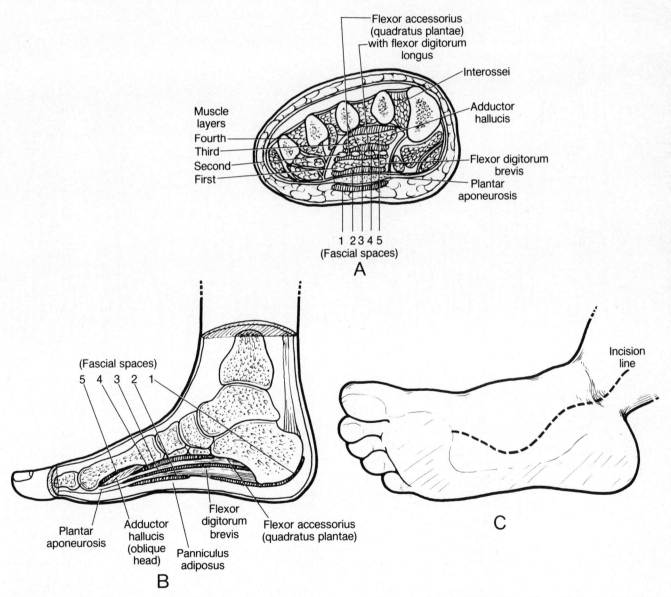

Figure 4.16. Plantar fascial spaces and surgical approach. (A) Cross section of the foot through bases of metatarsals demonstrating locations of plantar fascial spaces. (*Note that space number 1 occurs* *beneath the heel area.*) (B) Sagittal section of foot showing fascial spaces 1 to 5. (C) Single incision access to all five fascial spaces.

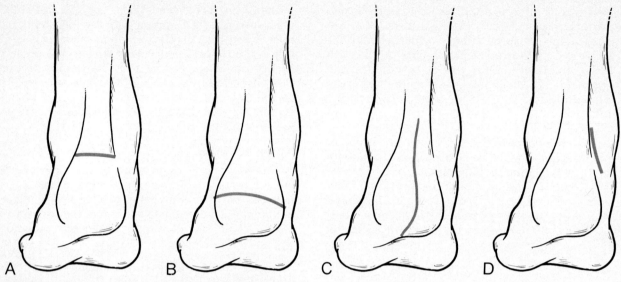

Figure 4.17. Some approaches to posterior heel. (A) Fowler and Philip, 1945. (B) Banks and Laufman, 1953. (C) Gaenslen, 1931; . Pridie, 1946. (D) Zadek, 1939.

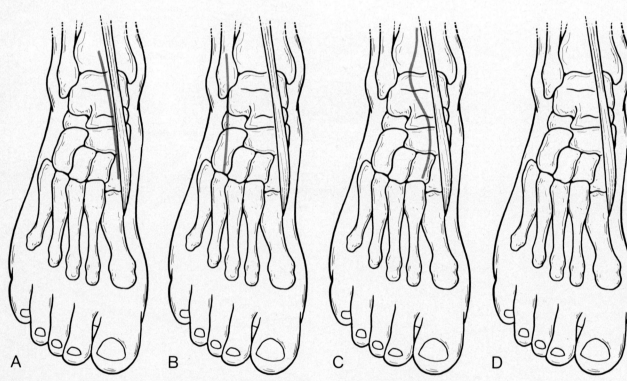

Figure 4.18. Approaches to anterior ankle. (A) Anteromedial—Nicola, 1945; Colonna and Ralston, 1951. (B) Anterolateral—Colonna and Ralston, 1951; Boyd, 1971.

curved to allow for scar contracture. Because of the friability of the skin in this area, prolonged retraction and flaps should be avoided. Care must be taken to preserve the superficial peroneal nerve and its branches plus the long saphenous vein in the imme-

diate area. The anterior tibial neurovascular bundle is best dissected free but kept together as one group still joined to the underlying tissues. It can then be retracted from side to side as a unit for maximum protection. This is especially important when a mid-

Figure 4.19. Approaches to medial ankle. (A) Simple medial—DuVries, 1973. (B) Posteromedial—Jergesen, 1959. (C) To posterior tibia— Broomhead, 1932. (D) Colonna and Ralston, 1951. (E) Koenig and Schaefer, 1929. (F) Anteromedial—Jergesen, 1959. (G) Couvelaire, 1938.

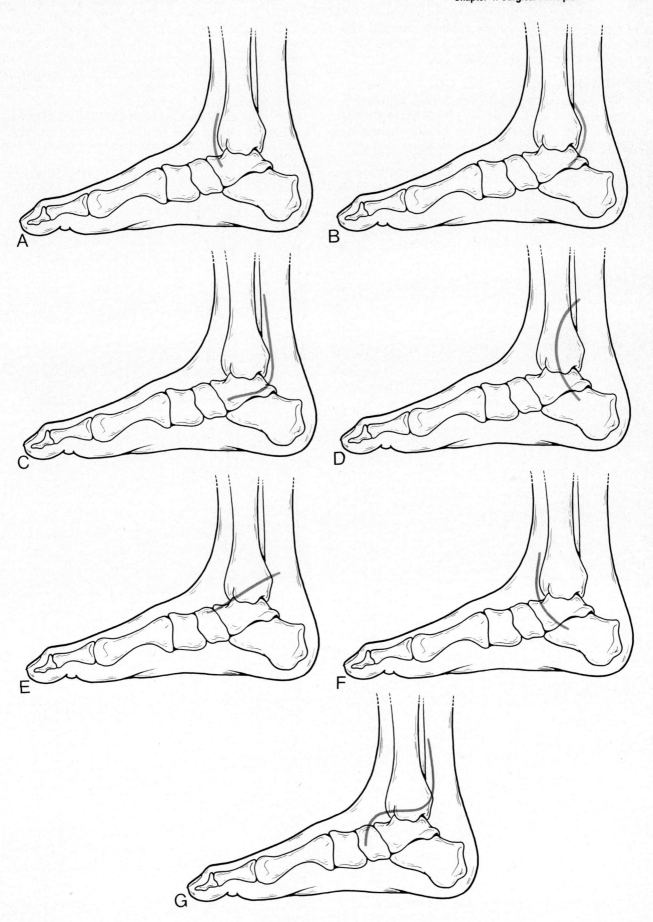

line anterior approach to the ankle is selected. The transverse crural and cruciate crural ligaments must be repaired after they are divided.

Medial Ankle

The principles applied to incisional approaches in the medial ankle involve adequate joint access while protecting and manipulating the laciniate compartment tendons and posterior tibial neurovascular bun-

dle. When these structures cannot be gently retracted posteriorly, they should be mobilized and reflected anteriorly, especially if combined access to the ankle and subtalar joint is anticipated. Both the middle and anterior facets of the subtalar joint can be approached medially (Fig. 4.19).

The incision may curve around the posterior aspect of the medial malleolus or may curve anteriorly directly across the bony prominence. When reflecting

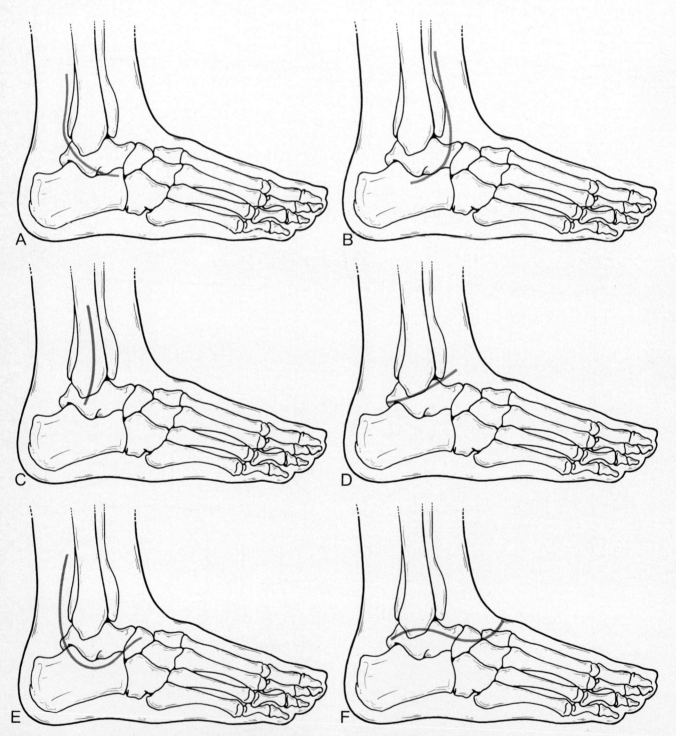

Figure 4.20. Approaches to lateral ankle. (A) Gatellier and Chastang, 1924; Henry, 1957. (B) Jergesen, 1959. (C) McLaughlin and Ryder, 1929. (D) Ollier, 1891. (E) Kocher, 1911. (F) Sutherland and Rowe, 1946.

the tissue, dissection must first be carried directly down through the subcutaneous tissue. A curved transverse incision is acceptable, but is better made parallel to the posterior tibial vessels when they must be crossed. Multiple arterial branches of the medial malleolar rete are found in this region. It is an anastomotic network supplied from two principle sources: the anterior medial malleolar artery arising from the dorsalis pedis artery and the posterior medial malleolar artery arising from the posterior tibial artery (28).

An osteotomy to reflect temporarily the medial malleolus has been advocated for better access to the talar dome (36, 42, 43). This can be repaired with a compression screw at the conclusion of the surgery.

The deltoid ligament and ankle capsule should be identified and repaired if violated by the dissection or previous trauma. They have both superficial and deep fibers.

Lateral Ankle

The lateral malleolar area is commonly entered for fracture repair, subtalar joint access, and ankle joint surgery including ligamentous repair or reconstruction. Vital structures in the immediate area are the sural nerve, peroneal tendons, and joint ligaments. A variety of curved longitudinal incisions can be used when keeping both anatomical landmarks and vital structures in mind whether entering posterolaterally or anterolaterally. Again, dissection must be carried down through subcutaneous tissue before the skin is reflected. Arterial branches of the lateral malleolar rete may be encountered here. Also, the anterior lateral malleolar artery coming off the dorsalis pedis artery is found in this area as it contributes to the perimalleolar transverse and sagittal arterial loops (29). A transverse incision in the ankle flexion creases

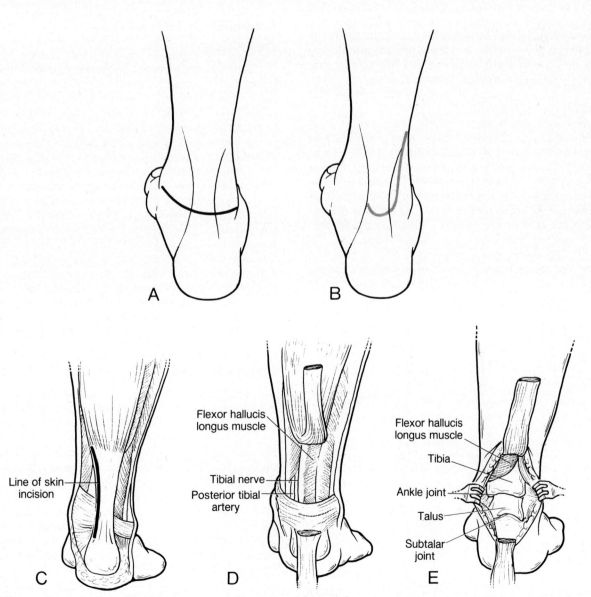

Figure 4.21. Posterior approaches to triceps surae, ankle, and subtalar joint. (A) Transverse approach (B) J approach—Picot, 1923.

(C) Longitudinal approach, medially placed. (D) Reflecting Achilles tendon. (E) Visualizing posterior ankle and subtalar joints.

provides good exposure to the subtalar joint and sinus tarsi, but the intermediate dorsal cutaneous nerve must not be damaged (Fig. 4.20).

For direct access to the ankle joint or posterior tibia, the fibula can be osteotomized about 10 cm proximal to the tip of the lateral malleolus. It can be reflected out of the wound with the ligaments left intact, then repaired by internal fixation at the conclusion of the surgery (44).

The ligaments about the lateral malleolus and the ankle joint capsule should be identified and carefully repaired when violated. The peroneal retinaculum must be repaired if the peroneal tendons are mobilized. Otherwise they can sublux or even dislocate on return to function.

Posterior Ankle and Triceps Surae

The tendo achillis or gastrocnemius aponeurosis can be approached posteriorly through a longitudinal medial, lateral, or central incision. However, a slightly medially placed longitudinal incision will make the scar less obvious and at the same time help avoid the sural nerve. Transverse incisions are acceptable because they are at right angles to the direction of pull of the underlying muscles. However, adequate exposure across the wound is not always present for lengthenings (Fig. 4.21).

Access to the posterior ankle and subtalar joint requires Z-plasty division of the tendo achillis and dissection through the crural fascia, as well as the adipose tissue in Kager's triangle (45). The posterior branch of the peroneal artery with its veins and the smaller medial posteromedial and lateral calcaneal arteries may be encountered in this area. The posterior tibial nerve and artery should be identified and protected as they run along the medial border of the incision. As dissection is continued deeper into the wound the musculotendinous flexor hallucis longus will be found to course across the posterior process of

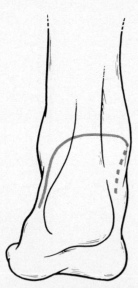

Figure 4.22. Cincinatti incision—comprehensive approach to posterior ankle and associated structures (Crawford, 1982).

the talus and disappear beneath the sustentaculum tali. It can easily be transected inadvertently if a capsulotomy need be performed. The periarticular fat in this area can make visualization difficult. A comprehensive posterior approach to the medial, lateral, and posterior rearfoot and ankle was devised by Crawford (46) for extensive procedures such as clubfoot release (Fig. 4.22).

It is obvious when dealing with incisions and surgical approaches that local circulation is as important as skin mechanics. Although the location of major arterial vessels is well detailed in anatomical textbooks, especially Sarrafian's (29), little is known about the fine circulation beneath the skin of the lower extremity. There is a definite need for studies such as that of Curtin (37) to understand these patterns in each anatomical area. Only then will the knowledge necessary for making intelligent incisions be more complete and available.

ANATOMIC DISSECTION
Definition

Anatomical dissection refers to the minimally traumatic technique of gently exposing tissues by carefully following natural cleavage lines, anatomical landmarks, and interfacing tissue planes. Whether using sharp or blunt instrumentation, this method seeks the pathways of least resistance causing limited disruption of lymphatic channels and blood vessels. Tissues are not torn wantonly, nor are they incised to excess, leaving behind an excess of necrotic cellular debris.

The existing anatomical architecture is not rearranged nor destroyed other than to fulfill the goals of the surgery. This allows for proper layer closure to restore the local anatomy. Thus, by minimizing the vascular and tissue disruption, the meticulous application of the principles of anatomical dissection will reduce postoperative bleeding, swelling, and disability. Blind dissection without visual reference not only increases local tissue destruction and bleeding, but can permanently interrupt nerves and blood vessels in the area.

Tissue Planes

The first principle of anatomical dissection revolves around the identification and use of tissue planes to separate anatomical layers. These planes are best described as the interface that occurs between histologically different tissues. Except for the epidermal/dermal interface and the periosteum/bone interface, each of these planes can be easily identified by the presence of loose areolar tissue that yields effortlessly to gentle blunt separation dissection techniques. By following these planes the least amount of cellular and structural damage is done. Blood vessels and nerves tend to run within tissue layers and seldom cross the planes or interfaces.

The epidermal/dermal interface is identified by a distinct basement membrane layer that is quite firm and resilient. This membranous tissue is readily identified during the blunt dissection of verrucae from the epidermis. It must be penetrated before a scar will form in the skin.

The dermal/subcutaneous interface has rather firm attachments so that direct dissection is difficult. There is good reason for this because the skin is supplied by vessels that run in and pass through the subcutaneous tissue. Excessive separation in this plane can result in ischemia and necrosis of the local skin.

On the deep side of the adipose subcutaneous layer, adjacent to the deep fascia, lies one of the easiest and safest planes in which to dissect. Only the perforating musculocutaneous arteries cross this interface and they do not supply the majority of the blood to the skin. Such nourishment travels via the direct cutaneous vessels that course in the subcutaneous layer and supply specific areas of skin by way of terminal subdermal arterial plexes (47, 48) (Fig. 4.23). Thus once surgical dissection is carried straight down through the skin and subcutaneous tissues, the majority of the blood supply to the skin has been preserved. The subcutaneous/deep fascial areolar interface can be followed across the entire surface of the foot or leg with minimal tissue disruption and loss of local circulation.

The plane between deep fascia and muscle or intermuscular septa and muscle is quite distinct and usually easy to separate. Care must be taken to observe for perforating arteries and veins that seldom accompany each other. The superficial peroneal nerve pierces the crural fascia in the lower third of the anterolateral leg.

The extensor digitorum brevis muscle belly lying on the dorsolateral tarsal bones is a good example of the muscle/periosteal interface. This is a very loose areolar layer that separates effortlessly. It is not present where muscle fibers arise from the bony surface. In fact the periosteum itself is absent in areas of muscle attachment. This is seen on stripping periosteum from the lesser metatarsal shafts as it disappears along the sides where the interosseous muscles arise.

Sometimes the subcutaneous tissue lies directly over the periosteum, as on the ankle malleoli and anteromedial tibial shaft, or immediately next to capsule, as on the medial side of the first metatarsophalangeal joint. The distal extensor and flexor tendons run just beneath the subcutaneous layer with their peritendonous structures. Easy access can be made by gently separating along the subcutaneous interface.

Periosteum has a loose enough attachment to bone that it can be freely stripped away as an intact layer, which tends to thin considerably in older patients. As periosteum nears capsular attachments it becomes firmly adhered to the bone. In dealing with the periosteal/bony interface it is important to recognize that a considerable amount of blood supply is carried to the bone through the periosteum. The tissue should be anatomically replaced as often as possible.

Anatomical landmarks provide guides for minimally traumatic tissue dissection. By gently following bony prominences, tendons, and other structures along tissue planes, there is limited disruption of local circulation, whether to skin, tendon, or bone. When using the same principle in toes, acral circulation is preserved. The digital neurovascular bundles travel within the subcutaneous tissue so once it is freed and protected, so are the vessels. Tissues are minimally disturbed resulting in limited postoperative edema and disability.

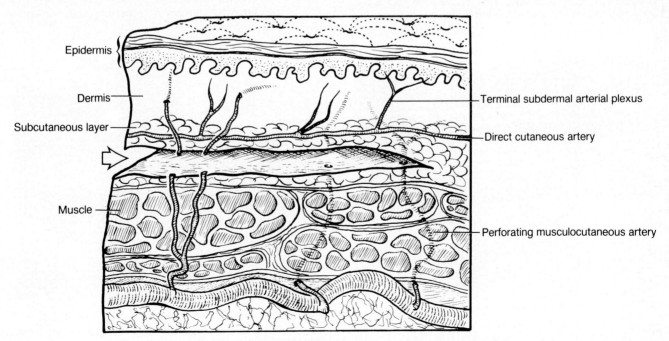

Figure 4.23.   Circulation to skin. Dissection plane is within subcutaneous layer.

Operative Techniques

Instrumentation

Selection of the appropriate instrument and its proper use are paramount to initiating good dissection. Specific application of this principle is discussed in detail in Chapter 7, Instrumentation.

Dissection Techniques

Tissue separation begins with the skin incision. It should be performed with one, smooth, gliding stroke using the belly of the scalpel blade. The scalpel should be kept vertical so as not to bevel or skive the skin. A beveled incision is difficult to reapproximate at closure and the superficial skin edge will necrose and slough. When making a curve in the incision the scalpel handle should be raised to allow the tip of the blade to cut cleanly around the corner.

Tension should be placed on the skin against the direction of scalpel movement (Fig. 4.24). The initial cut should almost but not completely penetrate the dermis. Finger tension should then be placed on either side of the wound so that the tissues fall apart with each scalpel stroke (Fig. 4.25). In this manner underlying tissue planes can be identified, as well as blood vessels before they are cut. Once severed these small structures can be difficult to locate and clamp.

As hemostasis is achieved dissection should continue straight down through the subcutaneous tissue by sharp and blunt technique until the underlying interface is reached. There should be little deviation until arriving at this level. Otherwise there can be much cellular damage and vascular interruption within the wound. This will only lead to more dead space and increased swelling, pain, and fibrosis during healing.

From this point on, anatomical landmarks and appropriate tissue planes will direct the dissection until the site for surgical intervention is reached.

There are several basic techniques for dissection.

Sharp dissection refers to the direct cutting with a scalpel blade or scissors. These instruments must be razor sharp to cut cleanly. Sometimes a scalpel can be used to push the tissue away from areolar attachments while following a plane. The edge of the blade should face the denser tissue. Blunt dissection is another method used to separate tissues. It can be done by spreading scissors or hemostats in the direction the wound is to be opened, not parallel with the incision. Other blunt techniques may involve the butt of a scalpel handle, a dissecting probe, the surgeon's finger, or a wet sponge to gently spread the tissues. Blunt dissection works best when mobilizing subcutaneous tissue.

Throughout the dissection the surgeon must be visually alert. Nerves, blood vessels, and tendons can easily be severed inadvertently if they are not identified during the dissection. Constant gentle probing with blunt instruments and digital palpation will help localize and direct the surgery. Blood vessels are identified by gently spreading the subcutaneous tissues and isolating them so they can be cleanly clamped without including surrounding structures or adjacent tissue. They are then cleanly severed and ligated or electrocoagulated, depending on their size. A hemostat should not be aimed in the general direction of a bleeder and then clamped for electrocoagulation. The result is needless cellular destruction. The bleeder should be covered with a sponge that is gently rolled back until a fresh show of blood gives away the vessel's location. It can then be accurately clamped.

Handling Tissues

The term "atraumatic technique" was coined by Bunnell (49) in 1921 to describe a system of operative technique designed to overcome the two great obstacles in reconstructive surgery of the hand: infection and excessive inflammatory reaction with resulting

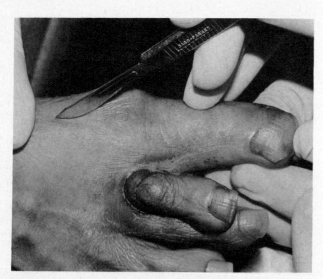

Figure 4.24. Proximal countertension against motion of scalpel allows for smoother stroke for initial incision.

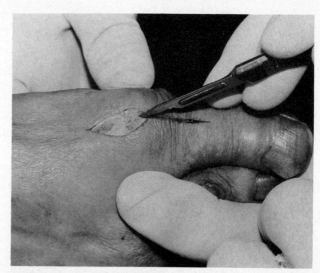

Figure 4.25. Side-to-side or lateral finger tension causes tissues to fall cleanly apart as they are incised. This makes for better layer separation as well.

fibrosis. It is a method of approach based on the careful and gentle handling of tissues, the reduced trauma through improved dexterity, and the expeditious use of instruments, tissues, and time (50).

Bunnell promoted the idea that the care and handling of skin and subcutaneous tissues should be based on a histological conception. Tissues should be conceived as a mass of living cells joined by a fine network of connective tissue and served by delicate nerve fibrils, blood vessels, and lymphatic channels. To minimize their destruction during surgery, they must be gently manipulated and treated with great respect. It is the surgeon's responsibility to develop a "feeling for tissue." In other words, the surgeon must be able to sense the cells beneath the scalpel or within the forceps (20). The tissues must not be pinched, crushed, torn, rubbed, dried, or strangled. Once they are gently divided and exposed they must be kept clean and moist with frequent irrigation using normal saline or Ringer's solution. Sponging should be accomplished by pressing the wound firmly in a down-and-out motion, because one wipe of the surface will damage thousands of cells.

By using atraumatic technique, there is a minimal disruption of the vessels and nerves, resulting in less postoperative pain, fibrosis, and disability. The reduction in local reaction and inflammation can be quite surprising because it leads to an easier convalescence and more rapid healing with fewer complications of edema, hematoma, and infection.

The expeditious and dextrous control of movement is also important in handling tissues. There should be a conservation of movement such that it is controlled by thought and anticipation while being gentle when manipulating tissues. Fewer motions and less repeated tissue contact will greatly reduce tissue trauma. Even the normal tremor of the surgeon's hand can be detrimental (47). The technique of bracing elbows against body or stabilizing hands or fingers on the patient will diminish such tremor. Bracing also slows muscle fatigue that can imperceptibly occur during intense hours of concentration over the surgical field.

Each tissue seems to have its own requirements for proper handling and manipulation. Skin is elastic, extensible, and resilient but can be easily damaged by too much tension on the wound edges particularly from unforgiving self-retaining retractors. It is frequently forgotten and inadvertently abused as dissection is carried on into the deep tissues. It should be handled only with skin hooks or delicate retractors. When manipulated with forceps the jaws or teeth should barely be closed, moving the skin as if by a retractor, to avoid pinching and crushing.

The key importance of subcutaneous tissue has already been discussed. As larger blood vessels, nerves, and tendons are exposed they should be protected and retracted with moistened umbilical tape or Penrose drains. They should not be grasped directly with crushing instruments and their tissue covers should be undisturbed. By localizing them they are more likely to be respected during dissection and not trapped in sutures during closure.

Fascia, ligaments, and periosteum are unyielding and without elasticity. They must be divided cleanly and not shredded. Little tension can be applied with sutures because these tissues can tear through easily. The capsule is quite resilient but can easily be frayed or perforated during dissection, especially when it is thin. It should be kept intact if possible and repaired at once if damaged.

Other Principles

Hemostasis is a critical surgical principle. The adage that "nature leaves no empty spaces and neither should the surgeon" (51) is best fulfilled by appropriate closure of the surrounding soft tissues. However, this is not always possible. When dead space remains or, more especially, hemostasis is not complete as in the bleeding of cancellous bone, then the principle of closed suction drainage should be implemented. (See Chapter 9, Postoperative Management).

Wound closure can best be described as "backing out of the wound." Anatomical dissection and atraumatic technique should allow for easy identification of tissue layers and, therefore, anatomical closure. Reestablishing the anatomical architecture will optimize healing and, later, function.

References

1. American College of Surgeons: *Manual of Preoperative and Postoperative Care*, ed 3. Philadelphia, WB Saunders Co, 1983, p 3.
2. Cruse PJE, Foord R: A five-year prospective study of 23,649 surgical wounds. *Arch Surg* 107:206–210, 1973.
3. Gerbert J: The indications and techniques for utilizing preoperative templates in podiatric surgery. *J Am Podiatry Assoc* 69:139, 1979.
4. Lowbury, EJL: Skin disinfection. *J Clin Pathol* 14:85, 1961.
5. Price PB: New studies in surgical bacteriology and surgical technic with special reference to disinfection of the skin. *JAMA* 111:1993–1996, 1938.
6. Lovell DL: Skin bacteria: their location with reference to skin sterilization. *Surg Gynecol Obstet* 80:174, 1945.
7. Bost TG: An experimental comparison of certain skin sterilizing agents: a preliminary report. *N Carolina Med J* 5:4, 1944.
8. Rodeheaver G, Bellamy W, Kody M, Spatafora G, Fitton L, Leyden K, Edlich R: Bactericidal activity and toxicity of iodine-containing solutions in wounds. *Arch Surg* 117:181–186, 1982.
9. Kaul AF, Jewett JF: Agents and techniques for disinfection of the skin. *Surg Gynecol Obstet* 152:677–685, 1981.
10. Peterson AF, Rosenberg A: Comparative evaluation of surgical scrub preparations. *Surg Gynecol Obstet* 146:63–65, 1978.
11. Ulrich JA: Clinical study comparing Hibistat (0.5% chlorhexidene gluconate in 70% isopropyl alcohol) and Betadine surgical scrub (7.5% povidone-iodine) for efficacy against experimental contamination of human skin. *Curr Ther Res* 31:27–30, 1982.
12. Aly R, Maibach HI: Comparative evaluation of chlorhexidene gluconate (Hibiclens) and povidone-iodine (E-Z Scrub) sponge/brushes for presurgical hand scrubbing. *Curr Ther Res* 34:740–745, 1983.
13. Nealon TF Jr: *Fundamental Skills in Surgery*, ed 2. Philadelphia, WB Saunders Co, 1971.
14. Johnson HA: Infiltration with epinephrine and local anesthetic mixture in the hand. *JAMA* 200:990, 1967.
15. Elliott GD, Stein E: Oral surgery in patients with atherosclerotic heart disease. Benign effect of epinephrine in local anesthesia. *JAMA* 227:1403–1404, 1974.

16. Steinberg MD, Block P: The use and abuse of epinephrine in local anesthetics. *J Am Podiatry Assoc* 61:341, 1971.

17. Kaplan EG: Disclaiming the myth of use of epinephrine local anesthesia in feet. *J Am Podiatry Assoc* 61:335, 1971.

18. Scarlett JJ, Walter JH Jr, Bachmann RJ: Digital blood perfusion following injections of plain lidocaine and lidocaine with epinephrine. A comparison. *J Am Podiatry Assoc* 68:339, 1978.

19. Green DR, Walter J, Heden R, Menacker L: The effects of local anesthetics containing epinephrine on digital perfusion. *J Am Podiatry Assoc* 69:397–409, 1979.

20. Roth RD: Utilization of epinephrine—containing anesthetic solutions in the toes. *J Am Podiatry Assoc* 71:189, 1981.

21. Inman VT (ed): *DuVries' Surgery of the Foot*, ed 3. St. Louis, The CV Mosby Co, 1973, pp 456–470.

22. Murray JE, Milliken JB: General plastic surgical principles. *Surg Clin North Am* 57:849–853, 1977.

23. Langer K: Cleavage of the cutis. In Bick EM(ed): *Classics of Orthopaedics*. Philadelphia, JB Lippincott Co, 1976, pp 424–433.

24. Cox HT: The cleavage lines of the skin. *Br J Surg* 29:234, 1941.

25. Borges, AF: Scar prognosis of wounds. *Br J Plast Surg* 13:47, 1960.

26. Gibson T: The physical properties of skin. In Converse JM(ed): *Reconstructive Plastic Surgery*, ed 2, vol 1. Philadelphia, WB Saunders Co, 1977, pp 69–77.

27. Compere EL: Avoiding unnecessary scars. *Clin Orthop* 91:13, 1973.

28. Peacock EE Jr, Van Winkle W Jr: *Wound Repair*, ed 2. Philadelphia, WB Saunders Co, 1976.

29. Sarrafian SK: *Anatomy of the Foot and Ankle*. Philadelphia, JB Lippincott Co, 1983, pp 233–373.

30. Przylucki H, Jones CL: Entrapment neuropathy of muscle branch of lateral plantar nerve, a cause of heel pain. *J Am Podiatry Assoc* 71:119–124, 1981.

31. Locke RK, Fryberg RG: An effective surgical technique in the treatment and prevention of intractable plantar scars. *J Am Podiatry Assoc*, 67:70–78, 1977.

32. Kuwada GT, Dockery GL, Schuberth JM: The resistant, painful plantar lesions; a surgical approach. *J Foot Surg* 22: 29–32, 1983.

33. Miller SJ: Surgical technique for resection of Morton's neuroma. *J Am Podiatry Assoc* 71:181–188, 1981.

34. Burns AE, Stewart WP: Morton's neuroma, preliminary report on neurectomy via transverse plantar incision. *J Am Podiatry Assoc* 72:135–141, 1982.

35. Hodor L, Dobbs BM: Pan metatarsal head resection, a review and new approach. *J Am Podiatry Assoc* 73:287–292, 1983.

36. Scurran B: Plantar approaches to foot surgery. *J Am Podiatry Assoc* 67:66–69, 1977.

37. Curtin JW: Fibromatosis of the plantar fascia. *J Bone Joint Surg* 47A:1605, 1965.

38. Burns AE, Harvey CK: Plantar fibromatosis, surgical considerations and a case report. *J Am Podiatry Assoc* 73:141–146, 1983.

39. Michetti ML, Jacobs SA: Calcaneal heel spurs: etiology, treatment, and a new surgical approach. *J Foot Surg* 22:234–239, 1983.

40. Loeffler RD Jr, Ballard A: Plantar fascial spaces of the foot and a proposed surgical approach. *Foot Ankle* 1:11–14, 1980.

41. Gaenslen, FJ: Split-heel approach in osteomyelitis of os calcis. *J Bone Joint Surg* 13A:759–772, 1931.

42. Banks SW, Laufman H: *An Atlas of Surgical Exposures of the Extremities*. Philadelphia, WB Saunders Co, 1953, pp 344–379.

43. Koenig F, Schaefer P: Osteoplastic surgical exposure of the ankle joint. In forty-first report of progress in orthopedic surgery. Abstracted from *Z Chir* 215:196, 1929, p 17. (Quoted in Edmonson AS and Crenshaw AH (eds): *Campbell's Operative Orthopaedics*, vol 1. St. Louis, The CV Mosby Co, 1980, p 107.)

44. Gatellier J, Chastang: La voie d'acces juxtaretro-peroniere dans le traitement sanglant des dractures malleolaires avec fragment marginal posterieur. *J Chir* (Paris) 24:513–531, 1924.

45. Lieber GA, Lemont H: The posterior triangle of the ankle, determination of its true anatomical boundary. *J Am Podiatry Assoc* 7:363–364, 1982.

46. Crawford AH: The Cincinnati incision: a comprehensive approach for surgical procedures of the foot and ankle in childhood. *J Bone Joint Surg* 64A: 1982.

47. McKinney P, Cunningham BL: *Handbook of Plastic Surgery*. Baltimore, Williams & Wilkins, 1981, p 39.

48. Grabb WC, Smith JW (eds): *Plastic Surgery*. Boston, Little, Brown and Co, 1973, pp 53–55.

49. Bunnell S: An essential in reconstructive surgery—atraumatic technique. *Calif State J Med* 19:204, 1921.

50. Boyes JH (ed): *Bunnell's Surgery of the Hand*. Philadelphia, JB Lippincott Co, 1970, pp 137–162.

51. Dobbs BM: A practical application of wound healing as applied to podiatric surgery. *J Am Podiatry Assoc* 69:310–315, 1979.

Additional References

Abbott LC, et al: Surgical approaches to the joints. In Cole WH (ed): *Operative Technique in Specialty Surgery*. New York, Appleton-Century-Crofts, 1949, pp 286–377.

American College of Foot Surgeons: *Complications in Foot Surgery. Prevention and Management*. Baltimore, Williams & Wilkins, 1976.

Betts LO: Morton's metatarsalgia: neuritis of the fourth digital nerve. *Med J Aust* 1:514–515, 1940.

Borges AF: Relaxed skin tension lines, Z-plasties on scars and fusiform excision of lesions. *Br J Plast Surg* 15:242, 1962.

Borges AF: The five single Z-plastics. *Va Med Monthly* 101:168, 1974.

Boyd HB: Surgical approaches. In Crenshaw AH(ed): *Campbell's Operative Orthopaedics*, ed 5, vol 1. St. Louis, The CV Mosby Co, 1971, p 60.

Brockman EP: *Congenital Club-Foot (Talipes Equinovarus)*. Bristol, Eng, J Wright and Sons, Ltd., 1930.

Broomhead R: Discussion on fractures in the region of the ankle-joint. *Proc Roy Soc Med* 25:1082–1087, 1932.

Brown IA: A scanning electron microscope study of the effects of uniaxial tension on human skin. *Br J Dermatol* 89:383, 1973.

Chang WHJ: *Fundamentals of Plastic and Reconstructive Surgery*. Baltimore, Williams & Wilkins, 1980.

Clayton ML: Surgery of the lower extremity in rheumatoid arthritis. *J Bone Joint Surg* 45A:1517–1536, 1963.

Colonna PC, Ralston EL: Operative approaches to the ankle joint. *Am J Surg* 82:44–54, 1951.

Converse JM: Introduction to plastic surgery. In Converse JM (ed): *Reconstructive Plastic Surgery*, ed 1, vol 1. Philadelphia, WB Saunders Co, 1964, p 16, Fig 1–17.

Converse JM: Introduction to plastic surgery. In Converse JM (ed): *Reconstructive Plastic Surgery*, ed 2, vol 1. Philadelphia, WB Saunders Co, 1977, pp 3–68.

Converse JM, McCarthy JG, Brauer RD, Ballantyne DL: Transplantation of skin: grafts and flaps. In Converse, JM (ed): *Reconstructive Plastic Surgery*, ed 2, vol 1. Philadelphia, WB Saunders Co, 1977, pp 152–239.

Courtiss EH, Longacre JJ, DeStefano GA, Brizlio L, Holmstrand K: The placement of elective skin incisions. *Plast Reconstr Surg* 31(1):1963.

Couvelaise R, Baumann J, Delinotte P: Technic of and indications for total tibiotarsal resection in therapy of traumatic lesions of the instep in adults. *J de Chir* 51:354–383, 1938.

Crenshaw AH: Surgical approaches. In Edmonson AS, Crenshaw AH (eds): *Campbell's Operative Orthopedics*. St. Louis, The CV Mosby Co, 1980, pp 32–41.

Daniel RK, Williams HB: The free transfer of skin flaps by microvascular anastomosis. An experimental study and reappraisal. *Plast Reconstr Surg* 52:16, 1973.

DuVries HL: *Surgery of the Foot*, ed 2. St. Louis, The CV Mosby Co, 1965, p 226.

Dwyer FC: Osteotomy of the calcaneum for pes cavus. *J Bone Joint Surg* 41B:80–86, 1959.

Fowler A, Philip JF: Abnormality of the calcaneus as a cause of painful heel: its diagnosis and operative treatment. *Br J Surg* 32:494–498, 1945.

Fujino T: Contribution of the axial and perforator vasculature to circulation in flaps. *Plast Reconstr Surg* 39:125, 1967.

Fulp MJ: Plastic surgery. In McGlamry ED (ed): *Reconstructive Surgery of the Foot and Leg*. New York, Intercontinental Medical Book Corp, 1974, pp 201–214.

Gatellier J: The juxtaretroperoneal route in the operative treatment of fracture of malleolus with posterior marginal fragment. *Surg Gynecol Obstet* 52:67, 1931.

Gibson T, Kenedi RM: Biochemical properties of skin. *Surg Clin North Am* 47:279, 1967.

Gibson T, Kenedi RM: The structural components of the dermis. In Montagna W, Bentley JP, Dobson RL (eds): *The Dermis*. New York, Appleton-Century-Crofts, 1970, p 19.

Gibson T, Stack H, Kenedi RM: The significance of Langer's lines. In Hueston JT (ed): *Transactions of the Fifth International Congress of Plastic and Reconstructive Surgery*. Sydney, Australia, Butterworths, 1971, p 1213.

Grice DS: An extra-articular arthrodesis of the subastragalar joint for correction of paralytic flatfeet in children. *J Bone Joint Surg* 34A:927–940, 1952.

Grodinsky M: A study of fascial spaces of the feet and their bearing on infections. *Surg Gynecol Obstet* 49:739–751, 1929.

Hainge F, Bucholtz JM: Principles and methods of clean surgical wound irrigation. *J Foot Surg* 21:241–246, 1982.

Hardy JD (ed): *Rhoad's Textbook of Surgery: Principles and Practice*. Philadelphia, JB Lippincott Co, 1977.

Henry AK: *Extensile Exposure*, ed 2. Baltimore, Williams & Wilkins, 1957.

Henry AK: *Extensile Exposure*, ed 2. Edinburgh, E & S Livingstone Ltd, 1966.

Hoadley AE: Six cases of metatarsalgia. *Chicago Med Rec* 5:32, 1893.

Hoffman P: An operation for severe grades of contracted or clawed toes. *Amer J Orthop Surg* 9:441–448, 1911.

Hunt TK, Dunphy JE: *Fundamentals of Wound Management*. New York, Appleton-Century-Crofts, 1979.

Inman, VT: Surgical approaches to the deep structures of the foot and ankle. In Inman VT (ed): *DuVries' Surgery of the Foot*, ed 3. St. Louis, The CV Mosby Co, 1973, pp 457–470.

Jergesen, F: Open reduction of fractures and dislocations of the ankle. *Am J Surg* 98:136–150, 1959.

Kaissel CJ: Selection of appropriate lines for elective surgical incisions. *Plast Reconstr Surg* 8:1–28, 1951.

Kamel R, Sakla F: Anatomic compartments of the sole of the human foot. *Anatomy* 140:57–60, 1961.

Kitting RW, McGlamry ED: Removal of an intermetatarsal neuroma. *J Am Podiatry Assoc* 63:274, 1973.

Kocher T: *Textbook of Operative Surgery*, ed 3. (Translated by HJ Stiles and CB Paul), London, A and C Black, 1911.

Langer K: Zur Anatomie und Physiologie der Haut. 1. Uber die Spaltbarkeit der Cutis. *S-B Akad Wiss Wien* 44:19, 1861.

Langer K: Zur Anatomie und Physiologie der Haut. 2. Die Spannung der Cutis. *S-B Akad Wiss Wien* 45:133, 1862.

Lowbury EJL, Lilly HA: The effect of blood on disinfection of surgeon's hands. *Br J Surg* 61:19–21, 1974.

Miller WE: Operative incisions involving the foot. *Orthop Clin North Am* 7:785–793, 1976.

McGregor IA: *Fundamentals and Techniques of Plastic Surgery*. New York, Churchill-Livingstone, 1980.

McKeever DC: Surgical approach for neuroma of plantar digital nerve (Morton's metatarsalgia) *J Bone Joint Surg* 34A:490, 1952.

McKinney P, Cunningham BL: *Handbook of Plastic Surgery*. Baltimore, Williams & Wilkins, 1981.

McLaughlin HL, Ryder CT: Open reduction and internal fixation for fractures of the tibia and ankle. *Surg Clin N Amer* 29:1523–1534, 1949.

Monroe CW: Basic operative technique. *Surg Clin N Am* 57(5):855–862, 1977.

Mulder JD: The causative mechanism in Morton's metatarsalgia. *J Bone Joint Surg* 33B:94–95, 1951.

Nicola, T: *Atlas of Surgical Approaches to Bones and Joints*. New York, MacMillan, 1945.

Nissen KI: The etiology of Morton's metatarsalgia. *J Bone Joint Surg* 33B:293, 1951.

Ober FR: An operation for the relief of congenital equino-varus deformity. *J Orthop Surg* 2:558–565, 1920.

Ollier L: *Traite des Resections et des Operations Conservatrices quon Peut Praticquer sur le Systeme Osseux*, vol 3. Paris, G. Masson, 1891.

Peacock EE: Repair and regeneration. In Converse JM (ed): *Reconstructive Plastic Surgery*, ed 2, vol 1. Philadelphia, WB Saunders Co, 1977, pp 78–103.

Picot G: L'intervention sanglante dans les fractures malleolaires. *J Chir* (Paris), 21:529–542, 1923.

Pirrucello FW: *Fundamentals of Plastic Surgery*. Oradell, NJ, Medical Economics Company, 1979.

Price PB: Fallacy of a current surgical fad; 3 minute preoperative scrub with hexachlorophene soap. *Ann Surg* 134:476, 1951.

Pridie KH: A new method of treatment for severe fractures of the os calcis: a preliminary report. *Surg Gynecol Obstet* 82:671–675, 1946.

Rutt A: *Surgery of the lower leg and foot*. (Translated by G Stiasny). In Hackenbroch M, Witt AN (eds): *Atlas of Orthopaedic Operations*, vol 2. Philadelphia, WB Saunders Co, 1980, pp 108–353.

Sabiston DC Jr(ed): *Davis-Christopher Textbook of Surgery*, ed 11. Philadelphia, WB Saunders Co., 1977.

Simmons BP: CDC guidelines for prevention of surgical wound infections. *Infection Control* 3:187–196, 1982.

Sutherland R, Rowe MJ Jr: Arthrotomy approaches in the lower extremity. *Am J Surg* 71:335–337, 1946.

Westin GW, Hall CB: Subtalar extra-articular arthrodesis: a preliminary report of a method of stablizing feet in children. *J Bone Joint Surg* 39-A:501–511, 1957.

Zadek I: An operation for the cure of achillobursitis. *Am J Surg* 43:542–546, 1939.

CHAPTER 5

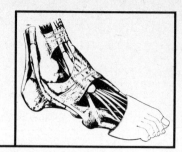

Suture Materials and Needles: Their Properties and Uses

Gerard V. Yu, D.P.M. and **Raymond G. Cavaliere, D.P.M.**

As the number, complexity, and sophistication of surgical procedures increase, so do the number of complications caused by suture failure. The development and introduction of new synthetic materials provide today's surgeon with a wide variety of suture materials and surgical needles. Too frequently, however, the choice of suture material or needle has been based on considerations other than objective, biological, or scientific data. Optimal surgical results are best achieved if selection is based on sound scientific knowledge. Although faults in the making of a suture or needle are the responsibility of the suture manufacturer, the errors in their use belong solely to the surgeon. Such error begins with improper selection.

This is a review of currently available suture materials and needles and summarizes more recently available comparative information to facilitate selection of the most appropriate suture material or needle for each specific surgical indication.

DEFINITION AND CLASSIFICATION

Surgical sutures are sterile filaments used to approximate and maintain tissues until the healing process has endowed the wound with sufficient strength to withstand mechanical stress. Attached to needles, they are employed for stitching wounds or surgical incisions and as ligatures to tie off severed tubular structures such as blood vessels and ducts to prevent bleeding or leakage of body fluids (1, 2).

The Food and Drug Act passed by the US Congress in 1906 recognized the United States Pharmacopeia (USP) as an official compendium, with its standards mandatory under federal law for products so labeled. The USP is presently the official compendium providing the description of suture materials. The USP sets the standards and guidelines under which sutures are manufactured, packaged, labeled, and sterilized. When a question arises concerning the

properties of a suture, it is the USP standards against which the product will be judged because they are the current standards (3–5).

Sutures are classified in the USP in separate monographs covering *absorbable surgical sutures* and *nonabsorbable surgical sutures*. These are the two groups into which sutures are conveniently divided (Table 5.1); they can be further divided into subgroups (Tables 5.2, 5.3).

The USP monograph on absorbable surgical sutures carries this description:

Flexible strand varying in treatment, color, size, packaging, and resistance to absorption, according to the intended purpose. The collagen suture is either Type A Suture or Type C Suture. Both types consist of processed strands of collagen, but Type C Suture is processed by physical or chemical means so as to provide greater resistance to absorption in living mammalian tissue.

Absorbable Surgical Suture is a sterile strand prepared from collagen derived from healthy mammals or from a synthetic polymer. Its length is not less than 95.0 percent of that stated in the label. Its diameter and tensile strength correspond to the size designation indicated on the label, within the limits prescribed herein. It is capable of being absorbed by living mammalian tissue, but may be treated to modify its resistance to absorption. It may be modified with respect to body or texture. It may be impregnated or coated with a suitable antimicrobial agent. It may be colored by a color additive approved by the Federal Food and Drug Administration (3).

Table 5.1
Classification of Surgical Sutures

Absorbable
Natural (derived from animals)
Synthetic (artificial)
Nonabsorbable
Natural filament
Metal
Synthetic

From Yu GV, Cavaliere R: Suture materials. *J Am Podiatry Assoc* 73:57, 1983.

Table 5.2
Classification of Absorbable Surgical Sutures

Generic Name	Raw Material	Trade Name
Natural collagens		
Plain gut	Submucosa sheep intestine	None
	Serosa of beef intestine	
Chromic gut	+Buffered chromicizing	None
Plain collagen	Bovine deep flexor tendon	None
Chromic collagen	+Buffered chromicizing	None
Synthetics		
Polyglycolic acid	Homopolymer of glycolide w/poloxamer 188 coating	Dexon-S
		Dexon-Plus
Polyglactin-910	Copolymer lactide-glycolide with calcium stearate coating	Vicryl
Polydioxanone	Polymer of paradioxanone	PDS

Modified from Yu GV, Cavaliere R: Suture materials. *J Am Podiatry Assoc* 73:58, 1983.

Table 5.3
Classification of Nonabsorbable Surgical Sutures

Generic Name	Raw Material	Trade Name
Natural fiber		
Surgical cotton	Twisted natural cotton	None
Surgical silk	Braided protein natural fiber	None
Virgin silk	spun by silk worm	None
Dermal silk		Perma-hand[®2]
Surgical linen	Twisted long-staple flax	None
Synthetic		
Nylon	Polyamide polymer-monofilament	Dermalon[®2]
		Ethilon[®1]
	Multifilament-braided	Nurolon[®2]
	Multifilament-braided-silicone treated	Surgilon[®1]
Polypropylene	Polymer of propylene-monofilament	Surgilene[®1]
		Prolene[®2]
Polyethylene	Thermoplastic synthetic resins	Dermalene[®1]
Polyester	Polyethylene terephthalate-multifilament	
	—Braided-plain	Dacron[®3]
		Mersilene[®2]
	—Braided-silicone coated	T1-Cron[®4]
	—Braided-polybutilate coated	Ethibond[®2]
	—Braided-PFTE {Teflon[®4]} coated	Polydek[®5]
		Ethiflex[®2]
	—Braided-heavy PFTE(Teflon) impregnated	Tevdek[®5]

From Yu GV, Cavaliere R: Suture materials. *J Am Podiatry Assoc* 73:58, 1983.

The diameter of each suture strand must fall within the minimum and maximum limits for its gauge, which differ for both collagen sutures and synthetic sutures. Metric size designations are now included along with USP size (gauge) to facilitate voluntary international uniformity in suture standards.

The USP monograph on nonabsorbable surgical sutures provides this description:

Flexible, monofilament or multifilament, continuous strand, placed in an envelope, tube or other suitable container or wound on a reel or spool. If it is a multifilament strand, the individual filament may be combined by spinning, twisting, braiding or any combination thereof.

Nonabsorbable Surgical Suture is classed and typed as follows:

Class I.   Suture is composed of silk or synthetic fibers of monofilament, twisted or braided construction.

Class II.   Suture is composed of cotton or linen fibers or coated natural or synthetic fibers where the coating forms a casing of significant thickness but does not contribute appreciably to strength.

Class III.   Suture is composed of monofilament or multifilament metal wire.

Nonabsorbable Surgical Suture is a strand of material that is suitably resistant to the action of living mammalian tissue. Its length is not less than 95.0 percent of that stated on the label. Its diameter and tensile strength correspond to the size designation indicated on the label, within the limits prescribed herein. It may be nonsterile or sterile. It may be impregnated or coated with a suitable antimicrobial agent.

Nonabsorbable Surgical Suture may be modified with respect to body or texture, or to reduce capillarity, and may be suitably bleached. It may be colored by a color additive approved by the Federal Food and Drug Administration (3).

From a practical perspective absorbable sutures are generally thought of as temporary sutures. Prepared from collagen derived from healthy mammals or synthetic polymers, they are absorbed by living mammalian tissues via digestion by lysosomal enzymes, in the case of surgical gut, and collagen sutures (plain or chromic), or by hydrolysis, in the case of polyglycolic acid (Dexon "S," Dexon-Plus), polyglactin 910 (Vicryl) and polydioxanone (PDS). They are monofilament or multifilament (braided) in construction and may be dyed or undyed, coated or uncoated. The newer synthetic sutures are available in braided multifilament form or in the more recently introduced monofilament form (Table 5.2).

From a practical perspective nonabsorbable sutures are generally thought of as permanent sutures. They are resistant to biodegradation by living mammalian tissue, and generally remain encapsulated when buried in tissue unless extruded or removed from the body. They may be multifilament (twisted, braided, or spun) or monofilament in construction, dyed or undyed, and coated or uncoated (Table 5.3). Only nylon and stainless steel are available in both forms. Nylon and silk, although classified as nonabsorbable sutures, actually undergo degradation at various rates and should be classified as slowly absorbed sutures (Fig. 5.1) (2, 6–10).

Capillarity refers to a process that allows the passage of tissue fluids along the strand, permitting infection (if present) to be drawn into the surgical wound. Type A sutures are untreated and capillary; type B are treated and noncapillary. The nature of the raw material and/or the specific processing establish type B sutures (3–5).

BIOLOGICAL PROPERTIES

All suture material, whether absorbable or nonabsorbable, is a foreign body to human tissue, and, as such, elicits reaction within tissues. The initial reaction is thought to reflect the amount of injury inflicted by passage of the needle and suture through tissue. The reaction lasts for approximately five to seven days, and is essentially the same for all suture materials (7). It is the subsequent reaction that is of interest and is dependent on the chemical and physical prop-

erties of the material used. The system of grading the reaction includes the size of the reaction zone, the type of reactive cells, and an estimate of their number. To date no evidence of neoplasia has been reported. In general the monofilament sutures elicit far less reaction than do multifilament sutures; uncoated sutures less than coated. Synthetic sutures cause significantly less tissue reaction than sutures derived from natural materials (9–12).

With respect to infection, the chemical nature of the suture appears to be of greater importance than its physical configuration (13). It has been suggested, however, that the interstices present in multifilament sutures may provide potential sites for the propogation and transmission of bacterial infection as well (14–16). All sutures should be avoided in dirty, contaminated, or infected wounds whenever possible because they have been shown to impair the ability of the wound to resist infection (17–19). When suture use is necessary, synthetic monofilament nonabsorbable sutures are recommended. Recent evidence indicates that synthetic absorbable sutures, although multifilament, may produce breakdown products that are potent antibacterial agents producing conditions unfavorable to bacterial multiplication (13, 20, 21). Nylon may also possess similar properties (13).

Absorbable Sutures

The degradation and absorption of surgical gut suture, plain or chromic, is mediated through cellular and tissue proteases. Processed from dead animal tissue, they elicit a wide range of biological reactions, depending on the type and condition of tissue in which they are implanted as well as the general health status of the patient. Both the surgeon and patient can be assured of little predictability with respect to absorption of tensile strength (9, 20). Many studies have demonstrated that surgical gut sutures elicit the highest degree of tissue reaction, often severe enough to impede tissue healing (2, 11, 14, 20, 22–25). Collagen sutures are also highly reactive. The use of gut or collagen sutures in skin closure is strongly discouraged because bacterial infection often occurs secondary to the inflammatory tissue response (2, 20). In addition, the presence of infection will accelerate the absorption with a loss of strength and an increase in the risk of wound dehiscence.

Present reports indicate that polyglactin 910 (Vicryl) and polyglycolic acid (Dexon "S", Dexon-Plus) sutures have virtually identical biological characteristics. Any differences in the literature can most probably be attributed to differences in investigational methods, diversity of tissue, and variables not related to the suture material itself. Polyglactin 910, however, does not meet the requirement for size as set forth by the USP and therefore is larger on a size for size comparison basis with polyglycolic acid sutures. Both are absorbed by a noncellular, nonenzymatic, virtually noninflammatory process at predictable rates. Minimal absorption is reported until the thirtieth to forty-fifth day and essentially complete absorption in 60 to

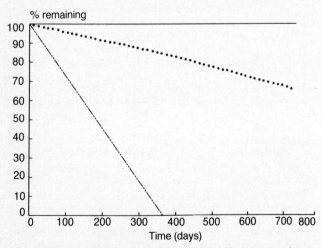

Figure 5.1. Graph demonstrating resorption of polyester, polypropylene, nylon, and silk sutures over time. Solid line, polyester polypropylene. Dotted line, nylon. Dashed line, silk.

90 days (Fig. 5.2). They incite far less tissue reaction and inflammation than their natural collagen counterparts (surgical gut and collagen) (4, 5). The synthetic sutures, unlike the natural collagens, can be used in skin closure. The manufacturers have indicated that skin sutures remaining in place longer than seven days may cause localized irritation requiring their removal.

Significant refinements have been made to the synthetic materials to alter their handling characteristics without changing their degree of tissue reaction. Polyglactin 910 contains a coating of calcium stearate whose components are present in the body and are constantly metabolized and excreted. Coated polyglycolic acid contains a surfactant called polaxamer 188, which is essentially eliminated from the body within three days. Both coating materials decrease tissue drag and enhance its handling properties (4, 5).

The more recently introduced synthetic monofilament, absorbable suture, polydioxanone (PDS), possesses slightly different characteristics. Data obtained from implantation studies in rats show that the absorption of these sutures is minimal until about the ninetieth postimplantation day. Absorption is considered to be essentially complete within six months, a considerable length of time. Tissue response has been reported to be of minimal to slight intensity. No evidence of acute or chronic toxicity and no evidence of tumorigenicity, teratogenicity, allergenicity, immunogenicity, or pyogenicity have been revealed in clinical or preclinical studies. Polydioxanone suture is a smooth monofilament with near optimum biological properties. Construction of this monofilament precludes the necessity of a coating to increase its lubricity and decrease tissue drag and decreases the likelihood of drawing fluids into the tissue when used in skin closure.

Nonabsorbable Sutures

Silk and cotton consistently incite more tissue reaction than their synthetic counterparts, and are responsible for the greatest incidence of infection among all sutures in this group (2, 7, 10, 13, 26) (Table 5.4). Silk, although classified as a nonabsorbable suture, undergoes degradation and absorption at variable rates and thus behaves as an absorbable suture (Fig. 5.1) (2, 6–10, 27, 28).

Monofilament nylon (Dermalon, Ethilon) is far from being chemically inert and undergoes absorption by slow hydrolysis over an extended period of time (14, 19) (Fig. 5.1). Tolerance to bacterial contamination is good, but inferior to that of polypropylene.

Polypropylene (Surgilene, Prolene) is an extremely inert material and is not subject to the tissue degradation shown by nylon and silk. It is highly resistant to bacterial contamination and is superior to both nylon and stainless steel in this regard (2, 10, 13, 17, 20). These properties make it an ideal suture material for skin closure and for closure of previously infected or contaminated wounds.

Polyester sutures in general are well tolerated with only mild tissue response reported, but they are associated with a higher incidence of infection in contaminated wounds than is nylon, but less than stainless steel. When they are coated or impregnated with polytetrafluoroethrae (Teflon or PFTE, Tevdek, Polydek, Ethiflex) or silicone (Ti-Cron), they tend to shed fragments over several months, giving rise to marked inflammatory responses (7, 10, 26). When they are coated with polybutilate (Ethibond), minimal cellular response is seen, even superior to that of uncoated polyester sutures (5, 9). The high affinity of the polyester for polybutilate results in virtually no flaking or shredding. Evidence suggests that coatings do not alter the incidence of infection in contaminated tissue (9, 13).

Stainless steel is not as inert as some of the pure synthetic polymers just mentioned. It elicits a tissue reaction similar to monofilament nylon sutures. Furthermore, metallic materials may undergo degradation by corrosion, especially at points of stress. Its physical properties prevent it from readily conforming to the topography of the suture pathway and impart considerable mechanical irritation and trauma to the tissue. These factors may be responsible for impairing the wound's ability to resist infection (10, 17).

MECHANICAL PROPERTIES
Absorbable Sutures

Synthetic absorbable sutures are far superior to and more dependable than surgical gut or collagen

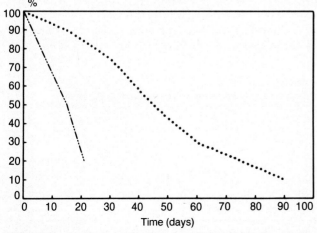

Figure 5.2. Graph demonstrating resorption and tensile strength loss of polyglycolic acid and polyglactin 910 sutures over time. Dotted line, resorption. Dashed line, tensile strength loss.

Table 5.4
Relative Tissue Reaction of Nonabsorbable Sutures

Monofilament polypropylene
Monofilament nylon
Stainless steel wire
Polybutilate coated polyester
Uncoated braided polyester
Teflon/silicone coated polyester
Natural fiber materials

Modified from Yu GV, Cavaliere R: Suture materials. *J Am Podiatry Assoc* 73:60, 1983.

sutures with respect to tensile strength loss or retention, knot security, and handling properties. The early tensile strength of the synthetic absorbable (Dexon "S", Dexon-Plus, Vicryl) sutures is reported to be greater than that of comparable surgical gut sutures. In vitro studies have shown that, at two weeks post-implantation, approximately 55% of the original tensile strength remains, whereas at three weeks approximately 20% of its original strength is retained. The tensile strength of synthetic absorbable sutures is not a function of absorption rate (Fig. 5.2). In addition, they are not influenced by exposure to aqueous tissue fluids, as is surgical gut, which may show a rapid loss of tensile strength and marked loss of knot security under such conditions. There is some recent evidence, however, that indicates tensile strength and its loss and retention may be affected by the pH of the surrounding environment (4, 5, 9, 28, 30, 31).

Coated polyglycolic acid (Dexon-Plus), the newest marketed synthetic absorbable suture, possesses excellent handling properties, but poor knot security with conventional tying methods. These characteristics are attributed to its extremely low coefficient of friction. The manufacturer has advised that several additional knots be thrown and that ear lengths be longer than in conventional knots. The tensile strength of Dexon Plus may be slightly greater than other absorbable sutures of comparable size.

Polydioxanone sutures have been formulated to provide prolonged wound support through an extended healing period. Available data indicate that polydioxanone retains its breaking strength in vivo healing twice as long as any other synthetic absorbable sutures. Implantation studies of polydioxanone sutures in animals indicate that approximately 70% of the original strength remains two weeks after implantation. At four weeks postimplantation approximately 50% of its original strength is retained, and at six weeks, approximately 25% of the original strength is retained. These sutures are particularly useful when the combination of an absorbable suture and extended or prolonged wound support (up to six weeks) is desirable. When such requirements are not desirable, polyglycolic acid (Dexon "S") or polyglactin 910 (Vicryl) suture are probably preferrable. Two clinical studies evaluating the performance characteristics of polydioxanone sutures rated the sutures as significantly better than surgical gut sutures with regard to visibility, pliability, strength, ease of passage, ease of tying, fraying, knot security, and overall handling. The final postoperative evaluation in these same studies rated polydioxanone suture as significantly better than surgical gut sutures in relation to the wound healing process.

Nonabsorbable Sutures

Tensile Strength

If the force necessary to break a strand of material is divided by its cross-sectional area, a constant known as the tensile strength is derived that permits comparison of relative strength between different suture materials (9). Stainless steel, in either monofilament or multifilament form, possesses the highest tensile strength, and natural fiber materials, such as cotton, silk, and linen, the least (30–33). The synthetic monofilament and multifilament sutures possess intermediate tensile strengths (Table 5.5) (31, 32). Silk and cotton, however, gradually lose tensile strength when implanted in tissue, as does nylon (11, 28). Nylon has been shown to retain virtually no tensile strength after six months (34). Polyester sutures are second only to metallic sutures in tensile strength, followed by monofilament nylon, polypropylene, and polyethylene. Only polypropylene and polyester sutures have been shown to retain their tensile strength for long periods of time (13, 28). Braided nylon sutures are somewhat weaker than monofilament nylon sutures (30–33).

Elasticity and Plasticity

The elastic behavior of a suture is the inherent ability of the internal tension (called stress) to return to the material to its original length after stretching (called strain). The material is considered to be relatively compliant or stiff. The plastic behavior of a suture refers to the tension increase seen when the material is stretched beyond its elastic limit up to the breaking point and is not reversible (9).

Compared with silk, polyester is stiff and brittle, whereas steel is very stiff but ductile (33, 35, 36). Nylon and polypropylene are clearly the most compliant and most ductile of all available suture materials. They possess the property of "memory," a built-in orientation of the polymer produced by stretching during the manufacturing process. This property permits elongation under tension and recovery to its original dimension when tension subsides or is removed. Polypropylene sutures in particular are noted for this property (36).

Knot and Knot Security

A knot may be defined as the fastening made by entangling together one or more cords so that any tension on the fastening results in increased contact pressure between the component parts of the knot. Unsecured knots result from slippage, a phenomenon that occurs to some degree with all knots, regardless of the material used. A secure knot is one that will

Table 5.5
Relative Tensile Strength of Nonabsorbable Sutures

Stainless steel wire
Coated braided polyester
Uncoated braided polyester
Monofilament nylon
Braided nylon
Monofilament polypropylene
Monofilament polyethylene
Natural fiber

From Yu GV, Cavaliere R: Suture materials. *J Am Podiatry Assoc* 73:61, 1983.

hold without slipping significantly until the suture breaks, and very closely correlates with the material's coefficient of friction. Other factors affecting knot security include the length of the cut ends or ears, the type of knot and, for some materials, the presence or absence of moisture or tissue implantation. Surgical technique in knot tying is another important factor (9, 17, 31).

The structural configuration of the knot is the most variable factor that critically affects knot security. Regardless of the material employed, square knots or a surgeon's knot with superimposed square knots are far superior to any other configuration (Fig. 5.3). The surgeon should tie secure knots with the fewest number of throws, thus ensuring the burial of the least amount of suture material. Increasing the number of throws increases the knot security further; however, the increment of additional security gained with each additional throw is decreased. It is the meticulous technique in the laying and setting of knots that is essential (17, 30, 31, 37).

The length of the cut ends or ears of the suture will affect knot slippage and thus knot security. Cutting the ears flush with the knot is hazardous and invites untying of the suture. It has been recommended that 3 mm at the cut ends be left intact. Long ears serve to provide an unnecessary abundance of foreign material in the surgical wound. Tension applied to a knot also influences the eventual slippage. Each throw should be snugged against the adjacent throw to prevent slippage (17).

The coefficient of friction is another critical factor affecting knot security (Table 5.6). Metallic sutures possess the highest coefficient of friction and the greatest knot security, regardless of the configuration or number of knots thrown. Uncoated polyester sutures (Dacron, Mersilene), lightly coated polytetrafluoroethylene (PFTE, Teflon), polyester sutures (Polydex, Ethiflex), and silk sutures are superior to both the polytetrafluoroethylene-impregnated polyester sutures (Tevdek) or silicone-coated polyester sutures (Ti-Cron) in knot security. Other materials are intermediate in knot security. Monofilament nylon sutures (Dermalon, Ethilon) possess the greatest proclivity for

knot slippage. Polypropylene sutures (Surgilene, Prolene), on the other hand, when carefully tied with square knots and set securely and firmly, show flattening wherever strands cross, which helps to lock the knot and then improve knot security. This is attributed to its softer construction. When the effects of implantation within tissues are considered, uncoated polyester sutures are unsurpassed in resisting the effects on knot failure. Cotton and linen sutures show increased knot security when wet (9, 30, 35).

THE SUTURES—A PRACTICAL OVERVIEW
Stainless Steel Wire

Stainless steel wire provides the greatest strength and knot security of all available nonabsorbable suture materials; however, its poor handling characteristics may result in kinking, fatigue, fracture, or deformation at points of stress. It incites mild to moderate tissue reaction, but is generally well tolerated in body tissues. The ends of the wire suture must be handled carefully to avoid puncture of gloves or tissue. Special instrumentation should be employed to cut the wire suture. Twisted multistrand steel wire sutures (Flexon) are more flexible and easier to handle and tie. However, they may be associated with a higher incidence of infection. Development of the Roto Grip needle minimizes twisting and kinking, and allows the needle and suture to swivel 360° on one another. Stainless steel sutures are particularly useful for bone fixation. Other uses include repair of tendon ruptures, as retention sutures, and less commonly in subcuticular skin closure. It is not currently available attached to plastic cuticular needles and thus is not strongly recommended over other suture materials possessing superior characteristics that are available attached to premium needles.

Polypropylene

Although only average in strength, polypropylene (Surgilene, Prolene) maintains its strength indefinitely when implanted in tissue, and will undergo stretch more than any other currently available suture material. In addition, it is highly resistant to flexural fatigue. It should not, however, be employed where strong coaptation of tissue is a critical or major requirement. Other absorbable and nonabsorbable sutures are superior in this regard. It is extremely inert,

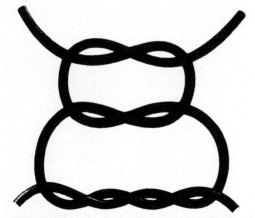

Figure 5.3.   Surgeon's knot with superimposed square knot.

Table 5.6
Relative Coefficient of Friction of Nonabsorbable Sutures

Stainless steel
Uncoated braided polyester
Uncoated braided nylon
Coated braided polyester
Coated braided nylon
Monofilament synthetics

From Yu GV, Cavaliere R: Suture materials. *J Am Podiatry Assoc* 73:62, 1983.

passes through tissues with minimal drag and trauma, and overall possesses excellent handling characteristics. When delayed or retarded healing is expected or contamination is present, closure with polypropylene will provide dependable wound support. As with other synthetic sutures, knot security requires the surgical technique of flat and square ties with additional throws, if indicated by surgical circumstances or the experience of the surgeon. It is the ideal skin closure material, whether used in a subcuticular (intradermal stitch) fashion or conventionally.

Nylon

In its monofilament form (Dermalon, Ethilon) nylon is superior to polypropylene in strength but inferior in elasticity; tissue reaction is somewhat greater than with polypropylene. It undergoes slow absorption by hydrolysis and loses tensile strength over a long period of time. Like polypropylene it is not recommended for application where permanent holding power is desired or required. In addition, it possesses the greatest proclivity for knot slippage. Its handling characteristics and knot-tying properties are otherwise similar to that of polypropylene. Multifilament (braided) nylon (Nurolon, Surgilon) offers no clinically significant advantages over the monofilament form. Monofilament nylon is an excellent suture material for skin closure second only to polypropylene sutures when a nonabsorbable suture is desired..

Polyester

Sutures made of polyester are the strongest nonabsorbable synthetic suture material available today, superior to both nylon and polypropylene and second only to stainless steel sutures. It undergoes very little stretch but elicits some degree of increased tissue reaction. This is an ideal suture material when strong coaptation of ligaments, capsule, or tendon is a critical requirement, and one desires a nonabsorbable suture.

Uncoated polyester sutures (Mersilene, Dacron) are somewhat rougher than coated sutures but allow unsurpassed knot security. Lightly coated polytetrafluoroethylene (Teflon, PFTE) polyester sutures (Ethiflex, Polydek) rank second in this regard and possess improved handling characteristics. The polytetrafluoroethylene-impregnated polyester sutures (Tevdek) and silicone-coated polyester sutures (Ti-Cron), although possessing excellent handling characteristics, demonstrate increased tissue reaction and decreased knot security. Polybutilate-coated polyester sutures (Ethibond) possess similar handling characteristics, but appear to have less tissue reaction than the uncoated or coated polyester suture materials and would appear to be the ideal polyester suture for use in podiatric surgery.

Polyethylene

Polyethylene (Dermalene) sutures are similar to polypropylene but appear to have less knot security. Clinical studies to date are very limited. They have no apparent significant advantages over nylon or polypropylene sutures.

Polyglycolic Acid and Polyglactin 910

Polyglycolic acid and polyglactin 910 sutures are very similar absorbable materials with biological and physical properties superior to that of surgical gut or collagen, but similar to each other. In addition to eliciting far less tissue reaction, they are generally superior in tensile strength, tensile strength retention and loss, knot security, and resisting the effects of tissue fluids or contamination, without possessing special handling restrictions imposed on the surgical gut sutures.

Both polyglycolic acid sutures and polyglactin 910 sutures lose their strength much faster than they are absorbed (Fig. 5.2). They can be used in skin closure without concern about increased infection rates, although localized topical irritation has been reported that has required removal of the material. Coated polyglycolic acid sutures (Dexon-Plus) show very poor knot security with conventional tying methods. Consequently their use in foot surgery is somewhat limited. The manufacturer has recommended the addition of several extra square knots and cutting ear lengths of 4 to 5 mm. It appears to be an excellent suture material in subcuticular (intradermal) skin closures.

The polyglycolic acid sutures are indicated when a permanent suture is not required or desired, as in muscle, fascia, capsule, paratendinous tissues, tendon, subcutaneous tissues, and subcuticular skin closure. Surgical gut has earned a most honorable place in the history of surgical sutures, but its use today should be limited. It is a suture that should be relegated to the past. It offers no advantages over any of the synthetic absorbable sutures available today.

Polydioxanone

Like Dexon-Plus, polydioxanone suture is one of the newer synthetic absorbable sutures. Unlike its counterparts that are multifilament, polydioxanone is the first synthetic absorbable suture to be prepared as a monofilament in a full range of sizes. It possesses a relatively high degree of flexibility that is achieved by the incorporation of an ether group into the backbone structure of polydioxanone.

Although clinical studies comparing this suture to its synthetic counterparts (Dexon "S", Dexon-Plus, Vicryl) are limited, it has been established that the retention of breaking strength of this new suture is superior to the other absorbable sutures: at four weeks postimplantation approximately 50% of its original strength is retained compared with that for polyglycolic acid or polyglactin 910 (Dexon "S", Vicryl), which is typically only 20% at three weeks postimplantation. In addition, infection at the site of suture implantation appears to have no effect on the breaking strength retention of polydioxanone sutures. The absorption profile of this suture is somewhat less than ideal, being minimal until about the ninetieth postimplantation day. Absorption can be considered essentially complete at about six months; a more rapid absorption profile is certainly more desirable. Tissue reaction is minimal.

Polydioxanone suture should not be routinely used as a substitute for other synthetic absorbable sutures. These sutures should be used when a combination of an absorbable suture and extended wound support are desirable. Examples of such situations would include medial capsulorrhaphy of the first metatarsophalangeal joint in bunion surgery; primary repair of ruptured tendons and ligaments; major tendon transfers and lengthenings; and certain deep fascial structures. In many circumstances this suture could be used in place of the various polyester sutures. It is hoped that additional clinical studies of the suture will be published in the near future.

SURGICAL NEEDLES

Surgical needles function to carry and deliver suture material through specific tissues. Like suture materials, they are available in a wide variety of designs. The inappropriate selection of a surgical needle may not only prolong the conduct of the operation but may also cause unnecessary damage to the specific tissues being sutured. Such needless damage to the structural integrity of tissues may produce necrosis of tissue with the subsequent development of infection and failure to maintain approximation. At times such failure may compromise the final outcome of a surgical procedure. Wound dehiscence, evisceration or herniation of tissues, adhesions, and the development of sinus tracts or fistulas may result depending on the tissues and the area of the body involved.

Like suture materials, the surgical needle chosen should be determined by the nature of the procedure being performed, the type and nature of the tissues being sutured, the location and accessibility of the tissue, and to a lesser degree the individual preference of the surgeon. There are, however, certain desirable features of all surgical needles deserving of discussion.

One basic assumption can be made regarding the most appropriate or ideal surgical needle for a given application, namely, that the tissues being sutured should be minimally altered because the only purpose of the needle is to provide delivery of the suture material through the tissues to be approximated. Apposition of the sutured tissues must then be maintained until sufficient tensile strength develops by normal biological processes of healing.

The surgical needle should be sharp enough to penetrate tissues easily with minimal resistance and minimal trauma, yet rigid enough to prevent excessive bending or alteration of the physical and architectural design while being flexible enough to bend before fragmenting or breaking. The needle should make a hole in the tissue just large enough to permit the introduction and passage of the suture material. The needle should be large enough and of appropriate shape and design to permit rapid, accurate, and precise suturing of tissues. Finally, the architecture of the

tissues being sutured should not be weakened to any significant degree during the process of wound approximation.

There is currently a paucity of information regarding and comparing similar needles of different manufacturers. However, recent surgical literature has presented many new needles, most of which have been modifications of needles in use for many years. One of the largest suture manufacturing companies in the world lists well over 100 various needles. It is important that the surgeon be aware of factors that are important in the selection of a particular shape, size, or type of needle, even before selecting a needle from the huge number available on the market today. Important factors that should be considered are the characteristics of the tissue and wound being sutured, as well as the characteristics of the needles themselves.

TISSUE AND WOUND CHARACTERISTICS

Although the mechanical aspects of wound closure seem insignificant by comparison, technical considerations, such as the broad apposition of raw tissues, avoidance of excessive tension on sutured wounds, preservation of adequate blood supply, accurate alignment of different tissue layers, and appropriate eversion or inversion of wound edges, as the case may be, are all clinically important and based on biological factors. The mechanical characteristics of any given specific type of tissue, such as tensile strength, weave, shear strength, penetrability, density, elasticity, and thickness would seem to be tissue factors that the surgeon should consider in choosing a surgical needle and suture. Because tensile and sheer strength of the tissue are probably more important than the ability of the suture material to maintain the sutured tissues in apposition, one should then concentrate on the characteristics of weave, penetrability, density, elasticity, and thickness of the tissue. Each of these characteristics will affect successful passage of a surgical needle through the tissues (38).

The fabriclike qualities of any given tissue are determined by the type of connective tissue that it contains. The subcutaneous tissue is primarily loose connective tissue or areolar tissue with cellular and reticular components. Its various cellular elements consist of fibroblasts, mesenchymal cells, macrophages, and fat cells. The subcutaneous tissue has little structural integrity and thus sutures passing through it would be incidental rather than purposeful in contrast to the sutures through denser connective tissues with significant substance and integrity. The type of needle will determine the ease with which one can readily penetrate the tissue and pass the sutures through (38).

In general, access to surgical wounds of the foot does not pose major problems for the surgeon, as is frequently encountered in general surgery, and thus has little direct influence on the insertion of sutures. Most problems regarding access to the wound can be readily resolved by proper positioning of the lower extremity (i.e. use of sandbags beneath the hip to facilitate internal rotation of the limb to improve access to the lateral aspect of the foot) and/or positioning of the surgeon.

The specific topography of the wound, however, is second in importance to the nature of the tissues in the wound. Specific factors such as the width, depth, and curvature may pose problems with suturing a wound. Every surgeon has encountered a situation where a given needle, because of inadequate or improper strength, curvature, and design, posed great difficulty in suturing. The medial capsulloraphy following a bunion procedure is but one example.

Both the depth and diameter of a given wound will be important in the selection of the most appropriate surgical needle. The overall geometrical configuration of a needle will greatly influence the amount of hand and wrist motion required during suturing. A straight needle or one-half curved needle may be more easily manipulated because very little pronation or supination motion will be required. These same needles, however, because of the larger arch of manipulation required, are either more ackward or simply cannot be used in deeper cavities or wounds. A one-half or five-eighths circle needle, on the other hand, although requiring more pronation and supination of the wrist, is much easier to use in confined or relatively inaccessible locations. At the same time, the additional arc of degrees required in manipulating these needles make them distinctly disadvantageous for use when suturing the skin or wide, superficial or shallow wounds or tissue layers. In such cases a three-eighths circle needle will be easier to manipulate. Regardless of whether the surgeon is suturing the skin edges or closing the deeper layers, the needle size and curvature will affect the ease with which the needle can be manipulated and thus have a direct bearing on the efficiency of wound closure (38).

NEEDLE CHARACTERISTICS
Materials

Current surgical needles are manufactured from high quality stainless steel wire chosen to provide such characteristics as strength, temper, hardness, malleability, ductility, and surface finish. The wire that comes from the supplier to the needle manufacturer is soft in nature. Various heat treating techniques provide strength to the needle, reflected by such characteristics as temper, hardness, malleability, and sharpness. The needles must be clean and corrosion resistant to minimize the risk of infection. Electropolishing of the needle will remove debris from the surface and eliminate surface defects. Special treatment of the needle surfaces with a microthin film of silicon increases their lubricity and allows greater ease of penetration and passage through the tissues. The manufacturing of needles today is so highly standardized that only the finest quality opthalmic and microsurgical needles are subject to individual scrutiny by an inspector. The majority of surgical needles are batch tested for quality assurance (4, 5, 38).

Larger manufacturers of needles have raised the technology of production to unbelievable standards of quality by developing machines and processes that, with minimal human intervention, perform each step of manufacture. The highly automated manufacturing process allows batches of 10,000 to 14,000 needles to pass through the successive manufacturing stages at one time. Various testing devices measure the ability of the needle to penetrate a given surface, measure compression or tension forces on a needle, as well as the strength, diameter, and even the ability of the needle to be bent and then straightened before breaking. The finest plastic surgery needles today undergo special honing processes to ensure precision points with sharpness that is retained even on repeated passage of the needle through the skin.

A fascinating book, *The History of Needlework Tools and Accessories*, provides the reader with a historical tracing of the needle manufacturing process from Tudor England where needles were first made by individual craftsmen from bronze wire (39).

Basic Design

All surgical needles have three basic components: the eye, the body or the shaft, and the point.

The Eye

There are three types of eyes for the surgical needle: closed eye, French (split or spring) eye, or swaged (eyeless). Until 1874, needles had been eyed. The suture material was threaded through the eye, usually positioned at the end of the needle. With time, a number of modifications of the needle eye were made to recess and lessen the bulk of the double strands of suture materials passing through.

The French eyed or spring needles are slotted from inside the eye to the end of the needle so that the suture material can be snapped into or out of the eye. Eyed needles possess several disadvantages. They require special threading of the desired suture material before use, a potentially tedious and time-consuming activity. Eyed needles also tend to become separated from the suture frequently. The excessive bulk of the double strand is cumbersome to handle and imparts greater injury to the tissues being sutured. Although tying the suture to the eye greatly lessens the possibility of separation, it further increases the bulk of the suture material being drawn through the tissues and the subsequent damage being imparted. The use of the eyed needle in podiatric surgery is quite limited except in special circumstances such as major tendon transfers and the repair of tendon ruptures where specific suturing methods are facilitated by such needles.

Today most of the different sutures have appropriate needles attached by the manufacturer. Sutures directly attached to eyeless needles are referred to as swaged sutures. Swaged needles do not require special handling, selection, or threading and permit a single strand of suture material to be drawn through the tissues. The smooth junction between the suture and the needle, which results in a smaller hole, causes less tissue damage than threaded eyed needles. The needle and suture strand diameters of a swaged needle are almost equal. A new unused and undamaged needle is provided with each strand of suture that does not become unthreaded with use. When the expense of manufacturing swaged needles as compared with the cost of individual needle preparation, packaging, and threading, swaged needles possess distinct advantages over eyed and reusable needles. The swaged or eyeless surgical needles are by far the most popular and commonly used and are currently manufactured under the trade names Astraloc and Atraumatic.

An adaptation and modification of swaged needles to permit the fast separation of the needle from the suture when desired by the surgeon has recently been made. The introduction of these Control/Release, D-Tach, or RN (removable needles) provides a needle and suture combination that allows the placement of many sutures rapidly with extremely easy separation of sutures from needles by holding the needles securely in a needle holder and grasping the suture securely just below the needle followed by a straight line gentle but firm tug. In instances where a French eyed needle would previously have been used or in which it is desirable to leave a number of long suture ends before or after tying, such quick release needle suture products may prove convenient and beneficial to the surgeon.

The Body

The body or shaft of the needle may vary significantly in its overall shape and configuration with respect to both its longitudinal and cross sectional geometry. With respect to the needle's longitudinal geometry, it may be straight, half-curved (sometimes referred to as a ski needle), or curved. The straight needle is of course typified by the Keith needle or the milliner's needle. The half curved or ski Needle is curved only at its sharp end with the remaining portion of the shaft straightening the configuration. The curved needle is used most frequently. Its designations correspond to the arcs of the various degrees of a circle. The curvature may be one-fourth circle, three-eighths circle, one-half circle, and five-eighths circle. The three-eighths and one-half circle needles are the most frequently used in podiatric surgery today. (Fig. 5.4)

The cross-sectional geometry of the body or shaft of the needle may also vary from round or oval to flat or triangular. Round or oval bodies usually taper from a large diameter at the eye end decreasing to a smaller diameter at the point end. Triangular bodies have one edge lying either on the concave or convex side of the needle depending on the needle point. Other special cross-sectional configurations are available for specific surgical specialities and are not within the scope of this chapter.

To these basic shapes may be added the ribbed needle, a modification developed and invented by Gladys Chrisman in 1964, presently added to needles as an exclusive feature by one manufacturer. The

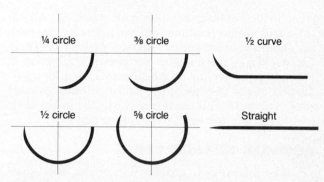

Figure 5.4. Diagrammatic representation of longitudinal geometry of surgical needle.

needle is fabricated with longitudinal ridges on the concave or convex surface, or both, to decrease undesirable angulational or rotational movements of the needle in the holder during the process of suturing. This is achieved by interdigitation of the longitudinal ribs with the serrations of the jaws of the needle holder. Ribbed needles give the surgeon the assurance of having a needle less likely to rock, twist, or turn while in the needle holder.

The Point

Each basic body may have one of several needle points that also vary in their geometrical configuration (Fig. 5.5). Each specific design is honed to the specific degree of sharpness to allow smooth penetration of a variety of tissues that are encountered in surgery. Basic shapes of the needle points are blunt, tapered, triangular, and diamond shaped. Each is used and recommended for specific purposes and specific tissues. Other shapes of needle cross sections are available but not relevant to extremity surgery. A more detailed description of needle point design and use is included within the section discussing the individual needles.

Size

Figure 5.6 illustrates the various parameters used in describing the size of a needle. The needle cord length represents the straight line distance from the point end of a curved needle to its eyed end. Needle length refers to the distance measured along the convex surface of the needle itself from point to end.

The diameter of the needle represents the caliber or thickness of the needle wire. Length-to-diameter ratio represents the ratio of the length of the needle to its diameter; a ratio greater than 8:1 renders the needle significantly more sensitive to loading and the needle will buckle or bend more easily. A lower ratio presents the disadvantage of wire diameter in relation to the diameter of the attached suture material and needlessly shortens the needle making it more difficult to pass through tissues and grasp with the needle holder or forceps.

Sterilization

Following packaging of the needle and suture combination, sterilization is accomplished with ethlyene oxide gas or irradiation with cobalt-60. All sutures and needle combinations are packaged dry with the exception of gut sutures that are packaged in fluid. The packaging method does not permit application of heat either by boiling or steam autoclaving for sterilization of the outside of the packet without damage to the contents. Foil packets may explode or the seals may become loosened in steam under pressure.

COMMON NEEDLE TYPES

The following is a discussion of the most commonly used needle types in podiatric surgery. Specific recommendations reflect the individual experience of both the authors and the staff of Doctors Hospital.

Taper Needle

The taper needle, the most commonly used noncutting needle in podiatric surgery, has no edges, thus preventing the likelihood of a portion of the needle behind the point cutting through tissues. The point of the needle is a rounded configuration and possesses minimal sharpness when compared to cutting needles and making its clinical use quite limited. Tapered needles are designed for the suturing of soft, friable, easily penetrable, tissues such as the paratenon, some tendon sheaths, some deep fascial tissues, and most commonly the superficial fascia or subcutaneous tissue layer. It is ideal for these tissue layers because it minimizes the accidental tearing or cutting during the suturing process. Penetration of more densely organized tissues such as the skin, ligaments, tendon, and capsule may be difficult with the use of a taper needle.

Although tapered point needles are sometimes referred to as round needles, inspection of their cross-sectional configuration will show them to be round only at the portion just behind the needle tip or point.

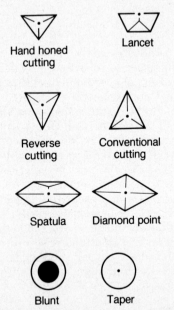

Figure 5.5. Diagrammatic representation of geometrical configuration of some of more commonly employed types of needle points.

The body or shaft of these needles will either be round or oval shaped, with or without ribbing depending on the manufacturer. The authors recommend the use of a T-5 or an SH for the suturing of superficial fascial tissues (subcutaneous tissue) on most areas of the foot, ankle, and lower leg. When a smaller needle is desired, such as when suturing the digits, a T-16 or SH-1 needle is recommended (Fig. 5.7).

Conventional Cutting Needle

The conventional cutting needle is one of two types of cutting needles that are ground and honed to provide edges that will cut through dense, difficult to penetrate, relatively thicker connective tissue layers. Because of the significant length of the needle's body or shaft's cutting edges, care must be taken in suturing those tissues with a thick layer of dense connective tissue to avoid inadvertently cutting through more of the tissue than is desired. Both conventional cutting and reverse cutting needles are triangular in shape and thus possess a total of three cutting edges.

The conventional cutting needle contains two opposing edges with a third cutting edge of the inner side or concave surface of the needle. Accidental enlargement of the hole made by the point of the needle

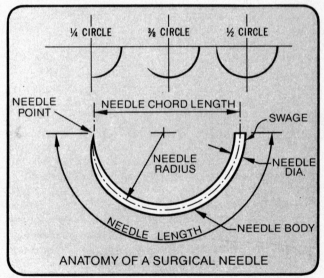

Figure 5.6. Diagram of some various parameters used in describing anatomy of surgical needle.

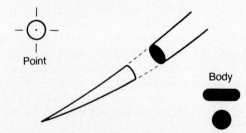

Figure 5.7. Geometrical configuration of point and body of taper needle. Note absence of cutting edges. Body of needle may be either round or oval in configuration.

may pose a problem during suturing. Several observations are deserving of comment. During suturing, greater force is usually directed toward the concave surface because the surgeon generally finds it easier to insert sutures with a forehand stroke of supination rather than a backhand stroke of pronation. As a result there is greater tendency to cause unnecessary and inadvertent cutting of tissues in the direction of the edge to be approximated. At times the tissue may be accidentally cut from its point of penetration to the edge of the tissue. This results in an increased incidence of "rethrow" or resuturing of the same area. In addition, because the third cutting edge on the inner or concave surface leaves a triangular hole whose apex is directed toward the edge of the tissue being sutured, there is a greater tendency for the sutures themselves to "pull through" as the suture is being worked or tied. Conventional cutting needles do not leave a hole with a flat surface paralleling the edge of the tissues being sutured and thus do not allow the suture to lay flat as it is being tied into position.

The authors do not recommend the use of a conventional cutting needle during the suturing of wounds or tissues in podiatric surgery. Its risks for potential damage of tissues far outweigh any potential benefits. Reverse cutting needles are preferred to conventional cutting needles when a cutting needle is desired by the surgeon (Fig. 5.8).

Reverse Cutting Needles

The reverse cutting needle, like the conventional cutting needle, is a multipurpose needle used to suture difficult to penetrate tissue, such as skin, and some dense, thick connective tissues such as tendon, ligaments, and capsule. It differs from the conventional cutting needle in that its third unopposed cutting edge is on the outer or convex surface of the needle. Because greater force is usually directed toward the concave surface as the surgeon inserts the needle with a forehand stroke of supination, less inadvertent damage and excess of cutting of the transfixed tissues is likely to occur. In addition, the triangular hole created with this needle has a flat surface paralleling the edge of the tissues and thus results in fewer rethrows or

resuturing of the wound, as well as fewer pull-throughs.

Reverse cutting needles for the most part have replaced conventional cutting needles as general multipurpose surgical needles. With care they can be used to suture virtually all types of tissues including the skin. They are, however, not the ideal needle for any given tissue or specific application. The authors recommend the use of a CE-6 or C-6 needle or a CP-2 or FS-1 for the surgeon desiring a general multipurpose needle. The C-6 or CP-2 and CE-6 or FS-1 differ only in their arc configurations, the first two being three-eighths of a circle and the latter being one-half circle. Ultimately the selection should be based on individual preference and the experience of the surgeon. These needles are preferred over their conventional cutting counterpart needles (Fig. 5.9).

Taper Cut, Diamond Point, or "K" Needles

The Taper Cut, Diamond Point, or "K" Needles represent the combination of a tapered needle and cutting needle. A Taper Cut needle possesses a reverse cutting point with a round needle shaft and an oval body. A Diamond Point needle employs a diamond point with four specially honed cutting edges and a round body. Both needles are ideally suited for penetration of virtually all tissues that are frequently difficult to penetrate and are composed of dense, thick, organized or unorganized connective tissue including tendon, capsule, ligament, and deep fascia. The only exception is skin. Although the cutting point provides ease of penetration, the remainder of the needle is a noncutting taper cross-section body that minimizes inadvertent damage or excessive cutting, slicing, splitting, or fraying of tissues. In addition there is less likelihood of accidental enlargement of the needle hole.

The authors recommend the use of this type of needle for closure of those tissues, except the skin, that may prove otherwise difficult to penetrate. Specific needle recommendations include the DT-19 or KC-5 for major ligament and tendon repairs; if a large needle is desired, the DT-12, KC-6, or V-34 may be preferred. The DT-5, KC-2, or V-7 are finer needles that are extremely useful for less dense tissues such

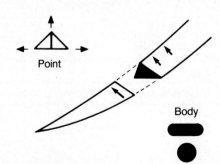

Figure 5.8. Goemetrical configuration of point and body of conventional cutting needle. Arrows on the point and body of needle indicate third unopposed cutting edge present on inner concave surface of needle and involves one half to two thirds of body. Remaining portion of body may be round or oval.

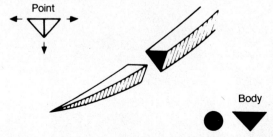

Figure 5.9. Geometrical configuration of point and body of reverse cutting needle. Third unopposed cutting edge is on outer concave portion of needle and involves one half to two thirds of body. Remaining portion of body may be round or oval.

as the deep fascia, smaller tendons, and some capsular tissues. The needles combine the best qualities of the taper and conventional or reverse cutting needles into one (Fig. 5.10).

Precision Point or Hand Honed Reverse Cutting Needles

Precision point or hand honed reverse cutting needles are especially designed reverse cutting needles which have undergone a special honing process of the point either by machine or hand to assure the smoothest passage through tissues, better placement of sutures, and a minute needle path that heals quickly. The cutting tip and point of one manufacturer are honed an extra 24 times to ensure the sharpest needles possible. These needles are particularly useful for skin closure and cosmetic and plastic reconstructive surgery. They are frequently referred to as plastic or cuticular needles. Because of their expense, they should not be employed for closing of tissues other than the skin because they offer no advantages over the previously described needles for closure of other tissues. Their routine use should be limited to reapproximation and closure of the skin edges.

The recently introduced slim blade edge (SBE) needles appear to be the slimmest, finest, and most precise needles for skin closure and leave an almost imperceptible hole. The authors strongly recommend the routine use of the SBE-4 (or SBE-3) for routine skin closure to aid in obtaining the finest cosmetic

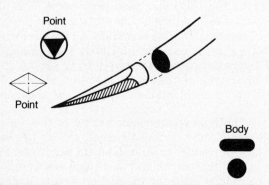

Figure 5.10. Geometrical configuration of point and body of Taper Cut or Diamond Point needle. Note this needle employs combination of taper needle body and reverse cutting needle point.

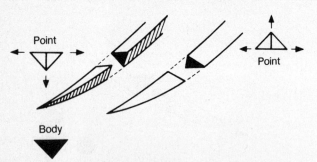

Figure 5.11. Geometrical configuration of point and body of a precision point or hand honed reverse cutting needle also known as plastic or cuticular needle. Note that point is similar to reverse cutting needle but has undergone extra honing. Body may be of conventional or reverse cutting configuration.

scars. Because of its fragility an alternative plastic surgery needle should be employed for closure of skin of the digits with an overlying hyperkeratotic lesion, as well as for skin of the plantar aspect of the foot. Alternative needles here would include the PS-2 or PRE-4. If a slightly smaller needle is desired, the PS-3 or PRE-3 may be preferred. The PRE-6 needle is a very beneficial needle for placement of larger retention type sutures particularly when suturing the plantar aspect of the foot (i.e. vertical mattress sutures). Plastic surgery needles that are of a conventional cutting needle configuration, although available, should not be employed for skin closure. They offer no advantages over the reverse cutting design. A limited selection of conventional cutting plastic surgery needles is available on the market today (Fig. 5.11).

NEEDLE CODING SYSTEM

The needle coding system presently employed by the three largest suture manufacturers is, unfortunately, one that has been described as being essentially without rhyme or reason. Each of the present manufacturers employs designations that consist of one or more letters alone or, more commonly, in combination with one or more numbers. These combinations, however, vary greatly among the manufacturers. In some instances the letter(s) may represent an abbreviation for a description of the needle itself; in other instances they may refer to a specialized surgical procedure in

Table 5.7
Common Letter Designations and Abbreviations of Swaged Atraumatic Needles

Letter or Abbreviation	Needle Description
SC or MC	Conventional cutting
C	Reverse cutting
PR	Hand honed reverse cutting
DT or DG	Diamond point
T	Taper point
Additional Letter	*Designation*
None	One-half circle
E	Three-eighths circle
O	One-fourth circle
Repeat first letter	Five-eighths circle
S	Straight needle

Table 5.8
Common Letter Designations and Abbreviations of Swaged Astralac Needles

Letter or Abbreviation	Needle Description
P	Plastic surgery
PS	Plastic surgery
CPS	Conventional plastic surgery
PC	Precision cosmetic
FS	For skin
FSL	For skin larger
FSLX	For skin large extra
SH	Small half
V	Taper cut needle
CP	Cutting point

which it has been found particularly useful; and in still other instances the letters may refer to the arc/ configuration or shape of the needle. The associated numbers most always refer to the length of the needle though there is no direct mathematical relationship between the number used in the needle designation and the actual length or size of the needle. One company employs a system of increasing size numbers corresponding with increasing arc length of the needle. Another employs a system of increasing size number corresponding to the decreasing size and length of its needles. Designations for needles commonly employed in podiatric and extremity surgery are listed in Tables 5.7 and 5.8.

One manufacturer employs letter designations to represent not only the type of needle (i.e. reverse cutting, taper point) but also the arc configuration (i.e. half-circle, one-fourth circle). For example, a PR needle is a half-circle hand honed reverse cutting needle whereas a PRE needle would be a three-eighths circle hand honed reverse cutting needle. The letter designations employed by another manufacturer represent either the type of needle (i.e. V for taper cut), size of the needle (i.e. SH for small half), or for what use the needle is intended (i.e. PS for plastic surgery). The differences in coding and lack of consistency have contributed greatly to the confusion over understanding the presently employed needle coding system. Standardization would be a welcomed change.

SUMMARY

The purpose of any surgical suture is to maintain approximation of severed tissues until endowed with sufficient strength to withstand stress without artificial or mechanical support. The purpose of the surgical needle is to deliver the selected suture material through the tissues undergoing reapproximation. Beyond this point sutures and needles generally serve no useful purpose and may serve as a source of irritation or a nidus for infection. The surgeon should understand that tissue support requirements vary extensively from a few days (skin, muscle, superficial fascia) to weeks and months (deep fascia, tendon, capsule, and bone).

In spite of continued progress and research, the ideal or perfect suture or needle has yet to be found and may in fact never be achieved. As a result today's surgeon has a wide choice of materials from which to select. Knowledge and understanding of the biological and physical properties of the various suture materials and needles, the healing capacity of various tissues, and the compatibility of the two, combined with sound judgment and careful surgical technique, will enhance the optimal outcome of any given surgical procedure. As new or improved suture materials and needles become available, the surgeon should be prepared to evaluate them to enhance operative skills and techniques.

References

1. Snyder CC: On the history of the suture. *Plast Reconstr Surg* 58:4, 1976.
2. "Sutures," in *Encyclopedia of Polymer Science and Technology*, Suppl No 1. New York, John Wiley & Sons Inc, 1976.
3. *United States Pharmacopeia XX*. Rockville, MD, The US Pharmacopceial Convention, Inc, 1980.
4. *Perspective on Sutures*. Pearl River NY, American Cyanamic Co, 1978.
5. Suture, Use Manual: *Use and Handling of Sutures and Needles*. Somerville NJ, Ethicon Inc, 1977.
6. Macht SD, Krifex TJ: Sutures and suturing: current concepts. *J Oral Surg* 36:710, 1978.
7. Postlethwait RW, Willigan DA, Ulin AW: Human tissue reaction to sutures. *Ann Surg* 181:144, 1975.
8. Peacock EE, Vanwinkle W: Repair of skin wounds. *Wound Repair*. Philadelphia, WB Saunders Co, 1976.
9. Clark DE: Surgical suture materials. *Contemp Surg* 17:40, 1980.
10. Postlethwait RW: Long-term comparative study of nonabsorbable sutures. *Ann Surg* 171:6, 1970.
11. Postlethwait RW: Wound healing: II. An evaluation of surgical suture material. *Surg Gynecol Obstet* 108:555, 1959.
12. Everett WG: Suture materials in general surgery. *Progressive Surg* 8:14, 1970.
13. Edlich RF, Paner PH, Rodenheaver GT: Physical and configuration of sutures in the development of surgical infection. *Ann Surg* 177:679, 1973.
14. Van Winkle W, Hastings C: Considerations in the choice of suture material for various tissue. *Surg Gynecol Obstet* 135:113, 1972.
15. Alexander JW, Kalplan JF, Altermeier WA: Role of suture materials in the development of infection. *Ann Surg* 165:192, 1967.
16. Blomstedt B, Osterberg B, Bergstrand A: Suture material and bacterial transport. *Acta Chir Scand* 143:71, 1977.
17. Thacker JG, Rodenheaver G, Kurtz L: Mechanical performance of sutures in surgery. *Am J Surg* 133:713, 1977.
18. Blomstedt B, Osterberg B: Suture materials and wound infections. *Acta Chir Scand* 144:269, 1978.
19. McGeehan D, Hunt D, Chaudhuri A: An experimental study of the relationship between synergistic wound sepsis and suture materials. *Br J Surg* 67:636, 1980.
20. Laufman H, Rubel T: Synthetic absorbable sutures. *Surg Gynecol Obstet* 145:597, 1977.
21. Stillman RM, Bella FJ, Seligman SJ: The effect of various wound closure methods on susceptibility to infection. *Arch Surg* 115:674, 1980.
22. Madsen ET: An experimental and clinical evaluation of surgical suture materials, part I. *Surg Gynecol Obstet* 97:439, 1953.
23. Madsen ET: An experimental and clinical evaluation of surgical suture materials, part II. *Surg Gynecol Obstet* 97:439, 1953.
24. Madsen ET: An experimental and clinical evaluation of surgical suture materials, part III. *Surg Gynecol Obstet* 106:216, 1958.
25. Forrester JC: Suture materials and their use. *Br J Hosp Med* 8:578, 1972.
26. Postlethwait RW: Five year study of tissue reaction to synthetic sutures. *Ann Surg* 190:54, 1979.
27. Van Winkle W, Salthouse TN: Biological response to sutures and principles of suture selection. Scientific Exhibit, American College of Surgeons 1975, Clinical Congress, San Francisco, CA.
28. Hermann JB: Changes in tensile strength and knot security of surgical sutures in vivo. *Arch Surg* 106:707, 1973.
29. Brantigan CO, Brown RK: The broken wire suture. *Am J Surg* 45:38, 1979.
30. Tera H, Aberg C: Strength of knots in surgery in relation to type of knots, type of suture material, and dimension of suture thread. *Acta Chir Scand* 143:75, 1977.
31. Hermann JB: Tensile strength and knot security of surgical suture materials. *American Surgeon, 37* 5:209, 1971.
32. Merchant LH, Knapp S, Apter JT: Effect of elongation, ratio on tensile strength of surgical suture materials. *Surg Gynecol Obstet* 139:231, 1974.
33. Becker H, Davidoff MR: The physical properties of suture materials as related to knot holding. *S Afr J Surg* 15:105, 1977.
34. Moloney GE: The effect of human tissue on the tensile strength of implanted nylon sutures. *Br J Surg* 68:528, 1961.
35. Holmlund DEW: Suture techniques and suture holding capacity. *Am J Surg* 134:616, 1977.

36. Holmlund DEW: Physical properties of surgical suture materials and stress-strain relationships, stress-relaxation and irreversible elongation. *Ann Surg* 184:189, 1976.

37. Thacker JG, Rodeheaver G, Moore JW: Mechanical performance of surgical sutures. *Am J Surg* 130:374, 1975.

38. Trier WC: Considerations in the choice of surgical needles. *Surg Gynecol Obstet* 149:84, 1979.

39. Graves S: *The History of Needlework Tools and Accessories.* Middlesex Eng, Hanlyn Publishing Group Ltd, 1966.

Additional References

Chu CC: A comparison of the effect of pH on the biodegradation of two synthetic absorbable sutures. *Ann Surg* 1:195, 1982.

Hardy JD: *Rhoads' Textbook of Surgery: Principles and Practices,* ed 5. Philadelphia, JB Lippincott Co, 1977, p 36.

Herman JB, Kelly RJ, Higgings GA: Polyglycolic acid sutures: laboratory and clinical evaluation of a new absorbable suture material. *Arch Surg* 100:486, 1970.

Herron J: Skin closure with subcuticular polyglycolic acid sutures. *Med J Aust* 2:535, 1974.

Laufman H: Is catgut obsolete? *Surg Gynecol Obstet* 145:587, 1977.

Lerwick E: Studies on the efficacy and safety of polydioxanone monofilament absorbable suture. *Surg Gynecol Obstet* 156:51, 1983.

Magilligan D Jr, DeWeese JA: Knot security and synthetic suture materials. *Am J Surg* 127:355, 1974.

Nora PF: *Operative Surgery, Principle and Techniques.* Philadelphia, Lea & Febiger, 1980, p 10.

Perey B, Watier A: Effect of human tissue on the breaking strength of catgut and polyglycolic acid sutures. *Chir Gastroenterol* 9:1, 1975.

Postlethwait RW: Polyglycolic acid surgical suture. *Arch Surg* 101:489, 1970.

Ray JA, Dodd N, Regula D: Polydioxanone (PDS): a novel monofilament synthetic absorbable suture. *Surg Gynecol Obstet* 153:497, 1981.

Rodeheaver GT, Edgerton MT, Smith S: Tissue containing suture implants. *Am J Surg* 133:609, 1977.

Rodeheaver GT, Thacker JG, Edlich RF: Mechanical performance of polyglycolic acid and polyglactin 910 synthetic absorbable sutures. *Surg Gynecol Obstet* 153:835, 1981.

Sabiston DC: *Textbook of Surgery,* ed 11. Philadelphia, WB Saunders Co, 1977, p 330.

Salthouse TN, Matlaga BR: Polyglactin 910 suture absorption and the role of cellular enzymes. *Surg Gynecol Obstet* 142:544, 1976.

Srugi S, Adamson J: A comparative study of tendon suture material in dogs. *Plast Reconstr Surg* 50:1, 1972.

Taylor FW: Surgical knots. *Ann Surg* 107:458, 1938.

Taylor TL: Suture material: a comprehensive review of the literature. *J Am Podiatry Assoc* 65:7, 1975.

Tera H, Aberg C: The strength of suture knots after one week in vivo. *Acta Chir Scand* 142:301, 1976.

CHAPTER 6

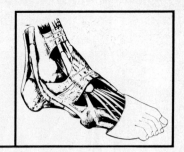

Materials and Products Used in Foot Surgery

David E. Marcinko, D.P.M.

There are many different intrinsic, extrinsic, permanent, temporary, and topically applied products used in reconstructive foot surgery. Each device may incorporate a variety of metallic, plastic, chemical, synthetic, or naturally occuring materials, the purpose of which is to facilitate surgery, minimize complications, and improve functional results. However, it is extremely important to understand the concepts, indications, and contraindications of each product to avoid indiscriminant use and technical complication. It is also important for the patient to understand how each of these products may affect postsurgical activity level, sequelae and convalescense. Therefore the following is a survey of current available materials and products used in foot surgery.

IMPLANT MATERIALS

Many different metals have historically been used in the construction of human joint implants. Metals used for prosthetic devices in foot surgery have included alloys of titanium, cobalt, chromium, molybdenum, vitallium, and durallium, as well as other compositions of stainless steel (1) (Fig. 6.1). Because metals seem to possess excellent biocompatibility and biodurability characteristics, the American Society for Testing Materials (ASTM) has established standards for metallic composition and quality (2). Unfortunately the biophysical response to these unyielding materials may often produce destructive in vivo complications because of the extensive osseous remolding they invoke (3). Therefore metals are currently not primarily used, but rather conjoined with softer materials to interface between component parts (4).

An example of this concept is the congruous constrained ankle joint implants of Scholz and Smith (5,6) that incorporate molybdenum and polyethylene components. Another example is the Richards Total First metatarsophalangeal joint implant arthroplasty system, which was introduced by Weil and Smith (7) in 1976 but has since been abandoned. Similarly, the Reginald ball and socket first metatarsophalangeal joint prosthesis fell into disuse because of dorsal migration of the metatarsal head component (8). Thus metals will probably have little relevance in foot surgery until modifications are developed to reduce destructive bone complications.

SILICONE ELASTOMER PRODUCTS

The development of medical grade silicone rubber was accomplished in 1962 and has been regularly used in the production and fabrication of various implant and product designs (9). Silicone elastomer is considered a material of choice because, according to Scales, (10) it is (a) chemically inert and incapable of a foreign body or hypersensitivity reaction, (b) noncarcinogenic, (c) capable of precise molding and shaping, (d) capable of resisting stress and strain as evidenced by its hookian curve ratio, and (e) capable of being sterilized. Silicone elastomer is manufactured from a high viscosity fluid with particles of silicone added for tensile strength (11). The elastomer itself is composed of a chain of silicone and oxygen atoms, to which organic side groups are attached, to achieve differing durometers. The resultant material is then vulcanized with a dichlorobenzaline catalyst, which links the polymer side chains without becoming a permanent part of the compound (12). Hence the heat cured conventional silicone Silastic elastomer contains only silicone polymer and silica fiber (13).

In 1975 medical grade high performance (HP) silicone elastomer was introduced for use in implantable materials (14). HP silicone differs from conventional silicone elastomer in that its propagation strength and fatigue resistance is increased six hundred fold (15). Its flexural durability and tear propagation are derived from excellent physical prop-

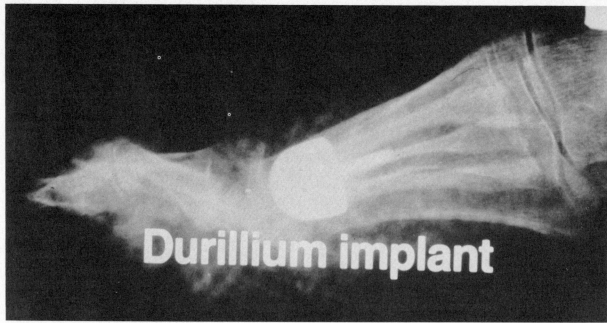

Figure 6.1. Seeburger type durallium extension prosthesis used to cap first metatarsal head.

Table 6.1.
Typical Physical Properties of High-Performance and Conventional Medical-Grade Silicone Elastomer

PROPERTY	METHOD	CONVENTIONAL	HIGH PERFORMANCE
Tensile strength	ASTM D 412[a]	1200 psi	1500 psi
Ultimate elongation	ASTM D 412	450%	700%
Modulus at 100% elongation	ASTM D 412	200 psi	300 psi
Tear-initiation strength, Die C	ASTM D 624	Varies widely	300 ppi
Tear-propagation strength, Die B	ASTM D 624	75 ppi	300 ppi
Crack-growth resistance	ASTM D 813	.42"/7000 cycles	.1"/10^6 cycles
Durometer, Shore A	ASTM D 2240	50	52
Specific gravity	ASTM D 924	1.14	1.15

[a] ASTM—American Society for Testing and Materials.
(From Frisch E: Biomaterials in foot surgery. In Weil LS (ed): *Clinics in Podiatry* 1:18, 1984.)

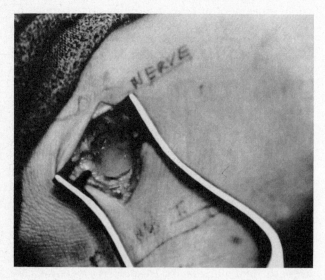

Figure 6.2. Hand carved cylindrical Silastic endoprosthesis, situated within canalis tarsalis, used as type of arthrodesis procedure. (Courtesy of Dr. M. Rappaport, Atlanta, GA.)

erties: tensile strength of 1400 psi, tear propagation strength of 300 psi, and a fatigue crack growth rate of only 0.1 inch per million cycles (16). HP silicone is radiopaque, nonadherent, biocompatible, and possesses excellent forced dampening properties (Table 6.1). It is also versatile, being supplied in both block form, which is shaped intraoperatively, and as the well-known intramedullary stemmed implants of Swanson, Weil, and others (17) (Fig. 6.2).

Other Silicone-Derived Products

One silicone-derived product is thin (.007 inch) flat, BaSo4-impregnated, flexible Incision Drain designed for the evacuation of blood and fluids from wound sites following minor procedures (18). It minimizes the potential for inflammation and sinus tract formation, is supplied sterile in 25-cm lengths (two drains per package), and is easily cut into the desired length at the time of surgery.

Another silicone-derived product is silicone Tendon Spacer, which is used as a temporary conduit to facilitate two-stage reconstruction of flexor or extensor tendons of the foot. At stage I the spacer is placed in the reconstructed tendon bed and attached at its insertion, while the proximal end is left free. Stage II surgery usually is done after an adequate pseudosheath is formed around the spacer, and a permanent active free tendon graft is attached to the spacer and drawn into the pseudosheath as the spacer is removed. A spacer sizing set is supplied for proper size determination during surgery (19).

A translucent (0.18 mm) Silastic sheet may be used for the formation of a pseudotendon sheath, in localized pedal sites, when conditions are present that might lead to excessive postoperative fibrous tissue (20) (Fig. 6.3).

A tubular Silastic nerve cap is designed to cover the end of an amputated peripheral nerve to aid in the prevention, or minimize the recurrence, of painful neuromata (Fig. 6.4). The closed end may also be cut off sharply and the tubular portion used as a nerve cuff in selected cases to protect the site of nerve repair (21).

Finally, although rare and relatively benign, many different complications have been associated with the use of silicone materials and products. These have included inflammatory reactions, fibrous tissue hyperplasia, microfragmentation, detritic synovitis, bone destruction, cyst formation, aseptic necrosis, and silicone lymphadenitis (22–27).

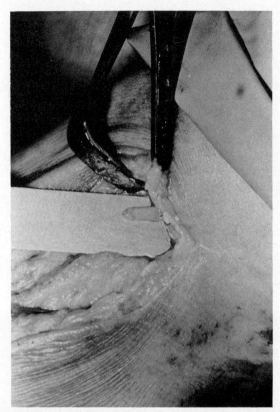

Figure 6.4. Tubular Silastic nerve cap used to cover end of stump neuroma of anterior tibial nerve of foot. (Courtesy of Drs. C. Frank and K. Weeber, Atlanta, GA.)

Injectable Silicone/Collagen

Percutaneously injected fluid silicone has been used as a soft tissue replacement substitute since it was first reported by Baronedes and associates in 1950 (28). In podiatric medicine it has been effectively used in the conservative treatment of helomata, tylomata, and recurring neurotrophic ulcerations, and to protect various skin sites from focal pressure by bony prominences (Fig. 6.5). Pioneering work in this field was done by Balkin (29) whose 19-year retrospective study revealed that the only adverse side effect was asymptomatic silicone migration.

Although the safety of injectable silicone has not been confirmed by the Food and Drug Administration, long-term necropsy and biopsy specimens have revealed no adverse tissue response (30). Successfully completed research, federal approval, and proper use could alleviate surgery and provide relief for millions of people who suffer from common but debilitating pedal disorders (Fig. 6.6A, B).

During the past two years carefully controlled and double-blind studies on the use of injectable cowhide (Zyderm Collagen Implant, ZCI) collagen have been performed by various researchers throughout the country (Dr. D. Elleby, personal communication). Injectable collagen differs from injectable silicone in that it is a highly purified and reconstituted dispersion that

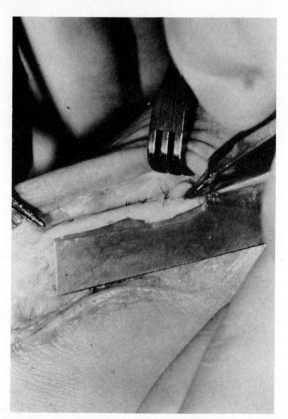

Figure 6.3. Translucent Silastic sheet material used to create pseudotendon sheath of the tendon of m. extensor hallucis longus. (Courtesy of Drs. C. Frank and K. Weeber, Atlanta, GA.)

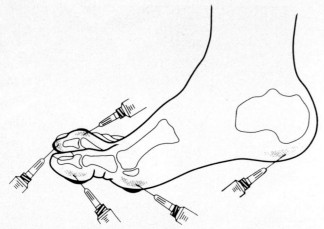

Figure 6.5. Digital and plantar pressure points benefited by fluid silicone injections between skin and bones. (From Balkin SW: The fluid silicone prosthesis. In Weil LS (ed): *Clinics in Podiatry* 1:145, 1984.)

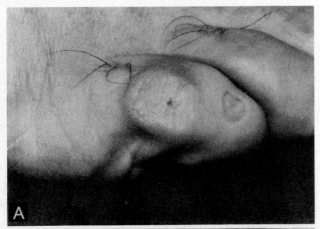

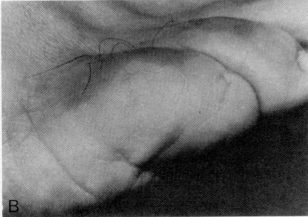

Figure 6.6. (A) Painful dorsolateral lesion of fifth digit before treatment with injectable silicone fluid. (B) Increased comfort with diminished lesion appearance, 10 years after injection of 0.4 ml silicone fluid prosthesis. (From Balkin SW: The fluid silicone prosthesis. In Weil LS (ed): *Clinics in Podiatry*. 1:145, 1984.)

serves as a matrix into which host fibroblasts and capillaries grow (31). The newly vascularized implant is subsequently incorporated by the host tissue into the soft tissue stroma of the implantation site (Fig.

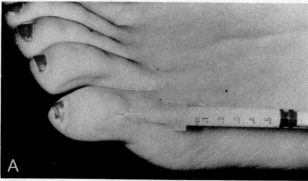

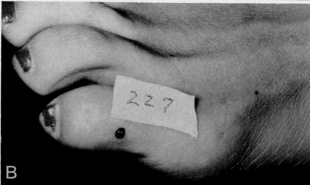

Figure 6.7. (A, B) Carefully controlled double-blind studies are being performed throughout the country by podiatric medical researchers to test efficacy of injectable collagen implant. (Courtesy of Dr. D. Elleby, Atlanta, GA.)

6.7A, B). Preliminary unreported results appear to parallel the work of Balkin but co-ordination of all studies must be completed before meaningful conclusions can be reached.

Pyrolytic Carbon

Pyrolytic carbon is formed in a fluidized bed by the pyrolysis of gaseous hydrocarbon at a temperature of 1000° to 1400° C and deposited on a polycrystalline graphite substrate. It has recently been under investigation for use as a possible synthetic material for tendon and ligament reconstruction, heart valve replacements, and as a dental implant in oral surgery. This is because of its inherent strength, frictionless drag and ability to withstand cylindrical load. According to Urist (32), pyrolytic carbon would allow osseous fixation to bone through a process of osteoinduction. This would make it an excellent material to combine with silicone elastomers without the use of bone cement or external devices (Fig. 6.8). Recently the role of pyrolytic carbon as a joint replacement in foot surgery has been extensively investigated by Hetherington and associates (33).

Polyethylene

Ultra high molecular weight polyethylene material is used as a primary implantable device in only one procedure commonly employed in foot surgery (Fig. 6.9). This is because the material has a tendency to undergo the phenomenon of cold flow or "creep"

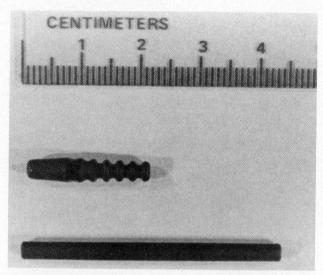

Figure 6.8. Pyrolytic carbon possesses excellent biocompatibility properties and appears to be promising material for construction of joint replacements in foot surgery. (From Hetherington VJ, Kavros SJ, Conway F, Mandracchia VJ, Martin W, Harbold AD: Pyrolytic carbon as a joint replacement in the foot: a preliminary report. *J Foot Surg* 21:160, 1982.)

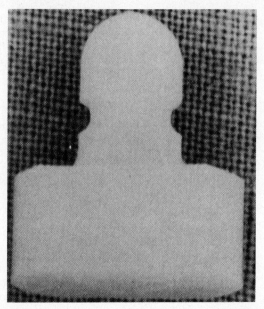

Figure 6.9. The STA peg is sub-talar joint endoprosthesis made of ultra-high molecular weight polyethylene. (From Smith SD: The STA operation for the pronated foot in childhood. In Weil LS (ed): *Clinics in Podiatry* 1:165, 1984.)

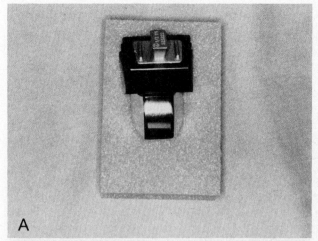

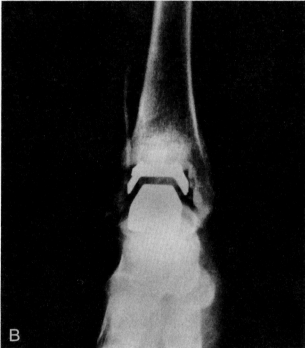

Figure 6.10. (A) Oregon total ankle replacement system with polyethylene tibial component and cobalt-chromium-molybdenum talar component. (B) Radiograph of intact Oregon ankle joint prosthesis. (From Marcinko DE, Lazerson A, Elleby D: Ankle joint arthrodesis or implant arthroplasty —a report of two cases. *J Am Podiatry Assoc* 74:559, 1984.)

when it is force loaded. However, when used as a subtalar joint endoprosthesis type peg, results have been encouraging (34). When used in joint replacement surgery, however, it is often interfaced with metal or other rigid components to augment strength. This is the concept used in the Zimmer Oregon Total Ankle Joint Replacement System. Polyethylene components are typically applied to concave joint surfaces and fixed with bone cement to avoid implant-induced bone absorption (Fig. 6.10A, B). Ultra high molecular weight polyethylene has enjoyed greater success in general orthopedic surgery than in foot surgery.

Porous polyethylene film, on the other hand, has been used by Stark and associates (35) and Williams and associates (36) since 1977 for the prevention of adhesions in tendon surgery of the hand. Similar work in foot surgery with other polyvinyl materials such as polyurethane and polyoelefin is currently in progress (37).

BONE IMPLANT MATERIALS

In the United States freeze dried human homogeneic graft material is available from strategically located tissue banks throughout the country. These institutions are functional because of the pioneering work of Krveze and associates (38) in 1951. Their manufacturing process is now the basis of graft preparation used by commercial tissue banks. It consists of cadaver bone harvesting under sterile conditions, followed by bacterial, viral, serological, and histocompatability antigen testing procedures (39, 40). The lengthy process is under the auspices of the Uniform Anatomical Gift Act adopted by the American Bar Association to protect the medical environment from legal entanglement (41). The harvested bone is sorted, sized, and then either frozen for use at −179° C using liquid nitrogen or lyophilized and freeze dried in a vacuum chamber. Bone moisture content is reduced and grafts can be indefinitely stored without the need for refrigeration (Fig. 6.11). Reconstitution in sterile saline takes place before surgery to avoid brittleness and to facilitate shaping (Fig. 6.12).

A review of the current status of bone grafting was performed by McGlamry and Miller (42) in 1977 and the availability of freeze dried bone has meant that sophisticated podiatric reconstructive procedures are possible without the perioperative complications associated with traditional graft harvesting. Included among these procedures are the Silver, Evans, and Valderamma type calcaneal osteotomies used in pes valgus surgery (43, 44) (Fig. 6.13A, B). Additionally, the hand fashioned cortical bone dowels of Eisenfeld and Bouchard have been used with good results internally to fixate other osteotomy sites (Dr. P. Eisenfeld and Dr. J. Bouchard, personal communication) (Fig. 6.14A, B). Homogenous bone has the capacity to be precisely cut for use in interlocking surfaces and may be preferred in conditions where bone is absent or when mechanical stability is of prime importance. Homogeneic bone grafts heal in much the same manner as autogenous grafts, only at a much slower rate, and may be visible on radiographic review for many years after implantation. Since Hutchinson (45),

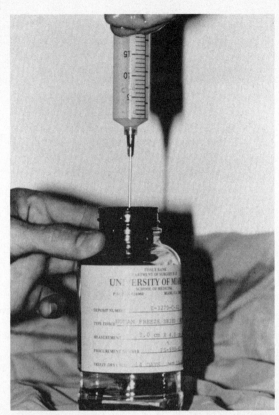

Figure 6.12. Human freeze-dried cadaver bone, packaged in vacuum-sealed sterile glass container for reconstitution with saline. (Courtesy of Dr. A. Shaw, Atlanta, GA.)

Chalmers (46), and Bonfiglio (47) have observed delayed hypersensitivity reactions with the absorption of bone implants, it has been recommended that freeze-dried bone not be re-autoclaved before use.

Most recently, Surgibone, a specially processed mature bovine heterograft for human implantation, has become available on the European market for use in place of homologous or autologous bone. It has been compression tested to withstand a minimum of 250 kg force to prevent postoperative collapse and is available in four different bone stock types: cortical plates, load-bearing cancellous blocks, non-load-bearing cancellous blocks, and corticocancellous combinations. Animal and controlled clinical tests, over a period of more than 15 years, have shown that Surgibone is not immunogenic or antigenic (48).

TOPICAL MATERIALS

Cutaneous lower extremity ulcerations continue to be a perplexing problem for the medical community. They are often a mirror of systemic disease, and treatment may continue for many months to the frustration of both physician and patient. In past years the use of homogenous skin grafting techniques were employed but proved cumbersome. Before that, heterografts were introduced by Reverdin (49) in 1869 and since then ulcerations have been treated with rabbit, frog, dog, and fowl skin grafts (50). The following is a survey of the currently available heterograft and syn-

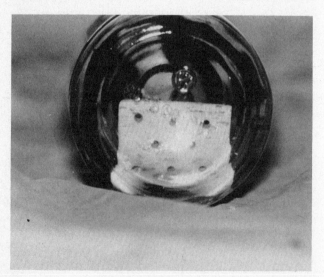

Figure 6.11. Homogeneic cortical bone graft that can be obtained preshaped for immediate use. (Courtesy of Dr. A. Shaw, Atlanta, GA.)

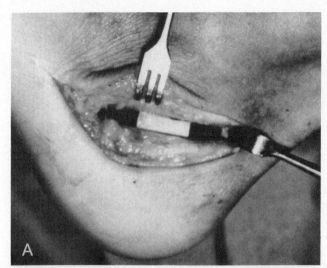

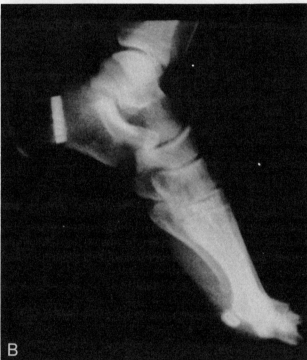

Figure 6.13. (A) Lateral opening wedge calcaneal osteotomy with in situ bone graft. (B) Radiograph of same patient demonstrating osteotomy site and graft placement. (From Marcinko DE, Lazerson A, Elleby D: Silver calcaneal osteotomy for flexible flatfoot; a retrospective preliminary report. *J Foot Surg* 23:191, 1984.)

thetic materials, which may prove useful in the treatment of chronic or acute ulcerations or skin defects.

Porcine Heterografts

One manufacturer has prepared four types of porcine skin grafts: fresh (refrigerated), frozen-irradiated, lyophilized-irradiated, and gluteraldehyde treated varieties. Successful use of these materials has been impressive. Silvetti and associates (51), Bromberg and associates (52), Burke and associates (53), Culliton and associates (54), Morris and associates (55), State and associates (56), and McCarthy and

Axler (57) have all promoted the use of porcine heterograft material. Additionally, conditions indicated for its use have been expanded to include treatment for burns, plastic reconstructive procedures, skin defects, and to promote healing following verrucae fulgeration. Porcine heterografts have even been used following toenail avulsion surgery when applied to the nail bed as a biological dressing. Further techniques for clinical application, dose schedules, evaluation of response, and follow-up care may be obtained from the work of Heifitz (58) and Elliot and Hoehn (59).

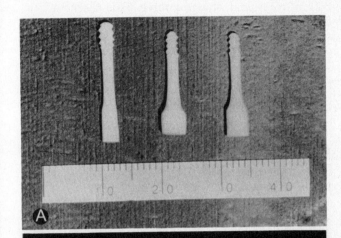

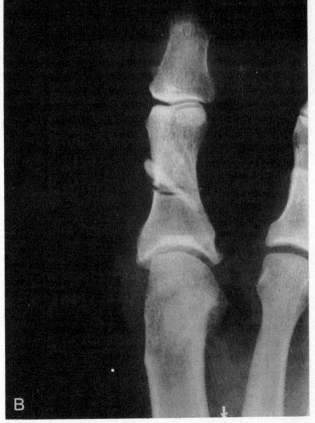

Figure 6.14. (A) Hand fabricated cortical dowels made from homogeneic bone graft material. (B) Radiograph of bone dowel used internally to fix osteotomy of hallux. (Courtesy of Drs. P. Eisenfeld and J. Bouchard, Atlanta, GA.)

Synthetic Skin Hydrophilic Colloid

Spenco Synthetic Skin is a hydrophilic colloid gelatin that possesses a consistency similar to human skin and absorbs the equivalent of its own weight in water, serum, or blood. Second Skin is inert and will not absorb stains, odors, or undergo chemical reactions in or on the body. It is centered by a low density polyethylene net that gives it strength but does not inhibit its properties as a semipermeable membrane. It is also backed on both sides by an inert film that controls osmosis.

The product will absorb 2 cm of transverse and 360° of rotational, shearing force. This characteristic makes Second Skin an excellent soft tissue supplement for defects that are subject to constant friction or delayed healing. In an extensive study performed by Cangialosi (60) in 1982 the rate of overall ulcer healing was considerably more rapid than that of control groups. Although this study was only a preliminary report the encouraging effects of this artificial colloid warrant further clinical study.

Amniotic Membrane Grafting

The use of a sterile, viable human amniotic membrane has proven to be a satisfactory adjunct in the treatment of lower extremity ulcerations since first used by Douglas in 1952 (61). Amniotic membranes are readily available, easily stored, and relatively inexpensive to use. They are efficacious as a biological dressing and serve to prevent fluid exudate and protein loss. Robson (62) has demonstrated that amniotic membranes are as effective as autografts but superior to both allografts and xenografts. The natural membrane adheres to wound surfaces and allows phagocytes and serum bacteriolytic factors to heighten host defenses. The material is bacteriostatic and detailed application techniques have been outlined by Rudnick (63). Amniotic membrane material is not only recommended as a primary mode of therapy, but also in those cases where standard methods have failed.

Op Site and Bioclusive Transparent Dressing

Op Site semipermeable membrane and Bioclusive Transparent Dressing are elastic film membranes that adhere only to dry surfaces yet still remain permeable to moisture vapor and air. They both conform completely to body contours and stretch liberally with patient movement. Because Op Site and Bioclusive Transparent Dressing are semipermeable, they can be left in place during the healing process of wounds, ulcerations, burns, and skin graft harvesting procurement procedures. They do not promote eschar formation or maceration of delicate tissue, leukocytosis continues uninhibited, and surface re-epithelization time is decreased because cells move directly across the wound surfaces. Cutaneous nerve endings remain covered by serous exudate, greatly reducing pain. Op Site and Bioclusive Transparent Dressing are available in a wide range of sizes to suit every dressing or draping need and can be hand cut to shape unusual application contours.

HEMOSTATIC AGENTS

Capillary or venous blood oozing from cut bone surfaces or soft tissue structures is often encountered following surgery and may create considerable complications. Various topically applied agents have been developed to retard this problem. A quantitative comparison of the following agents was performed by Harris and associates (64) in 1978.

Topical Thrombin

Topical thrombin (Thrombostat) is a protein substance of bovine origin produced through a conversion reaction in which prothrombin is activated by tissue thromboplastin in the presence of calcium chloride. The product requires no intermediate physiological agent because it clots the fibrinogen of blood directly. Clotting time is proportional to concentration. Five hundred units of topical thrombin will clot 5 cc of blood in less than one second or 1000 cc in less than one minute. It is available in 1000, 5000, or 10000 units and is designed to be used as a powdered agent or as a prepared solution. Thrombin must not be injected or extensive intravascular clotting can occur. Topical thrombin is contraindicated in patients with a known hypersensitivity to any of its components. Because this provides a mechanism for antigenicity, precautions for allergic manifestations must be undertaken (65).

Absorbable Gelatin Sponge

Absorbable gelatin sponge (Gelfoam) is a hemostatic agent prepared from purified animal protein. It is capable of controlling blood oozing by absorbing many times its own weight in whole blood. It is completely absorbed in four to six weeks without scar formation, and will completely liquify in two to five days (65). Gelfoam is available in many different sizes or in jars containing 1 gm of the powdered substance. In addition to its primary indicated use Gelfoam has been found to be a valuable adjunct in the treatment of lower extremity ulcerations. Freeman and Joyner (66) reported ulcerative wound healing in an average of 30 days and Burke and associates (67) reported similar results when Gelfoam was used in conjunction with Betadine. It is thought that Gelfoam stimulates granulation tissue by providing a lattice framework into which viable tissue may grow. It may also be capable of inducing epithelialization.

Microfibrillar Collagen

Microfibrillar collagen hemostat (Avitene) is an agent prepared as a fibrous, water insoluble, partial hydrochloric acid salt of bovine corium. Microfibrillar collagen hemostat (MCH) tenaciously adheres to blood-soaked surfaces. However, excess material not involved in the hemostatic process may be removed without resuming bleeding. The product works by attracting platelets that adhere to fibrils in the interstices of its fibrous mass. Avitene is inactivated by autoclaving and ethylene oxide sterilization. (It has been shown to be effective in patients on aspirin therapy.) Its effect on platelet adherence is not affected by heparin. It is supplied in 1 to 5 gm jars with 1 gm being sufficient for a 50 cm² area. MCH does not interfere with bone healing but it should not be used on skin incisions. Additionally, MCH induces a mild inflammatory response that takes approximately 84 days to resolve (65).

Oxygen Regenerated Cellulose

Oxygen regenerated cellulose (Surgicel) is an absorbable knitted fabric prepared by the controlled oxidation of cellulose. The material is white with a caramel-like aroma and is strong enough to be sutured without fraying. It differs from other agents in that it depends on physical rather than chemical properties to effect hemostasis. Actual blood absorption depends on factors such as degree of saturation, amount of exudate, and tissue type. Surgicel is supplied in four different sized envelopes and has been shown to be bacteriocidal against a wide variety of gram positive and gram negative organisms including both aerobes and anaerobes. Because this agent may interfere with bone healing, it is not popular among surgeons dealing with bony reconstruction or trauma (65).

Bone Wax

Historically, bone wax was first prepared and used by the British neurosurgeon Horsley (68) in 1892. Its hemostatic action is physical (tamponade) rather than chemical and it is supplied in sterile 2.5 gm packettes. Its assets include availability, ease in preparation and handling, and quick results. However, it is not a hemostatic agent of choice because it was found to inhibit bone healing (69).

TEMPORARY DISPOSABLE DEVICES

Many temporary disposable devices are useful during the intraoperative or perioperative period of surgery. These include active and passive drain systems and various transcutaneous electrical nerve stimulating units. An ingenious new drug delivery system has also been developed using polymethylmethacrylate beads, which offers therapeutic benefits within the realm of infection control.

Drain Systems

Regardless of design or type, the prophylactic or therapeutic advantages associated with external drain systems have been documented by McFarlane (70), Buchanan and Lambley (71) and Radcliffe (72). These include the evacuation of fluid, reduction of hematoma or necrotic tissue formation, reduced pain, increased rate of healing, and reduced treatment costs.

These goals are achieved by three classes of drain systems currently in vogue.

Overflow Gravity Drains

The Penrose overflow gravity drain is a rubberized sterile tube that is inserted directly into a wound and left to protrude partially from the incision site. It can be preperforated to increase efficiency and is a static device that depends on postural attitude for function. Its flexibility makes it ideal for small wounds or contorted incision sites.

Closed Suction Drains

The TLS Closed Surgical Wound Drainage System was developed by Kalish and is marketed in several different sizes. Its efficiency in foot surgery was documented in a 35-case investigative study by Miller (73) in 1981. Similar devices were originally described by Josephs (74) in 1977 and Jacoby (75) in 1978. It is designed for use in small procedure surgery when less than 20 cc of fluid is anticipated over a 48-hour time period. Because the collection tube and vacuum source are sterile, they can be transported for cultural examination without the need for transferral to another container.

The TLS system essentially consists of a 30 cm fenestrated silicone drain catheter connected to a plastic hub. The hub is fitted with an 18 gauge needle for piercing the collection tube stopper. A curved metallic trochar is provided for precise positioning of the catheter through a separate stab exit portal placed away from the primary surgical site. A graduated protective housing facilitates routine periodic fluid evacuation when necessary. A new Bulb Drainage System is now available in applications where a larger fluid reservoir is needed (Fig. 6.15).

Several other closed suction drain systems are available in the United States. These include the Hemovac and Jackson-Pratt systems. They are designed for the drainage of large surgical areas (Fig. 6.16). Additionally the Mini-Flap Drain System is applicable to foot surgery because of its small caliber.

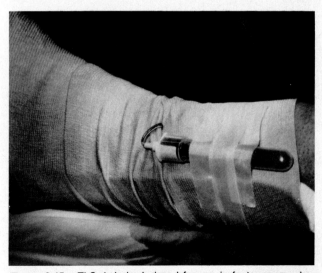

Figure 6.15. TLS drain is designed for use in foot surgery when less than 20 cc of fluid is anticipated over a 48-hour time period. (Courtesy of Dr. A. Lazerson, Atlanta, GA.)

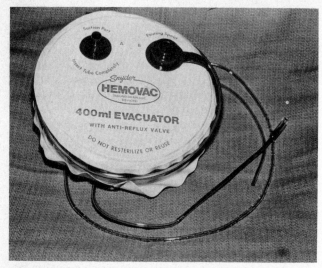

Figure 6.16. Hemovac drain may be used for evacuation of fluid from large surgical wounds in ankle and leg surgery. (Courtesy of L. Barnett, Atlanta, GA.)

Closed Suction Irrigation Drains

Closed suction irrigation drainage systems incorporating antibiotic solutions that are instilled into a wound and withdrawn by vacuum suction have been used with varying degrees of success for many years (76). It was not until 1970, however, that Willenegger (77) advocated the general use of suction irrigation devices on a larger scale. Since then Pressman (78) has devised a continuous closed irrigation system that he used in the treatment of osteomyelitis following first metatarsophalangeal joint hemiimplant arthroplasty in 1977. Similarly in 1978 Green and associates (79) fashioned a device using a preexisting Hemovac drain that was used in the treatment of other osseous pedal infections. Sorto (80) has even modified the Kritter type one-tube-in-out drain system that may serve as a substitute for traditional methods of open wound packing. Unfortunately, these homemade devices have often proved too impractical for routine podiatric use.

In 1984 Schwartz and Marcinko (81) constructed and patented a closed suction irrigation drainage system specifically designed for the treatment of acute pedal infections. Excellent results were obtained in 16 cases of serious soft tissue infections and 19 cases of osteomyelitis.

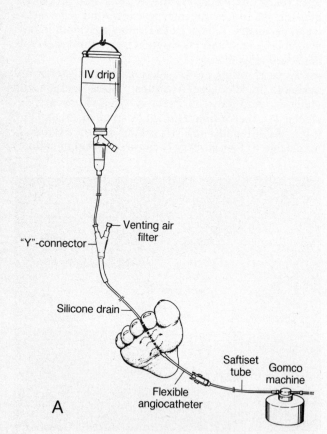

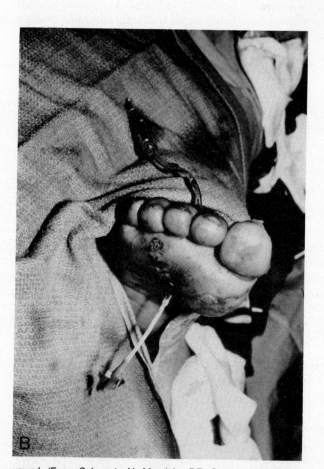

Figure 6.17. (A) Schematic representation of assembled component parts of Blajwas-Schwartz-Marcinko Closed Suction Irrigation Drainage System. (B) Intraoperative placement within contaminated pedal wound. (From Schwartz N, Marcinko DE: Suction irrigation—construction and use of a dependable closed system. *J Am Podiatry Assoc* 24:216, 1984.)

The Schwartz-Marcinko Closed Suction Irrigation Drainage System consists of five parts: trochar with drain, flexible angiocatheter, "Y" adapter, extension tube, and standard intravenous infusion set (Fig. 6.17A, B). Suction is established by a Gomco-type negative pressure suction machine and when fully assembled the result is a drain passing completely through the contaminated body part for treatment fluid delivery and mechanical agitation (Fig. 6.18A, B).

Transcutaneous Electrical Nerve Stimulation Units

Transcutaneous Electrical Nerve Stimulation (TENS) is sent as a peripheral signal from a generating electrode and is often used to alter the message of pain transmitted to the brain. Its significance and application to foot surgery was first detailed by Alm and associates (82) in 1979. The Neuromode Pulse Generator Unit is used for an average duration of 20 to 40 minutes, with amplitude, pulse width, and rate settings set at a medium level for the device.

One hundred and twenty-five patients reported that postoperative subjective and objective relief of pain was significant and resulted in an overall decrease in use of analgesic medications. Grosack and associates (83) reported that postoperative use of the same model TENS unit resulted in a 63% improvement in pain control. Additionally they urged that patients be evaluated before use and cautioned that the modality be used with care in heart patients, patients with cardiac pacemakers, pregnant women, and patients with problems within the neck region.

Since 1965 the gate theory of pain has been used to explain the mechanism of pain relief through TENS stimulation. In more recent years this mechanism has been disputed in light of the endorphin hypothesis (84). Apparently the electrical effects of TENS stimulate morphinelike substances and raise the pain threshold. Based on these studies the application of TENS to a number of other podiatric conditions seems plausible. These include various types of neuritis, vasculitis, fasciitis, strains, sprains, and fractures.

TENS is also helpful in patients who should limit their amount of analgesic intake, whether they are medically compromised, allergic, or simply hypersensitive to pain. TENS may also be used in conjunction with other pain relief modalities such as hypothermia therapy (85). Thus TENS therapy, although not without hazard, is highly recommended when applicable.

Methylmethacrylate

Polymethylmethacrylate (PMMA) is an acrylic polymer that has been used in orthopedic surgery for many years. This self-curing bone cement and grouting agent is supplied in a package that contains a portion of methylmethacrylate and a compatible amount of liquid acrylic monomer, the latter having a

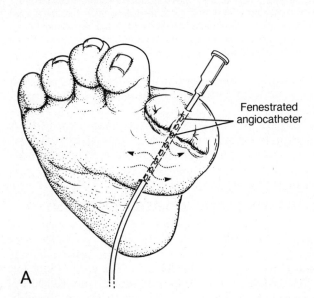

Fenestrated angiocatheter

A

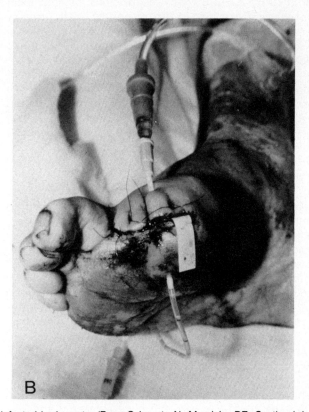

B

Figure 6.18. (A) Schematic illustration of Alternative Blajwas-Schwartz-Marcinko Irrigation Drain system incorporating fenestrated flexible angicatheter. (B) Functioning of same system useful in smaller infected body parts. (From Schwartz N, Marcinko DE: Suction irrigation—construction and use of a dependable closed system. *J Am Podiatry Assoc* 74:216, 1984.)

chemical configuration similar to chloroform. When the two ingredients are mixed a white dough is formed that sets in 5 to 10 minutes following an exothermic reaction with a temperature range of 17° to 48° C. The most successful use of methylmethacrylate has been in the bonding of various prostheses into bone for artificial joint replacement surgery.

In foot surgery methylmethacrylate has had relatively limited application in implant arthroplasty techniques of the first metatarsophalangel joint, the talonavicular joint, and the ankle joint. It has also been used as a leuting agent to anchor the previously mentioned Smith (86) subtalar joint peg arthroeisis implant. However, the use of PMMA has not been without complication. Recent studies have shown that the monomer may leak from the polymerizing cement and produce toxic effects on the cardiovascular and respiratory systems. It may also compromise the immune system by decreasing leukocytic phagocytosis. Additionally, incomplete radiolucent lines are frequently seen between bone and methylmethacrylate cement, and uncertainty continues about what implications this has for subsequent implant loosening. A lack of firm fixation may also lead to increased stress on the implant-cement complex (87).

An exciting new therapeutic development in the treatment of wound sepsis is the use of gentamicin-impregnated PMMA beads, which are locally implanted following surgical decompression (of soft tissue) and debridement of infected bone. First developed in 1972 by Klemm (88) the principles of high local antibiotic tissue levels are combined with primary wound closure (Klemm K, personal communication).

The beads are marketed under the trade name Septopal and allow protracted release of the aminoglycoside into the surrounding tissues with only trace amounts detectable in the systemic circulation (89). Individual 0.2 gm beads have a diameter of 7 mm and each bead contains 7.5 mg gentamicin sulfate, as well as 20 mg of zirconium dioxide used as a contrast medium. The beads are available for use individually or strung on multifilament strands of stainless steel wire in the form of chains.

Minibeads have also been handmade by Asche (90) for use in smaller infected parts such as the foot and hand. These minibeads are 3 × 5 mm in diameter, are packaged in a sterile double pouch (Fig. 6.19A, B) and are immediately available for temporary implantation. Because local gentamicin levels are 10 to 1000 times higher than those achieved through parenteral routes, such levels are bacteriocidal against organisms previously resistant in the routine antibiotic administration. Because the Septopal beads have been precured, no exothermic heat reaction is expected and the possibility of deleterious side effects is reduced. Wound healing takes place as in an aseptic procedure.

Although these beads are not yet currently available for general use in this country, Grieben (91) and Taglang and Jenny (92, 93) have pioneered and recommended their use in the treatment of catastrophic osseous and soft tissue infections (Jenny G, Taglang,

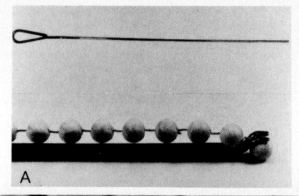

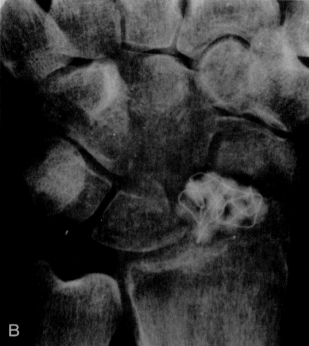

Figure 6.19.   (A) Flexible metallic insertion implement used to introduce gentamicin-PMMA beads into medullary cavity through a small aperture. (B) Gentamicin-PMMA minibeads used in treatment of infected nonunion of carpal scaphoid bone. (Courtesy of Dr. K. Klemm, Frankfurt, West Germany.)

G, personal communication). Finally, results reported from the 1980 Amsterdam Symposium on local antibiotic treatment in osteomyelitis and soft tissue infections have confirmed the use of gentamicin-PMMA beads in the treatment of chronic postoperative osteomyelitis, hematogenous osteomyelitis, infected pseudarthrosis, infected osteosynthesis, and infected soft tissue structures (94).

BONE GROWTH STIMULATION UNITS

An interesting development in recent years has been the rapid progress in the study of bioelectrical stimulation of new bone growth. The concept is not new however, and dates back to the early 1800s. In 1953 Yasuda (95) first reported that he induced osteogenesis adjacent to an electrical cathode implanted in laboratory rabbits treated with continuous microamperage for three weeks.

The widespread clinical use of direct current stimulation to treat osseous nonunions began in 1971 when Friendenberg (96) successfully treated a nonunion of the medial malleolus. Since then Brighton and associates (97) have become leaders in this field of research. Through their work and the work of others two possible explanations for this phenomenon have been postulated. First, a direct cellular effect may be caused by the activation of cyclical AMP in the osteoblastic system. Second, indirect changes in the cellular environment may be related to lower tissue oxygen levels and increased cathode alkalinity (98).

From these early investigations three commercially available systems have been developed for clinical use in the treatment of nonunions, delayed unions, failed arthrodeses, and congenital pseudarthroses. The systems were reviewed in detail by Mahan (99) in 1983. The manufacturers claim an 80% success rate, although each system possesses unique intrinsic advantages and disadvantages.

Zimmer Usa

Zimmer USA manufactures a semiinvasive bone stimulating unit that has enjoyed great popularity among podiatric surgeons. The system requires percutaneous placement of four Teflon-coated cathode pins, which makes it ideal for use in patients with poor skin coverage. A power source, the Quadpack, is used by the patient to monitor each cathode, which recieves 20 mA of current. A disposable anode pad is placed on the patient's skin and changed every day to avoid irritation and optimize conductivity (Fig. 6.20).

The extremity is immobilized in a non-weight-bearing cast. The standard treatment period is six weeks, and if evidence of bone healing has not occurred, an additional waiting period of three months should be observed before a second trial with the Zimmer system. Brighton (100) has reported results comparable with bone grafting: 83.7% success with patients treated in a University of Pennsylvania series. Fox and Smith (101) have also reported success in the treatment of metatarsal nonunions using this system.

Electro-Biology, Inc

Electro-Biology, Inc has developed a noninvasive external treatment coil unit that incorporates an indirectly coupled pulsating electromagnetic field. The system is available for use on a home rental basis and, because surgery is not involved, there is no risk of related complications. A protocol for use has been developed by Bassett and associates (102) and it is essential to situate the unit around the immobilized body part creating a magnetic field that is perpendicular to the device. The system is used for 10 to 16 hours a day and the patient progresses to gradual weight bearing, following evidence of bone healing. Results of Electro-Biology systems have revealed a success rate of 77%, including 82% for nonunions of the tibia with either active or recent infection (103).

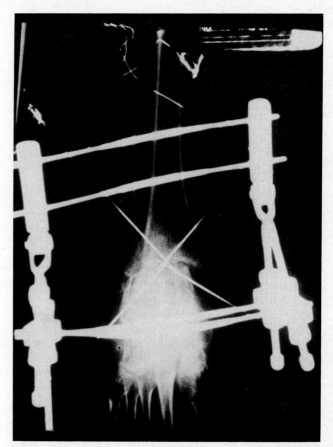

Figure 6.20. Correct cathode placement of Zimmer semiinvasive bone growth stimulation device. Disposable anode pad is placed on patient's skin and changed daily. (From Marcinko DE, Lazerson A, Elleby D: Ankle joint arthrodesis or implant arthroplasty—a report of two cases. *J Am Podiatry Assoc* 74:559, 1984.)

Failure with pulsating electromagnetic field treatment may be attributed to inadequate immobilization, a large fracture gap, or the presence of a synovial pseudarthrosis.

DePuy

The DePuy invasive direct bone growth stimulating unit requires two operative procedures (i.e. implantation and removal) for use. The device consists of a generator and an anode sealed into a titanium case, with a wound helical cathode that is implanted directly into the nonunion site. The unit delivers 20 mA of current and does not necessarily require a non-weight-bearing status. Osteomyelitis is a contraindication to the use of this system, which is left in place for five to six months and then removed. Although Peterson and associates (104) reported a healing rate of 86%, podiatrists have not extensively employed this device.

EXTERNAL FIXATION DEVICES

External fracture or osteotomy fixation is a method of osseous immobilization that employs percutaneous metal transfixing pins in bones that are attached to a rigid external frame support. The concept can be traced back to Malgaine and Levi in the mid-nineteenth century (105). Since then pioneers such as Lambotte (1907), Anderson (1934), Stader (1937), Hoffman (1939), and Charnley (1951) have attempted to develop and use similar devices. In the 1960s Vidal (106) and Adrey (107) examined and further refined the original Hoffman system. The device was modified to include a double external frame support that is still employed today.

Devices particularly suited for the foot, ankle, and leg include the Charnley-Hoffman systems, the Jaquet Miniature External Fixation Device, and the Calandruccio Triangular Compression Device.

Charnley-Hoffman Systems

The Charnley Compression Apparatus and Hoffman External Fixation Device are available in different sizes that permit use in pediatric and adult cases. Each unit consists of four parts centered about a stainless steel or titanium frame. These parts include threaded transfixation pins, longitudinal slide bars for distraction or compression, and articular couplers with ball joints, which secure the transfixation pins to the apparatus itself (Fig. 6.21).

Most authors believe that the primary application of external fixation is for fractures that are comminuted or associated with massive soft tissue injuries or infections (108). The Charnley clamp has also been used by Reinherz and associates (109) in a case of primary ankle joint fusion, whereas Wright and Jones

(110) used a Hoffman apparatus to fuse an ankle following previous attempts and pseudarthrosis formation. These two devices may be employed to achieve optimal immobilization in such diverse cases as arthrodesis following infected total joint implants, fractures associated with complex neurovascular damage, and extensive limb lengthening procedures (111).

Jaquet Miniature Device

The Jaquet Miniature External Fixation Device is a fully adjustable apparatus that is useful in the treatment of selected fractures, nonunions, and osteotomies of pedal long bones. The device was introduced approximately eight years ago and has proven to be versatile because of swivel clamps and pin holders that produce osseous compression by means of a calibrated wheel. Rigid stabilization is maintained when adjustable locks are secured by hexagonal tightening screws. The apparatus is composed of five basic parts, with supplemental attachments available depending on parameters of use (Fig. 6.22).

Podiatric use of the Jaquet Device was first reported in 1981. Walter and Pressman (112) used the device in conjunction with autogenous corticocancellous bone grafting techniques for the treatment of painful metatarsal nonunions. Later, Duke and Walter (113) used the device as a means of osteotomy fixation in the surgical repair of hallux abducto valgus deformity. In all reported cases the apparatus was

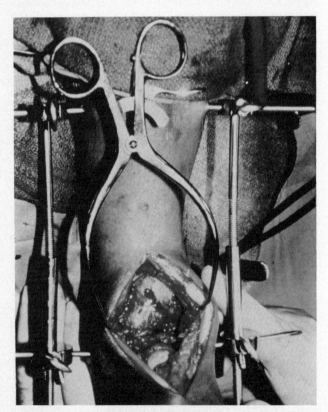

Figure 6.21. Four structural components of this Charnley compression apparatus are visible along with Charnley clamp. (Courtesy of Drs. J. Bouchard and M. Dollard, Atlanta, GA.)

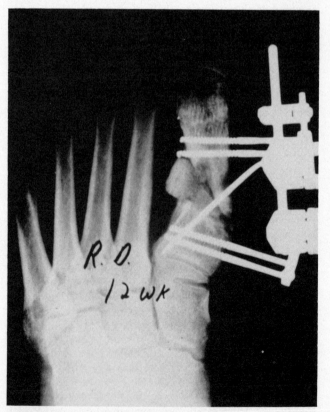

Figure 6.22. Jaquet miniature external fixation device used in conjunction with autogenous bone graft to salvage nonunion of first metatarsal. (Courtesy of Dr. E. D. McGlamry, Atlanta, GA.)

removed in four weeks without additional surgery or anesthesia. All osteotomies were clinically healed in six weeks, and radiographic evaluation revealed little callus formation, suggesting a primary bone healing process. None of the surgical osteotomies became displaced and no other surgical complications were encountered.

Calandruccio Triangular Fixation Device

The Calandruccio Triangular Compression Fixation Device is an external frame appliance that was described by Williams and associates (114) in 1983. It provides compression, rigidity, and deformity correction of the distal tibia. Triplanar mobility is accomplished by providing for placement of two or three horizontal rods placed in the frontal and transverse body planes (Fig. 6.23). Compression and angulation may be further adjusted by tightening hexagonal compression nuts located on a transverse strut. A unique pivot hinge system allows correction of angulational deformities in the lateral and anteroposterior planes. Because the Calandruccio Device incorporates two pins in the talus and two in the tibia, the possibility of movement between the two surfaces is minimized (Fig. 6.24A, B, C). Therefore this feature makes the Calandruccio Triangular Compression Fixation Device the external fixator of choice for arthodesis of the talotibial joint (114).

MISCELLANEOUS MATERIALS FOR FIXATION

Kirschner wires, Steinmann pins, flexible monofilament wire, and bone or skin staples are traditional materials used in foot surgery. Their purpose is to provide a means of fixation for osteotomy, fracture,

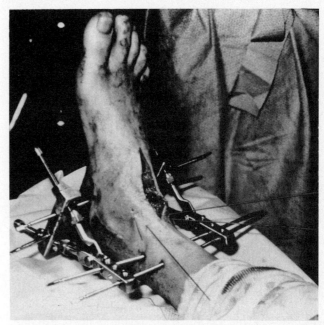

Figure 6.23. Intraoperative photograph of Calandruccio Triangular Compression Device used to fuse ankle joint. (From Marcinko DE, Lazerson A, Elleby D: Ankle joint arthrodesis or implant arthroplasty—a report of two cases. *J Am Podiatry Assoc* 74:559, 1984.)

or fusion sites. They may also be used to stabilize soft tissue structures, such as tendon and ligament, and technique modifications are being used with increasing success.

Kirschner Wires and Steinmann Pins

Kirschner wires were introduced through a principle of engineering applied to the bicycle wheel in 1909 (115). By 1940 Taylor (116) advocated the use of

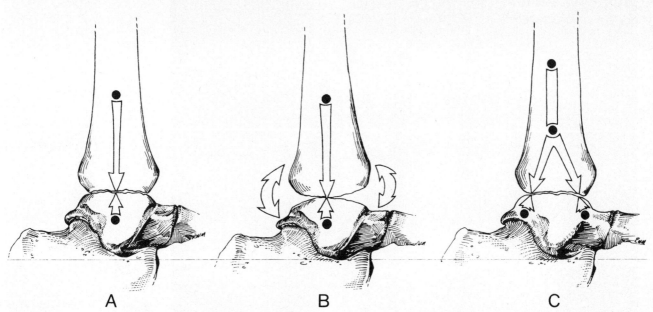

A   B   C

Figure 6.24. (A) Two-hole fixation technique used in conventional external fixation devices. (B) Nonreciprocating osseous surfaces may allow motion with employment of two-pin devices. (C) Calandruccio device achieves increased osseous stability with triangular three-hole configuration. (From Williams JE, Marcinko DE, Lazerson A, Elleby D: The Calandruccio Triangular Compression Device—a schematic introduction. *J Am Podiatry Assoc* 73:536, 1983.)

Kirschner wires for the fixation of bone tissue. Today Kirschner wires and Steinmann pins are made of medical grade stainless steel and differ only in size. Kirschner wires are available in 0.028, 0.035, 0.045, and 0.062 inch diameter sizes. Steinmann pins are available in ⁵⁄₆₄, ³⁄₃₂, ⁷⁄₆₄, ¹⁄₈, ⁹⁄₆₄, ⁵⁄₃₂, and ³⁄₁₆ inch diameters. They are both manufactured in two styles with either a round end or a diamond-trocher tip. They may be smooth or threaded and range in length from 9 to 18 inches (117). Reichert and Caneva (116) have reviewed their many possible uses in foot surgery and insertion is usually by means of a hand, electric, gas, or pneumatic wire driver. Removal of smooth wires or pins require no additional equipment, although threaded pin removal may require hand tools or power equipment (Table 6.2).

Disadvantages in the use of Kirschner wires and Steinmann pins include pin tract infections and accidental breakage that may leave a portion of the wire inside the foot. Some surgeons elect to bury wires and pins into the bone in an effort to avoid these complications, but this method is not recommended. Finally, it is important to realize that Kirschner wires and Steinmann pins do not produce active compression and may actually serve to distract fixated segments.

An exception to this guideline is their use in combination with Arbeitsgemeinschaft fur Osteosynthesefragen/Swiss Association for the Study of Internal Fixation (AO/ASIF) tension band fixation, or in forefoot surgery using the modified tension band technique described by Schwartz and Buchan in 1984 (unpublished data) (Fig. 6.25A, B).

Flexible Monofilament Wire

Internal monofilament wire may be used as a means of primary fixation or combined with other forms. Flexible wire is available in both monofilament or multifilament (119) braided styles and is supplied in individual strands, with or without needle attachments, or on 1 oz spools (120). Additionally, all forms of wire are manufactured in a number of different gauges; 27, 28, and 30 being popular sizes in foot surgery. Perhaps the most common use of flexible stainless steel Austenic wire, which contains molybdenum to resist corrosion, is for the fixation of osteotomy sites that have one cortical hinge remaining intact. A two-hole, three-hole, box-lock, or figure-of-eight technique is commonly employed, and a sterile crochet hook or Johnson-tucker instrument may be used to manipulate the wire through preplanned drill

Table 6.2.
Comparison of Suture Wires

						SIZE								
	6-0	6-0	5-0	4-0	4-0	000	00	0	1	2	3	4	5	7
B & S Gauge	40	38	35	34	32	30	28	26	25	24	23	22	20	18
Diameter in inches	.0031	.0040	.0056	.0063	.0080	.0100	.0126	.0159	.0179	.0201	.0226	.0254	.0320	.0403
Diameter in millimeters	.079	.102	.142	.160	.203	.254	.320	.404	.455	.511	.574	.643	.813	1.016

(From Digiovanni J, Martin R: Pin, wires, staples in foot surgery. In Weil LS (ed): *Clinics in Podiatry* 1:212, 1984.)

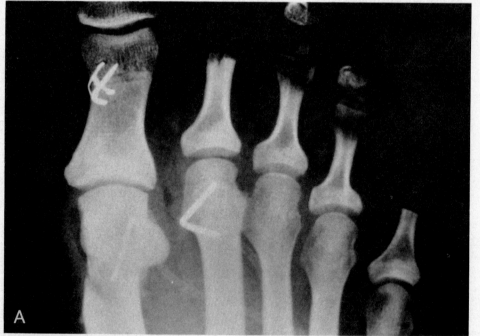

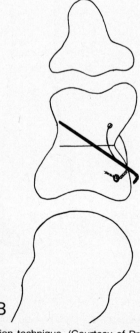

Figure 6.25.   (A) Internal tension band fixation of hallucal osteotomy using 0.35 Kirschner wire and 30 gauge monofilament wire. (B) Diagrammatic representation of same radiograph demonstrating modified internal tension band fixation technique. (Courtesy of Drs. N. Schwartz and D. Buchan, Atlanta, GA.)

holes (121). However, if no opposing cortical bone hinge remains intact, flexible internal wire fixation is not adequate (Fig. 6.26).

Surgical Staples

There are two classes of surgical staples: Bone staples, used internally to splint osseous sites but achieving no real compression, and removable soft tissue staples that are used to coapt incision margins.

Bone Staples

Bone staples are generally used in rearfoot arthrodesing procedures such as a triple tarsal fusion or calcaneal osteotomy. They may also be used to achieve tenodesis when major tendon transpositions or transfers are performed. Although round staples are available in many different sizes and types, only two are generally applicable to podiatric foot surgery: 19 × 22 × 2 mm and 19 × 22 × 1.7 mm sizes. They are made of stainless steel and have smooth or barbed prongs. Insertion involves a staple holder, used for precise placement, and a driver, used to seat the staple across the bone. Holes may be predrilled to countersink the staple and prevent adjacent soft tissue irritation. When necessary, staple removal is performed using a special remover; however, barbed staples may be more difficult to extract and cause significant bone destruction (Fig. 6.27).

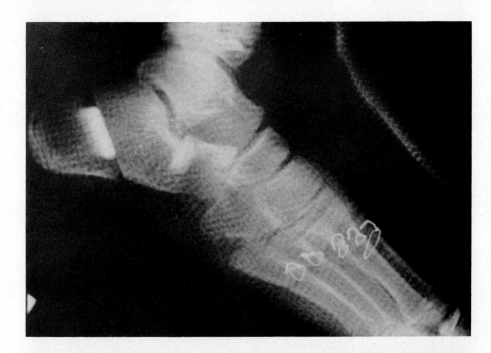

Figure 6.26. Metatarsus adductus repair using internal monofilament wire fixation of all five closing abductory base wedge metatarsal osteotomies. Note double calcaneal osteotomy with homogenous bone graft implantation.

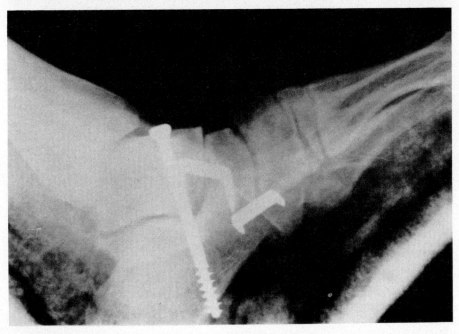

Figure 6.27. Bone staple fixation of midtarsal joint in triple arthrodesis. (Courtesy of Dr. D. E. Marcinko, Atlanta, GA.)

The Stone staple is a square or pentagonal shaped staple that has been developed to aid in the difficult fixation of displaced, intra-articular, calcaneal fractures. Classically, the staple is placed across the superomedial fracture line, to prevent posterior facet joint rotation (Fig. 6.28A, B). Using this device, Stephenson (122) has reported good results in 12 of 24 fractures reviewed after a 22-month retrospective valuation.

Another highly specialized staple, the osteoclasp, has been used by Levitsky (123) in an ingenious fashion. First developed by Zlotoff to fixate hallux wedge osteotomies, the osteoclasp is a modified staple with two legs that are angulated at 15° and placed on each side of an Akin osteotomy site (124). By stretching the clasp from one fourth to one third of its length, compressive force is exerted across the surgical site. The neck portion of the staple may then be left percutaneously exposed to keep the osteoclasp away from the skin surface. It is removed without anesthesia when bone healing has occurred. Osteoclasp fixation has not enjoyed wide support by most foot surgeons and its use remains somewhat of a novelty (Fig. 6.29).

Finally, the Richards Scaphoid Compression Device may be adapted for use in foot surgery (125). Predrilled holes are first made across an osteotomy site with a template and then a corresponding Richards' staple is driven into place with a driver-distractor device. The Richards' clamp and staple have been suc-

cessfully used in fractures of the fifth metatarsal and osteotomies of the first metatarsal. Continued evaluation will determine its usefulness in other podiatric surgical procedures.

Skin Staples

Stainless steel skin staples are used in surgery to decrease tissue reactivity and operating room time. Through the development of new technology two manufacturers have manufactured two of the most popular sterile and disposable stapler units (Proximate and Auto Suture). The Appose skin stapler features a precocking automatic release system that allows placement regardless of stapler direction or movement. All three instruments are available in two sizes, regular and wide staples, although Kerman and Arnold (126) have recommended the regular staple size for most podiatric procedures. Skin staples can be ordered in 12, 25, and 35 staples per unit sizes. The size of a regular staple is 0.51 mm in diameter and the staple span is 10.2 mm before closure and 3.4 mm high after closure. The stapler instruments themselves have locating arrows imprinted at their implantation ends to allow easy placement. Staples are generally placed two to four to the inch according to the size and location of the incision site. Staple removal is easily and quickly accomplished with an extractor supplied with each unit. Time of removal depends on wound tensile strength and patient compliance.

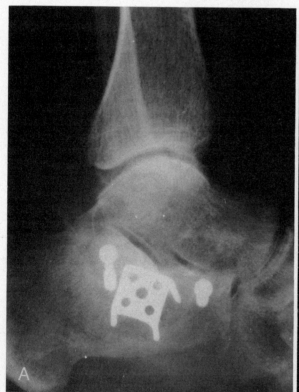

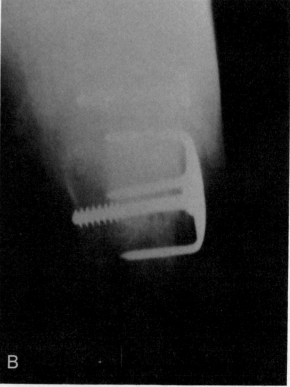

Figure 6.28. (A) Stone staple placement following ORIF of joint depression, intra-articular, calcaneal fracture. Notice cancellous screw fixation and anatomical realignment of subtalar joint. (B) Axial view of same patient demonstrating prongs of Stone staple. (Courtesy of Drs. G. Gumann and A. Studebaker, Columbus, GA.)

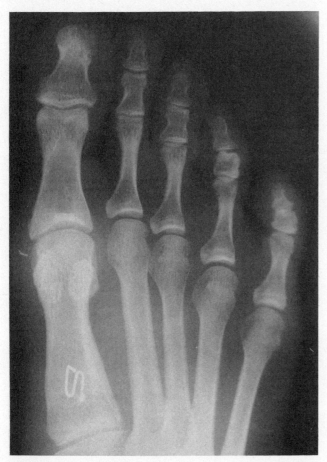

Figure 6.29. Osteoclasp used internally to fixate closing basewedge first metatarsal osteotomy.

CONCLUSION

The materials and devices described here serve as useful adjuncts in the practice of podiatric medicine and surgery. All products should be used with precise technique and careful attention to patient selection and goals of surgery. When appropriately applied they are a welcomed addition to the foot surgeon's armamentarium.

References

1. Seeburger RH: Surgical implants of alloyed metals in joints of the feet. *J Am Podiatry Assoc* 54:391, 1964.
2. *ASTM Annual Book of Standards: Medical Devices*, vol 13.01, Section 13. Philadelphia, American Society for Testing and Materials, 1983.
3. McGlamry ED: *Reconstructive Surgery of the Foot and Leg.* Miami, Intercontinental Medical Book Corp, 1974.
4. Frisch EE: *Functional Considerations in Implant Design*, vol 3. Santa Monica, CA, Medical Device and Diagnostic Industry, 1981.
5. Scholz KC: Total ankle replacement arthroplasty. In Bateman JE (ed): *Foot Science.* Philadelphia, WB Saunders Co, 1976.
6. Smith RC: *Smith Total Ankle Surgical Procedure.* Arlington TN, Wright Laboratories Product Information Bulletin, 1976.
7. Weil LS, Smith SD: *Total First.* Richards Manufacturing Corporation, Product Information Bulletin, Memphis, TN, 1976.
8. Weil LS, Pollak R, Goller WL: Total first joint replacement

9. Swanson JW, Lebeau JE: The effect of implantation on the physical properties of silicone rubber. *J Biomed Mater Res* 8:367, 1974.
10. Scales J: Implant materials. In Owen R, Goodfellow J, Bullough P (eds): *Scientific Foundations of Orthopedics and Traumatology.* London, William Heinemann Medical Books Ltd, 1980, p 465.
11. Swanson AB, Meester WD, Swanson G, Rangaswamyl L, Schut, GED: Durability of silicone implants—An in vivo study. *Orthop Clin North Am* 4:1097, 1973.
12. Swanson AB: Silicone rubber implants for replacement of arthritic or destroyed joints of the hand. *Surg Clin North Am* 48:1113, 1968.
13. Swanson AB: *Dow Corning Wright Data Sheet LO83-6217.* Arlington TN, Dow Corning, April 1983.
14. Kashuk K, Haber E: Tendon and ligament prostheses. *Clin Podiatry* 1:131, 1984.
15. Swanson AB: *Dow Corning Wright Data Sheet 83-5*, Arlington TN, Dow Corning, 1979.
16. Braley S: The chemistry and properties of medical-grade silicones. In Rembraum A, Shen M (eds): *Biomedical Polymers.* New York, Marcel-Dekker, 1971.
17. Sutter Biomedical Inc: *The Sutter Hinged Great Toe Joint Implant (LaPorta Design) Data Sheet.* SUT 56, 1982.
18. Frisch E: Biomaterials in foot surgery. *Clin Podiatry* 1:11, 1984.
19. Hunter JM, Salisbury RE: Flexor tendon reconstruction in severely damaged hands: a two stage procedure using a silicone-dacron reinforced gliding posthesis prior to tendon grafting. *J Bone Joint Surg* 53A: 829, 1971.
20. Holtz M, Midenberg ML, Kirschenbaum SE: Utilization of a silastic sheet in tendon repair of the foot. *J Foot Surg* 21:253, 1982.
21. Swanson AB, Boeve NR, Lumsden RM: The prevention and treatment of amputation neuroma by silicone capping. *J Hand Surg* 2:70, 1977.
22. Aptekar RG, Davie JM, Cattell HS: Foreign body reaction to silicone rubber: complication of a finger joint implant. *Clin Orthop* 98:231, 1974.
23. Vanore JV, O'Keefe RG, Pikscher I: Silastic implant arthroplasty: complications and their classification. *J Am Podiatry Assoc* 9:423, 1984.
24. Arenson DJ, Weil LS: Aseptic necrosis: an unusual cause of silastic (Swanson) implant failure: a case report. *J Am Podiatry Assoc* 69:616, 1979.
25. Worsing RA, Engber WD, Lange TA: Reactive synovitis from particulate silastic. *J Bone Joint Surg* 64A:581, 1982.
26. Caneva RG: Postoperative degenerative changes of the metatarsal head following use of the Swanson implant: four case reports. *J Foot Surg* 16:34, 1977.
27. Lim WT, Landrum K, Weinberger G: Silicone lymphadenitis secondary to implant degeneration. *J Foot Surg* 22:243, 1983.
28. Barondes R de R, Judge WD, Towne CG, Baxter ML: The silicones in medicine: new organic derivatives and some of their unique properties. *Mil Surg* 106:379, 1950.
29. Balkin SW: Silicone augmentation for plantar callouses. *J Am Podiatry Assoc* 66:148, 1976.
30. Balkin SW: Plantar keratoses: treatment by injectable liquid-silicone, report of an eight year experience. *Clin Orthop* 87:235, 1972.
31. Kaplan EN, Falces E, Tolleth H: Clinical utilization of injectable collagen. *Ann Plast Surg* 10:437, 1983.
32. Urist MR: Practical applications of basic research on bone graft physiology. *AAOS Instructional Course Lectures* 25:1, 1976.
33. Hetherington VJ, Kavros SJ, Conway F, Mandracchia VJ, Martin W, Haubold AD: Pyrolytic carbon as a joint replacement in the foot: a preliminary report. *J Foot Surg* 21:160, 1982.
34. Smith SD, Millar EA: Arthrosis by means of a subtalar polyethylene peg implant for correction of hindfoot pronation in children. *Clin Orthop* 181:15, 1983.
35. Stark HH, Boyes JH, Johnson L, Ashworth CR: An evaluation

in hallux valgus and hallux rigidus. *Clin in Podiatry* 1:103, 1984.

of the healing process of paratenon, polyethylene film and
silastic sheeting to prevent adhesions to tendons in the hand.
J Bone Joint Surg 59A:908, 1977.

36. Williams CW, Dickie WR, Colville J: Silastic sheeting in hand
surgery. *Hand* 4:273, 1972.
37. McCarthy DJ, Montgomery B: Polyurethane in the management of ulcerating lesions of the lower extremities. *J Am
Podiatry Assoc* 73:1, 1983.
38. Krvez FP, Hyatt GW, Turner TC, Bassett AL: The presentation and clinical use of freeze-dried bone. *J Bone Joint Surg*
33A:863, 1951.
39. Tomford WW, Doppelt SH, Mankin HJ, Friedlaender GE:
1983 bone bank procedures. *Clin Orthop* 174:15, 1983.
40. Friedlaender GE: U.S. navy tissue bank. *J Am Podiatry Assoc*
67:38, 1977.
41. Sadler AM, Sadler BL, Stason EB: The uniform anatomical
gift act: a model for reform. *JAMA* 206:2501, 1968.
42. McGlamry ED, Miller IH: A review of the current status of
bone grafting. *J Am Podiatry Assoc* 67:42, 1977.
43. Marcinko DE, Lazerson A, Elleby DH: Silver calcaneal osteotomy for flexible flatfoot: a retrospective preliminary report.
J Foot Surg 23:191, 1984.
44. Dollard MD, Marcinko DE, Lazerson A, Elleby DH: The
Evans calcaneal osteotomy for correction of flexible flatfoot
syndrome. *J Foot Surg* 23:291, 1984.
45. Hutchinson J: The fate of experimental bone autografts and
hemografts. *Br J Surg* 39:552, 1952.
46. Chalmers J: Transplantation immunity in bone hemografting.
J Bone Joint Surg 41B:160, 1959.
47. Bonfiglio M, Jeter WS: Immunological responses to bone. *Clin
Orthop* 87:19, 1972.
48. Taheri F, Monoucher G: Experience with calf bone in cervical
interbody spinal fusion. *J Neurosurg* 36:67, 1972.
49. Reverdin JL: De la Gireffe epidermique. *Bull Soc Imper Chir*
10:483, 511, 1869. Cited in Rogers BO: Historical development
for free skin grafting. *Surg Clin North Am* 39:289, 1959.
50. Raven TF: Skin grafting from the pig. *Br Med J* 1:623, 1871.
51. Silvetti AH, Cotton C, Byrne RJ, Berrian JH, Menendef AF:
Preliminary experimental studies on bovine embryo skin
grafts. *Transplantation* 4:24, 1957.
52. Bromberg BE, Song C, Mohn MP: The use of pig skin as a
temporary biological dressing. *Plast Reconstr Surg* 36:80, 1965.
53. Burke HB, Confer HE, Kutlick DA, Reister G, Vidt L: The
use of porcine xenografts in treatment of chronic ulcerations.
J Am Podiatry Assoc 69:345, 1977.
54. Culliton P, Kwasnik RE, Novicki D, Corbin P, Patton G,
Collins W, Terleckyj B, Axler DA: The efficacy of porcine skin
grafts for treating non healing cutaneous ulcers. Part I. *J Am
Podiatry Assoc* 68:1, 1978.
55. Morris PJ, Bondor C, Burke JF: The use of frequently changed
skin allografts to promote healing in the non healing infected
ulcer. *Surgery* 60:13, 1966.
56. State D, Peter M: Clinical use of porcine xenografts in conditions other than burns. *Surg Gynecol Obstet* 13B:13, 1974
57. McCarthy DJ, Axler DA: The efficacy of porcine skin grafts
for treating non-healing cutaneous ulcers. Part II. *J Am Podiatry Assoc* 68:86, 1978.
58. Heifitz NM: Podiatric evaluation of pig skin graft. *J Am
Podiatry Assoc* 67:573, 1977.
59. Elliot R, Hoehn J: Use of commercial porcine skin for wound
dressings. *Plast Reconstr Surg* 52:401, 1973.
60. Cangialosi CP: Synthetic skin—a new adjunct in the treatment
of decubitus ulcers. *J Am Podiatry Assoc* 72:48, 1982.
61. Douglas B: Homografts of fetal membranes as a covering for
large wounds—especially those from burns. *J Tenn Med Assoc*
45:230, 1952.
62. Robson MD, Krizek TJ: Amniotic membranes as a temporary
wound dressing. *Surg Gynecol Obstet* 136:904, 1973.
63. Rudnick SS: The use of amniotic membrane grafting in podiatric office practice. *J Am Podiatry Assoc* 71:679, 1981.
64. Harris WA, Crothers OD, Moyen BJ, Bourne RB: Topical
hemostatic agents for bone bleeding in humans. *J Bone Joint
Surg* 60A:454, 1978.
65. *Physician's Desk Reference.* Oradell NJ, Medical Economics
Co, 1986.

66. Freeman LW, Joyner JE: Absorbable gelatin sponge in the
treatment of decubitus ulcers. *JAMA* 184:784, 1963.
67. Burke HB, Kuglar W, Oriti J, Seidenspinner C, Lockwood B,
Buskey A: The use of gelfoam powder and betadine saturated
gauze in treatment of chronic ulcerations. *J Foot Surg* 20:76,
1981.
68. Howard TC, Kelley RR: The effect of bone wax on the healing
of experimental rat tibial lesions. *Clin Orthop* 63:226, 1969.
69. Geary JR, Frantz VK: New absorbable hemostatic bone wax,
experimental and clinical studies. *Ann Surg* 132:1128, 1950.
70. McFarlane RM: The use of continuous suction under skin
flaps. *Br J Plast Surg* 11:77, 1958.
71. Buchanan JM, Lambley D: The advantages of wound suction
drainage in general surgery. *J Intern Coll Surg* 34:701, 1960.
72. Radcliffe A: Continuous suction in neck surgery. *J Laryngol
Otol* 78:1114, 1964.
73. Miller SJ: Surgical wound drainage system using silicone tubing. *J Am Podiatry Assoc* 71:287, 1981.
74. Josephs RL: Vacudrain system for foot surgery. *J Foot Surg*
16:97, 1977.
75. Jacoby RP: Closed sterile suction system. *J Am Podiatry Assoc*
68:834, 1978.
76. Smith-Petersen MN, Larson CB, Cochran W: Local chemotherapy with primary closure of septic wounds by means of
drainage and irrigation cannulae. *J Bone Joint Surg* 27A:562,
1945.
77. Willenegger H: Klinik und therapie der Pyogenen Knochen-
infektionen. *Chirug* 41:215, 1970.
78. Pressman M: Continuous closure suction irrigation following
post operative infection of silastic implant. *J Am Podiatry
Assoc* 67:746, 1977.
79. Green R, Pitzer S, Mann I, Kaplan E: A suction irrigation
technique utilizing a hemovac system in treatment of osteomyelitis. *J Foot Surg* 17:22, 1978.
80. Sorto LA: The infected implant. *Clin Podiatry* 1:199, 1984.
81. Schwartz NH, Marcinko DE: Suction irrigation—construction
and use of a dependable closed system. *J Am Podiatry Assoc*
74:216, 1984.
82. Alm WA, Gold ML, Weil LS: Evaluation of TENS in podiatric
surgery. *J Am Podiatry Assoc* 69:537, 1979.
83. Grosack MA, Gibbons RW, Cohen G: TENS: its significance
and application in podiatry. *J Foot Surg* 20:127, 1981.
84. Melzack R, Wall PD: Pain mechanisms: a new theory. *Science*
150:971, 1965.
85. Lanham RH, Powell S, Hendrix BE: Efficacy of hypothermia
and TENS in podiatric surgery. *J Foot Surg* 23:152, 1984.
86. Smith SD: The STA operation for the pronated foot in childhood. *Clin Podiatry* 1:165, 1984.
87. Hugh P, Cole P, Lettin A: Cardiovascular effects of implanted
acrylic bone cement. *Br Med J* 23:460, 1971.
88. Klemm K: Gentamicin PMMA kugeln in der behandlung
abszedieren der Knochen und Weichteilinfektionen. *Zentralbl
Chir* 104:934, 1979.
89. Wahlig H, Dingeldein E, Bergman R, Reuss K: The release of
gentamicin from polymethylmethracrylate beads. *J Bone Joint
Surg* 60B:270, 1978.
90. Asche G: Spulsaugdrainage oder gentamicin-PMMA-kugeln in
der Therapie infizierter Osteosynthesen. *Unfallheilkunde*
81:463, 1978.
91. Grieben A: Results of septopa in more than 1500 cases of bone
and soft tissue infections—a review of clinical trials. *J Bone
Joint Surg* 62B:275, 1980.
92. Jenny G, Taglang G: Lokale knocheninfektions behandlung
mit gentamicin PMMA-kugelketten. *Beitr Orthop Traumatol*
27:3, 1980.
93. Taglang G, Jenny G: Clinical experience with the use of
gentamicin PMMA beads and chains in 200 cases of bone and
soft tissue infections; early and late follow-up results. In Van
Rens TJG, Kayser FH (eds):*Local Antibiotics and Treatment
in Osteomyelitis and Soft Tissue Infections.* Amsterdam, Excerpta Medica, 1981.
94. Van Rens TJG, Kayser FH: *Local Antibiotic Treatment in
Osteomyelitis and Soft Tissue Infections.* Amsterdam, Excerpta
Medica, 1981.
95. Yasuda I: Fundamental aspects of fracture treatment. *J Kyoto*

Med Soc 4:395, 1953.

96. Friendenberg Z, Harlow M, Brighton C: Healing on nonunion of the medial malleolus by means of direct current. A case report. *J Trauma* 11:883, 1971.

97. Brighton C, Adler S, Black J, Itada N, Friedenberg FB: Cathode oxygen consumption and electrically induced osteogenesis. *Clin Orthop* 107:277, 1975.

98. Sharrard WJ, Sutcliffe ML, Robson MJ, Maceachern AG: The treatment of fibrous non-union of fractures by pulsating electromagnetic stimulation. *J Bone Joint Surg* 64B:189, 1982.

99. Mahan K: Electrical stimulation of bone—a practical review. *J Am Podiatry Assoc* 73:86, 1983.

100. Brighton C: Current concepts review: the treatment of non unions with electricity. *J Bone Joint Surg* 63A:847, 1981.

101. Fox IM, Smith SD: Bioelectric repair and metatarsal non unions. *J Foot Surg* 22:108, 1983.

102. Bassett C, Mitchell S, Gaston SR: Pulsating electro magnetic field treatment in ununited fractures and failed arthrodesis. *JAMA* 247:623, 1982.

103. Brighton GT, Black J, Friedenberg FB, Esterhai JL, Day L, Connolly JF: A multicenter study of the treatment of nonunions with constant direct current. *J Bone Joint Surg* 63A:2, 1981.

104. Peterson D, Lewis G, Cass CA: Treatment of delayed union and non union with an unpaired direct current stimulator. *Clin Orthop* 148:117, 1980.

105. Mears DC: History of external fixation. In Booker AF Jr, Edwards CC (eds): *External Fixation: the Current State of the Art.* Baltimore, Williams & Wilkins, 1979.

106. Vidal J: Notre experience de F.E. d'H a propos de forty-six observations. Les indications de son emploi. *Montpellier Chir* 14:451, 1968.

107. Adrey J: Le fixateur externe d'hoffmann couple. In *Cadre*, Paris, Gead, 1970, p 11.

108. Jackson RP, Jacobs RR, Neff JR: External skeletal fixation in severe limb trauma. *J Trauma* 18:201, 1978.

109. Reinherz RP, Sharon SM, Schwartz R, Pitzer S, Knudsen HA: Modification of the Charnley approach to ankle arthrodesis. *J Am Podiatry Assoc* 69:265, 1979.

110. Wright JC, Jones RO: Revisional left ankle arthrodesis for pseudoarthrosis. *J Foot Surg* 22:57, 1983.

111. Said E, Hunka L, Siller TN: Where ankle fusions stand today? *J Bone Joint Surg* 60B:211, 1978.

112. Walter JH, Pressman MM: External fixation in the treatment of metatarsal non unions. *J Am Podiatry Assoc* 71:297, 1981.

113. Duke HF, Walter JH: External fixation in hallux abducto valgus surgery. *J Am Podiatry Assoc* 72:443, 1982.

114. Williams JE, Marcinko DE, Lazerson A, Elleby DH: The Calandruccio triangular compression device—a schematic introduction. *J Am Podiatry Assoc* 73:536, 1983.

115. Kirschner M: Verbesserungen der Drahtextention. *Arch Klin Chir* 148:656, 1927.

116. Taylor RG: An operative procedure for the treatment of hammer toe and claw toe. *J Bone Joint Surg* 22:608, 1940.

117. *Reference Guide for Pins and Wires.* Warsaw, Zimmer Inc, 1982.

118. Reichert K, Caneva RG: The use of kirschner wire fixation in forefoot surgery. *J Foot Surg* 22:218, 1983.

119. Estersohn HS, Stanoch JF: A simplified technique for internal wire fixation. *J Am Podiatry Assoc* 73:593, 1983.

120. DiGiovanni JE, Martin R: Pins, wires and staples in foot surgery. *Clin Podiatry* 1:211, 1984.

121. Vega MR, Wishiew J, Johnson TE: Johnson-Tucker: instrumentation for better internal wire fixation. *J Foot Surg* 23:121, 1984.

122. Stephenson JR: Displaced fractures of the os calcis involving the sub-talar joint: the key role of the superomedial fragment. *Foot Ankle* 4:91, 1983.

123. Levitsky DR: Percutaneous osteoclasp fixation of Akin osteotomy: an alternative fixation technique. *J Foot Surg* 20:163, 1981.

124. Shaw AH: The Akin procedure for correction of hallux valgus. In McGlamry ED (ed): *Reconstructive Surgery of the Foot and Leg.* New York, Intercontinental Medical Book Corp, 1974, p 57.

125. Floyd EJ, Perillo JT, Dailey JM: The scaphoid compression staple: an effective form of fixation. *J Foot Surg* 23:56, 1984.

126. Kerman BL, Arnold D: Skin staple usage in podiatric surgery. *J Am Podiatry Assoc* 73:212, 1983.

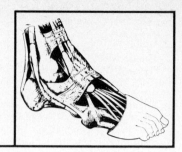

CHAPTER 7

Instrumentation

Scot Malay, D.P.M.

Surgical instrumentation is highly specialized and it has been said that there is a tool for every job. In many instances there are multiple instruments serving the same function, and each surgeon will develop his or her own preferences. Students and residents should familiarize themselves with the basic set of podiatric surgical instruments. A thorough understanding of the design and proper use of the basic tools will enable the surgeon to become comfortable and proficient with his or her skill.

SURGICAL BLADES

The scalpel is the instrument of choice for precise, atraumatic division of tissue. The scalpel consists of a handle portion and the blade portion. Blades may be detachable and thereby replaceable, or the scalpel may consist of a solid piece of steel that requires periodic sharpening of the blade. The handle portion of the scalpel may differ in size. The #3 handle is most commonly used for podiatric surgery. The handle should have an engraved metric scale on one side. The scalpel can be held between the thumb, third, and fourth fingers with the index finger placed along the back of the blade when incising glabrous areas of tissue. The pencil grip is frequently used in podiatric surgery because it provides greater control when making precise incisions on small areas of the foot.

Scalpel blades (Fig. 7.1) are also available in various sizes and shapes. Blades are constructed of high quality surgical steel, with the cutting edge honed to a width of approximately 0.015 inch. The scalpel blade is designed strictly for incising tissues, and the belly of the blade should be used more than the tip. Scalpel blades should never be used for prying because they may easily break within the wound. Reversing one's grip and prying with the handle portion of the scalpel is acceptable. Separate blades are usually used for incising the skin and deeper tissues. The broad #10 blade functions well as the "skin knife" in most cases, although the smaller #15 blade may be desirable for making precise skin incisions on the digits. The #15 blade is also most commonly used as the "deep

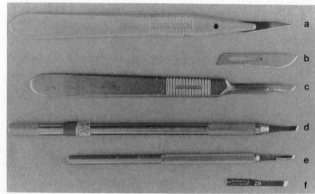

Figure 7.1. Surgical blades. (a) Disposable #11, (b) #10, (c) #15 blade on #3 handle, (d) #81 blade on minihandle, (e) #67 blade on minihandle, (f) #62 blade.

knife." The #11, or bayonet, blade is useful when performing the frontal plane Z-plasty tendo achillis lengthening, as well as when incising superficial abscesses for drainage. Some surgeons find the smaller Beaver blades (#64, #67, #81) and matching handle useful for digital arthroplasty and occasional nail plate and bed incisions.

SCISSORS

Except for the scalpel, scissors (Fig. 7.2A, B) are the instruments most commonly used for tissue dissection. Scissors also serve as the general purpose instrument for cutting sutures, bandages, and other materials. Tissue scissors are finely constructed of surgical steel, and are of lighter weight compared to the heavier suture cutting and utility scissors. Dissecting scissors are designed to cut soft tissues only and should never be used to cut other materials. Scissors are best grasped with the thumb and ring fingers in the finger rings, the index finger stabilizing the hinge region of the scissors, and the middle and little fingers on either side of the lesser digital finger ring (Fig. 7.3). The tips of the scissors are best used for spreading and cutting the tissues, and a thumb

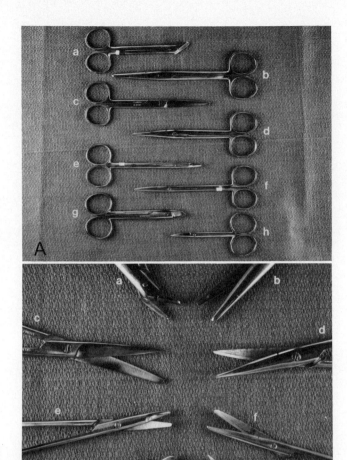

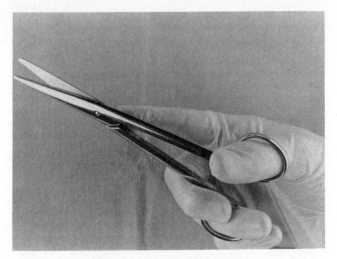

Figure 7.2. (A, B) Scissors. (a) Wire cutting, (b) large Mayo, (c) utility or suture cutting, (d) small Mayo, (e) short blade Metzenbaum, (f) long blade Metzenbaum, (g) crown-and-collar or Sistrunk, (h) iris.

Figure 7.3. Grasping the scissors.

forceps is usually held in the other hand to aid dissection. The blades of the scissors should never be closed without first visualizing the tips. Straight blades are used near the wound surface whereas curved blades aid deeper dissection. The heavier blunt-tipped Mayo scissors are used for cutting thick bands of fascia and ligament, and are available with either straight or curved blades. The lighter Metzenbaum scissors have narrow, slightly curved, blunt-tipped blades that are ideal for subcutaneous dissection and cutting lighter fascial and capsular structures. The fine cutting blades of the lightweight iris scissors are only suited for delicate tissue dissection. The short, broad-bladed collar-and-crown, or Sistrunk, scissors are occasionally used for accurate dissection of osseous structures such as sesamoid bones.

Suture scissors usually have straight blades with blunt tips, thereby reducing the chance of inadvertent injury to nearby tissues. When cutting deep sutures the tips of the scissors are placed about the suture and the blades slid down to the level of the knot, turned approximately 25° and, with the tips in full view, the scissors are closed. When cutting deep sutures that are under a large amount of tension a small tag of suture should be left above the knot. A larger tag is left when cutting skin sutures that will be removed at a later date. Often the general utility scissors, which come in various sizes, are used for cutting sutures. Stainless steel monofilament wire sutures are cut with wire cutting scissors.

Bandage scissors are designed with a flat, plowlike lower blade tip that protects the patient from inadvertent injury during bandage application or removal. Ideally a wound should be undressed without cutting the bandages. Nonetheless, all house staff and medical students should carry, and have readily available, a clean, sharp pair of bandage scissors.

HEMOSTATIC FORCEPS

Hemostats (Fig. 7.4A, B) are hinged instruments composed of a set of jaws, finger rings, and a locking mechanism. They are the primary means of acquiring hemostasis during anatomical dissection, and are also useful for bluntly spreading tissues. There are many types of hemostatic forceps, and those most commonly used in podiatric surgery include the mosquito (Halstead), Crile, and Kelly designs. Hemostatic jaws are straight or curved, with serrations that run either perpendicular or parallel to the long axis of the jaws. The forceps close with force about the vessel and lock, thereby crushing the contained tissue that will be ligated and no longer viable. If the clamped portion of vessel is to remain functional, such as in vascular reconstruction, a noncrushing or controlled-closure hemostat must be used.

THUMB FORCEPS

Thumb forceps (Fig. 7.5) consist of two pieces of surgical steel attached at one end and are used to pick up or grasp tissues. The forceps are held between the thumb, middle, and index fingers of either hand. The tips may be flat or have teeth or fine serrations, and they vary in width. Forceps with teeth (Brown-Adson, rat-tooth or one-two) are usually narrow and allow the surgeon to hold structures with a sure grip while

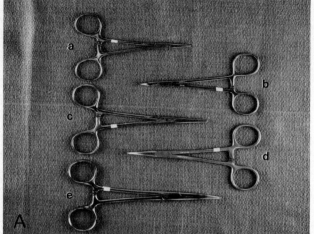

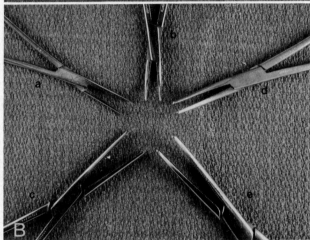

Figure 7.4. (A, B) Hemostatic forceps. (a) Straight mosquito, (b) curved mosquito, (c) straight Crile, (d) curved Crile, (e) curved Kelly.

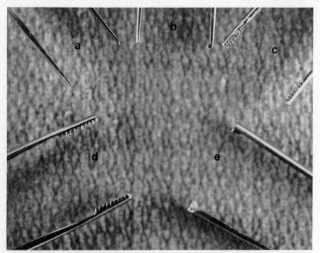

Figure 7.5. Thumb forceps. (a) Atraumatic, (b) one-two or rat-tooth, (c) Brown-Adson, (d), (e) large toothed pick-ups.

applying a minimum of tension. Flat-tipped or finely serrated narrow forceps (atraumatic forceps) are used delicately to grasp vital structures, pull sutures and needles, and, with great care, gingerly to manipulate

skin during closure. The one-two (rat-tooth) pick-up is frequently used for skin closure, depending on the surgeon's preference. A wide tipped atraumatic forceps (Potts-Smith) can also be useful for the application and removal of surgical dressings.

TRACTION FORCEPS

Traction forceps (Fig. 7.6) are of heavier construction than hemostats and consist of a locking mechanism and finger rings, as well as jaws for grasping tissues. The grasping portion of each jaw typically has teeth, or a single sharp point, that provides traction without undue pressure or crushing force.

The Backhaus towel clamp provides a double-sharp set of jaws and is used for draping the operative field and, occasionally, for grasping bone. The Allis clamp is available with narrow or wide jaws, each jaw composed of opposing serrated edges or short teeth. These are effective for grasping and retracting fascia and the subcutaneous layer, and are occasionally used for clamping towels while draping. The Kocher forceps have two long bladed jaws displaying transverse serrations with opposing sharp, interlocking teeth at the tips. These are useful for placing traction on heavy fascia, although care must be taken to avoid crushing tissues. Uterine packing forceps have gently curved, long jaws that make them ideal for passing tendons along tendon sheaths during tendon transfer procedures. The sesamoid clamp and phalangeal forceps are specifically designed for grasping small ossicles and bony fragments. The sponge clamp has two opposing circular jaws with transverse serrations used to hold a folded gauze sponge while prepping the surgical area.

RETRACTORS

Retractors are used to hold tissues aside, thereby increasing exposure and protecting vital structures.

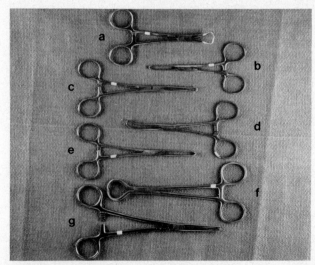

Figure 7.6. Traction forceps. (a) Backhaus towel clamp, (b) small Allis, (c) phalangeal forcep, (d) sesamoid clamp, (e) large Allis, (f) Lewin, (g) Kocher.

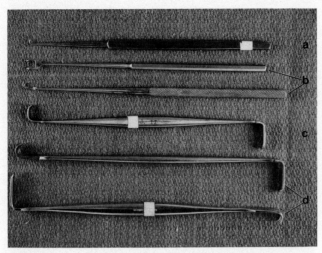

Figure 7.7. Hand-held retractors. (a) Single-prong skin hook and (b) double-prong skin hooks, (c) Ragnell, (d) Senn.

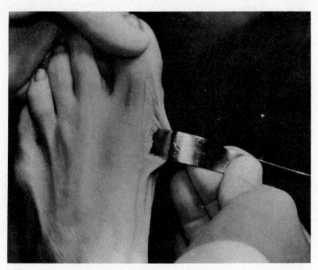

Figure 7.8. Seeburger hand-held malleable retractor used at medial aspect of first metatarsophalangeal joint.

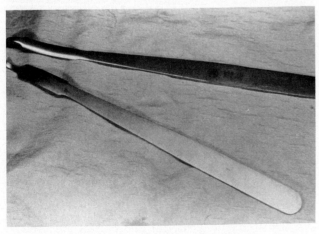

Figure 7.9. Mini-Hohmann retractors.

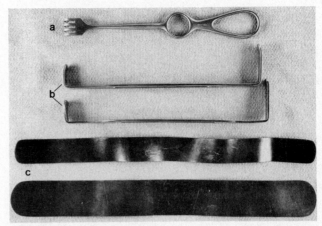

Figure 7.10. Retractors. (a) Large rake, (b) Army-Navy or right angle, (c) large malleable ribbon.

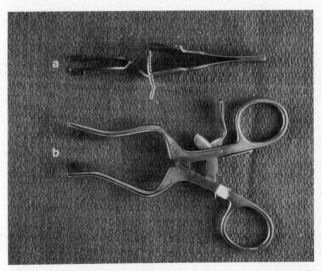

Figure 7.11. (a) Digital self-retaining or Holzheimer retractor, (b) three-two Weitlaner retractor.

The blade portion of the retractor can be fixed or malleable, and the retractor itself can be hand-held or self-retaining. Hand-held retractors enable the assistant to control the force with which tissues are held, and to intermittently release tension as necessary. On the other hand, self-retaining retractors free the assistant to perform duties that may expedite the procedure. Nonetheless, self-retaining retractors should be intermittently released during long procedures to avoid tissue necrosis or excessive retraction trauma.

A wide variety of retractors are necessary for proper exposure of the many different surgical areas of the foot and leg (Table 7.1, Figs. 7.7–7.13).

PERIOSTEAL ELEVATORS

Periosteal elevators (Figs. 7.14–7.16) are used to separate periosteum from underlying bone and, occasionally, to provide leverage for retracting deep fascia and periosteum. These instruments have smooth, broad blades that vary in sharpness. The Freer elevator is commonly used in podiatric surgery and is

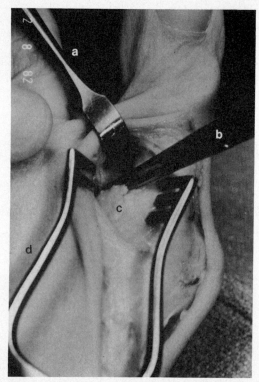

Figure 7.12. Dissection in first interspace. (a) Deep end of Senn retractor, (b) curved Crile, (c) grasping conjoined tendon of adductor hallucis, (d) three-two Weitlaner.

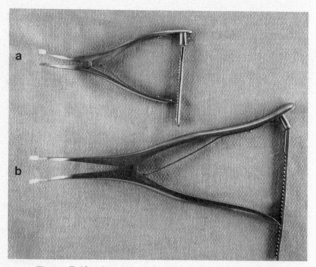

Figure 7.13. Lamina spreaders (a) small and (b) large.

Table 7.1
Retractors

Hand-held (Figs. 7.7–7.10)	*SELF-RETAINING* (Figs. 7.11–7.13)
Skin Hook (single or double prong)	Digital (Holzheimer, Heis)
Senn Double-end (sharp or blunt rake)	Alm
Ragnell (double-end, blunt)	Weitlaner (3-2, 4-3)
Meyerding finger ring	Lamina spreader
Seeburger (malleable)	
Mini-Hohmann	
Volkmann rakes (sharp, blunt)	
Right angle, or Army-Navy	
Malleable ribbon	

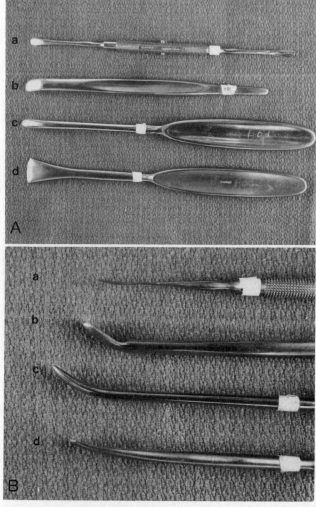

Figure 7.14. (A, B). Periosteal elevators. (a) Freer, (b) Sayre, (c) narrow Langenbeck elevator, (d) wide Langenbeck elevator.

ideal for reflecting periosteum from the shaft of a metatarsal. One end of the Freer elevator is semisharp whereas the other is blunt. The Sayre elevator has a short, heavy, rounded blade frequently employed to distract the sesamoid apparatus from the first metatarsal head. Key elevators are excellent for rapidly reflecting periosteum from glabrous bony surfaces, as are the narrow- and broad-ended Langenbeck elevators. Crego elevators expedite periosteal reflection around curved surfaces such as the talar neck and posterior aspect of the calcaneus, and are essential in performing triple arthrodesis and other rearfoot procedures.

OSTEOTOMES, CHISELS, GOUGES, AND MALLETS

Osteotomes (Lambotte) and chisels are used to resect prominent portions of bone, and the cutting

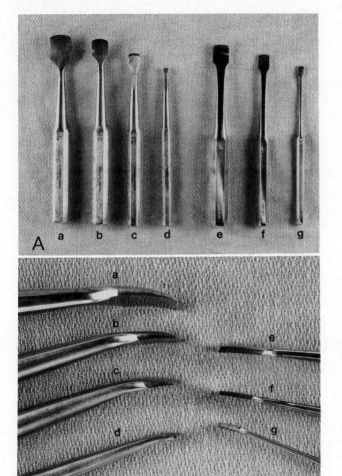

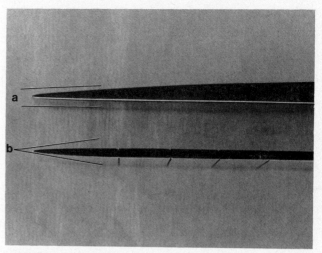

Figure 7.17. Comparison of (a) chisel configuration to that of (b) osteotome. Note that one surface of chisel converges on opposing horizontal surface, whereas both surfaces of osteotome converge to meet at cutting edge.

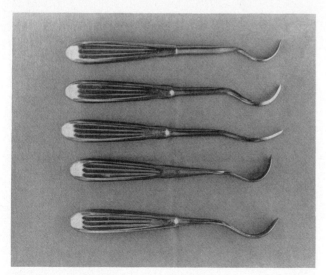

Figure 7.15. (A, B) Assorted Key elevators.

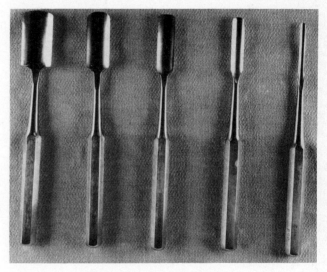

Figure 7.18. Set of large gouges.

Figure 7.16. Set of curved Cregos.

edge of these instruments must be periodically sharpened to assure proper function. Osteotomes differ from chisels in that both surfaces of an osteotome taper to form a fine cutting edge, whereas one surface

of a chisel tapers to meet the opposite flat surface at the cutting edge (1) (Fig. 7.17).

Straight osteotomes should be available in an assortment of widths ranging from 4 to 22 ml. At least one curved osteotome of medium width, and one chisel (18 ml US Army pattern) should be available in the basic instrument set.

Osteotomes and chisels are held firmly in one hand and driven with deliberate, repetitive blows from the surgical mallet. Mallets are available with stainless steel heads, as well as heads capped with synthetic material (Delrin) for quieting the blow. The small and medium sized mallets are best suited for podiatric surgery.

Gouges (Fig. 7.18) are similar to chisels; however, the cutting edge is curved. These come in various widths and are useful in smoothing curved surfaces and rounding flat surfaces of bone. Gouges can also be used to free metatarsal heads from surrounding soft tissue structures. The metatarsal elevator (Fig. 7.19) is a specialized gouge with a broad, curved, scooplike blade set on a curved handle. This instrument is ideal for freeing metatarsal heads from adherent soft tissues, and exposing the plantar surface of the head for observation.

BONE CUTTING FORCEPS AND RONGEURS

Bone cutting forceps and rongeurs are used to incise through and reduce bone, or for resecting cartilaginous surfaces. Hinged instruments used for osseous work (Fig. 7.20) are frequently of the multihinge design, and function on the so-called double-action principle. This increases mechanical advantage, reduces strain, and provides increased accuracy. Double-action bone cutting forceps have straight or slightly curved jaws that are ideal for transecting phalanges and other small diameter portions of bone. Rongeurs have strong, heavily constructed opposing jaws, each of which is scooped out like the tip of a curette. Rongeur jaw designs include broad or narrow (needlenose) and straight or curved. The sharp cutting edges of the rongeur are ideal for reducing bony prominences, such as spurs and spicules, and sharp edges. The Kerrison rongeur (Fig. 7.21), with its long and narrow design, is suitable for reducing sharp edges of bone in hard-to-reach areas.

TREPHINES AND CURETTES

Trephines (Fig. 7.22) display a circular cutting edge at the tip of a hollow tube that enables the operator neatly to remove plugs of bone (Fig. 7.23) for biopsy, graft procurement, or osseous reduction. Assorted trephines and corresponding obturators should be available. Curettes (Fig. 7.24) consist of a curved, scooplike blade on a handle. Heavy curettes are used for reducing rough bony surfaces and gouging into broad areas of bone. They are also useful for debriding infected or necrotic bone. Dermal curettes, on the other hand, are of lighter construction and are used for the debridement of soft tissues and nail beds and grooves.

BONE HOLDING CLAMPS AND REDUCTION FORCEPS

Clamps (Figs. 7.25, 7.26) used to grasp bone or hold bony fragments together are of heavy construction and are capable of applying large amounts of pressure. Some bone clamps and reduction forceps have a hinge with a locking ratchet, whereas others close on tightening of a locking nut. Small fragments

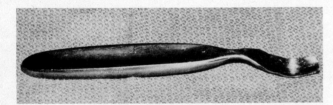

Figure 7.19.   Metatarsal elevator.

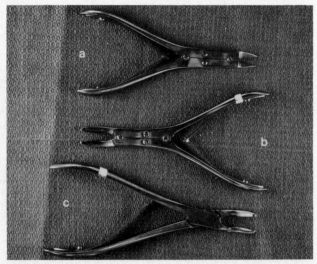

Figure 7.20.   Bone cutting instruments. (a) Double-action bone cutting forceps, (b) double-action curved rongeur, (c) single-hinged curved rongeur.

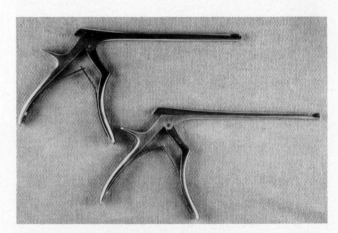

Figure 7.21.   Kerrison rongeurs.

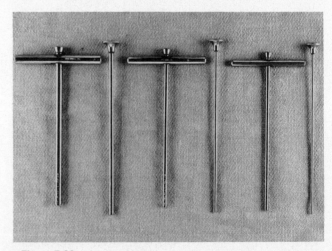

Figure 7.22.   Assorted trephines and corresponding obturators.

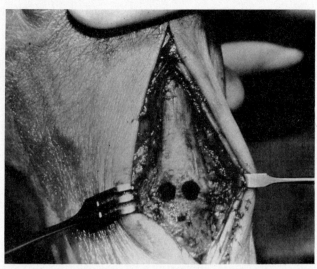

Figure 7.23. Trephine holes in metaphysis of first metatarsal, left foot dorsal aspect.

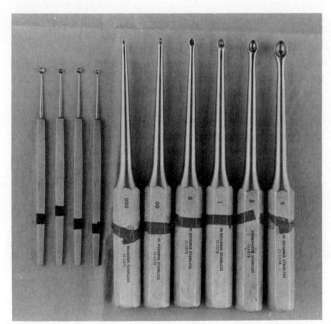

Figure 7.24. Dermal (small set) and bone (large set) curettes.

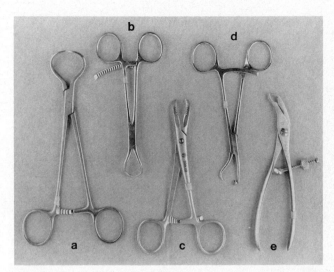

Figure 7.25. Bone reduction forceps. (a) Lewin, (b) ASIF double-sharp, (c) ASIF "alligator" small fragment, (d) ASIF small plate forceps, (e) ASIF small fragment self-centering clamp.

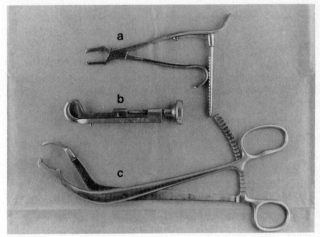

Figure 7.26. Large fragment reduction forceps. (a) "Baby" Lane, (b) Lowman, (c) Verbrugge.

of bone and small ossicles such as sesamoids or phalanges can be grasped and manipulated with the sesamoid and phalangeal clamps. The double-sharp and "alligator" tip bone reduction forceps are ideally suited for reducing and maintaining small and medium sized fragments. Larger fragments encountered in calcaneal, tibial, and fibular fractures require heavier reduction forceps such as the Lewin, "baby" Lane, Lowman, and Verbrugge.

RASPS

Rasps (Fig. 7.27) are used to reduce and smooth bony surfaces. Rasps are usually used after a bony prominence has been grossly reduced by means of an osteotome and mallet, rongeur, or power saw. The cutting surface of a rasp presents serrations of fine

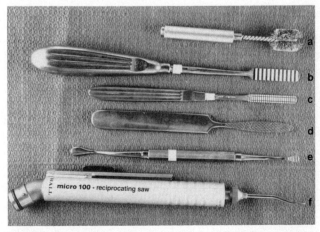

Figure 7.27. Rasping instruments. (a) Wire brush, (b) Parkes coarse rasp, (c) Maltz rasp, (d) Joseph's nasal or beaver-tail rasp, (e) Bell rasp, (f) pneumatic reciprocating rasp.

teeth running in a parallel or cross-cut pattern (Fig. 7.28). The Bell rasp is double-ended with two small elliptical rasping surfaces. The Joseph's nasal rasp, also known as the beaver-tail rasp, has a single, long, elliptical cutting surface with a double cross-cut pattern for fine smoothing of broad surfaces. The Maltz and Parkes rasps each present a single, coarse cutting surface ideal for rapid reduction of large osseous prominences. Rasping surfaces are also available for reciprocating power instrumentation. A stainless steel wire brush should be available for periodic intraoperative cleansing of the rasp surface.

NEEDLE HOLDERS

Needle holders consist of finger rings, a locking mechanism, and jaws, and come in a wide variety of sizes and shapes (Fig. 7.29). The individual surgeon will pick the design that he or she prefers for each specific task. Long-handled needle holders are used for closing deeper layers whereas shorter designs are used superficially. Jaw designs vary from smooth, to cross-cut or parallel serrations, to channeled jaws for holding specific needles and those modified for twisting wires. Needle holders with heavy jaws are used to hold large needles, and vice versa. Examples of commonly used needle holders include Mayo-Hegar, Sarot, Ryder, and Halsey.

POWER INSTRUMENTATION

Practically any aspect of osseous surgery can be performed with power instrumentation. Power saws, both oscillating and reciprocating, drills, burs, rasps, wire drivers, osteotomes, and screwdrivers are commercially available. Power sources may be pneumatic or electrical (alternating or direct current). Power instrumentation varies with respect to size, strength, maneuverability, precision, and durability, and the decision as to which set is to be used varies with the surgical site and surgeon's preference. Both the Zimmer (Fig. 7.30) and Stryker (Fig. 7.31) pneumatic arrangements are frequently used for podiatric surgery. A hand drill should always be available as a

backup should the power instrumentation fail (Fig. 7.32).

INSTRUMENTS FOR FIXATION OF BONE AND OTHER TISSUES

Fixation of bony fragments can be obtained in many ways. Bony fixation is probably best obtained following standard Association for Osteosynthesis/Association for the Study of Internal Fixation (AO/ASIF) principles and techniques. Fixation devices include stainless steel wire sutures (26, 28, and 30 gauge)

They also include Kirschner wires ranging in size from 0.035 inch to 0.062 inch in diameter, both threaded and smooth, with tips varying from tapered to trocar or bayonet for easy penetration of hard cortical bone. These can be used to fixate bony fragments via direct pinning or intramedullary nailing, as well as providing anchoring for skeletal traction. A

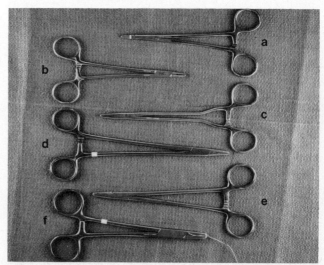

Figure 7.29. Assorted needle holders. (a) Ryder or vascular, (b) small Mayo-Hegar, (c) Sarot, (d) large Mayo-Hegar, (e) Halsey, (f) channeled wire twister/needle driver.

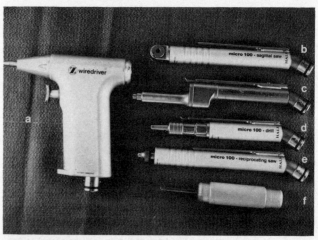

Figure 7.30. Zimmer pneumatic power instrumentation. (a) Wire driver, (b) sagittal saw, (c) oscillating saw, (d) rotary drill, (e) reciprocating saw, (f) Allen wrench for sagittal and oscillating saws.

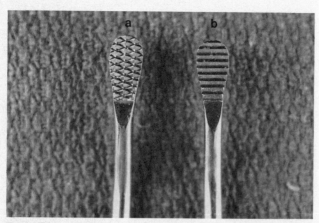

Figure 7.28. Comparison of (a) cross-cut and (b) parallel-cut rasping surfaces.

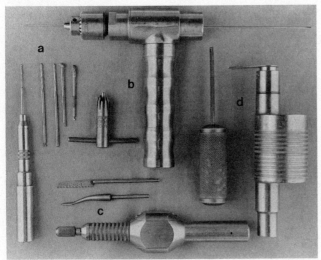

Figure 7.31. Stryker penumatic power instrumentation. (a) Rotary drill and burrs, (b) large drill and wire driver with chuck key, (c) reciprocating saw and rasp, (d) oscillating saw with Allen wrench.

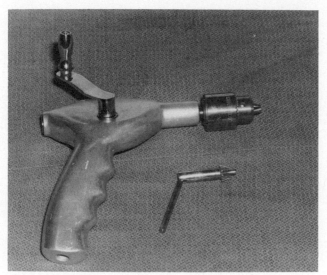

Figure 7.32. Hand drill/wire driver and chuck key.

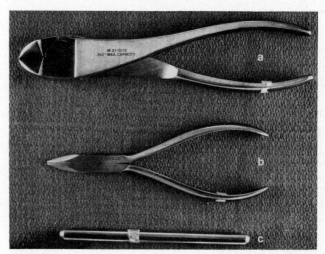

Figure 7.33. (a) Side-cutting wire cutter, (b) needle-nose pliers, (c) tubular wire bender.

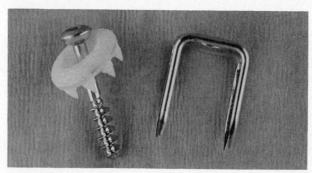

Figure 7.34. (a) Polyacetyl spiked washer with ASIF compression screw and (b) Blount staple.

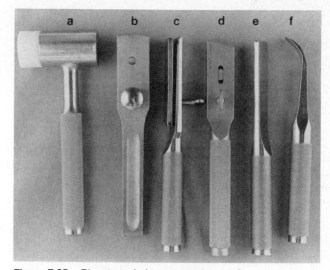

Figure 7.35. Blount staple instrumentation. (a) Surgical mallet, (b, c, d) assorted staple holders, (e) driver, (f) staple puller.

specialized wire holder is available. A hand-held wire bender, a wire cutter, and a pair of needle-nose pliers are also necessary (Fig. 7.33).

Steinmann pins $5/64$ inch in diameter and larger are used in much the same way as Kirschner wires, when larger bones are involved.

Small and large fragment sets with a complete assortment of cortical and cancellous screws, plates, and associated specialized instrumentation (2, 3, 4) are also available.

Assorted Blount and Stone staples (Fig. 7.34) are used for fixation of bony fragments. Polyacetyl spiked washers combined with a compression screw (Fig. 7.34) can be used to anchor tendon to bone, or a single Stone staple may be applicable. Instrumentation for use with the Blount staples can be seen in Figure 7.35.

Miscellaneous fixation devices may be useful in a limited number of specific situations. These include the osteoclasp, Bilos pins, external fixatures, and other devices depending on the surgeon's preference.

SUCTION APPARATUS

A continuous suction source should be available on most podiatric surgical cases. The amount of suc-

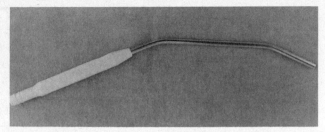

Figure 7.36. Malleable Frazier tip suction catheter.

tion should be variable and controlled by the assistant operating the suction catheter. The malleable Frazier-tip suction catheter (Fig. 7.36) is ideal for use in podiatric surgery.

CONCLUSION

It can be seen that a wide variety of surgical needs mandates the availability of a large array of instrumentation (5). Not every instrument is needed on every case, and for this reason the basic instruments are divided into a forefoot pack and a rearfoot pack. The forefoot pack supplies instrumentation for a typical bilateral forefoot case. For rearfoot surgery, the rearfoot pack is opened along with the forefoot pack. Division of instrumentation into reduced sets also allows more efficient sterilization and storage. Instruments that may be needed at any time, regardless of surgical site, are packed separately. Basic instrument packs for specific surgical application include the following.

I. Forefoot Pack
  A. Blade handles
    1. #3 scalpel handle (6)
    2. Long and short Beaver handles (one each)
  B. Scissors
    1. Iris, small (1)
    2. Crown and collar (1)
    3. Curved and straight Mayo (1 each)
    4. Metzenbaum (2)
    5. Large utility (2)
    6. Lister bandage (1)
    7. Monofilament wire cutter (1)
  C. Hemostatic forceps
    1. Curved and straight mosquito (12 and 4, respectively)
    2. Curved and straight Crile (2 each)
    3. Curved and straight Kelly (2 each)
  D. Thumb forceps
    1. Brown-Adson (4)
    2. Rat tooth (one-two pickup) (2)
    3. Atraumatic (2)
    4. Large toothed (2)
    5. Large atraumatic (2)
  E. Traction forceps
    1. Backhaus towel clamp (6)
    2. Allis clamp, large and small (2 each)
    3. Kocher (2)
    4. Sesamoid clamp (1)
    5. Phalangeal forceps (1)
    6. Sponge clamp (1)
  F. Retractors
    1. Digital self-retaining (1)
    2. Weitlaner 3-2 and 4-3 (2 and 1, respectively)

    3. Skin hooks, single and double prong (2 and 4, respectively)
    4. Ragnell (4)
    5. Senn (4)
    6. Seeburger (2)
    7. Mini-Hohmann (4)
    8. Rakes (4-prong, sharp) (2)
    9. Army-Navy (2)
    10. Malleable ribbon (2)
  G. Periosteal elevators
    1. Freer (4)
    2. Langenbeck, narrow and broad (1 each)
    3. Sayre (1)
  H. Osteotomes, Chisels, Mallets
    1. Lambotte osteotomes (2 mm to 22 mm) (1 each)
    2. Curved osteotome (8 mm) (1)
    3. US Army #18 chisel (1)
    4. Medium sized surgical mallet (1)
  I. Bone Cutting Forceps, Rongeurs
    1. Double-action bone cutting forceps (1)
    2. Large and small curved double-action rongeurs (1 each)
    3. Needle-nose rongeur (1)
  J. Bone holding clamps
    1. Lewin (1)
  K. Rasps and wire brush
    1. Bell rasp (2)
    2. Joseph's nasal (beaver tail) (2)
    3. Maltz and Parkes (1 each)
    4. Wire brush (1)
  L. Needle holders
    1. Assorted sizes and jaw configurations depending on surgeon's preference
  M. Miscellaneous
    1. Ruler (stainless steel)
    2. Wire cutter (1)
    3. Wire bender (1)
    4. Needle-nose pliers (2)
II. Rearfoot Pack
  A. Retractors
    1. Large ribbon (2)
    2. Large rakes (2)
    3. Lamina spreader (1)
  B. Periosteal elevators
    1. Key (one set)
    2. Crego (one set)
  C. Osteotomes, gouges, mallets
    1. Large osteotomes (one set)
    2. Gouges (one set)
    3. Large surgical mallet (1)
  D. Bone cutting forceps and rongeurs
    1. Large double-action bone cutting forceps (1)
    2. Large double-action rongeur (1)
    3. Kerrison rongeur (2)
  E. Curettes and trephines
    1. Bone curettes (one set)
    2. Trephines (one set)
  F. Miscellaneous
    1. Blount staple holder, driver, puller (one set)
    2. Large pin cutter (1)
III. Minor Surgical Pack
  A. Blade handles
    1. #3 scalpel handle (2)
  B. Scissors
    1. Iris (1)
    2. Crown and collar (1)
    3. Curved and straight Mayo (1 each)
    4. Metzenbaum (1)
    5. Utility scissors (1)

C. Hemostatic forceps
  1. Curved and straight mosquito (4 and 2, respectively)
  2. Curved and straight Crile (1 each)
  3. Curved and straight Kelly (1 each)
D. Thumb forceps
  1. Brown-Adson (1)
  2. Rat tooth (one-two) (1)
  3. Atraumatic (1)
E. Traction forceps
  1. Bachaus towel clamps (2)
  2. Allis clamp (2)
F. Retractors
  1. Digital self-retaining (1)
  2. Weitlaner 3-2 (1)
  3. Skin hooks, double prong (2)
  4. Senn (2)
  5. Seeburger (2)
G. Periosteal elevators
  1. Freer (2)
H. Rasps
  1. Bell (1)
  2. Joseph's nasal (1)
I. Needle holders
  1. Large and small (1 each)
J. Miscellaneous
  1. Large bone curette (1)
  2. Straight nail nipper (1)
  3. Curved tissue nipper (1)
  4. Glass medicine cup (1)
  5. Stainless steel bowl (3 inch diameter) (1)
  6. Bandages
    (a) 4 × 4 inch gauze (10)
    (b) 2 and 3 inch Kling (1 each)
IV. Nail Surgical Pack
A. Blade handles
  1. #3 scalpel blade (1)
  2. Beaver blade handle (1)
B. Scissors and nippers
  1. Iris (1)
  2. Utility (1)
  3. Large and small nail nippers (1)
  4. English anvil nail nipper (1)
C. Hemostatic forceps
  1. Straight mosquito (2)
  2. Straight Kelly (1)
D. Thumb forceps
  1. Brown-Adson (1)
E. Elevators and Curettes
  1. Freer (2)

  2. Nail plate elevator, large and small (1 each)
  3. Medium sized dermal and bone curette (1 each)
F. Needle holder
  1. Small (Mayo-Hegar jaw) (1)
G. Miscellaneous
  1. Glass medicine cup (1)
  2. Cotton tip applicators (10)
  3. Bandages
    (a) 2 × 2 inch and 4 × 4 inch gauze (10 and 6, respectively)
    (b) 2 inch Kling (1)
V. Ulcer Debridement Pack
A. Blade handles
  1. #3 scalpel handle (2)
B. Scissors and nippers
  1. Iris (1)
  2. Utility (1)
  3. Nail nipper (1)
  4. Tissue nipper (1)
C. Hemostatic forceps
  1. Curved and straight mosquito (1 each)
D. Thumb forceps
  1. Brown-Adson (1)
  2. Atraumatic (1)
E. Elevators and curettes
  1. Freer (1)
  2. Medium sized dermal and bone curette (1 each)
F. Miscellaneous
  1. Bandages
    (a) 4 × 4 inch gauze (10)
    (b) 2 inch Kling (1)
VI. Podiatry Dressing Pack
  1. 4 × 4 inch gauze (10)
  2. Kling
    (a) two inch (1)
    (b) three inch (1)
  3. Tube gauze (2 ⅝ inches × 36 inches) (2)

References

1. Edmonson AS, Crenshaw AH (eds): *Campbell's Operative Orthopedics*, ed 6. St. Louis, The CV Mosby Co, 1980, pp 1–20.
2. Heim U, Pfeiffer KM: *Small Fragment Set Manual*. Berlin, Springer-Verlag, 1974.
3. Muller ME, Algower M, Schneider R, Willeneggar H: *Manual of Internal Fixation*, ed 2. Berlin, Springer-Verlag, 1979.
4. Sequin F, Texhammar R: *AO/ASIF Instrumentation Manual of Use and Care*. Berlin, Springer-Verlag, 1981.
5. Nealon TF: *Fundamental Skills in Surgery*, ed 3. Philadelphia, WB Saunders Co, 1979, pp 12–24.

CHAPTER 8

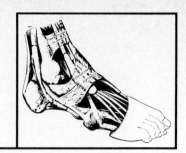

Principles of Rigid Internal Compression Fixation and its Application in Podiatric Surgery

John A. Ruch, D.P.M. and Thomas Merrill, D.P.M.

The surgical management of fractures and techniques of internal fixation have been employed since the mid-1800s. Lister (1860) originated aseptic surgical technique and used silver wire suture for the fixation of fractures (1). Gurlt (1862) advocated the use of open reduction as an initial form of treatment in acute injury instead of waiting until conservative methods had failed (1). Ollier (1870) introduced plaster cast immobilization treatment in the management of fractures (1). Hansmann (1886) first used nickel-plated screws and plates for fixation of fractures (1). Roentgen (1895) discovered x-rays, and fracture reductions that previously appeared to be clinically satisfactory were seen to be unacceptable (1).

Advances in surgical technique, instrumentation, and asepsis stimulated research into the operative management of fractures. Lambotte (1907) realized the importance of reduction of intraarticular fractures and early postoperative joint motion (1). He was also one of the first to use a compression device. Smith-Peterson (1931) designed an improved fixation nail and Kuntscher (1940) introduced the intramedullary nailing technique (1). Danis (2) was an advocate of internal fixation and postulated the theory of primary bone healing.

Unfortunately many of these early surgical attempts were associated with a high failure rate and often devastating results of nonunion, infection, and loss of limb. In 1958, fifteen Swiss surgeons including Muller and associates joined together to form the AO — Arbeitgemeinschaft fur Osteosynthesisfragen; English translation — Association for the Study of Internal Fixation (ASIF) — study group. The AO group realized the necessity to identify the causes of failure associated with internal fixation and to develop an approach to prevent these complications. Failure of operative management of fractures was initially attributed to a physiological component of inadequate bone healing or failure of the internal fixation device. The Swiss group directed their efforts initially to determine how bone healed under various conditions of internal fixation and through these studies began to appreciate the influences of fixation on the physiological process of bone healing. Their studies further revealed the need for the development and standardization of instrumentation and techniques used in the operative management of fractures.

Out of their efforts the Swiss developed a basic objective of early return to function of the injured limb. This goal was achieved by the application of the four following biomechanical principles outlined in the *Manual of Internal Fixation* by ME Muller and associates (4).

Atraumatic Operative Technique

The first principle, atraumatic operative technique, relates to the preservation of the viability of bone and soft tissues. The techniques of surgical dissection become paramount in preserving the vascular supply needed to heal bone and soft tissue. The techniques of anatomical dissection are no more appropriately applied than in trauma surgery and the sophisticated techniques of reconstruction of deformities of the foot and ankle.

Accurate Anatomical Reduction

Accurate anatomical reduction contributes not only to the gross alignment and apposition of the fracture, but also to the mechanical soundness of the fixation process. This concept is of particular importance when dealing with intra-articular fractures.

Rigid Internal Compression Fixation

The third principle encompasses the mechanical science of the principles and techniques of rigid compression fixation. These mechanical functions are the basis for the successful operative management of fractures and osteotomies.

Avoidance of Soft Tissue Damage

The fourth of the basic principles brings together all of the four principles to accomplish the primary goal of early return to function of the injured limb. Avoidance of soft tissue damage is described as the prevention of fracture or cast disease. Early range of motion of the injured part is made possible by the stable fixation of the fracture. Healing of the viable injured tissues can continue even during rehabilitation because the fracture or osteotomy is held securely by the internal fixation device. This early rehabilitation decreases the atrophy and loss of motion in the injured limb and promotes an early return to normal function.

EARLY OBJECTIVES OF THE SWISS STUDIES

The early objective of the Swiss studies was to determine how bone heals under various conditions of internal fixation. Their basic research evolved into a complex and sophisticated study of bone healing and the variety of factors that influenced it. From their investigations came six fundamental areas of research that are the foundation for the AO philosophy (5): (a) biocompatibility of implant materials; (b) mechanical and physiological requirements for primary bone healing; (c) histology of primary bone healing; (d) scientific experimentation and definition of the bioengineering principles of primary bone healing; (e) standardization of instrumentation and implants; and (f) documentation and analysis of clinical experience.

Biocompatibility of Implant Materials

One of the earliest recognized causes for failure of internal fixation was the rejection of the implant device by the human body and the deterioration of many of the implant materials when subjected to human body tissues and fluids. Early materials included gold, silver, lead, platinum and iron (6). Although foreign body reaction and corrosion were seen in varying degrees with all of these materials, their physical properties were also a source of failure when used as internal fixation devices. Biocompatibility was therefore dependent on both a biologic and physical relationship between bone and the fixation device.

As the science of metallurgy matured, success came with the sophistication of iron based alloys with the ultimate development of a surgical grade of stainless steel. This austenitic material was found to be extremely inert when implanted into body tissues (5). A cellularly motivated foreign body response is essentially nonexistent with the exception of the individual demonstrating a true allergy to nickel based substances. Chemical corrosion of the implant surface is inhibited by the formation of a protective passification layer that spontaneously develops over the surface of the implant in the presence of oxygen (4).

The physical properties of the surgical grade stainless steel have been found to be most compatible with the physical requirements of fixation of the osseous skeleton (5). Keeping in mind that the effect of the implant is only temporary, the degrees of hardness, strength, ductility, malleability, and memory exhibited by stainless steel have been found to be quite compatible with the physical requirements of a fixation device used to stabilize osseous tissues during a prescribed period of healing.

The Swiss developed AISI 316L type surgical stainless steel is a chromium nickel molybdenum steel alloy (5).

Even though the implant material is relatively corrosion resistant, significant erosion can occur with chronic in situ abrasion of the implant surfaces. Movement between a loose screw and fixation plate will create chronic breakdown of the passification layer and promote a chemical erosion of the implant material by the body fluids (5).

An internal fixation device is again only intended to stabilize a fracture for a short period of time while the bone healing process continues to a point where the bone itself is able to withstand load forces. Should the fracture fixation be subjected to excessive forces or bone healing be delayed, metal fatigue may precipitate failure of the fixation with fracture of the implant. Absorption of bone at the implant-bone interface may also produce loosening of the implant and loss of stable fracture fixation.

Whereas research continues for the ideal fixation material, surgical stainless steel remains the standard for internal fixation devices.

Mechanical and Physiological Requirements for Primary Bone Healing

Schenk and Willeneger (7) pursued the original postulation of Danis (2) of primary bone healing. They defined the two basic requirements for consistent healing of bone without callus formation. This primary intention healing of bone occurred when viable fracture fragments were apposed and rigidly fixated. The significance of an intact vascular supply and rigid fixation of the fracture fragments became the guiding model for further research and clinical management of fractures.

Histology of Primary Bone Healing

The cellular process of secondary or callus bone healing has been thoroughly researched and described. The previously unidentified process of primary bone healing however, was yet to be described on a cellular level. Schenk and Willenegger (8) performed exhaustive studies to demonstrate clearly and to define the cellular processes of primary intention healing of bone.

Scientific Experimentation and Definition of the Bioengineering Principles of Primary Bone Healing

Just as the cellular processes required study and description, the mechanical aspects of accomplishing rigid fixation needed extensive study and definition. The engineering of fracture fixation was a key and integral part of the overall AO concept. Perren et al performed extensive research evaluating the effectiveness of various designs of fixation devices and techniques of fixation (9). The basic concepts of rigid internal compression fixation evolved from a mechanical understanding of what was actually required to perform and maintain stable, rigid fixation.

Standardization of Instrumentation and Implants

As the mechanical requirements of rigid compression fixation became more clearly defined, it became apparent that specific instrumentation and implant devices were required to accomplish consistent techniques of internal fixation (5). The standard AO instrument and implant set was initially designed and followed by the small fragment set and other specialized instruments and implants.

Documentation and Analysis of Clinical Application

With the sound development of basic science, mechanical engineering, and clinical application, the AO research was just beginning. The credibility of the concept was dependent on close evaluation of the clinical application and experience. The AO surgeons formed an extensive network for documentation of the AO experience (4). Results and observations continue to guide the on-going research and development of the AO concepts, philosophy, and technique.

Through a dedicated and sophisticated process, the Swiss developed a unique concept in the management of fracture. They took the process of bone healing as it was classically understood and manipulated the physical environment of healing fracture. Study of the cellular and mechanical processes required consistently to produce primary intention bone healing led to a new appreciation of the management of fractures. The principles and techniques developed by the AO group are now the basis for rigid internal compression fixation. If these principles and techniques are fully understood and mastered by the individual surgeon, his or her experience with fracture, osteotomy, and arthrodesis will be more controlled, predictable, and rewarding.

PROCESS OF BONE HEALING

The process of bone healing has been observed and investigated by physicians for centuries. Nature has uniquely combined fracture immobilization and the cellular processes of repair successfully to mend broken bones since the evolution of the osseous skeleton. Although the process may be dependable, the end functional result often left the victim with disability and impaired function of the injured part. Historically the efforts of the physician have been to assist the healing process and accomplish a more functional result.

Immobilization is the key to understanding the healing process of bone. The body naturally attempts to prevent motion of fractured segments by the physiological processes of pain, edema, and muscle splinting. The resultant disuse of the part significantly decreases the motion between the fracture fragments and allows for further immobilization through an intrinsic cellular process. This intrinsic process has classically been known and described as callus formation. Callus serves to unite the bone ends and provides a mechanism ultimately to eliminate motion between the fracture fragments. Indeed, Charnley (10) even described callus as nature's own internal fixation device. Once motion has been arrested, the callus itself serves as a scaffold for bony remodeling and the restoration of normal bone architecture and function (Fig. 8.1).

The classic descriptions of callus formation relate to cortical fractures in long bones (11). This type of callus formation exhibits an extraosseous component that is radiographically detectable and easily monitored to evaluate the progress of bone healing. This expanding type of callus formation is related to the periosteal activity and mechanical forces associated with fracture and the instability of diaphyseal bone (12).

Endosteal callus, however, plays a significant role in fracture healing even though it is difficult radiographically to appreciate. The healing of cancellous bone in metaphyseal regions and in short bones similarly fails to exhibit the classic exuberant external callus in the bone healing process (10). The lack of visible callus formation in these bony areas is related to their internal relationship. There is intimate bone contact because of the impaction of the softer and more numerous contact points of trabecular bone (13). Any endosteal callus that would form then serves only

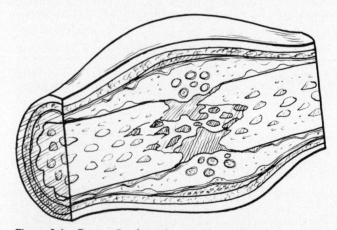

Figure 8.1. Bone callus formation provides stabilization of mobile bone edges and serves as framework for bone remodeling.

to fill in the gaps and further to obscure the void or defect between bone surfaces.

The basic process of callus formation that occurs in diaphyseal bone begins with the hemorrhage created by osseous and periosteal vessels that are torn with the bone fracture (14). Hematoma invades and fills the space between fracture fragments and torn soft tissues. As the hematoma organizes it is invaded by a multitude of cells with varying form and function. Macrophages from the vascular compartment invade the area to remove necrotic blood and tissue debris (15). This inflammatory phase is similar to that seen in skin and other soft tissues.

Within several days fibroblasts from the surrounding periosteal and mesenchymal tissues invade the organized clot and begin the deposition of collagen fibrils and fibrocartilage (16). These substances serve to stiffen the organized clot, making it a more effective tissue for limiting motion between the ends of the fracture fragments.

Necrosis at the surface of the fracture fragments is described as a result of the retraction of the interrupted vascular network and of the relatively low oxygen tension of the interposing hematoma (15). This same low oxygen tension of the organized hematoma dictates the production of fibrocartilage as the basic ground substance in the initial phases of callus formation. Resorption of necrotic bone occurs as the haversian system begins the process of remodeling with removal of nonviable osseous tissue (Fig. 8.2).

At the same time vascularization of the maturing hematoma or procallus is occurring from three specific areas (4, 17, 18). Capillary infiltration migrates from the external periosteal vessels and internally from those of the endosteal tissues. The third avenue of vascular migration comes from the haversian system of the cortical bone itself. This intercortical blood supply accompanies the haversian structure with its leading osteoclastic cells and trailing deposition of osteoblastic cells.

As the oxygen tension of the procallus increases the product of the osteoprogenitor cells becomes that of osteoid (15, 19). This phase of bone healing becomes radiographically visible because the primary makeup of the deposited osteoid is that of the relatively radiopaque calcium hydroxyapatite. The physical properties of the osteoid render the tissue more rigid and the effective stiffening of the callus increases (10). The ultimate elimination of motion between the fracture fragments or clinical bone union is accomplished by this intermediary osseous tissue. The size or extent of callus formation is dependent on the mechanical requirements of the fracture segment (20). The size of the callus or the extent of callus formation is a reflection of the mechanical function of nature's internal fixation device. Relative instability of the apposed fracture fragments creates greater mechanical requirements of the fixation medium (i.e. the more motion across the fracture, the larger the callus needed to stop that motion).

Conversely, with less motion across a fracture the size of callus needed to block that motion will be smaller. Theoretically, if there were no motion across the fracture site there would be no callus formation (Fig. 8.3).

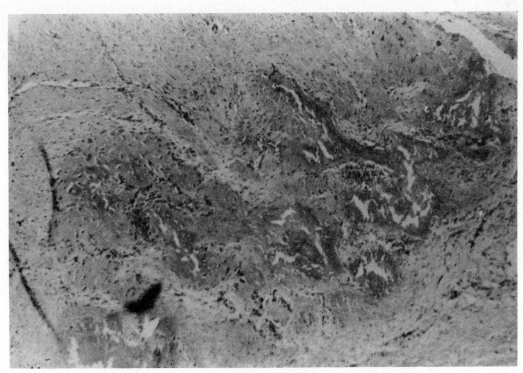

Figure 8.2.   Fibrocytes can be seen in this photomicrograph of callus fibrocartilage.

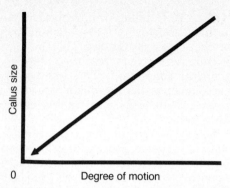

Figure 8.3. Graph shows relationship between motion and callus formation. Decreasing motion decreases stimulus for callus formation.

The mature callus creates clinical union of the bone fragments. It is a temporary tissue and is gradually replaced with the normal architecture of the primary osseous structure. The woven bone of the fixation callus is remodeled as the haversian network invades and resorbs this intermediary tissue replacing it with the mature lamellar osseous structure (10, 21).

PRIMARY BONE HEALING

Danis (2) was the first to consider the possibility of primary bone healing. His pioneering work with internal fixation was directed to accomplishing a stable internal fixation that would essentially be secure long enough for the bone to heal. Obviously, many of the earlier failures of internal fixation were considered to be a direct result of weakening or breakdown of the internal fixation device. His observations of a lack of external callus formation and complete bone union in circumstances of successful internal fixation led to the postulation of a new type of bone healing process, primary bone healing.

Beginning with the formation of the AO study group in 1958, an intense investigation was initiated to understand primary bone healing, its physical and biological requirements, and its significance in the management of skeletal injury (5). Schenk and Willenegger (7) documented the process of primary bone healing and the mechanical and biological factors that were necessary for consistent reproduction of this healing process.

The two basic requirements for primary bone healing are an intact vascular supply to the bone and stable rigid fixation of the fracture fragments (4). The significance of the combination of these two fundamental concepts has had a tremendous impact on all those who deal with the osseous skeleton. The changes in philosophy and technique spawned by the Swiss research have been met with both acceptance and rejection. The process of understanding begins with a sound knowledge of the biological and mechanical principles proposed by the AO research. With these tools in hand the surgeon can more aptly integrate these principles and technqiues to clinical practice

and both the physician and patient will benefit from the application of science to the art of surgical fixation.

The process of primary bone healing begins with the surgical manipulation of the fracture. All efforts are made to preserve the vascular supply to the segments as the fracture fragments are reduced into close apposition and anatomical alignment. The application of fixation is based on mechanical engineering principles and effects a rigid and stable reduction of the fracture that is able to withstand external forces within certain stress limitations. As the Swiss pursued this process in experimentation and research, they were able to accomplish the healing of a fracture without the formation of an external callus (5). Close histological evaluation revealed a significantly different cellular process in the repair of the rigidly fixated fracture. The process of primary bone healing was identified and even referred to as a side effect of the stable rigid fixation.

Primary bone healing has been extensively studied and basically consists of simultaneous remodeling and formation of new bone at the fracture site (22, 23). The intermediary phase of fibrocartilage formation, as seen in callus bone healing, is actually bypassed as new bone is formed intentionally at the fracture margins. Primary bone healing or contact healing is the direct reconstruction of the fragment edges by haversian remodeling (23). This is the same homeostatic mechanism that occurs in the living intact osseous skeleton on a daily basis. This process is carried on at an intensified level stimulated by the intrinsic environment of the fracture (4, 17).

Even with an anatomically reduced fracture, there are microscopic gaps between macroscopic areas of contact along the fracture surfaces. Primary bone healing demonstrates two patterns of repair in the regions of contact and the areas of gap (23). The hematoma that immediately fills the microscopic gaps is rapidly penetrated with capillaries and osteoblastic cells. The area is then rapidly filled with woven bone because the formation of connective tissue and fibrocartilage is completely absent. These regions of irregular woven bone will ultimately be reoriented as the haversian remodeling process continues.

Cutting Cone

Healing at points of contact along the fracture surface begins with the advance of a capillary bud from the haversian canal. The advancing column is formed of an intricately arranged and specifically functioning group of cells. This organized structure advances in a linear direction and crosses the fracture line depositing lamellar new bone along its path (23). The tip of the complex is a group of large multinucleated cells that function as osteoclasts. They cut their way through existing osteoid and cross the fracture line into the surface of the opposite fracture fragment. The term "cutting cone" has been applied to this highly specialized cellular organ (Fig. 8.4 A–C).

Osteon

The osteoblasts are followed closely by a capillary loop as the cutting cone creates a tunnel in the existing bone substrate. The wall of this tunnel is lined by cells with osteoblastic activity. These cells produce a concentric pattern of new lamellar bone as the cutting cone passes and and this is loosely deposited along the course of the haversian canal to exist as mature osteocytes within the lacunae of mature lamellar bone (23). The mature organization of concentric layers of lamellar bone and osteocytes is described as the osteon. The direction of motion of the cutting cone is usually in the longitudinal orientation of the bone; however, individual segments have been demonstrated actually to divert into the perpendicular orientation of a fracture gap as they deposit lamellar bone within the confines of the separated fracture surfaces. This function is limited to gaps of microscopic dimensions in the region of 0.2 to 0.4 mm (23). Ultimately the entire fracture line is welded with new lamellar bone as multiple haversian systems cross between the fracture fragments.

Schenk (23) has demonstrated the process of haversian remodeling with tetracycline labeling techniques (24). The cutting cone has been demonstrated to advance by 70 to 100 μm per day with regeneration of approximately 60% of the preexisting osteons in the osseous segment within an eight-week period of time.

Irritation Callus

The importance of rigid stability between fracture fragments in this delicate microscopic environment of capillaries and bone forming cells is readily appreciated. Instability and motion at the fracture surface would readily disrupt the migration of the cutting cone and the haversian structure resulting in additional hemorrhage (21, 23, 25). This continued disruption of the healing process would favor a process of fibrocar-

tilage formation and the ultimate formation of callus or secondary bone healing. Continued motion or irritation of a healing fracture produces a healing process that could be described as irritation callus (4).

By appreciating the basic process of primary bone healing seen with rigid fixation, it is easy to understand that when external callus is identified in fractures that have been fixated in any given fashion, motion or irritation of the fracture exists (26). Failure to maintain a rigid relationship between fracture fragments, for whatever reason, will lead to a disruption of the primary bone healing process and produce secondary bone healing or the formation of an irritation callus (Fig. 8.5). The mechanical process of rigid fixation now becomes the next science to understand and apply to the healing process of bone.

MECHANICAL BASIS OF RIGID INTERNAL FIXATION

Rigid fixation of bone can be observed from a purely mechanical point of view. The science of structural relationships and mechanical forces are of ultimate importance in the execution of rigid and stable fixation of the osseous skeleton.

The accomplishment of mechanical stability is dependent on both intrinsic and extrinsic factors. Once these factors are understood and appreciated, a

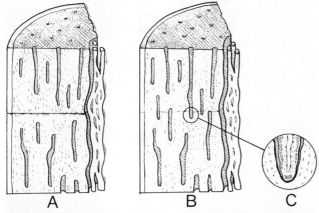

Figure 8.4. (A, B) Primary bone healing is seen at fragment margins as haversian canal remodeling is taking place without the intermediate callus formation. (C) Microscopic cellular organ, the cutting cone. Osteoclasts lead capillary loop lined with osteoblasts. Cutting cone can cross fracture line in proper microscopic environment.

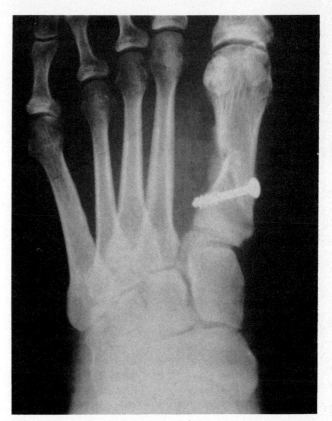

Figure 8.5. Irritation callus is radiographic sign of unstable fracture or osteotomy. Result of this interfragmentary movement is secondary bone healing.

sound mechanical system can be designed to create and maintain a secure fracture fixation.

Intrinsic Factors of Stable Fracture Reduction

The intrinsic factors of stable fracture reduction include the physical qualities and relationships of the fracture fragments. These basic factors are almost casually referred to in the Swiss literature, but are nonetheless of vital importance in the overall success in the operative management of fracture. These factors have been described as basic principles in the conservative management of fractures. Charnley (10) describes a classification of fractures based on the intrinsic stability of the reduced fracture to withstand telescoping forces that would serve to shorten the segment and render the fracture unstable. The fracture classification is based upon the orientation of the fracture line and is broken down into the unstable, stable, and potentially stable fracture (Fig. 8.6) (10).

Unstable Fracture

The unstable fracture is either a long oblique or spiral fracture or a comminuted fracture (10). These fractures are unable to withstand telescoping or load-bearing forces because of the mechanical instability created by the planes of the fracture. The long oblique or spiral fracture will easily shift and shorten on itself (Fig. 8.7). The comminuted fracture has no intrinsic stability because the fracture fragments readily displace with any loading force. The long oblique or spiral fracture demonstrates a fracture length that is greater than twice the diameter of the bone. This is because of the orientation of the fracture line. The plane of the fracture is angulated more than 45° from the transverse axis of the bone. This relationship has its obvious significance in the lack of intrinsic stability of the fracture and is also very significant in the selection of the most effective type of internal fixation of the fracture.

Stable Fracture

The stable fracture category includes transverse fractures (10). This fracture configuration readily resists telescoping of the fragments as long as forces

that would create angular deformity are controlled. These relationships will have their impact on the selection of the technique of internal fixation as well.

Potentially Stable Fracture

The potentially stable fracture is a short oblique fracture with the orientation plane of the fracture less than 45 100° from the transverse axis of the bone. The mechanical significance of this relationship allows the fracture to be stable with the application of a tension band type of fixation. The application of this principle will have a significant bearing on the choice of an effective fixation device for the short oblique fracture (Fig. 8.8).

The quality of the bone and fracture fragments is also of importance in the intrinsic stability of any fracture. Factors of density will have a significant bearing on the selection of the type of fixation device that can securely maintain the reduction of the fracture and not loosen or strip out of the bone when loading forces are applied. Dense cortical bone is obviously the most amenable to internal fixation; however, the surgeon must be able to deal with softer cancellous and even osteoporotic bone by modifying the technique and even the fixation device to accomplish a secure fixation.

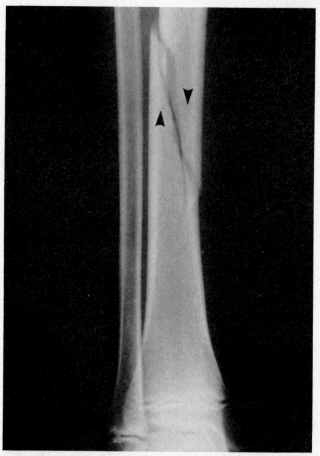

Figure 8.7. Long oblique fracture is unstable and fragments will telescope on each other as arrows show direction of movement of tibial fracture.

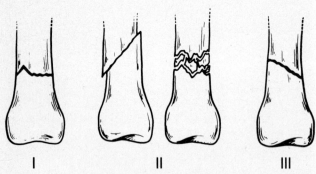

I   II   III

Figure 8.6. Charnley's classification of fractures is based on intrinsic stability of fracture to withstand forces that tend to telescope the fragments. (I) Stable. (II) Unstable. (III) Potentially stable.

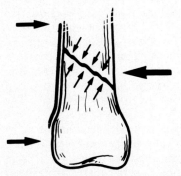

Figure 8.8. Potentially stable fracture pattern allows tension band type fixation to be very applicable. Arrows show three-point pressure technique with intact soft tissue hinge and compression that is produced.

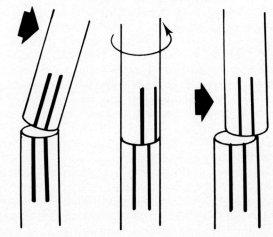

Figure 8.9. Three mechanical forces tend to disrupt stable fixation: bending, torsion, and shear. Each force must be controlled.

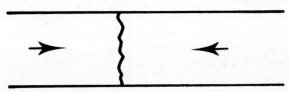

Figure 8.10. Compression between two fragments can be used to control all three disruptive mechanical forces.

Extrinsic Factors of Stable Fracture Reduction

The next concept to appreciate is a basic understanding of the mechanical forces that can act to disrupt the fixation device, apposition, alignment, and stability of any fracture fixation. These disruptive mechanical forces are bending, shear, and torsion (5).

Bending, Shear, and Torsion

A basic understanding of these simple mechanical relationships is essential in the formulation and implementation of an effective fixation (Fig. 8.9). The surgeon needs to understand the forces that must be counteracted when designing and applying the surgical implant or internal fixation device to any given fracture.

Control of these forces is based on the two mechanical principles of interfragmental compression and splinting (4). Interfragmental compression, when applicable, is superior to splintage.

Properties of Interfragmental Compression. The application of a compressive force between two fracture fragments increases the stability of the fracture fixation by increasing the friction between the two fragments (Fig. 8.10) (5). This increased friction at the surface of the fracture resists the motions of shearing and torsion. Bending forces are countered by the resistance to separation of the surfaces of the fracture fragments.

The force of compression has previously been credited with having some stimulating influence on the bone healing process. This concept was extrapolated from Wolff's law where increased stress on the osseous skeleton led to an intensification of haversian remodeling with the balance shifted in the favor of osteoblastic activity and the result of thicker cortices and trabecullar bone (24). Additional research correlates piezo electrical potentials and an unidentified bone morphogenic protein with enhanced repairing powers (27, 28). The Swiss research does not refute these influences, but demonstrates the effect that compression does have on the healing fracture.

Muller and associates (4) state that "compression does not exert any mystical osteogenic effect on bone." It is through the enhancement of rigid fixation and the elimination of motion between fracture fragments that compression has its influence on the healing process of bone. Mears (6) states that "compression does not itself enhance the rate of healing or remodeling of bone." It is through the contact of apposing surfaces of fracture fragments and the elimination of movement between those fragments that the bone healing process is altered. The cellular process of healing is transformed into the phenomenon described as primary bone healing. The rate of healing, although not accelerated, is not delayed by the irritation and breakdown of the intermediary granulation process as seen with an unstable fracture reduction. Compression is an integral component of the mechanical process of rigid fixation.

MECHANICAL BASIS OF STABLE FIXATION

Types of Interfragmental Compression

Static

Interfragmental compression can be applied in either a static or dynamic state for the fixation of osseous skeleton (5). Static interfragmental compression is a constant and uniform force. It is accomplished by placing the fixation device under tension and transmitting this force across the two fracture fragments with the result of compression at the contact surface of the two fragments. Static interfragmental compression of the osseous skeleton is usually accomplished by the insertion of a screw in a lag technique, or the application of an external fixator or a preloaded plate. Under favorable conditions of bone healing this static compressive force will gradually decrease by approximately 50% over a two-month period of time (4). This gradual loss of compression is caused by the remodeling of the haversian system rather than bone resorption or loosening of the implant.

Dynamic

Dynamic interfragmental compression is the combination of a statically loaded fixation device to a functionally loaded fracture configuration. The degree of compression is therefore dependent on the amount of functional loading applied to the part. This technique will be described as the tension band concept.

Splintage

Splintage or splinting is a basic concept of protection (5). It is a principle and technique that is applied when interfragmental compression is not possible and is used in combination with interfragmental compression when it alone is not adequate to provide a stable fixation. There are a multitude of applications of this basic concept that will be delineated under the section on technique.

Combinations

The combination of techniques of interfragmental compression and splintage is a common modification in the application of rigid internal compression fixation (5). Often, because of the configuration of the fracture, the single lag screw may not be adequate for providing stable rigid fixation. In many cases the fixation of the lag screw is reenforced or protected by the application of a plate. The plate may serve a basic function of neutralizing deforming forces or in specific circumstances may also adopt a load-bearing function, as in a buttress application. The combination of interfragmental compression and splintage may take a variety of forms, all intended to optimize the degree of stable rigid fixation.

TECHNIQUES OF STABLE FIXATION

Static interfragmental compression involves the use of a lag screw, an external fixator, and a preloaded plate. Dynamic interfragmental compression uses tension band techniques. Load-bearing splintage uses a buttress plate and an external fixator (distraction). Non-load-bearing splintage uses an intramedullar nail and Kirschner wires for apposition. Combinations include a neutralization plate with lag screw, buttress plate with lag screw, and Kirschner wire with tension band wire.

LAG SCREW

Screws are the most commonly used AO internal fixation devices in surgery of the foot and ankle (29). Their size and function readily lend them to the

creation of secure rigid compression fixation of the small bones of this region of the human anatomy (30). A screw can be placed through two apposed fragments of bone in such a manner as to create a significant degree of compression between the two fragments. The concept of the lag screw is a technique rather than a specific type or screw or device. The AO system uses primarily two types of screws, a cortical or fully threaded screw and a cancellous or spongiosa screw with threads only on the distal portion of the screw shaft (5). Both screws can be used to create interfragmental compression between two fracture fragments if they are applied with the proper techniques. However, both may be ineffective at producing the desired compression if the technique of insertion is not appropriate for the given clinical circumstance in which they are applied.

Technical Principles of the Lag Effect

A cortical screw can function as a lag screw only if the hole in the first or near cortex is overdrilled to prevent purchase of the screw threads in the proximal segment of bone (4). The cortical screw is fully threaded and prevents any sliding of the bone fragment along the axis of the screw without rotation of the screw. Two fragments of bone suspended on the threads of a screw would move in the same direction at the same time when the screw is rotated (Fig. 8.11). No relative movement between the two fragments would occur and no compression can be created.

By overdrilling the hole in the near cortex, the screw will glide through the hole without contact of the screw threads with the bone. The threads of the screw will engage the bone on the distal side of the fracture and the screw will advance in a linear direction (Fig. 8.12). Because there is no contact of the screw threads in the proximal cortex, the screw is literally gliding through the proximal segment of bone without exerting any force or movement on that fragment. As the head of the screw contacts the surface of the near cortex, it pulls the proximal segment along with the linear movement of the screw and literally presses the proximal segment of bone against the distal segment of bone. The result of overdrilling in the near cortex is the creation of interfragmental compression as the screw is tightened.

In contrast a cancellous screw does not require overdrilling of the near cortex to create interfragmen-

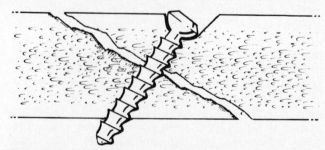

Figure 8.11. Cortical screw is fully threaded and will cause distraction between fragments as it crosses fracture line. Threads thus prevent compression.

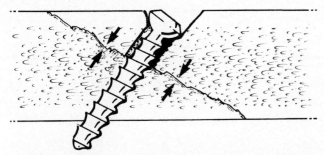

Figure 8.12. When near cortex is overdrilled, glide hole eliminates contact of threads with proximal fragment. As screw is turned, threads will pull far cortex toward screw head and interfragmentary compression is produced.

tal compression. The cancellous screw has threads only on the distal portion of the screw, whereas the proximal shaft is smooth. Because of the technical design of this screw, a gliding hole is not required in the near cortex to allow the unrestricted linear movement of the screw. The technical point that must be observed when using a cancellous screw for interfragmental compression is the requirement that all threads of the screw must be on the distal side of the fracture to effect the lag technique (4). If the screw threads spanned the fracture line, threads would engage bone on both sides of the fracture and the effect would be the same as using a cortical screw without overdrilling the near cortex. This is of particular importance when dealing with dense cancellous bone, i.e. fixation of the posterior malleolus from an anterior approach or tarsal arthrodesis (Fig. 8.13 A, B).

Mechanical Principles for Use of a Lag Screw

The basic principles for the use of lag screws as the sole means of producing interfragmental compression involve the dimensions of the fracture, quality and consistency of the fracture fragments, and the type and number of screws used to obtain a stable and secure rigid internal compression fixation. Each of these factors must be evaluated in every fracture or fixation situation to assure the most effective means of accomplishing a rigid and stable internal fixation.

General considerations in the use of a lag screw are: multiple screw fixation (Fracture length, number of screws, and angle of screw insertion); single screw fixation; and miscellaneous considerations.

RIGID INTERNAL FIXATION USING MULTIPLE SCREWS IN A LAG TECHNIQUE

Rigid internal compression fixation using screws alone is one of the most common techniques employed in the lower extremity. There are several basic principles that will make this type of fixation most appropriate and also most effective.

Fracture Length and Number of Screws

The first consideration is that of the length of the fracture. The most appropriate situation includes a

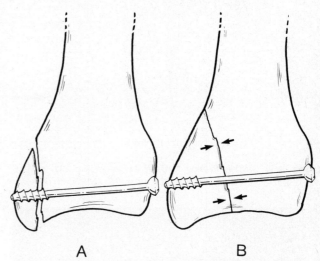

A   B

Figure 8.13. Even when using cancellous screw, all threads must be distal to fracture line. (A) When screw threads span fracture line, distraction occurs. (B) Fracture line is spanned by smooth shaft and interfragmentary compression is produced.

long oblique or spiral fracture where the length of the fracture is at least twice that of the diameter of the diaphyseal bone involved (5). In this circumstance, even though the fracture is unstable by its configuration, the mechanical relationships of the fracture create a situation where rigid and stable fixation can be readily accomplished with lag screws alone. Because of the length of the fracture in relation to the width of the bone it is possible to fixate the fracture with at least two or more individual screws. The mechanical security of this type of fixation with multiple points of interfragmental compression creates a stable and rigid internal fixation that will readily withstand the controlled forces of postoperative rehabilitation.

Angle of Screw Insertion

A commonly misunderstood principle is properly discussed in fixation of the long oblique fractures. The angle of the screw is placed halfway between the perpendicular to the plane of the fracture and the cortex of the bone (5). This principle has specific bearing on the fixation of long oblique fractures; however, its significance must be appreciated by defining the appropriate context of the application of the principle.

When fixating a long oblique fracture with multiple interfragmentary screws, the first interfragmental screw should be centrally placed and perpendicular to the cortex of the diaphyseal bone (Fig. 8.14) (4). This orientation places the points of contact of the fixation screw so that they will resist shift of the fracture fragments (Fig. 8.15). Should this first screw be placed perpendicular to the plane of the fracture, interfragmental compression would be lost with telescoping of the fracture fragments under a loading force. The head of the screw would simply back out of the proximal cortex with the shift of the fragments (Figs. 8.16 A, B, 8.17 A, B) (4). With the screw perpendicular to the surface of the cortex, interfrag-

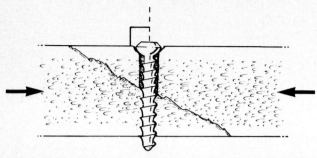

Figure 8.14. When fixating fracture or osteotomy with several screws, at least one screw should be perpendicular to both cortices.

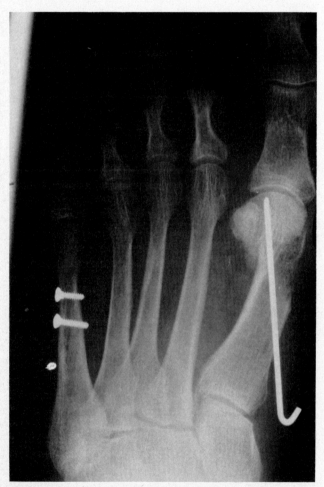

Figure 8.15. Oblique osteotomy was fixated with distal screw perpendicular to both cortices and proximal screw angulated.

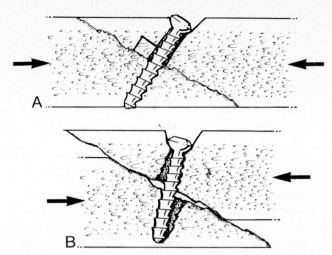

Figure 8.16. (A, B) When screw is placed perpendicular to fracture line and oblique to cortex, loading force can cause loosening of screw and telescoping of the fragments.

The second point of reference for the secondary screws is that of the longitudinal relationship to the shaft of the bone. The screws are inserted so that they bisect an angle between the perpendicular of the fracture and the perpendicular of the cortical surface of the bone. This placement serves to enhance the rigidity of the fixation by creating binding of the compression forces exerted by each individual screw (Fig. 8.19).

RIGID FIXATION WITH A SINGLE LAG SCREW

A single screw applied in a lag fashion can create adequate interfragmental compression to allow primary bone healing (5). The single screw fixation, however, is not able to withstand the heavier loads of shearing and bending that a multiple screw fixation technique can tolerate (29). Therefore the fixation must be protected against excessive loading to avoid disruption of the fracture reduction. Should the fixation be lost, the screw then serves as an axis of rotation for the fracture fragments and could create additional problems in the healing of the fracture (Fig. 8.20 A–D) (5).

When considering a single screw for fixation, local factors and manipulation of the fracture fragments by the action of the screw can be used to enhance the stability of the fracture fixation. These factors can be used especially in osteotomy techniques.

A single lag screw creates a force of compression in line with the direction of the screw. If the screw angle is perpendicular to the fracture plane, the force of compression is relatively static with no tendency to shift the fragments in relation to each other. This circumstance commonly exists with the fixation of avulsion fractures, such as those of the medial malleolus or base of the fifth metatarsal (Figs. 8.21, 8.22).

If the angle of the screw deviates from the plane of the fracture, there is a shift of the near fragment in the direction of the course of the screw as the screw is tightened and compression is created. This shift may create a gross movement of the fracture frag-

mental compression can only be lost if the head of the screw pulls through the near cortex or the threads strip through the far cortex. The second and third screws are secondary points of fixation and are placed on either side of the primary screw. Several points of reference need to be considered (4). Primarily, they are placed perpendicular to the plane of the fracture when observed in a cross-sectional reference to the shaft of the bone and the fracture plane (Fig. 8.18 A–C). This prevents a frontal plane shift of the longitudinal relationship of the fracture fragments and creates a uniform pressure along the plane of the fracture, especially in the long spiral oblique fracture.

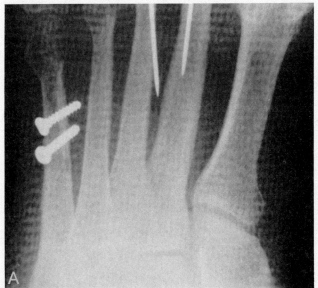

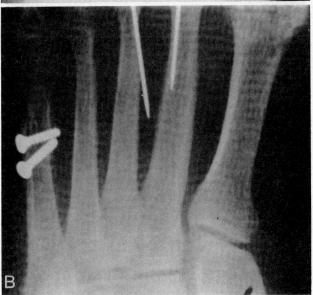

Figure 8.17. (A) Both interfragmentary screws are perpendicular to fracture line. (B) Two weeks later screws have loosened and fragments have telescoped on each other.

ments if there is no other stabilizing point of fixation. If a point of fixation or stabilization exists primarily, no gross shift of the proximal fragment will occur and an internal static pressure will be created that can actually enhance or jeopardize the overall fixation.

The gross shift of the fragments may be a technical complication in the fixation of fractures because it can actually create the loss of anatomical reduction. This is of critical significance especially when dealing with intra-articular fractures.

SHEAR EFFECT IN MULTIPLE SCREW FIXATION

In the long oblique fracture, the primary screw of fixation is placed perpendicular to the cortices of the bone. This places the angle of the screw at an oblique path across the fracture. Overtightening of this fixation screw would have the tendency to cause a shift of the near fragment so as to elongate the fracture segment. This force is obviously countering the natural forces of the unstable fracture, which would tend to cause shortening or telescoping of the segment. But once the screw is tightened properly it exists to resist shift of either fragment in either direction. The placement of the secondary screws is again at an angle that is a bisection between the perpendicular to the plane

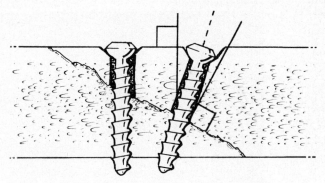

Figure 8.19. Secondary screws are also placed in specific relationship to fracture line in longitudinal plane. Screws are aligned to bisect perpendicular of cortex and perpendicular of fracture line.

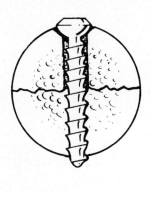
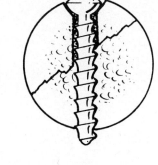
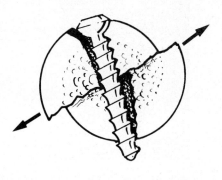

A   B   C

Figure 8.18. (A–C) Several points of reference need to be considered when fracture line is long, oblique, and possibly spiral in config-

uration. Screws must be oriented perpendicular to fracture line in a cross sectional reference.

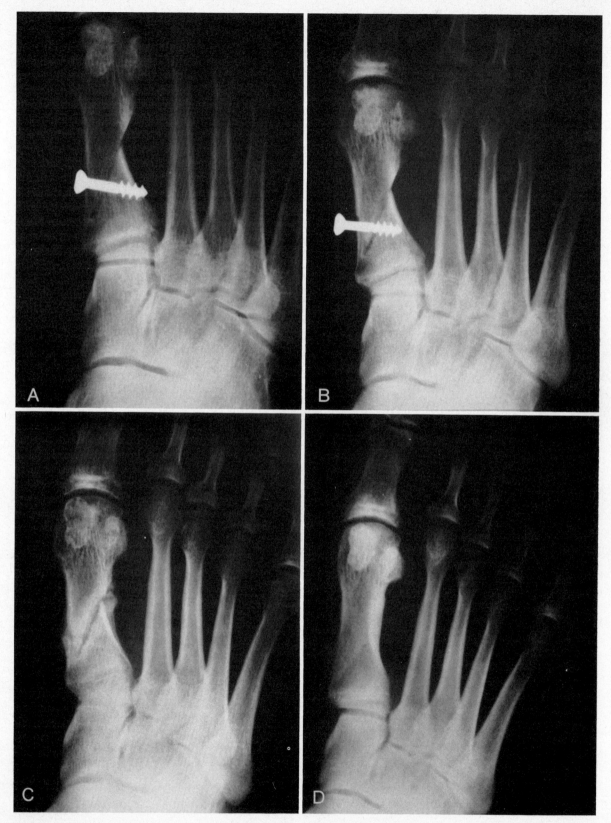

Figure 8.20.   (A–D) Failure of single screw fixation will allow rotation of fragments about screw and subsequent secondary bone healing.

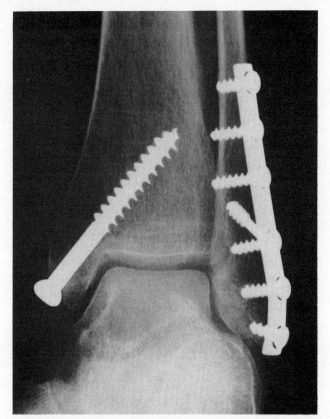

Figure 8.21. Medial malleolus fracture is fixated with single cancellous bone screw. Fibular fracture is fixated primarily with lag screw technique and secondarily with plate.

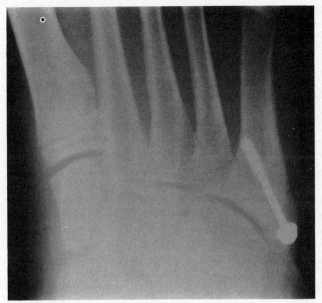

Figure 8.22. Transverse avulsion fracture of fifth metatarsal base is fixated with single lag screw.

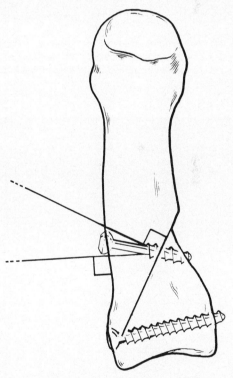

Figure 8.23. Intact cortical and soft tissue hinge of base osteotomy acts as primary point of fixation. This hinge will prevent rotation of fragments around fixation screw.

of the fracture and the cortex of the bone (4). This angle also serves to create a lengthening of the fracture segment. This shift is restricted by the natural configuration of the fracture and then by the primary fixation screw. A binding tension is then set up between the two screws and adds another dimension to the overall stability of the fixation.

In the specific circumstance of single screw fixation of an oblique osteotomy, the intact cortical hinge acts as the primary point of fixation (Fig. 8.23). If the path of the screw bisects the angle formed by the perpendiculars of the cortex and the plane of the osteotomy, a distal shift of the near fragment will be created by the compression of the lag screw (Fig. 8.24) "Pearls of Base Wedge Osteotomy", lecture by J. Ruch). The cortical hinge will be placed under tension and a binding force converts this tension into additional compression at the surface of the osteotomy. An inappropriate angle of fixation of the oblique wedge would create a proximal shear and a fragile fixation at best. Additional shear from the screw itself or a loading force could easily disrupt the cortical hinge and create shortening along the plane of the fracture (Fig. 8.25). The screw head would back out of the proximal cortex and all compression at the osteotomy surface would be lost. The screw would then serve as an axis of rotation of the fracture fragments and displacement would easily occur (Fig. 8.26 A, B).

MISCELLANEOUS CONSIDERATIONS

In most cases the use of two smaller screws is preferred to the use of a single larger screw (Fig. 8.27)(5). The use of two screws provides two points of fixation and more evenly disperses the compression forces across the surface of the fracture. Two screws also act to resist rotation of the fracture fragments.

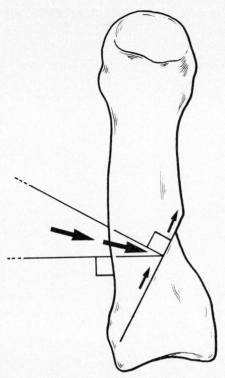

Figure 8.24. As compression screw is tightened, angle of screw will produce distal shift of near fragment. Cortical hinge will serve as tension band device and be placed under tension that is converted to binding force.

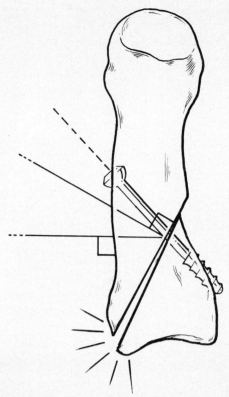

Figure 8.25. If compression screw is placed at angle that will shift near fragment toward hinge, fracture of hinge will occur and fixation will be lost.

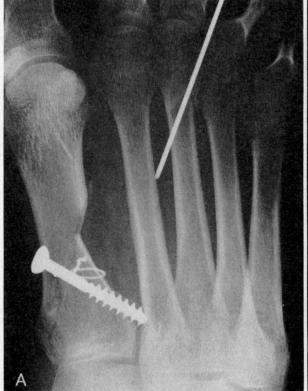

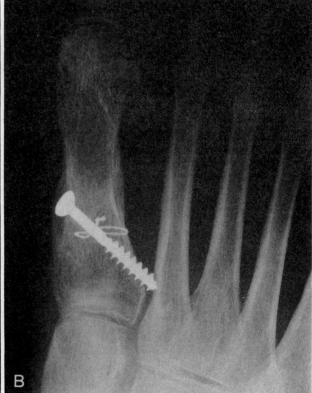

Figure 8.26. Properties of small cancellous screw and 3.5 mm cortical screws. (A) Cancellous screw in base osteotomy was directed toward cortical hinge. Near fragment shifted toward hinge and hinge was fractured. (B) Cerclage wire was used to reinforce fixation though six weeks postsurgery bone callus can be seen.

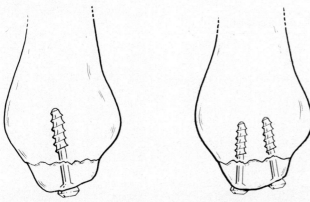

Figure 8.27. Two screws provide more stable fixation with more even dispersion of compression while preventing rotation between fragments.

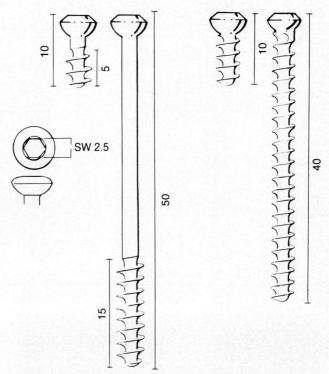

Figure 8.28. Cancellous screws have smooth shaft and contain threads only at distal aspect. Cortical screws are fully threaded. Each screw has advantages depending on clinical situation.

Obviously, the size of the fracture fragments, the consistency and quality of the bone, and the orientation of the fracture line need to be considered in the final selection of the fixation device. Certain unique and devised mechanical situations also lend to successful application of interfragmental fixation with the use of single or multiple lag screws. The surgeon must be aware of many factors in the final and successful application of the screw as a rigid internal fixation device.

SCREW ANATOMY

Early basic research into bone healing and fixation techniques expanded into all areas of the operative management of fractures. As the research continued it soon became apparent that new instrumentation was needed to implement the new principles of internal fixation (5). A uniform and integrated system of AO/ASIF instrumentation was developed with standardization of implant material, dimension, and application.

The AO/ASIF instruments are arranged into two basic sets, each with specific capabilities and set compatibilities (5). The basic organization includes the standard set with individual instrument, screw, and plate sets and the small and minifragment sets with the smaller screws and plates.

The AO/ASIF surgical stainless steel screw is the basic element for achieving rigid interfragmental compression fixation. Extensive research and experimentation have gone into the development of this specialized surgical implant (5). Every aspect of the screw's technical design has been used to maximize its technique of insertion and performance. The two basic screw designs include the cortical screw and the cancellous screw (including the self-tapping malleolar screw) (4). The cortical screws are fully threaded whereas the cancellous and malleolar screws are only partially threaded. Each screw has mechanical advantages depending on the specific technical and clinical situations in which they are employed (Fig. 8.28).

Technical Aspects of Screw Design (Table 8.1)

Screw Head

The diameter of the screw heads range from 3 to 8 mm. The miniscrew head measures 3 mm (1.5 mm screw) and 4 mm (2.0 mm screw) (5). The miniscrew heads use a cruciform recess with a centering hole that provides secure implant-to-screwdriver contact (Fig. 8.29).

The small fragment screws use a 5.0 mm head diameter on the 2.7 mm cortical screw and a 6.0 mm head diameter on the 3.5 mm cortical screw and the 4.0 mm cancellous screw (5). The diameter of the standard fragment screws, both cancellous and cortex, is 8 mm. A hexagonal slot is used in both the small and standard screws for a more secure insertion and contact of the screwdriver with the screw head. The hexagonal socket and stud-type screw driver configuration provides a large surface contact between the implant and the screwdriver that obviates the need for axial pressure to effect a controlled insertion or removal of the screw. The exact linear contact of this unique design also creates a directional relationship between the screw and the handle of the screwdriver.

The surfaces of the screwdriver tip and the slot in the head of each screw should be examined before use. Should shear or wear of the surface be identified, the instrument or implant should be replaced.

All AO/ASIF screws feature a spherical contour of the underside of the screw head. This shape creates

Table 8.1
AO/ASIF Small Fragment Set and Standard Set Screws and Related Instrumentation (mm)

Thread Dia.	Spherical Head Dia.	Hexagonal Screwdriver Dia.	Shaft Dia.	Core Dia.	Drill Bit Thread Hole	Drill Bit Gliding Hole	Tap Dia.
Small fragment							
1.5	3.0	(phillips)	(cort.)	1.0	1.1	1.5	1.5
2.0	4.0	(phillips)	(cort.)	1.3	1.5	2.0	2.0
2.7	5.0	2.5	(cort.)	1.9	2.0	2.7*	2.7
3.5	6.0	2.5	(cort.)	1.9	2.0	3.5•	3.5
4.0	6.0	2.5	2.3	1.9	2.0	(canc.)	3.5
Standard set							
4.5	8.0	3.5	(cort.)	3.0	3.2	4.5★	4.5
4.5	8.0	3.5	3.0	3.0	3.2	(canc.)	4.5
6.5	8.0	3.5	4.5	3.0	3.2	(canc.)	6.5

Straight Drill Sleeve	*	•	★
Gliding Hole	2.7	3.5	4.5
Drill Bit Hole	2.0	2.0	3.2

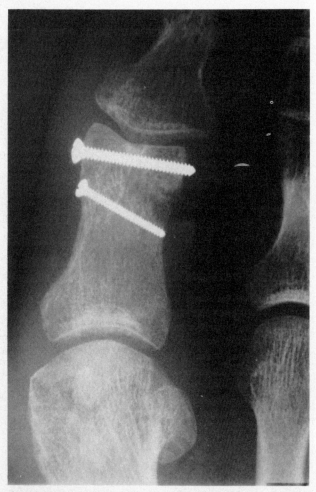

Figure 8.29. Minifragment screws are well suited for fractures of proximal phalanx of hallux.

consistent and even pressure at the contact surface between the screw head and the cortical bone. This relationship is dependent on a properly countersunk cortical surface.

Screw Shaft and Core

The shaft of the screw refers to that portion of the screw without a thread pattern (5). This is only seen on the cancellous screws. The diameter of the shaft is slightly greater than the thread hole used for the insertion of the cancellous screw to squeeze or press into the smaller thread hole creating an external pressure on the shaft, which serves to resist motion of the implant under load of the fixated fracture.

The core of the screw is the portion of the shaft that extends into the thread pattern (5). The core diameter is slightly smaller than the diameter of the thread hole to allow for clean purchase of the screw threads into cortical and cancellous bone without resistance of contact from the core surfaces.

Screw Thread

The AO/ASIF screw thread is designed to maximize the stability of the purchase of the screw thread in the bone substance (5). The thread pattern is asymetrical with the compression side of the thread being flat and relatively perpendicular to the shaft of the screw (Fig. 8.30). The cancellous thread pattern is wider or has relatively more space between threads to allow purchase of a greater mass of bone per thread. The cortical screw is designed with a greater number of threads and a shorter thread for a greater number of purchase points in the harder cortical bone.

The insertion of the cortical screw requires the use of a tap to cut the exact thread pattern and remove bone debris from the screw channel (5). In cancellous bone a tap is routinely used but may not be necessary in certain circumstances. Softer cancellous bone will readily deform with the pressure of the cancellous screw thread and allow firm thread purchase with only the use of a thread hole.

The specific mechanical design of the cortical and cancellous screws makes each screw a unique internal fixation device. The surgeon must understand the basic configuration and intended uses of each screw

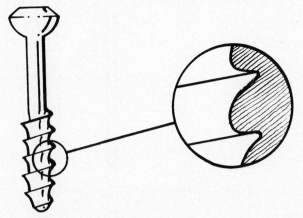

Figure 8.30. ASIF screw thread pattern is asymmetrical to afford stability and produce even compression between bone substance and screw shaft.

to take advantage of its fullest capabilities. Specific fracture patterns, quality of bone substance, and type of fixation all will influence the selection of the appropriate screw for internal compression fixation (31).

TECHNIQUE OF LAG SCREW INSERTION
Cortical Screws

The technique for insertion of a cortical screw as a lag screw is based on the creation of a gliding hole in the proximal or near cortex (4). This gliding hole prevents purchase of the screw threads in the near cortex and allows the screw head to press the near fragment against the far fragment to create compression at the fracture surface.

There is no one technique for insertion of the cortical screw. There are, however, several basic points common to a variety of techniques that can effectively be used to insert the cortical screw. The modification of techniques is dictated by the physical circumstances of the fracture fragments. One given technique may be more advantageous in a specific situation and allow for an easier or more exacting insertion of the screw.

The 3.5 mm cortical screw* will be illustrated. The 3.5 and 2.7 mm screws are probably the most common cortical screws used in the foot and ankle. Minor variation in technique may be indicated for use of the standard 4.5 mm cortical screw and the mini-screws.

Technique 1 (3.5 mm Cortical Screw)

Technique 1 is the standard or basic technique for insertion of the 3.5 mm cortical screw as a lag screw. Each step executes a particular function that is critical in the proper technique of insertion. All steps of the fixation process should be performed with

---

* For the purposes of this text the 3.5 mm cortical screw is the originally described 3.5 mm cortical screw of the small fragment set. The Swiss now refer to this screw as a fully threaded cancellous screw (5).

the fracture fragments held securely apposed with a bone clamp or other protective device. This particular technique is indicated for an uncomplicated fragment configuration where the path of the screw is relatively perpendicular to the surfaces of the bone.

Thread Hole

A 2.0 mm drill is used initially to create the thread hole in the near and far cortices (Fig. 8.31A). Because the drill is penetrating the surfaces of the cortices in a perpendicular orientation, there is little tendency for shift of the tip of the drill as it attempts to engage or bite into the cortex. The path of the drill is relatively easy to control as it penetrates both the near and far cortices.

Countersink

The countersink for the small fragment set is then used to recess the surface of the near cortex for the head of the screw (Fig. 8.31B). The tip of the countersink is a 2.0 mm nub that centers the countersink as it cuts into the cortex (5). The angle at which the countersink is held while cutting is critical and must be in line with the thread hole and the final path of the screw. Excessive countersinking should be avoided to prevent the head of the screw from pulling through a relatively thin cortex.

Countersinking obviously reduces the prominence of the head of the screw, but also serves two very important mechanical functions in the screw insertion process ("Pearls of Base Wedge Osteotomy," lecture by J. Ruch). Countersinking increases the surface area for contact of the head of the screw and the cortex of the bone. This decreases the likelihood of creating stress risers, microfractures, or even macrofractures in the cortex of the bone as the head of the screw presses into the near cortex. The second function of countersinking creates a concentric relationship between the countersink pattern and the thread hole of the screw. This prevents shift or lateral movement of the head of the screw as it engages the cortex. Any lateral movement of the head and shaft of the screw would obviously create a split or fracture within the near cortex and seriously compromise the stability of the fixation.

Gliding Hole

The third step in this fixation process involves creating the gliding hole in the near cortex with a 3.5 mm drill (Fig. 8.31C). The effect of overdrilling has been thoroughly discussed. However, the technique is most important. The near cortex has already been drilled with the 2.0 mm drill and contoured with the small countersink. The path or angle of the 3.5 mm drill must similarly be cut so that it is concentric and in line with the preceding maneuvers. The drill bit is self-centering as long as it is cutting into a smaller hole and allowed to cut cleanly in line with the previous instrumentation. Any angulation or deviation of this drill could alter the configuration of the process and cause threads of the cortical screw to bind or

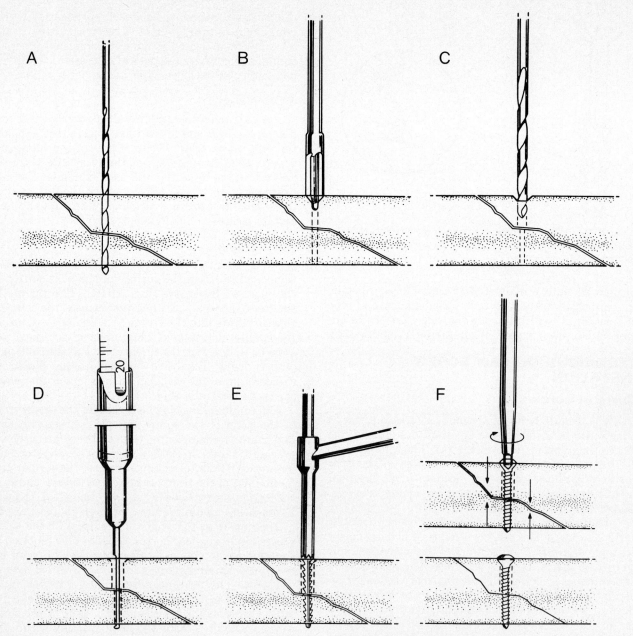

Figure 8.31. Basic technique for insertion of 3.5 mm cortical screw. (A) 2.0 mm thread hole. (B) Countersink 2.0 mm hole near cortex. (C) 3.5 mm gliding hole. (D) Depth gauge. (E) 3.5 mm tap far cortex. (F) 3.5 mm cortical screw.

engage the proximal cortex and prevent the gliding effect and ultimate compression of the fracture surfaces. The gliding hole is cut through the near cortex to the level of the fracture line. In cortical bone such as the first metatarsal, penetration of the near cortex is usually felt and is adequate for creation of the gliding hole. In denser compact bone, however, it may be necessary to monitor the depth of the gliding hole. The gliding hole must cut to the level of the fracture, but must avoid penetration into the distal fragment. A gliding hole in the distal fragment would prevent purchase of the screw threads and eliminate any component of fixation.

Depth Gauge

The depth gauge of the small fragment set is then used to measure the distance between the surfaces of the bone along the path of the screw (Fig. 8.31D). The tip of the depth gauge is inserted through both cortices and drawn back to engage the hook of the tip in the external surface of the far cortex. The barrel of the depth gauge is reduced to the surface of the near cortex and the length of the screw is determined. With the depth gauge essentially perpendicular to the surfaces of the bone, the length measured should be relatively uniform regardless of the orientation of the tip of the measuring device. This orientation will be significant, however, when the screw is passing obliquely to the cortex (16 mm motion picture film, "Base Wedge Osteotomy," Produced by J. Ruch, Doctors Hospital Podiatry Institute, Tucker, GA).

Tap

The final step before insertion of the fixation screw is the use of the 3.5 mm tap to cut the flutes or thread pattern in the far cortex ("Pearls of Base Wedge Osteotomy," lecture by J. Ruch) (Fig. 8.31E). The instrument is inserted through the gliding hole without purchase or cutting of the proximal cortex. The tip of the tap will engage the distal cortex and the thread pattern is cut with a clockwise rotation of the instrument. The instrument is rotated several times or until the cutting motion begins to bind. Binding is caused by a buildup of bone debris from the cutting threads. The debris is collected in the longitudinal channels of the tap and may be cleared with a simple counterclockwise rotation of the tap. Cutting of the thread pattern continues with periodic reversal to clear debris and create a clean thread pattern in the far cortex. Once the tap penetrates the far cortex fully there is no further restriction of the cutting action and the tap is reversed and removed. Tapping or cutting of the screw thread pattern should always be the final step of instrumentation before insertion of the fixation screw. This will avoid disruption of the delicate thread pattern by other instrumentation or manipulation of the fracture configuration.

Care must be taken to avoid excessive penetration into soft tissues as the tap exits the distal cortex. Similarly, a tap sleeve is recommended to prevent damage to soft tissues from the proximal tap threads at the wound surface (5).

Screw Insertion

Finally, the appropriate 3.5 mm cortical screw is inserted (Fig. 8.31F). The specific screw is identified in the screw rack. It is retrieved by inserting the hexagonal tip of the screwdriver into the screw head slot and reducing the brace on the screw drive to secure the head of the screw to the tip of the screwdriver (5). The screw is then lifted from the rack and measured to confirm its actual length.

The 3.5 mm cortical screw is then inserted into the gliding hole and advanced until it contacts the distal cortex. The technique of overdrilling allows the screw to advance without the need for rotation of the screw or purchase of the screw threads in the near cortex. Once the tip of the screw engages the far cortex it is delicately turned to engage the threads of the screw into the pattern of the cortical bone. The screw is advanced until the head of the screw contacts the near cortex. At this point care must be taken not to overtighten the screw and strip the threads from the far cortex. A two-finger technique or delicate control is used to tighten the screw for the maximum degree of compression without stripping the screw thread purchase in the opposite cortex.

Technique 2 (3.5 mm Cortical Screw)

Glide Hole and Thread Hole

The second basic technique for insertion of the 3.5 cortical screw as a lag screw simply reverses the order of sequence for the thread hole and the gliding hole (Fig. 8.32A). Initially the gliding hole is created in the near cortex by overdrilling with the 3.5 mm drill. The far cortex must then be drilled with a 2.0 mm drill, but it is critical that a concentric relationship between the two holes be maintained. This relationship would be difficult to accomplish if executing the 2.0 mm thread hole by hand control alone. A straight drill sleeve with an outside diameter of 3.5 mm and an inside diameter of 2.0 mm is inserted into the gliding hole and advanced until the teeth of the sleeve contact the far cortex (Fig. 8.32B)(5). The 2.0 mm drill is then inserted into the sleeve and the far cortex is drilled. This technical step accurately keeps the thread hole centered and in line with the proximal 3.5 mm gliding hole. If the drill path is relatively perpendicular to the cortices of the bone, the drill sleeve serves primarily to keep the concentric relationship between the two drill holes. If, however, the drill path is significantly oblique to the cortical surface, the drill sleeve can actually be used to control the penetration of the thread hole in the far cortex.

Countersink

The countersink is then used to shape the near cortex (Fig. 8.32C). The tip of the countersink, however, has a 2.0 mm guide tip that must be inserted into the 3.5 mm gliding hole. If the angle of approach is relatively perpendicular to the cortex, the countersink will tend to center itself with the rotation of the instrument. If, however, the angle is significantly oblique, the guide tip of the countersink will tend to shift to the edge of the glide hole and create an off-center countersink pattern. This malalignment can have significant bearing on the success of the internal fixation. An off-center countersink will cause the head and shaft of the screw to shift as the screw head engages the near cortex and result in fracture or splitting of the near cortex. Once countersinking has been performed, the instrumentation sequence remains the same.

Extenuating Circumstances

In those circumstances where the fixation screw approaches the cortical surface of the bone in an oblique path, there is a natural tendency for the drill bits and even the countersink to shift off-center as they bite into the cortical surfaces. It is for these situations that a significant modification of technique 2 can be most beneficial in the successful insertion of a lag screw (Fig. 8.33).

If a drill bit is held perpendicular to the surface it is attempting to penetrate, there is little shift of the bit. If, however, the drill bit is held oblique to the surface, the natural tendency of the bit is to skip down or along the surface of the bone (Fig. 8.34). This is

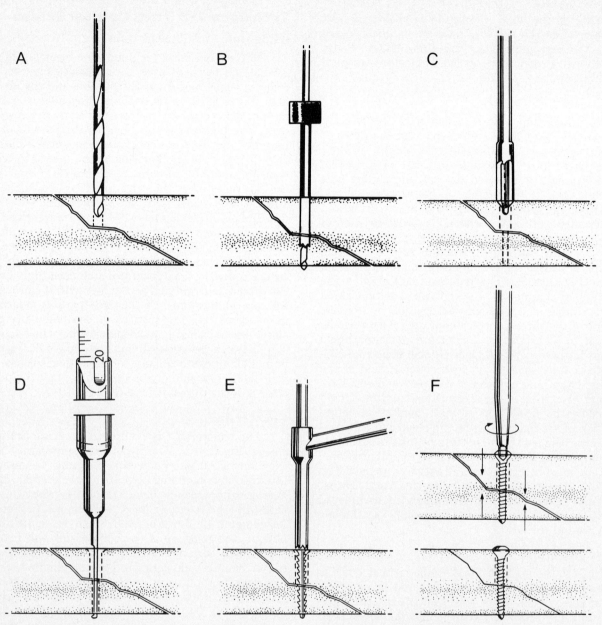

Figure 8.32. Technique 2 for insertion of 3.5 mm cortical screw. (A) 3.5 mm gliding hole. (B) Drill sleeve and 2.0 mm thread hole. (C) Countersink 3.5 mm hole near cortex. (D) Depth gauge. (E) 3.5 mm tap far cortex. (F) Insert 3.5 mm cortical screw.

encountered whether the drill bit is attempting to penetrate the near or the far cortex (16 mm motion picture film, "Base Wedge Osteotomy", producef by J. Ruch, Doctors Hospital Podiatry Institute, Tucker, GA).

If a 2.0 mm drill is used obliquely to penetrate the near cortex, it will readily skip along the surface of the bone. This problem can be overcome by holding the drill bit perpendicular to the surface initially and penetrating the cortex. The bit is then withdrawn and reinserted at the desired angle. It will then penetrate the first cortex at the desired angle without deviating from the intended point of penetration.

If the drill is then advanced to the far cortex it will similarly approach this cortex at an oblique angle.

The natural tendency again will be for the tip of the drill to migrate along the internal surface of the cortical bone. Because the shaft of the drill is held firmly in the first cortex, there is a significant bending pressure applied to the drill bit as the tip of the bit migrates along the internal bone surface (Fig. 8.35 A, B). The drill bit can easily be broken within the medullary aspect of the bone (Fig. 8.36). This situation can occur whether the hole in the near cortex is a thread hole or a larger gliding hole.

One technique that can be used to avoid this complication is the use of power instrumentation to penetrate the cortices of the bone. The high rpm of a rotary drill can be used to penetrate a cortex even at an oblique angle without migration of the penetrating

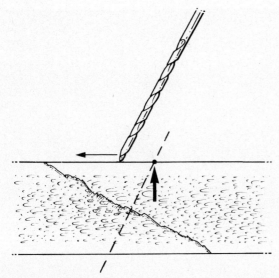

Figure 8.33. When fixation screw is to approach cortex at oblique angle there is tendency for drill bit or countersink to shift off-center and migrate down surface.

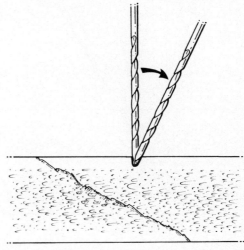

Figure 8.34. Problem of drill bit or countersink migration is overcome by initially attacking cortical surface at perpendicular and then withdrawing and reinserting at desired angle.

tip of the bit. This technique will be illustrated later in specific techniques of lower extremity surgery.

The second method to control accurately the penetration of the drill bit, to maintain a concentric relationship between drilling and countersinking patterns, and to avoid complications incorporates a slight modification of technique 2 previously described. The technique initially concentrates on the near cortex to create a concentric configuration for the gliding hole and the countersink pattern. Once this relationship has been produced the straight drill sleeve (3.5 mm × 2.0 mm) is used accurately to place and control the penetration of the 2.0 mm drill as it creates the thread hole in the far cortex.

Technique 2′ (3.5 mm Cortical Screw)*

Preliminary Thread Hole

Initially only the near cortex is penetrated with the 2.0 mm drill. The drill penetrates the cortex at the intended point of entry by holding the drill perpendicular to the surface of the bone. The bit is then withdrawn and redrilled at the desired angle (Fig. 8.37A).

Countersink

At this point, if the drill was advanced to the far cortex, bending and fracture of the drill bit would be likely (Fig. 8.37B). Instead of continuing to the far cortex, manipulation of the near cortex is completed. The 2.0 mm guide tip of the countersink is inserted into the preliminary thread hole and an accurately aligned and concentric countersink pattern is cut into the near cortex. Considerably more bone will be sculpted by the lower side of the countersink. Countersinking should be continued at least until the upper edges of the cutting blades contact the near cortex.

---
* Oblique line of approach to cortical surfaces.

Care should be taken not to penetrate the thin cortex with excessive countersinking.

Gliding Hole

The 3.5 mm drill is then used to cut the gliding hole into the near cortex (Fig. 8.37C). The self-centering quality of the drill bit will keep the 3.5 mm drill in line with the countersink pattern and the intended path of the fixation screw.

The deviation from standard sequence is created by the circumstance and the shape of the countersink. The small fragment countersink has only a 2.0 mm guide tip. The problem arises when attempting to countersink through a large glide hole. The standard fragment set uses only a 4.5 mm cortical screw and has two different countersinks. One of the countersinks has a 3.2 mm guide tip and is intended to be used when the hole in the near cortex is a thread hole. The second countersink has a 4.5 mm guide tip for use in the larger gliding hole (5).

Thread Hole

Once the near cortex has been accurately drilled and countersunk, the straight drill sleeve (3.5 mm × 2.0 mm) is inserted through the glide hole (5). The teeth of the drill sleeve are then pressed into the internal surface of the far cortex to anchor the drill sleeve in the appropriate angle. The 2.0 mm drill is then advanced through the drill sleeve and cuts through the far cortex. The drill sleeve is actually used to maintain a concentric relationship of the glide hole and the thread hole and effectively prevents migration of the tip of the 2.0 mm drill as it penetrates the far cortex (Fig. 8.37D).

The remaining steps for insertion of the screw remain the same with the use of the depth gauge, tap, and insertion of the screw. Several specific points, however, must be kept in mind with the completion

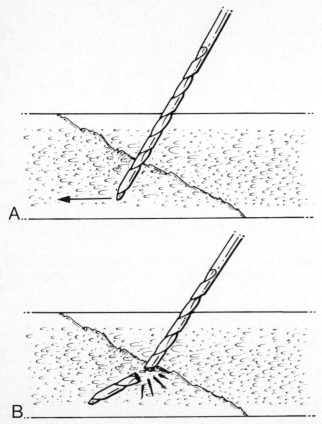

Figure 8.35. (A) As drill bit approaches far cortex at oblique angle, there is tendency for bit to slide down inside of bone shaft. (B) Drill bit can easily be broken within medullary cavity.

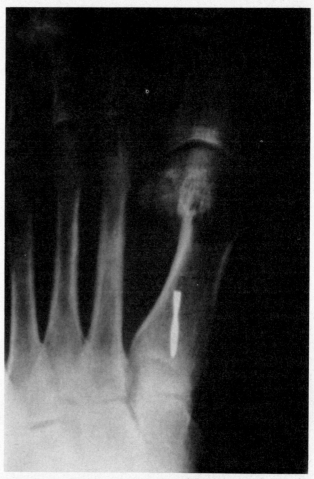

Figure 8.36. Broken drill bit that has fallen into medullary cavity. Drill bit was being used to fixate distal osteotomy and broke as it encountered far cortex and migrated down inside of bone.

of the fixation process when the screw is coursing obliquely to the cortical surface.

Depth Gauge

The depth gauge can measure two different lengths when an oblique screw is to be inserted (Fig. 8.37E). The proximal edge of the distal hole will measure shorter than a measurement taken if the tip of the depth gauge engages the distal side of the hole in the far cortex (31). If a screw is selected based on the shorter measurement, there may be a very tenuous fixation with only one thread engaging only one side of the thread hole in the far cortex. The longer measurement should be used so that there will be at least one thread penetrating the distal side of the thread hole in the far cortex and several threads visible at the proximal side of the thread hole. This technique will ensure secure purchase of the far cortex with as many threads as possible.

Tap and Screw Insertion

The tap and even the tip of the screw can glance off of the internal surface of the far cortex as they attempt to penetrate the thread hole (Fig. 8.37F). Care must be taken when an oblique screw path is used to ensure that the tap and the screw both engage and penetrate the far cortex. If the tap or screw should migrate and purchase the internal contents of the

bone, less than desired fixation may be obtained (Fig. 8.37G).

Technique 3 (3.5 mm Cortical Screw)

A third technique is described that can be useful in situations where the distal fragment may be difficult to visualize once the fracture is reduced (e.g. oblique fibular fracture.) The technique is initiated by drilling the thread hole in the distal fragment before reduction of the fracture and under full exposure of the internal surface of the distal fragment. The fracture is then reduced and a C guide or aiming device is used to place the gliding hole in the near cortex (Figs. 8.38 A–C). This technique allows for accurate placement of the thread hole in a fragment that may be difficult to visualize or contact if the fracture is initially reduced. Once the thread hole and gliding hole have been made the remaining steps of countersinking, measuring, and tapping are performed.

The actual technique of inserting a cortical screw as a lag screw may be modified in a variety of ways to take advantage of certain technical situations and avoid possible compromising circumstances. The basic components of the technique involve the gliding hole in the near cortex and the thread hole in the far

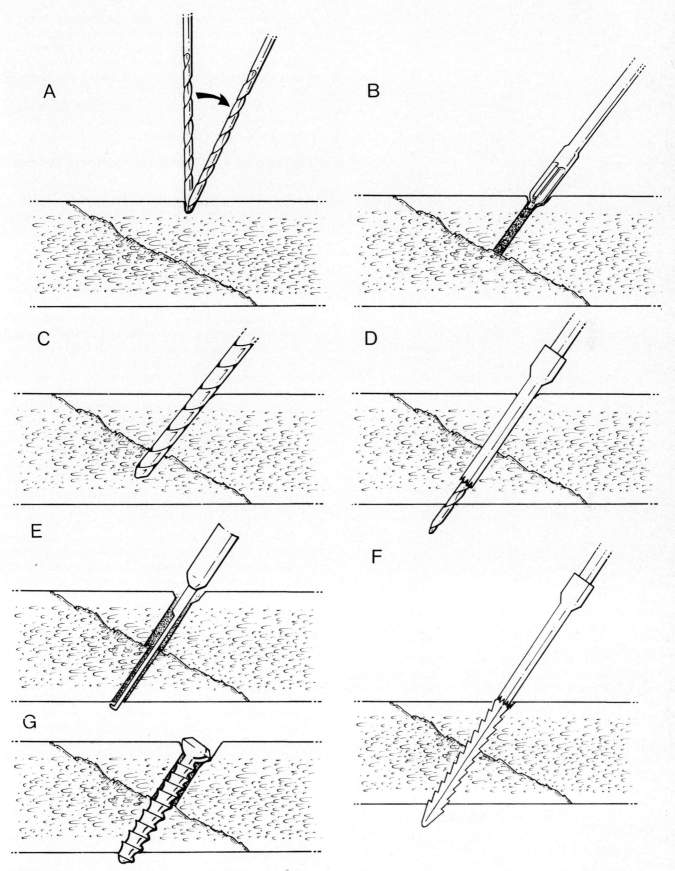

Figure 8.37.   Technique 2 for insertion of 3.5 mm cortical screw at oblique angle. (A) 2.0 mm drill hole near cortex only. (B) Countersink. (C) 3.5 mm gliding hole near cortex only. (D) Drill sleeve and 2.0 mm thread hole. (E) Depth gauge. (F) 3.5 mm tap far cortex. (G) 3.5 mm cortical screw.

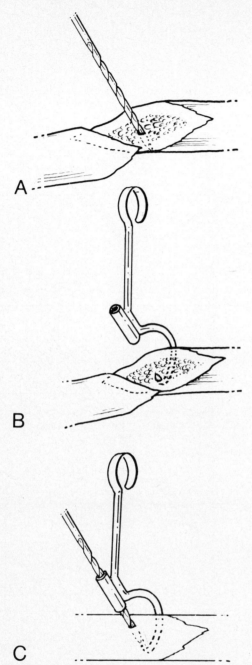

Figure 8.38. Technique 3 used C guide aiming device to place gliding hole in near cortex. (A) Distal cortex is drilled. (B) C guide is placed in distal hole. (C) Fragments are reduced and gliding hole is drilled.

cortex. If these techniques are accurately performed along with the remaining steps of screw insertion, a cortical screw can provide effective interfragmental compression and fixation.

TECHNIQUE OF LAG SCREW INSERTION

Cancellous Screw

The effective insertion of a cancellous screw as a lag screw is dependent on the purchase of the cancellous threads only in the distal fracture fragment (5).

If the threads of the screw span the fracture line and engage both the near and far fragment the screw will not act as a lag screw. No compression can be created at the fracture surface and separation of the fragments is actually created as the screw crosses the fracture line.

The proper sequence for insertion of the cancellous is similar to that of the cortical screw with the exclusion of the gliding hole.

Technique 4 (4.0 mm Cancellous Screw)

Thread Hole

Ideally a hand drill with a 2.0 mm bit is used to cut the thread hole (Fig. 8.39A). Hand instrumentation allows for a more precise cut with respect to the diameter of the thread hole. Hand instrumentation may have its disadvantages in certain situations, however. A high speed rotation is necessary to cut into an oblique or extremely hard cortical surface. Power instrumentation must be used judiciously to avoid burning and necrosis of the cortical bone and overreaming of the dimensions of the thread hole. Intimate thread and core contact of the screw with adjacent bone substance is critical in obtaining and maintaining secure purchase of the screw threads. Overreaming and resorption of necrotic bone will decrease surface contact between the bone and the screw and result in a less secure or stable fixation.

The cancellous screw is designed to be used in cancellous or soft bone, but can also be used in a variety of situations where it actually purchases the far cortex of the distal fragment (32). The thread hole therefore may penetrate only into the internal cancellous bone of the distal fragment or, when necessary, penetrate the far cortex of the distal fragment (33).

Overdrilling of the near cortex is not necessary for the insertion of the cancellous screw. In fact the swaging effect of pressing the 2.3 mm diameter smooth shaft of the cancellous screw into the 2.0 mm thread hole in the near cortex adds to the tight fit of the screw and the stability of the fixation (Fig. 8.39B).

Countersink

Countersinking serves the same function for insertion of the cancellous screw and the cortical screw. The two main purposes include increasing the surface area of contact between the head of the screw and the near cortex and the creation of a concentric linear channel for longitudinal migration of the head of the screw with tightening and compression. This technique helps to prevent split or fracture of the near cortex with the pressure from the head of the screw or from lateral shift of the head of the screw with an inexact contact at the cortical surface. Reducing the prominence of the head of the screw, although helpful, is of secondary importance (Fig. 8.39C).

Depth Gauge

The use of the depth gauge in the sequence of insertion of a cancellous screw that will purchase the far cortex is the same as that for insertion of a cortical

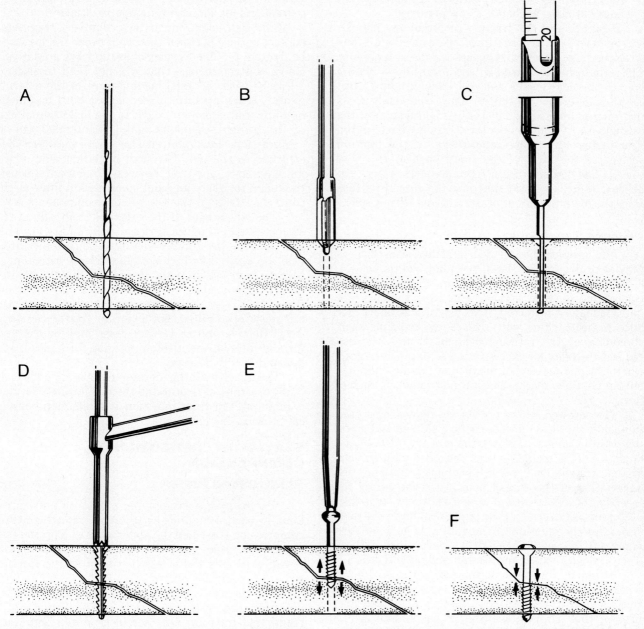

Figure 8.39. Basic technique for insertion of 4.0 mm cancellous screw. (A) 2.0 mm thread hole. (B) Countersink. (C) Depth gauge. (D) 3.5 mm tap both cortices. (E) Threads may distract fragments until threads cross fracture line. (F) 4.0 mm cancellous screw.

screw. Care must be taken accurately to engage the far cortex with the tip of the guide wire and obtain an accurate measurement by measuring the farthest point of the distal cortex. When the threads of the cancellous screw will only engage the internal cancellous bone of the distal fragment, the tip of the depth gauge is advanced to the end of the thread hole for the measurement of the screw length (Fig. 8.39D).

Tap

The 3.5 mm tap will cut a thread pattern in the near cortex, as well as the distal fragment and far cortex when appropriate. The same care must be taken with this instrument to feel the cutting action of the tap as it penetrates the osseous tissues. Special atten-

tion is given while tapping cancellous bone when the thread hole has not penetrated the far cortex. If the tap is inserted too far the tip of the tap will not penetrate the far cortex and all of the thread pattern will be stripped from the internal content of the bone as the tap is rotated.

Screw Insertion

Insertion of the 4.0 mm cancellous screw follows the final step of tapping. As the screw is inserted, slight resistance is appreciated as the 4.0 mm thread pattern presses into the 3.5 mm tapped pattern in the near cortex. This action again swages the thread into the softer bone for which the cancellous screw is intended. This action insures a greater surface contact between the thread and core surfaces of the screw and the adjacent bone for better screw purchase.

Separation of the fracture or osteotomy may be felt or even seen as the tip of the cancellous screw attempts to penetrate and engage the distal fragment. This separation is caused by the absence of a gliding hole in the near cortex and will be maintained until the threads of the cancellous screw completely cross the fracture line (Fig. 8.39E). The smooth shaft of the cancellous screw allows the screw to slide freely in the near cortex and create compression at the fracture surface as the head of the screw engages the near cortex. The screw is again tightened with a firm but delicate touch to avoid stripping the thread pattern from the distal fragment of the fracture (Fig. 8.39F).

Drill and Tap Sleeves

The primary use of drill and tap sleeves is to provide protection for the surrounding soft tissues (5). The drills and taps are very sharp and can readily engage and damage adjacent soft tissues if they are not adequately retracted. The use of the sleeve not only protects these soft tissues by avoiding their shredding by the rotating drill bit or tap but also reduces the need for excessive retraction in situations where the oblique line of the drill or tap may impinge on the confines of the incision and judicious retraction.

The serrated end of the sleeves may also be used to anchor the sleeve to the cortical surface and guide the drill bit as it penetrates the cortex at an oblique angle (5). This technique was described with the use of the straight drill sleeve (3.5 mm × 2.0 mm) for penetration of the thread hole in the far cortex for insertion of a cortical screw as a lag screw. It is also useful for penetration of the larger drill bit in the near cortex for the creation of the gliding hole. There are many other uses for the drill sleeves that will be discussed with axial compression and plate fixation.

Although the basic techniques for insertion of cortical and cancellous screws as lag screws are relatively simple, there are many subtle and refined maneuvers that must be mastered in the skillful use of these devices. A thorough understanding and working knowledge of these techniques is a basic requirement for any surgeon who intends successfully to use this type of rigid internal compression fixation (Figs. 8.40 A–E).

STATIC INTERFRAGMENTAL FIXATION
External Fixator

An external fixator can be used in many different ways in the fixation of the osseous skeleton. The function of interfragmental compression and fixation is one of its applications; however, its use in this fashion is rather limited and has several specific requirements for successful implementation.

The first requirement is a relatively transverse contact surface between the two osseous fragments to be fixated (5). This relationship produces a relatively stable contact surface that will not tend to shift or telescope with the axial loading force of the external fixator. Large pins are placed across both fragments in a line that is perpendicular to the longitudinal axis of the osseous segments and the intended line of compression. The external fixation devices are then attached to the pins that exit on either side of the limb or part and the devices are simultaneously tightened to create an axial compression force at the contact surfaces of the two osseous components (4).

The advantages of the external fixator lie in the extreme stability of the device and the ability to adjust and increase the compressive load at periodic intervals. Its basic uses include metaphyseal osteotomies of large bones such as the proximal tibia and arthrodesis of major joints such as the knee and the ankle (Figs. 8.41, 8.42 A, B). Although its appropriate uses are relatively limited, the external fixator can be a very effective and in certain cases may be the best form of interfragmental compression for fixation of a demanding situation (4).

Drawbacks of the device include its relatively bulky external apparatus and the special aftercare that it requires. Pin tract infection is a common complication with this technique.

STATIC INTERFRAGMENTAL COMPRESSION
Prestressed Plate

The technique of applying a plate to a fractured bone in such a manner as to create interfragmental compression is termed the application of a prestressed plate. The stress that the plate exhibits is that of tension whereas the stress delivered to the fracture surface is compression.

The concept can be illustrated by using a wooden doll that has been transected in the fashion of a transverse fracture. One screw is driven into each fragment an equal distance from the fracture line. A rubber band (shorter than the distance between the two screws with the fracture reduced) is stretched to loop over each screw. As the rubber band is stretched it is placed under tension. When the rubber band is suspended over the two anchor screws, it is still stretched beyond its resting length and is still under tension. As the rubber band is released, its tension is transferred to the anchor screws and the fracture fragments. The tension in the rubber band is transferred to the fracture fragments resulting in compression at the surface of contact between the two fragments.

Figure 8.40. Several examples of ASIF screw fixation. (A) Navicular fracture fixated with two minifragment screws. (B) Closing base wedge osteotomy with one 4.0 mm cancellous screw and intact cortical hinge. (C) Distal osteotomy fixated with single cancellous screw. (D) Interfragmentary lag screw reinforced with plate to fixate bone graft of first metatarsal. (E) Cortical screw overdrilled in distal phalanx to fixate hallux interphalangeal joint arthrodesis.

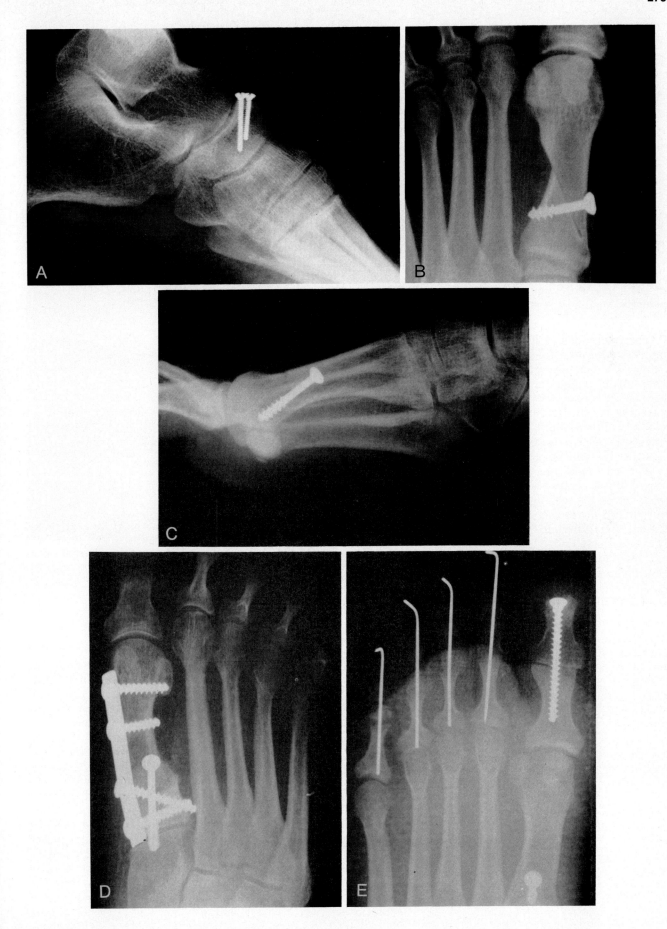

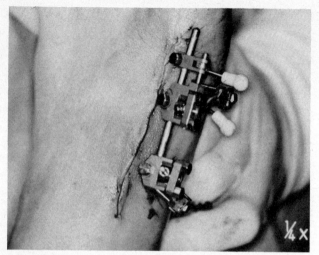

Figure 8.41. Nonunion of first metatarsal osteotomy required bone graft, and external fixator was used to increase the stability and compression.

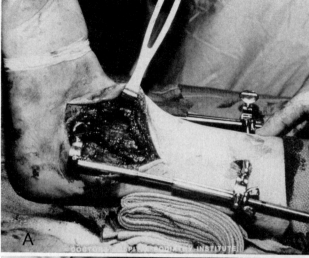

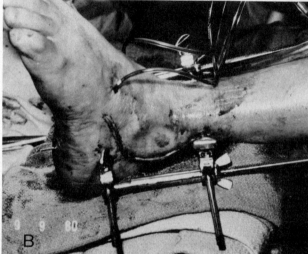

Figure 8.42. (A, B) Ankle fusion was fixated with external fixator to maintain alignment and provide axial compression for transverse osteotomy.

This technique is obviously mechanically most appropriate for an axial force that is to be applied to a transverse fracture configuration. Under circumstances of an oblique or comminuted fracture, axial compression alone would simply cause a shift and shortening of the fracture fragments with resultant instability of the fixation. Because of the linear design of the plates used in this type of fixation, the technique is best used in long bone fractures or osteotomy.

The axial load created by a prestressed plate is a form of static compression, but its static nature is dependent on the technique of application and on the external load forces that may involve the end fracture fixation. The technique of applying a static axial load with a prestressed plate can be accomplished by three basic techniques: (a) load screw technique, (b) dynamic compression plate, and (c) tension device.

Load Screw Technique

The load screw technique is the most common plate technique applied in the foot and ankle region, basically because of the dimensions of the plates used. The plates are relatively thin and flexible tension plates with semi-, third-, and quarter-tubular design. They are intended to be used under tension and alone* do not offer the strength or rigidity against bending that is seen with the thicker dynamic compression plate implant (5).

The load screw technique is performed by using an off-set or eccentrically drilled hole for the initial screws used to fixate the plate to the two fracture fragments (Fig. 8.43 A, B). With the fracture reduced, the plate is secured to the fragments by clamps. The plate is centered over the transverse fracture (5). The

two plate holes closest to the fracture are selected for the insertion of the load screws.

The thread hole for the fixation screw is drilled at the far side of the plate hole or at the edge of the hole farthest from the fracture. This may be performed by the use of an off-set guide or by manual means. No countersinking or overdrilling is performed and the thread hole is measured and tapped for the appropriate cortex screw.

As the screw is inserted, the head of the screw contacts the edge of the plate hole at its distal margin. The screw head will seat itself into the center of the hole in the plate by shifting the screw and the bone fragment in the direction of the fracture. This motion is countered by a similar motion from the opposite fragment and as the two fragments are pushed toward each other interfragmental compression is created.

Because of the simple spherical design of the plate holes in the relatively thin tension plates, only the two initial screws may be used as load screws (5). If a

---

* Excellent rigidity, however, can be obtained by using the tension plate in combination with another form of interfragmental compression such as a lag screw.

third or more distal screw were inserted in an off-set technique, it would have to push the previous screw head out of the plate hole to cause any additional longitudinal shift of the fracture fragment.

The load screw technique can provide a very significant degree of interfragmental compression to an anatomically reduced transverse fracture of a long bone (34). However, the technique can create an effect that is undesirable. In the example of the wooden doll model, if the apparatus were placed freely on the table surface, the tension of the rubber band would cause the fracture surface to separate or gape at the side opposite the tension device (Fig. 8.44). This same effect can occur with the tightening of the load screws in the fixation of a transverse fracture. The basic principle causing this condition is that the prestressed plate creates compression only at the cortex adjacent to the plate itself.

This technical complication can be avoided by the execution of a technique of prebending the plate before the load screws are inserted and tightened (35). The off-set holes are initially drilled with the plate in the straightened attitude. The plate is removed and slightly bent at its center to lift the center of the plate away from the surface of the bone. As the load screws are inserted the bone fragments are drawn up against the undersurface of the plate and the opposite cortices come in contact before the surface of the fracture that is adjacent to the plate. As the load screws are tightened the fragments are drawn closer together and

the gap at the adjacent cortex decreases. As the gap reduces the plate is bent back into a straightened position with even contact and pressure now existing along the entire fracture surface. The prebent plate acts as a leaf spring and resists gap of the opposite cortex ("The Principles of AO and the Tension Band Concept", lecture by J. Ruch) (Fig. 8.45).

Axial compression can also be used in the fixation of short oblique fractures of long bones. However, this unique situation requires a specific sequence in the fixation of the fracture fragments and provides the unique opportunity to combine interfragmental compression with a lag screw. This technique will be discussed in detail in the section dealing with combination forms of fixation.

The load screw concept and the technique of prebending are fundamental principles for the creation of axial compression with plate fixation. The use of this technique alone has relatively few applications in surgery of the foot and ankle. However, the basic principles can be used in many different areas and situations. Possible use of the prestressed plate alone might include arthrodesis of the first metatarsocunei-

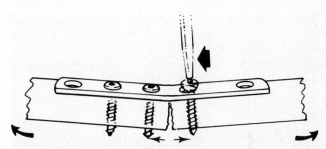

Figure 8.44. As load screws are tightened, tension will create compression at cortex adjacent to plate, but opposite cortex will separate.

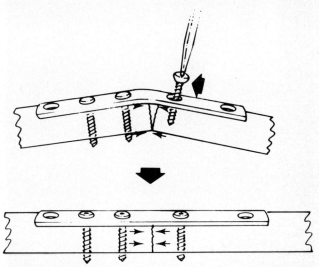

Figure 8.45. Separation of opposite cortex can be avoided by drilling off-set holes and then prebending plate. As load screws are tightened through bent plate, even interfragmentary compression is produced.

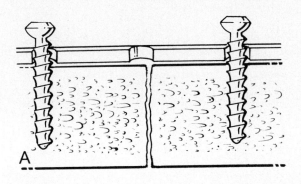

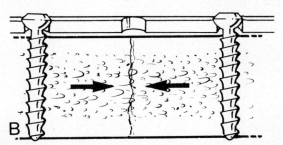

Figure 8.43. Load screw technique can produce rigid compression fixation. (A) Fracture is manually reduced and screw holes are drilled eccentrically away from fracture line. (B) As screw head contacts plate and seats itself, fragments are compressed together.

form joint and transverse fracture of the metatarsals or fibula (Figs. 8.46, 8.47).

Dynamic Compression Plate

The dynamic compression plate incorporates the load screw technique with the added effect of geometrically designed slots within the body of the fixation plate (36). The plate is significantly thicker and stiffer than the tension plates. The uniquely designed slots of the plate have two specific features that enhance the load screw application. The holes in the plate are oblong and longitudinally oriented to allow for longitudinal shift of individual screws. The shape of the slot has two different slopes for different functions of the fixation screw. As demonstrated in the load screw technique, the first and second fixation screws are eccentrically placed at the far side of the slot or plate hole. The incline or slope of the first portion of the slot is steep to give mechanical advantage to linear motion with the vertical seating of the screw head (37). Once the screw head has come to rest on the floor of the plate hole, there remains an additional millimeter of linear motion within the longitudinal shape of the plate hole. The slope on the remaining segment of the slot is relatively flat. The first acute slope is the compression slope whereas the second slope is a gliding slope.

This design allows the first and second screws to be inserted as load screws and then to be followed by a third and fourth screw that may also function as load screws for additional movement or compression of the fracture fragments. The first and second screws do not restrict additional compression because they have the space to glide in the direction of the axial compression.

The dynamic compression plate is more suitable as a solitary fixation device of a transverse fracture because of its additional rigidity. Its use in the foot is very limited because of the relative thinness of subcutaneous tissues. In those circumstances where a compression plate may be appropriate, the combination of a lag screw with the tension plate can provide excellent rigidity. There are individual dynamic compression plates for use with the standard 4.5 mm cortex screw, the 3.5 mm cortex screw, and the smaller 2.7 mm cortex screw (5). Each of these plates is specifically designed to accept the specific screw head with relatively smaller overall dimensions for each of the smaller screws.

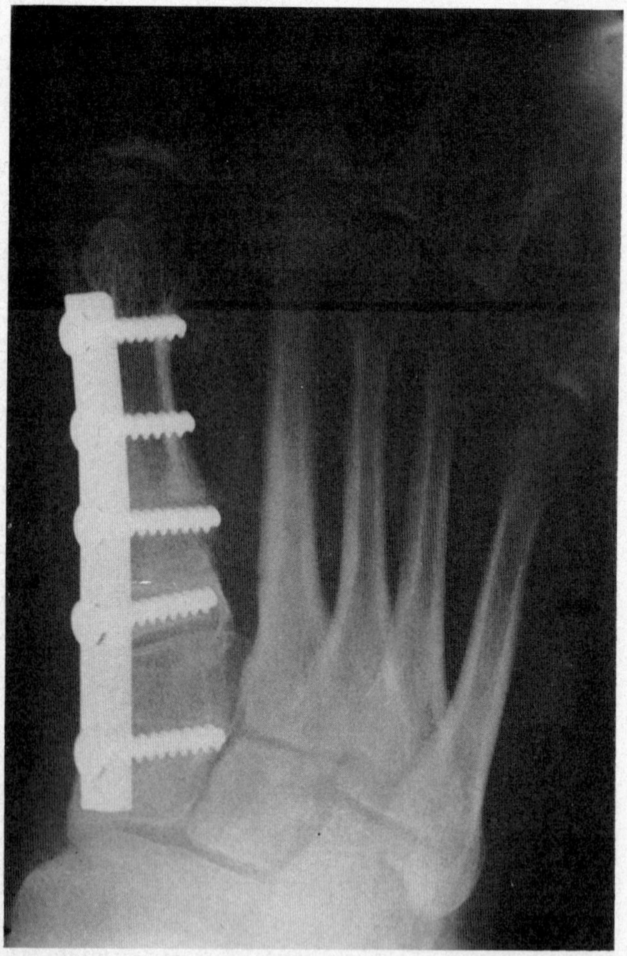

Figure 8.46. Prestressed plate with load screw technique and prebending can be used to provide interfragmentary compression as in this first metatarsal cuneiform arthrodesis.

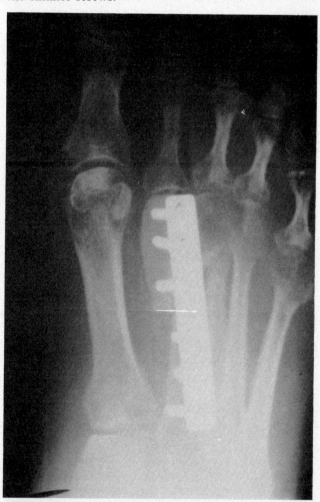

Figure 8.47. Load screw concept and prebent plate can create axial compression as in bone graft to second metatarsal.

Tension Device

A plate may also be applied for axial compression with the use of a tension device. This technique is applicable for large bones and the use of only the standard plates (5). The fracture is reduced and the plate is anchored to one fragment with the use of fixation screws. The tension device is then anchored to the second fragment and attached to the free end of the plate. The tension device is tightened, drawing the plate and opposite fragment toward the tension device creating axial compression at the fracture surface. The appropriate amount of tension is obtained, and the free end of the plate is anchored to the second fragment capturing the tension within the plate and retaining the interfragmental compression of the fracture fragments (Fig. 8.48).

The techniques of creating static interfragmental compression with a plate include the use of the load screw concept, the unique design of the dynamic compression plate, and the application of a tension device. The addition of axial compression significantly adds to the stability of fracture fixation in long bone fractures whereas the longitudinal arrangement of the fixation device adds to the ability of the fixation device to resist forces of bending and torque (38). Although the isolated use of the prestressed plate is intended for transverse fractures of long bones, the principles and mechanical aspects of this type of fixation are extremely important in the successful application of plates for any fracture fixation. The mechanical maneuvers created by plate application can serve to enhance the rigidity of the fixation if employed properly (4). They can also cause shift, angulation of the fracture, and can jeopardize the integrity of the overall fixation if their effects are not fully understood or are applied inappropriately.

DYNAMIC INTERFRAGMENTAL COMPRESSION

The Tension Band Concept

The previous discussion of plate application dealt with the intrinsic forces created by the application of the plate and the use of axial compression. This technique was described for a relatively neutral mechanical environment as might be expected with an isolated forearm or fibular fracture. In these instances the side of the bone where the plate is to be applied is dictated by anatomical considerations. In many cases, however, the extrinsic loading forces that will cross a reduced and fixated fracture will create a consistent pattern of bending so as to dictate a mechanical need for the specific application of the fixation device best to neutralize and counter those forces that may disrupt the fracture fixation. These forces may be created by the shape of the bone itself or by the overall shape of the limb with axial loading from muscle activity or even partial weight bearing (4).

When load forces to a longitudinal segment of bone are not in line with the segment of the bone itself or eccentric to the structure, a moment of bending is introduced to the segment that creates a tension side and a compression side of the bone. The cortex on the tension side or convex surface is subjected to tensile forces whereas the internal or concave surface is subjected to compressive loading (Fig. 8.49). The concept of eccentric loading was first appreciated and described by Pauwels (39) in 1935 and applied to fixation techniques of skeletal fractures. This principle is critical to the successful planning and execution of internal fixation. The extrinsic load forces that a fracture fixation must resist must be fully appreciated. Successful fixation is dependent on a mechanically sound technique designed to resist specific forces and even use these forces to enhance the stability of the fracture fixation.

Dynamic interfragmental compression indicates a changing or additive effect on the degree of com-

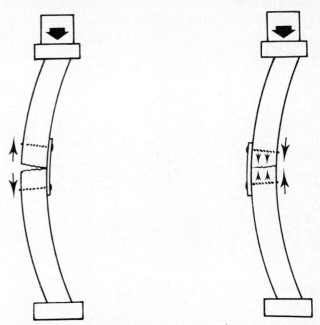

Figure 8.49. When load forces are applied eccentrically, compression side and a distraction side are produced. Tension band device is placed to prevent distraction and direct load force to produce compression.

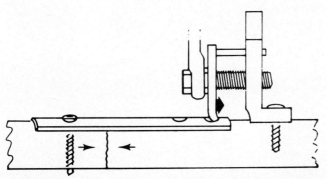

Figure 8.48. Tension device can be used for large bones to create static interfragmental compression. Tension device is anchored to one of fragments and used to pull plate and screw to compress fracture line.

pression (4). The tension band concept uses the mechanical features of eccentric loading actually to enhance the stability of a static fixation technique rather than allowing the bending forces to disrupt the fracture reduction. The tension banding concept is the combination of a static interfragmental compression technique with the functional loading of the part to create a dynamic degree of interfragmental compression (40).

The two basic components of the tension band technique are the load beam or the osseous segment and the tension band device. The tension band device is applied to the tension side of the bone to resist separation of the fracture (4). The implants usually employed include the tension band plate or even a dynamic compression plate in long tubular bones and a cerclage wiring technique applied to the tension surface of short bones or smaller fragments.

The tension device is applied to resist the tension of the eccentric bending force, but is dependent on this functional load to effect a dynamic degree of interfragmental compression. If the tension band device were tightened without the opposing force of eccentric loading, it would actually cause the opposite cortex to separate or gap as demonstrated in the load screw technique. Therefore the bending force of the eccentric load is critical to establish even compression across the entire fracture surface (Fig. 8.50).

Classic examples of the application of this technique in the lower extremity include the fixation of avulsion fractures of the medial and lateral malleoli and of the base of the fifth metatarsal (40, 41). In the example of the fifth metatarsal the tension band is applied to the lateral surface of the base of the metatarsal to counter the pull of the tendon of m. peroneus brevis (42). It is also dependent on the pull of this tendon and a position of slight adduction of the foot

to effect the dynamic compression of the fracture fragments (43). The avulsion fractures of the malleoli are dependent on the intact structure on the opposite side of the ankle to resist the tension band effect (4) (Figs. 8.51, 8.52 A–C).

Although these fractures may be fixated with the cerclage wire alone, the degree of stability is usually enhanced by the addition of Kirschner wires as a combination form of fixation.

The load beam depends on the stable and solid contact of the fracture fragments to accept and transmit the compressive load forces. The optimal fracture configuration for this technique is a clean transverse fracture with solid and intact cortices. Short oblique fractures may be amenable to this technique; however, the sequence of fixation of the fragments is critical to the success of stable fixation. Because of the mechanical effect of telescoping, long oblique fractures are not amenable to the tension band technique and are preferably fixated with the static interfragmental technique with the insertion of two or more lag screws. Similarly, comminuted fractures, butterfly fragments, or missing cortical segments are not well suited to fixation by the tension band technique (5). To be stable the load beam must be able to withstand the compressive forces of eccentric loading.

The concept of tension banding is an integral technique in the successful practice of rigid internal fixation. The mechanical principles illustrated have a significant bearing on many fracture situations. Eccentric loading forces must be respected and in turn used to ensure a more stable surgical reduction. The principles and techniques of tension banding have many uses, especially in combination with other forms

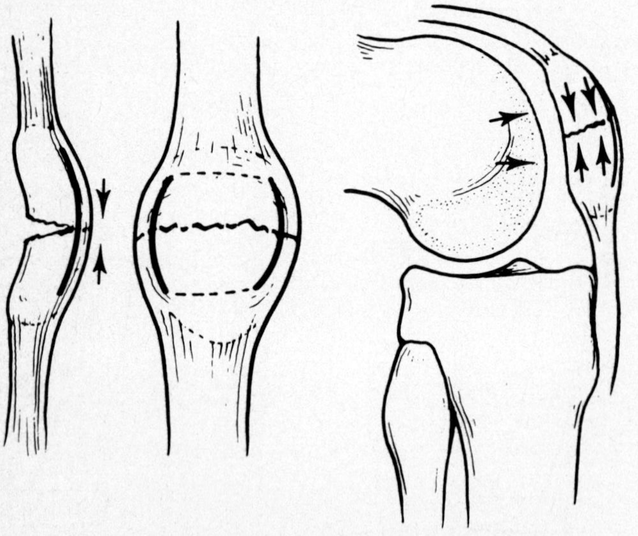

Figure 8.50. Fixation of patellar fracture with cerclage wire shows principles of tension band fixation. Tightening of tension band device will cause separation of opposite cortex. Eccentric loading will produce dynamic compression across fracture line.

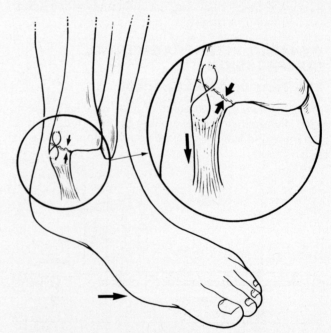

Figure 8.51. This example of tension band concept shows how movement of foot and intact deltoid ligaments can produce dynamic interfragmentary compression because of eccentric position of cerclage wire.

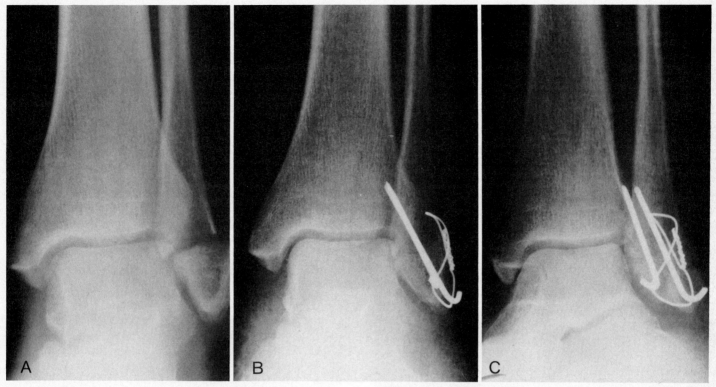

Figure 8.52. (A–C) Transverse avulsion fracture of fibula with deltoid ligaments and calcaneofibular ligament intact provides classic example of tension band fixation technique. Kirschner wires add stability to cerclage wire band.

of fixation such as the lag screw and splintage techniques.

SPLINTAGE

Splintage is a concept or technique used to splint or protect a reduced fracture. By itself splintage is not a form of rigid internal fixation and cannot be expected to produce primary bone healing. The technique, however, is important and has many applications in the overall practice of internal fixation.

The three primary uses of splintage are: (a) when interfragmental compression cannot be used (severe comminution or bone loss — buttress technique); (b) special situations (Kuntscher nail, epiphyseal fractures, secondary fixation); and (c) to protect a tenuous interfragmental fixation (combination techniques of interfragmental compression and splintage).

Splints have two basic functions; one load bearing and the other non load-bearing (5). The load bearing function is used when the fixation device is required to accept physiological loading of the bone to maintain length and alignment. This technique is referred to as buttressing. In a long bone fracture with severe comminution or even bone loss where interfragmental compression is not feasible, a buttress device is necessary to maintain anatomical alignment whereas a bone graft is used to restore the damaged segment. A buttress plate may be applied to maintain the length and alignment or an external fixator may be used. The external fixator would function as a distractor to maintain alignment and prevent shortening of the segment (Fig. 8.53) (5).

Non-load-bearing splints are used to maintain apposition of fragments and prevent displacement by extrinsic forces. The bone fragments themselves are required to sustain any compressive forces of physiological loading. The fracture configuration and quality of bone therefore become of ultimate importance in this type of fixation. The classic example of this type of fixation is the Kuntscher nail used to maintain reduction of midshaft fracture of the tibia or femur (5). The unique mechanical circumstances of this fracture are the key to successful healing even though a less than rigid form of fixation is used. The fracture must be transverse and noncomminuted. This allows the physiological loading forces to be transmitted by the bone and bending forces controlled by the intramedullary nail. A comminuted or oblique fracture pattern would doom this type of fixation because loading of the bone would produce shear, shortening, and instability with the ultimate fracture of the fixation device.

Epiphyseal fractures may be adequately fixated with splintage techniques. Kirschner wires may be used when the fixation device is to cross the growth plate and must avoid compression of the fracture surfaces (4). Interfragmental compression with a lag screw, however, may be used for fixation of opposing metaphyseal or epiphyseal segments as long as the screw does not cross the epiphyseal plate. The technique of the fixation of a fracture or osteotomy by the

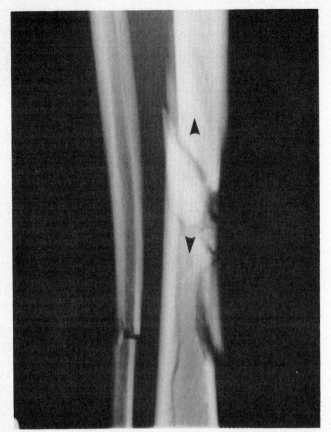

Figure 8.53. External fixator was used in comminuted fracture of tibia and arrows show direction of distraction needed to maintain length and prevent shortening.

insertion of Kirschner wires alone is a form of splintage and has certain value in the fixation of small or difficult to fixate fractures. This is a secondary form of internal fixation commonly employed by many surgeons in elective procedures and even in the reduction and fixation of common fractures. Although these techniques are less rigid than those using screws and plates, they may be used effectively if employed properly and adequately protected from disruptive forces. The addition of cerclage wiring techniques may add to the stability of this type of fixation and in some cases even lead to primary bone healing.

The use of Kirschner wire, however, in combination with other forms of compression fixation can provide a very stable and even rigid form of fixation. Similarly, a plate or even cerclage wire may be used in combination with other forms of fixation for the mutual enhancement of a stable fixation.

One of the most common applications of the splintage techniques comes in the protection of a tenuous interfragmental fixation. Even though interfragmental compression may have been accomplished, it may not be strong enough to withstand the extrinsic loading forces to which the reduction may be subjected. Combination of the various techniques and principles of rigid internal compression fixation brings together all of the skills and ingenuity of the surgeon to effect the most stable form of fixation for any given fracture situation.

COMBINATION OF THE TECHNIQUES OF RIGID INTERNAL COMPRESSION FIXATION

The use of the various techniques of internal fixation can be grouped into four basic categories for specific use in fracture management. A sound understanding of the principles and techniques of each of the individual concepts must precede the successful combination of these skills for the successful application of rigid internal compression fixation (5).

The two basic concepts of internal fixation, interfragmental compression and splintage, are combined to make up four combinations of fracture fixation: (a) lag screw and neutralization plate, (b) lag screw and buttress plate, (c) lag screw and tension band plate, and (d) Kirschner wires and tension band wire.

Lag Screw and Neutralization Plate

A short oblique fracture of a long bone may be fixated with a single lag screw for effective interfragmental compression. This single screw, however, may be inadequate to protect the fracture from extrinsic forces. A plate may be applied in the longitudinal axis of the bone to withstand the extrinsic forces that would otherwise disrupt the primary fixation. The plate would be applied with a neutral technique by contouring it to the surface of the bone and securing it to the bone with centrally drilled screws. This neutralization plate would have no dynamic effect on the fracture, would not incorporate the lag screw, and would only serve to protect the interfragmental fixation. If possible the plate should be placed on the tension side of the bone (Fig. 8.54).

The relationship of the lag screw to the plate can provide a unique fixation situation. Commonly the neutralization plate is oriented 90° or oblique to the axis of the lag screw so that the screw is not incorporated within a hole of the plate (4). This circumstance demands that the plate be applied neutrally to avoid shift or disruption of the primary fixation by a dynamic function of the plate (i.e. load screw technique) (Fig. 8.55).

In the unique situation where the lag screw lies in such a position as to be incorporated within one of the holes of the plate, additional interfragmental compression may be obtained by using the load screw technique (5) (Fig. 8.56 A, B). The sequence of fixation is critical in this situation to avoid shift and displacement of the oblique fracture with the axial compression force of the prestressed plate. The first fragment to be fixated to the plate is the fragment that forms an acute angle of less than 90° between the fracture surface and the undersurface of the plate. This acute angle will capture the tip of the opposite fragment as it is advanced with the tightening of the load screw. Once interfragmental compression has been applied in this fashion, the lag screw may be inserted in the appropriate hole of the plate to add additional interfragmental compression at the surface of the fracture. Accurate positioning of the plate is critical for successful placement of the lag screw.

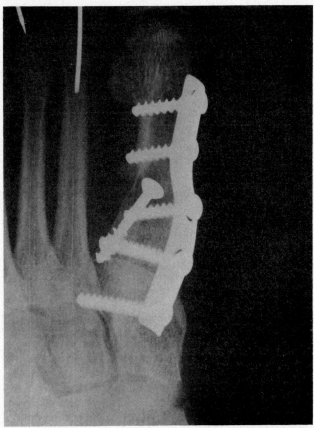

Figure 8.54. Single lag screw affords interfragmentary compression of bone graft and neutralization plate contoured to first metatarsal and cuneiform is used with centrally drilled screws.

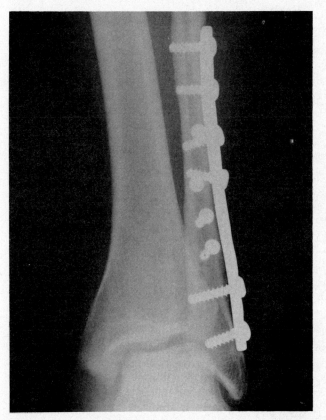

Figure 8.55. Long, spiral oblique fracture of fibula is fixated with lag screw technique and plate is oriented 90–100° to insertion of lag screws.

These techniques are quite useful in the lower extremity. Short oblique fractures of the fibular malleolus are well suited to interfragmental compression with a single lag screw and reinforcement with a neutralization plate (5, 43). Similar fractures of the metatarsals may be encountered and a variety of osteotomy and arthrodesing techniques are significantly improved by the combination of these principles (44). Arthrodesis of the first metatarsocuneiform joint and revision of nonunion of the first metatarsal are common examples.

Lag Screw and Buttress Plate

The lag screw and buttress plate may have application in severe comminuted fractures of the ankle. However, its use in the foot would require considerable imagination and ingenuity. Comminuted fractures of the metatarsals may provide the opportunity for this technique, however, interfragmental compression with lag screws is much more common.

Lag Screw and Tension Band Plate

The lag screw and tension band plate incorporates interfragmental compression of a lag screw and the additional compression and/or protection of a plate applied in a tension band function. The technique that uses a lag screw within a plate hole and crosses the fracture as well may be considered in this classification.

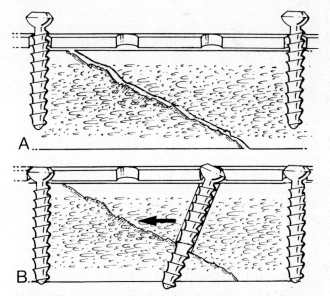

Figure 8.56. In unique situation where lag screw can be incorporated into holes of plate, load screw technique is initially used. (A) As load screws are tightened, bone edges are compressed against each other and plate. (B). Interfragmentary lag screw can then be introduced to produce additional compression.

Kirschner Wire and Tension Band Wire

The use of Kirschner wires has long been common for the fixation of fractures and osteotomies. Whereas Kirschner wires can afford apposition and alignment in fracture reduction, they cannot by themselves provide interfragmental compression. The unique combination of fracture apposition and alignment reinforced by a tension band wire technique can significantly enhance the rigidity of fixation for certain fractures.

This technique is most useful in avulsion type fractures where the fragments may be too small or their bone consistency is not amenable to interfragmental fixation with a lag screw or tension band plate. Avulsion fractures of the medial and lateral malleoli and of the base of the fifth metatarsal are common fractures that may be securely fixated with this technique (4, 43).

The technique involves the reduction of the fracture and the insertion of two Kirschner wires for maintenance of reduction and apposition (5). The two wires also prevent rotation of the fracture fragment. The wires are inserted perpendicular to the fracture plane and parallel to each other. A cerclage wire loop is then applied over the external cortex by looping the wire over the two Kirschner wires on one side of the fracture and through a drill hole in the opposite cortex. The wire is tightened to create compression at the external cortex and the tension band effect of resistance from proximal muscle or ligamentous pull disperses the compression evenly across the fracture. The exposed ends of the Kirschner wires are bent and embedded into the bone surface (4).

This technique has many applications in surgery of the foot and ankle. The success of the fixation is dependent on a sound understanding of the principles of the technique and the proper selection of the fracture or osteotomy. The critical requirement of the fracture complex is a definite mechanism of counterpull or resistance to the compressive forces of the tension band wire.

DISCUSSION

The principles and techniques of rigid internal compression fixation introduced and refined by the Swiss AO group have had a major impact on the surgical treatment of fractures and osteotomies. The implications of this surgical concept have significant bearing on surgery of the lower extremity, especially when postoperative management and the forces of weight bearing are considered.

The two basic premises of successful fracture healing, preservation of vascular supply and mechanically stable fixation, have been thoroughly researched and described in the AO literature (7). The application of these principles will have a monumental influence on the commonly accepted and practiced techniques and procedures for the foot and ankle.

Evaluation of the following concepts of rigid internal compression fixation from a clinical point of view has some very interesting findings that will have direct bearing on surgery of the lower extremity.

Mechanical Factors

The evaluation of the mechanical factors involved in the management of fractures and osteotomies can be broken down into three main areas (45): Stable fixation, intrinsic factors, and extrinsic factors.

Stable Fixation

The principles and techniques of rigid internal compression fixation have been soundly developed by the Swiss AO group. A review of these factors has been presented with an attempt to correlate their use with the specialized surgery of the foot and ankle. A study of these principles and techniques will lead the surgeon to a much greater understanding of the significance of sound mechanical engineering principles and techniques in the surgical management of fractures and osteotomies. It is the responsibility of each surgeon to master the basic techniques and then apply them properly in his or her own unique area of practice. These principles will have a dynamic effect on surgery of the foot.

One of the most significant areas that has evolved from our study of internal fixation is the mechanical function of osteotomy techniques (29). The proper use of the axis-hinge concept has had a dramatic influence on the elective osteotomy techniques of the lower extremity, especially in the area of hallux valgus surgery (32).

Although the significance of stable fixation has been fully explored, the importance of vascular supply cannot be overlooked. Successful bone healing is dependent on preservation of the blood supply to all tissues of the fracture complex.

Intrinsic Factors

The mechanical factors of stable fixation usually draw most of the attention in the discussion of internal fixation. The intrinsic factors of the bone itself, however, must always be considered in the total evaluation and management of fractures or osteotomies. Fracture configuration (i.e. stable, unstable, potentially stable, transverse, long oblique or comminuted, short oblique) has significant mechanical bearing on the type of fixation required to provide stable fixation (10). Bone stock, dimension, density, cortical, or cancellous also have to be considered in the complete approach to internal fixation of the osseous skeleton.

Extrinsic Factors

One of the primary goals of the Swiss concept is early rehabilitation of the limb or part without the need of cast immobilization for the maintenance of reduction of the fracture. This practice is designed to avoid or reduce the atrophy and complications of prolonged cast immobilization (4). The rehabilitative process, however, introduces a greater degree of the forces that can disrupt a fracture reduction and fixation. Bending, shear, and torsion are all forces that must be considered in the design and implementation of a stable internal fixation. These forces are produced from a relatively gentle active range of motion of the part, passive range of motion, and in some cases even partial weight bearing.

The basic guideline, however, must be understood and observed. No implant is designed to withstand the unsupported stresses of weight bearing (46). The forces of weight bearing are the most potentially damaging influences to a stable internal fixation (Fig. 8.57).

Early active and passive range of motion are encouraged in fractures fixated with rigid internal compression techniques (4). The potential hazards of any activity, however, must be fully appreciated and avoided to ensure the stability of the fracture fixation and the successful healing of the fracture itself.

Bone Healing

The process of primary bone healing has been discussed with respect to its basic requirements and its actual cellular process. Although primary bone healing is no more rapid than an uncomplicated secondary form of bone healing, its occurrence implies that the reduction obtained at surgery has been maintained. If the surgical reduction has been anatomical, and there are no other complicating factors of the injury or the surgery itself, full recovery can be anticipated. In elective surgical procedures such as osteotomies, the surgical result has been produced and maintained if the fixation is stable and primary bone healing ensues. The surgeon can then better evaluate the end surgical result as a direct reflection of the initial surgical manipulation and not some alteration created by partial loss of correction or alignment produced by a secondary form of bone healing.

Callus formation identified in relation to a fracture fixation or osteotomy technique can now be directly related to motion and an unstable fracture fixation. The continued movement of the fracture fragments is a disruptive process that produces an inflammatory healing response. This new view of secondary bone healing can redefine the nomenclature of the fixation callus as that of an irritation callus. Callus formation in association with internal fixation indicates the loss of rigid fixation and a potentially compromising situation for maintenance of surgical correction and successful bone healing.

Irritation callus is also directly reflected in the clinical presentation of the local part. Soft tissue edema, erythema, tenderness, and pain are all increased when the underlying fracture fixation is not stable or is not able to withstand those forces unto which it is being subjected. This clinical observation is a very important aspect in the practical evaluation and management of fractures or osteotomies treated by the principles of rigid internal compression.

Insight Into Failure

Surgical management of fractures has been historically criticized as unnecessary, exotic, overaggressive, and even unwise when it did not work. Many excuses and unsound conjectures have been volunteered in the aftermath of a failed internal fixation. A sound working knowledge of the principles and techniques of rigid internal compression fixation can provide the surgeon with a new scale by which he or she can evaluate the success and failure of the surgical techniques that he or she employs. The primary goals of the AO system provide the framework for an intel-

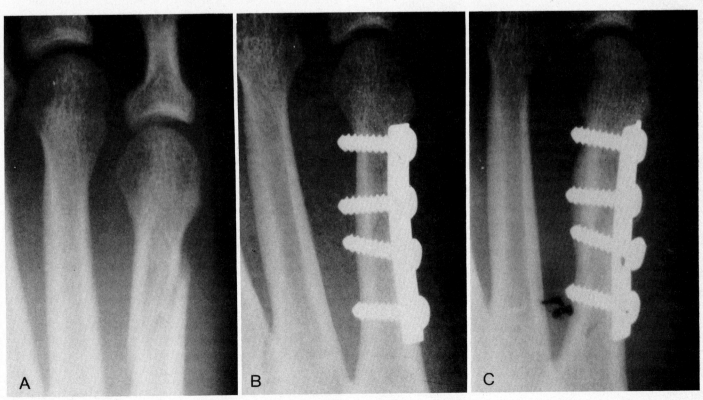

A B C

Figure 8.57. (A–C) No implant is designed to withstand unsupported stresses of weight bearing. Fifth metatarsal appears to be more than adequately fixated with four screws and plate, though weight bearing loosened screws and bone callus formation is evident.

ligent evaluation of the results of surgical management of fractures and osteotomies (4). These include (a) atraumatic surgical technique (vascularity and viability), (b) anatomical reduction, (c) rigid internal compression fixation, and (d) early rehabilitation.

These principles give the surgeon a new appreciation of bone healing and the factors that influence it. Vascular supply has always been of paramount importance. The techniques of anatomical dissection are never more beneficially applied than in trauma, fractures, and osteotomies (46). The mechanical engineering principles of rigid fixation include not only a thorough knowledge of stable fixation techniques but also include a functional appreciation of the configuration and quality of the fracture and its fragments. Once rigid internal fixation has been accomplished, it must be protected even in the environment of early range of motion and rehabilitation. Internal fixation has specific limitations that must be understood and respected. No implant is designed to withstand the unsupported stresses of weight bearing.

Consistent Procedures

The secret to producing consistent success in surgical management of fractures and osteotomies is an appreciation of those factors that can disrupt a stable internal fixation. If these disruptive forces and situations are identified and avoided, success will follow (4).

Successful Innovation

A sound basis in the principles and techniques of rigid internal compression fixation has opened the door for new and more effective surgical techniques in trauma surgery and reconstructive techniques of the foot and ankle. A mastery of these skills provides the surgeon with an exceptional tool. Respect for tissue through the principles and techniques of anatomical dissection and an unprecedented facility for manipulation of the osseous skeleton through the principles of internal fixation allow the surgeon fully to use creative talents for the improvement of surgical techniques and the development of new avenues in his or her surgical practice (Fig. 8.58 A, B).

PRINCIPLES AND USES OF KIRSCHNER WIRES AND CERCLAGE WIRE TECHNIQUES

Kirschner wires and loops of wire have been used for internal fixation of fractures and osteotomies for many years. In most cases each individual surgeon has developed a technique of fixation based on the ease of application and its relative success in his or her own clinical experience. The merits of the fixation technique were a result of the surgeon's own instinctive skills and an appreciation of not necessarily understood mechanical relationships. Occasionally a fundamental technique or some form of principle was identified and handed down through lectures, writing, and residency training. It was not until the organized

efforts of the AO group, however, that a systematic appreciation for the fundamental principles of rigid internal fixation was employed and applied to the use of Kirschner wires and cerclage wire fixation techniques.

The principles of rigid internal compression fixation have been discussed in detail in the preceding pages. The specific use of Kirschner wire fixation was demonstrated as a form of splintage for maintenance of apposition of epiphyseal fractures and in combination with cerclage wire to form a splintage and tension band type of fixation. This section is a discussion of some general principles and mechanical relationships important in the traditional use of Kirschner wires and loops of wire suture in the fixation of the osseous skeleton. These relationships are essential to the successful use of the more traditional forms of fixation in the foot and ankle. There are several fundamental principles that have been demonstrated and defined for the use of Kirschner wires and loops of wire that can lead to a stable form of internal fixation.

Kirschner Wires

Kirschner wires have been used for the fixation of fractures and osteotomies for many years. Several studies have been performed testing the strength and rigidity of a variety of configurations of Kirschner wire fixation techniques (47, 48, 50, 51). These techniques have included the single wire, parallel wires, and the crossed Kirschner wire technique (30).

Most authors will agree that a single Kirschner wire rarely provides rigid stability by itself (47, 49). Although the wire will tend to maintain apposition and alignment of the fracture fragments, it will offer little resistance against separation of the fragments along the axis of the pin. Its protection against bending forces is dependent on its purchase, angle of insertion, and its own inherent stiffness (Fig. 8.59).

Two parallel Kirschner wires improve the fixation by resisting rotation of the fracture fragments but offer little resistance again from separation of the fragments. Consistently the crossed Kirschner wire technique has been demonstrated to be the most secure of the Kirschner wire techniques (49). The use of two wires prevents rotation of the opposed fragments and the divergent path of the fixation devices resists separation of the fracture once the pins are inserted (50) (Fig. 8.60).

The strength of fixation has been demonstrated to correlate to the gauge of the fixation wire with Vanik and associates (47), describing the use of crossed 0.045 inch Kirschner wires to be the most stable. The authors' studies agree and demonstrate correlation of the gauge of the wire with the strength of fixation. The 0.062 inch wire produced the most stable fixation of experimental first metatarsal osteotomies (52).

The crossed Kirschner wire technique is not, however, without shortcomings. There is a potential for distraction of the fracture fragments with the divergent directions of insertion of the two crossing wires

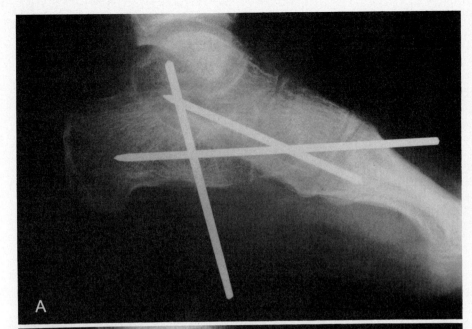

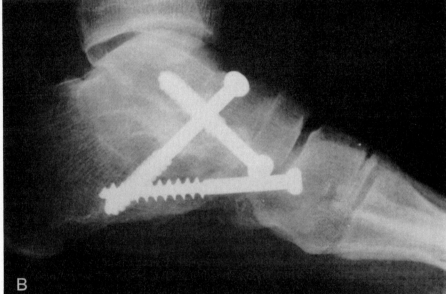

Figure 8.58. (A–B) Use of ASIF concepts and instrumentation have advanced techniques and mastery of these skills has improved results.

(49, 51). Should distraction of the fragments occur, the relationship is locked because the fragments cannot glide along two different axes at the same time (Figs. 8.61, 8.62).

Single Kirschner wires do offer stability when used in combination with intraosseous loop techniques to resist bending forces that would tend to disrupt the fracture fixation (47, 49).

Threaded Kirschner wires are rarely used because their inherent design leaves them mechanically unsound. The diameter of the threaded wire is measured as the thread diameter of a screw. The solid portion of the wire is then the core segment. Therefore a 0.045 inch threaded wire has a significantly thinner core diameter and is inherently weaker. Threaded wires tend to be brittle and fracture easily with bending.

Fracture may be encountered on insertion, removal, or with movement of the fracture fragments during the postoperative course. The insertion of the threaded wire also causes separation of the fracture or osteotomy as the tip of the wire attempts to penetrate the distal fragment. The same separation is seen with insertion of a cortical bone screw if it is inserted without overdrilling the proximal cortex.

Kirschner wire fixation techniques alone do not afford interfragmental compression (53). Only modification of their insertion technique in uniquely designed osteotomies or fractures can add some force of compression (54). The AO principles of splintage and tension band wiring can combine the use of Kirschner wires and wire loop techniques to afford rigid interfragmental compression fixation (4, 5, 55).

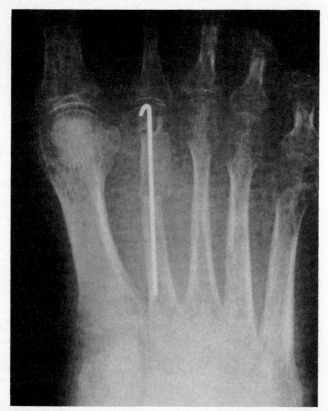

Figure 8.59.   Single Kirschner wire can be used to maintain apposition and alignment as in this bone graft of second metatarsal. Bone graft can still rotate around axis of wire and little compression is afforded.

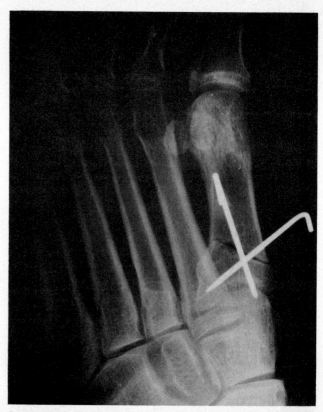

Figure 8.61.   Kirschner wires used in crossed fashion can cause distraction of bone edges as wires are driven in divergent directions.

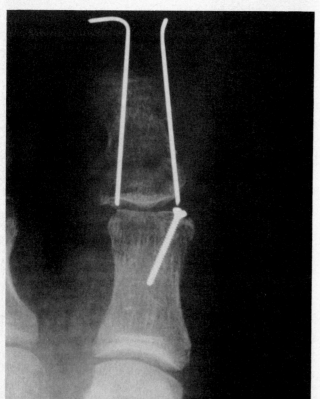

Figure 8.60.   Comminuted fracture of distal phalanx was best fixated with two Kirschner wires and fracture of proximal phalanx was well reduced with minifragment screw.

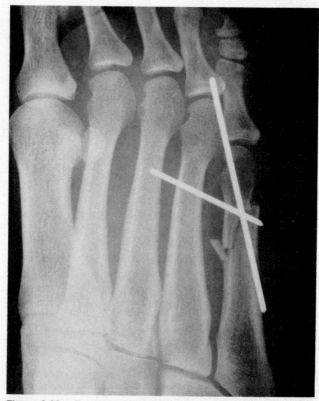

Figure 8.62.   Fracture of fifth metatarsal was fixated with crossed Kirschner wires and fragment separation and distraction can be seen.

Cerclage Wire Fixation and Intraosseous Wire Loop Techniques

The use of wire sutures for the fixation of osteotomies and fractures has been popular in surgery of the foot and ankle for many years. Whereas many applications have been relatively successful, there has been little application of sound mechanical principles to the techniques of internal fixation using wire suture and cerclage techniques. The classic use of wire loops in podiatric surgery has involved the dorsal loop technique for the abductory base wedge osteotomies of the first metatarsal, dorsiflexion osteotomies of the lesser metatarsals, and a dorsomedial loop for the Akin osteotomy (48, 56, 57). Although these techniques appear to provide adequate apposition of the osteotomy surfaces, they in fact add little strength to the fixation of the osteotomy (Fig. 8.63). The principles of mechanically sound fixation by the use of cerclage wire and wire loop techniques are relatively simple and straightforward. A working knowledge of these principles will enable the surgeon to apply rigid internal fixation with Kirschner wires and cerclage wiring that can rival that of the AO system (47).

The dorsal loop technique, when compared to a variety of intraosseous loop and Kirschner wire techniques, was consistently found to be the weakest form of internal fixation (47). The fixation suture applied to only one cortex offered little resistance to the disruption of experimental osteotomies. Dorsiflexion was literally unrestricted by the dorsal loop because the disrupting force created gaping at the plantar aspect of the osteotomy and compression at the dorsal aspect. The dorsal loop had no effect on the plantar aspect of the osteotomized segment and the stability of the fixation was literally dependent on the strength of the intact cortex alone (Fig. 8.64). The dorsal loop would offer resistance to the forces of plantarflexion of the distal segment; however, these forces are not naturally encountered in the postoperative management of metatarsal osteotomies. The dorsal loop technique for osteotomies of the metatarsals may provide maintenance of apposition of the osteotomy surfaces but offers little more to the stability of the reduction against disrupting forces. Weight bearing can be considered a significant risk to the stability of an osteotomy or fracture fixated by a single cortex fixation or dorsal loop technique (Fig. 8.65).

The most stable forms of wire suture fixation were accomplished with the use of intraosseous wire loop techniques (47). The basic configuration of this type of fixation involves the purchase of two cortices on each side of the osteotomy or fracture with the mattress type wire loop. The plane of the loop should be oriented perpendicular to the plane of the osteotomy and can be performed in a relatively vertical or horizontal configuration. Regardless of the orientation of the loop, the central location and the fact that the loop engages both cortices on opposite sides of the osseous segment produces a fixation technique that resists bending in all directions (Fig. 8.66). A horizontal loop will resist both dorsiflexion and plantarflexion as the bending force in either direction is resisted by the central horizontal loop (tension band). Compression is created at the dorsal cortex with dorsiflexion of the distal segment and at the plantar cortex with plantarflexion. An intact lateral hinge would be encircled and protected by this horizontal configuration.

A vertical or sagittal loop would similarly resist dorsiflexion and plantarflexion because the wire loop itself would resist separation of the opposed surfaces of the dorsal and plantar cortices.

The most secure fixation is actually accomplished by the combination of two loops in a 90° orientation to each other (47, 52).

The first and fifth metatarsals are amenable to a true sagittal and transverse plane relationship. The internal lesser metatarsals, however, may be fixated

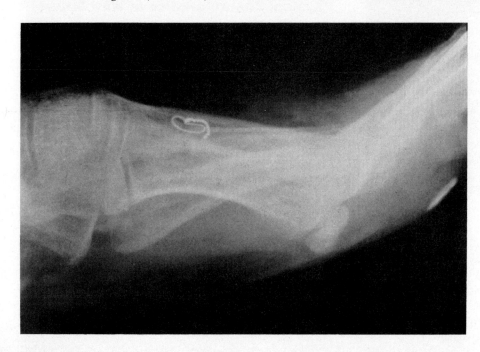

Figure 8.63. Classical use of dorsal wire loop as fixation of base wedge osteotomy.

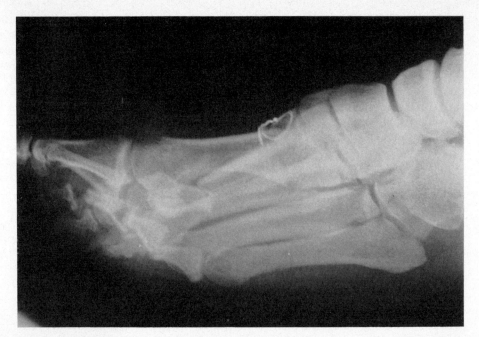

Figure 8.64. Dorsiflexion with weight bearing is unrestricted and result is fractured hinge with gaping of osteotomy.

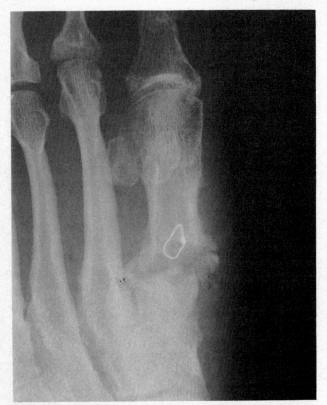

Figure 8.65. Significant bone destruction can take place with fractured osteotomy if patient is allowed to bear weight on unstable osteotomy.

by a 45° rotation of the fixation complex to create a dorsomedial to plantar-lateral orientation of one loop and a dorsolateral to plantar-medial orientation of the second loop.

A very important relationship must be kept in mind when considering this type of fixation, that being the requirement of a relatively transverse osteotomy

or fracture. This type of fixation is quite applicable to many of the elective osteotomies performed on the metatarsals.

FAILURE OF WIRE LOOP FIXATION

As with the development of the AO concepts, the secret to successful techniques of internal fixation is an understanding of the reasons for the failure of internal fixation. There are several important features of wire fixation techniques that can significantly add to the level of success. The two most common reasons for the failure of wire loop fixation are fracture of the wire and failure of the bone, with the wire loop pulling through the bone substance.

Physical Characteristics of Wire Suture

The physical properties of wire suture can add to the success of an internal fixation or they can cause its failure. The first basic consideration is the gauge of the wire suture. Smaller gauge wire (e.g. 30) is more flexible and easier to maneuver and manipulate. The smaller gauge wire, however, is proportionately weaker and is easily fractured with tightening of the loop and tension on the suture. Thicker gauge wire (20 to 22) is extremely strong but relatively stiff and difficult to bend and maneuver in and around delicate osteotomies and bone. If a wire loop can be made with a relatively thick and strong wire suture, failure of the fixation can still occur with tightening of the wire loop. The stronger wire can actually cut through the cortex of the osseous fragments with the simple tightening of the wire loop (Fig. 8.67).

The strength of the fixation can also be influenced by the gauge of the wire in another perspective. The thinner wire has a smaller surface area of contact with bone substance and therefore has a finer cutting edge. Thicker wire has a greater surface area of contact and

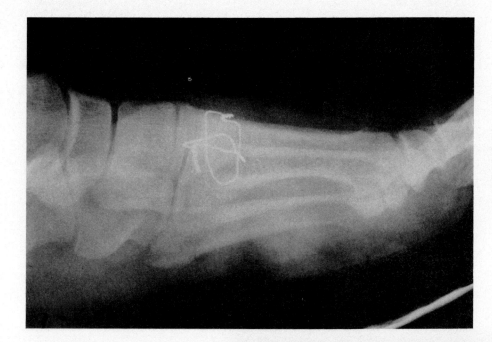

Figure 8.66. Ninety degree orientation of stainless steel wire fixation of base wedge osteotomy can provide stable, rigid fixation. Hinge concept for closing base wedge osteotomy was used to prevent elevatus of first metatarsal.

Figure 8.67. Care must be taken when tightening cerclage fixation. In this case 90–100° stainless steel wire fixation was used to fixate base wedge osteotomy and sagittal plane wire has been pulled through plantar cortex.

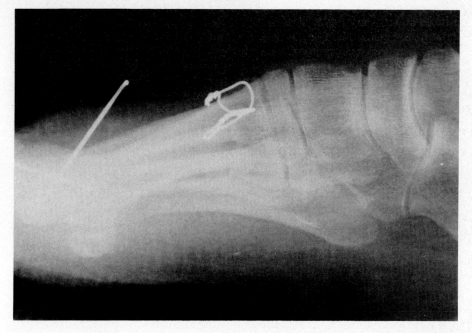

is duller and less likely to cut through bone in similar circumstances.

There is a fine balance between strength of the fixation wire and the malleability of the wire that enables ease of insertion. Each particular situation will dictate the specific gauge of wire that will provide the best fixation. The quality of bone and the mechanical requirements of the insertion technique must be considered when selecting the appropriate wire suture. In the authors' experience 20–22 gauge wire is more appropriate for thicker cortical bone and the tension band techniques employed in the repair of malleolar fractures. A 24 to 26 gauge wire adds strength and is still flexible enough to be successfully employed in osteotomies of the first metatarsal base.

The thinner 26 to 28 gauge wire is better suited for the smaller lesser metatarsals and phalanges. Thirty gauge wire is relatively thin and usually indicated in extremely delicate situations.

In general the thicker and stronger wire creates a stronger fixation. A basic rule would recommend the use of the thickest wire suture that could be successfully manipulated and secured without disrupting the fracture or osteotomy or cutting through the cortices when tightened.

Failure of wire loop fixation can also be related to the instrumentation and handling of the wire suture during insertion. Wire suture maintains its strength relatively well with bending in one direction. Repeated bending of the wire in opposite directions significantly

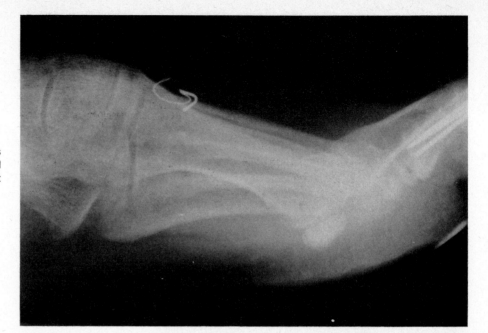

Figure 8.68. Fracture of wire fixation is usually caused by repeated bending and manipulation, producing stress riser that progresses to fixation failure.

weakens the wire and can readily lead to fatigue fracture (58).

One of the most common causes for fracture of the wire suture on stress is a nick or cut in the wire caused by instrumentation (58). This defect acts as a stress riser and is readily propagated into complete failure and fracture of the wire as the wire is stressed with tightening at insertion or tension of functional loading (Fig. 8.68).

The wire loop should always be secured and tightened with a twisting technique (59). This technique places a one-directional bend in the wire and is the most secure form of tying a wire suture. Surgical knots are strongly contraindicated for securing a wire suture. The site of the knot is consistently the site of failure.

Tightening and securing a wire loop are delicate maneuvers that require a significant degree of feel or tactile perception of the strain being applied to the wire. The use of instruments that are excessively large and heavy will significantly decrease the surgeon's ability to appreciate the forces that are being applied to the wire suture. The wire can be easily fractured or even pulled through the bone if heavy instruments are used.

CERCLAGE WIRE TECHNIQUES

The technique of cerclage or encircling long oblique fractures to afford internal fixation has been performed from the initial attempts at the surgical management of fractures. The technique, however, has been tainted with a poor reputation. The technique of cerclage has been credited with a relatively high rate of failure because of the conception that the cerclage technique actually strangled the distal tips of the fracture fragments (10). This concept has been questioned by Boehler (60) and Mears (1,) who suggest that the cause of nonunion associated with cerclage

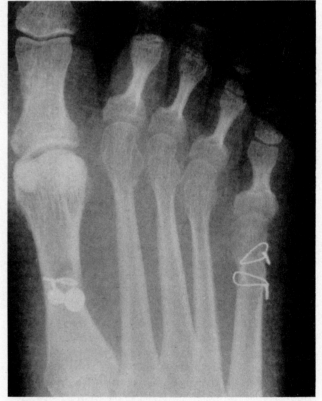

Figure 8.69. Cerclage wiring was used to salvage fractured fifth metatarsal osteotomy.

techniques is more likely caused by excessive and indiscriminate stripping of periosteum and soft tissue blood supply to the bone fragments.

Excessively traumatic soft tissue technique with loss of periosteum can obviously deprive fracture fragments of their vital blood supply. A deliberate and exacting technique, however, can maintain the periosteum as an intact layer that can be reapproximated to

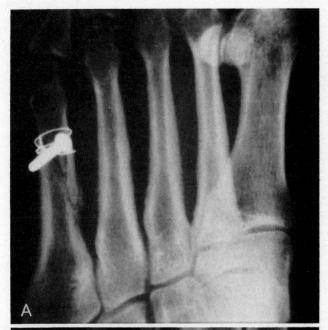

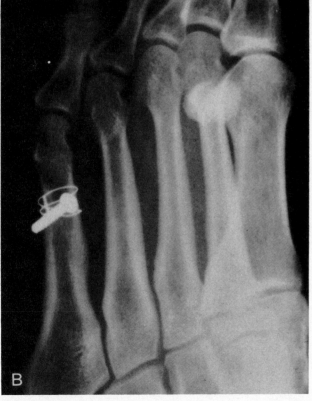

Figure 8.70. (A) Cerclage wire fixation was used in combination with cortical bone screw to reduce fifth metatarsal fracture. (B) Six weeks posttrauma the fracture has healed.

the bone surface and provide direct revascularization of fracture or osteotomy fragments.

Cerclage techniques also may have been doomed to failure from a mechanical standpoint. Although the mechanical effectiveness of the cerclage technique is appreciated in its ease of application and immediate reduction of fracture fragments, especially in long oblique fractures, the mechanical strength of the technique may not be adequate to resist the loading forces that are inherent in the relatively unstable type of

fracture in which it has been commonly employed (Fig. 8.69).

The basic premises of consistent and successful fracture healing described by the AO group require maintenance of vascular supply and the application of stable rigid fixation (4). The cerclage technique is more logically associated with complications because of the disruption of blood supply by shredding of periosteal tissues and the mechanical weaknesses of the technique. Certain cerclage applications simply

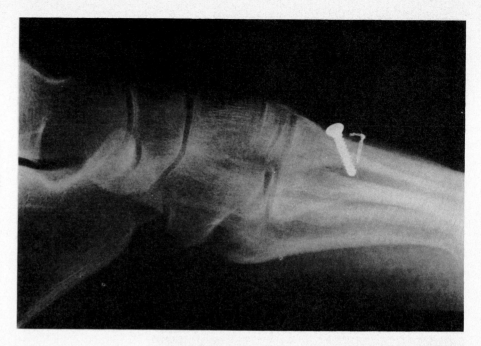

Figure 8.71. Elevating osteotomy of second metatarsal was initially fixated with cortical bone screw. Cortex was fractured and single cerclage wire loop was used for additional strength.

may not be strong enough to maintain rigid fixation of the fracture fragments when the fracture is subjected to functional loading.

Cerclage techniques, however, have been successfully employed when meticulous dissection technique has maintained vascular supply to the fracture fragments and when the strength of the fixation was adequate to withstand the disrupting forces of the stable fixation. Cerclage wiring may be used successfully in combination with other techniques such as splintage or even with interfragmental compression with screws and plates (Figs. 8.70 A, B, and 8.71).

References

1. Mears D: Introduction. *Materials and Orthopaedic Surgery.* Baltimore, Williams & Wilkins, 1979, pp 6–319.
2. Danis R: *Theorie et Pratique de l'Osteosyntheses.* Paris, Masson & Cie, 1947, p 9.
3. Muller M, Allgower M, Willinegger H: *Techniques of Internal Fixation of Fractures.* Berlin, Springer-Verlag, 1965, p 3.
4. Muller M, Allgower M, Willenegger H: *Manual of Internal Fixation.* New York, Springer-Verlag, 1979, pp 1–289.
5. Willenegger H: Medical and scientific directives. In Sequin F, Texhammer R (eds): *AO/ASIF Instrumentation, Manual of Use and Care.* New York, Springer-Verlag, 1981, pp 1–168.
6. Mears D: *Materials and Orthopaedic Surgery.* Baltimore, Williams & Wilkins, 1979, pp 2–160.
7. Schenk R, Willenegger: Zur histologie der primaren knochen neilung. *Langenbecks Arch Chir* 308, 440, 452, 1964.
8. Schenk R. Willenegger H: Morphological findings in primary fracture healing. *Symp Biol Hung* 7:75–86, 1967.
9. Perren S. Matter P, Ruedi T, Allgower M: Biomechanics of fracture healing after internal fixation. In Nyhus LM (ed): *Surgery Annals.* New York, Appleton-Century Crofts, 1975, p 361.
10. Charnley J: Conservative versus operative methods. In *The Closed Treatment of Common Fractures.* London, Churchill Livingstone, 1974, pp 3–50.
11. Elkouri E: Review of cancellous and cortical bone healing after fracture or osteotomy. *J Am Podiatry Assoc* 72:464–466, 1982.
12. Rhinelander F, Baragry R: Microangiography in bone healing in undisplaced closed fractures. *J Bone Joint Surg* 44A:1273–1298, 1962.
13. Uhtoff H, Rahn B: Healing patterns of metaphyseal fractures. *Clin Orthop* 160:295–303, 1981.
14. Rhinelander F: The normal microcirculation of diaphyseal cortex and its response to fracture. *J Bone Joint Surg* 50A:784–800, 1968.
15. Healing and repair of bone. In Peacock E: *Wound Repair.* Philadelphia, WB Saunders Co, 1984, pp 398–402.
16. Bryant W: Wound healing. *Clin Symp* 29:23–26, 1977.
17. Rhinelander F: Vascular proliferation and blood supply during fracture healing. In Uhthoff H, Stahl E (eds): *Current Concepts of Internal Fixation of Fractures.* Berlin, Springer-Verlag, 1980, p 9.
18. Rhinelander F, Phillips R: Microangiography in bone healing II. Displaced closed fractures. *J Bone Joint Surg* 50A:643–662, 1968.
19. Bassett C, Herrman I: Influence of oxygen concentration and mechanical factors on differentiation of connective tissue in vitro. *Nature* 190:400, 1961.
20. Rhinelander F, Baragry R: Microangiography in bone healing. *J Bone Joint Surg* 44A:1273–1298, 1962.
21. Bagby G, Janes J: The effect of compression on the rate of fracture healing using a special plate. *Am J Surg* 95:761–771, 1958.
22. Perren S, Cordey J: The concept of interfragmentary strain. In Uhthoff K, Stahl E (eds): *Current Concepts of Internal Fixation of Fractures.* Berlin, Springer-Verlag, 1980, pp 63–77.
23. Schenk R: *Histology of Fracture Repair and Non-Union.* Bern, Switzerland, Buchdruck-Offset, 1978, pp 14–28.
24. Jimenez AL: Technical principles and management of bone grafts. In Schlefman B (ed): *Doctors Hospital Podiatry Institute Seminar Manual.* Atlanta, GA, 1982, pp 62–65.
25. Rittman W, Perren S, Allgower M, Kayser F, Breunwald J: *Cortical Bone Healing After Internal Fixation and Infection.* Berlin, Springer-Verlag, 1974, p 70.
26. Jassen MR: Primary bone healing vs callus bone healing. In Schlefman B (ed): *Doctors Hospital Podiatry Institute Seminar Manual.* Atlanta, GA, 1982, pp 15–20.
27. Reynolds F, Key J: Fracture healing after fixation with standard plates, contact splints and medullary nails. *J Bone Joint Surg* 36A:577–587, 1954.
28. Yasuda I: Fundamental aspects of fracture treatment. *Clin Orthop* 124:5–19, 1977.
29. Ruch JA: First metatarsal osteotomies in the treatment of

hallux abducto valgus. Rigid internal fixation techniques. Results and complications. In Schlefman B (ed): *Doctors Hospital Podiatry Institute Seminar Manual*. Atlanta, GA, 1982, pp 89–99.

30. Fenton CF: Arthrodesis of the hallux interphalangeal joint. In Schlefman B (ed): *Doctors Hospital Podiatry Institute Seminar Manual*. Atlanta, GA, 1982, pp 105–110.

31. Downey MS, Kalish S: Clinical tips on AO fixation. In McGlamry ED, McGlamry R (Eds): *Doctors Hospital Podiatry Institute Seminar Manual*. Atlanta, GA, 1985, pp 150–154.

32. Ruch JR: Muscle tendon balance and first metatarsal osteotomy for hallux valgus repair. In McGlamry ED, McGlamry R (eds): *Doctors Hospital Podiatry Institute Seminar Manual*. Atlanta, GA, 1984, pp 11–22.

33. Ruch JR: Rigid internal fixation in triple arthrodesis. In McGlamry ED, McGlamry R (eds): *Doctors Hospital Podiatry Institute Seminar Manual*. Atlanta, GA, 1984, pp 45–48.

34. Perren S, Cordey J: Mechanics of interfragmentary compression by plates and screws. In Uhthoff H, Stahl E (eds): *Current Concepts of Internal Fixation of Fractures*. Berlin, Springer-Verlag, 1980, pp 184–191.

35. Gotzen L, Hutter K. Haas N: The prebending of AO plates in compression osteosynthesis. In Uhthoff M, Stahl E (eds): *Current Concepts of Internal Fixation of Fractures*. Berlin, Springer-Verlag, 1980, pp 201–210.

36. Allgower M, Matter P, Perren S, Ruedi T: *The Dynamic Compression-Plate DCP*. Berlin, Springer-Verlag, 1978, pp 1–32.

37. Matter P, Brennwald J, Perren S: *The Effect of Static Compression and Tension on Internal Remodelling of Cortical Bone*. Basel, Switzerland, Schwabe & Co, 1975, p 42.

38. Perren S, Cordey J: The concept of interfragmentary strain. In Uhtoff M, Stahl E (eds): *Current Concepts of Internal Fixation of Fractures*. Berlin, Springer-Verlag, 1980, p 75.

39. Pauwels F: *Der Schenkelhalsbruch, em Mechanisches Problem*. Stuttgart, Enke, 1935, p 25.

40. Ruch JR: Principles of AO and the tension band concept. In McGlamry ED, McGlamry R (eds): *Doctors Hospital Podiatry Institute Seminar Manual*. Atlanta, GA, 1985, pp 129–135.

41. Vogler HW: Basic bioengineering concepts. *Clin Podiatry* 2:161–190, 1985.

42. Laurich L, Witt C, Zielsdorf L: Treatment of fractures of the fifth metatarsal bone. *J Am Podiatry Assoc* 22:207–211, 1983.

43. Maxwell JR: Open reduction of lesser metatarsal fractures. Indications and techniques. In Schlefman B (ed): *Doctors Hospital Podiatry Institute Seminar Manual*. Atlanta, GA, 1982, pp 25–26.

44. Yu GV: Iatrogenic complications of first metatarsal osteotomies. In Schlefman B (ed): *Doctors Hospital Podiatry Institute Seminar Manual*. Atlanta, GA, 1983, pp 1–5.

45. Ruch JR: Principles of closed reduction and the conservative management of fractures. In McGlamry ED, McGlamry R (eds): *Doctors Hospital Podiatry Institute Seminar Manual*. Atlanta, GA, 1985, pp 189–193.

46. Heim U, Pfeiffer K: *Small Fragment Set Manual*. New York, Springer-Verlag, 1974, pp 1–42.

47. Vanik R, Weber R, Matloub M, Sanger J, Gingrass R: The comparative strengths of internal fixation techniques. *J Hand Surg* 9A:216–221, 1984.

48. Fyfe I, Mason S: The mechanical stability of internal fixation of fractured phalanges. *Hand* 11:50–54, 1979.

49. Green D: The hazards of internal fixation in podiatry. *Clin Podiatry* 2:95–119, 1985.

50. Massengill J, Alexander H, Parson J, Schecter M: Mechanical analysis of Kirschner wire fixation in a phalangeal model. *J Hand Surg* 4:351–356, 1979.

51. Gingrass R, Fehring B, Matloub H: Intraosseous wiring of complex hand fractures. *Plast Reconstr Surg* 66:383–394, 1980.

52. Cavaliere RG, Ruch JR: Fixation of first metatarsal osteotomies. In McGlamry ED, McGlamry R (eds): *Doctors Hospital Podiatry Institute Seminar Manual*. Atlanta, GA, 1985, pp 136–139.

53. Yu GV, Ruch JR: A new approach to the tailor's bunion deformity (intramedullary nailing). In Schlefman B (ed): *Doctors Hospital Podiatry Institute Seminar Manual*. Atlanta, GA, 1983, pp 84–89.

54. Cain T: Fixation of fifth metatarsal osteotomies. In McGlamry ED, McGlamry R (eds): *Doctors Hospital Podiatry Institute Seminar Manual*. Atlanta, GA, 1985, pp 140–142.

55. Marcinko DE: Modified tension band technique in forefoot surgery. In McGlamry ED, McGlamry R (eds): *Doctors Hospital Podiatry Institute Seminar Manual*. Atlanta, GA, 1985, pp 143–146.

56. Sgarlato T: *A Compendium of Podiatric Biomechanics*. San Francisco, California College of Podiatric Medicine, 1971, p 408.

57. Gerbert J, Melillo T: A modified Akin procedure for the correction of hallux valgus. *J Am Podiatry Assoc* 61:132, 1971.

58. Oh I, Sander T, Treharne R: The fatigue resistance of orthopaedic wire. *Clin Orthop* 192:228–236, 1985.

59. Estersohn H, Stanoch J: A simplified technique for internal wire fixation. *J Am Podiatry Assoc* 73:593–597, 1983.

60. Buhler J:Percutaneous cerclage of tibial fractures. *Clin Orthop* 105:276–282, 1974.

Additional References

Brighton C: Editorial comment, bioelectrical effects on bone and-cartilage. *Clin Orthop* 124:2–4, 1977.

DiGiovanni J, Martin R: Pins, wires and staples in foot surgery. *Clin Podiatry* 1:211–223, 1984.

Duke H, Walter J: External fixation in hallux abducto valgus surgery. *J Am Podiatry Assoc* 72:443–447, 1982.

Floyd E, Perrillo J, Dailey J: The scaphoid compression staple: an effective form of fixation. *J Foot Surg* 23:56–59, 1984.

Friedenberg Z, French G: The effects of known compression forces on fracture healing. *Surg Gynecol Obstet* 94:743–748, 1952.

Gerbert J: Digital arthrodesis. *Clin Podiatry* 2:81–94, 1985.

Ginsburg A: Arthrodesis of the first metatarsophalangel joint. *J Am Podiatry Assoc* 69:367–369, 1979.

Green D: The hazards of internal fixation in podiatry. *Clin Podiatry* 2:95–120, 1985.

Green D, Anderson J: Closed reduction and percutaneous pin fixation of fractured phalanges. *J Bone Joint Surg* 55A:1651–1654, 1973.

Gumann G, Engle A, Snowdy H: Comminuted intra-articular fracture of the first metatarsal base. *J Am Podiatry Assoc* 72:521–524, 1982.

Jacobs A, Oloff L: Podiatric metallurgy and the effects of implanted metals on living tissues. *Clin Podiatry* 2:121–142, 1985.

Jolly G, Novicki D: Treatment of delayed union of a fifth metatarsal by compression osteosynthesis. *J Am Podiatry Assoc* 70:449–453, 1980.

Lister G: Intraosseous wiring of the digital skeleton. *J Hand Surg* 3:427–435, 1978.

Mahan K: Electrical stimulation of bone. *J Am Podiatry Assoc* 73:86–92, 1983.

Maxwell J: Open or closed treatment of metatarsal fractures. *J Am Podiatry Assoc* 73:100–106, 1983.

Ognibene F, Siegel R, Galorenzo R, Sharon S, Gensheimer R: The utilization of the Richards scaphoid compression device in performing abductory base wedge osteotomies. *J Foot Surg* 21:247–249, 1982.

Rahn B, Gallinaro P, Baltensperger A, Perren S: Primary bone healing. *J Bone Joint Surg* 53A:783–786, 1971.

Schatzker J, Horne J, Sumner-Smith G: The reaction of cortical bone to compression by screw threads. *Clin Orthop* 111:263–265, 1975.

Smith G, Green A: Cerclage wiring of metatarsal fractures. *J Am Podiatry Assoc* 73:25–26, 1983.

Smith T: Bone graft physiology. *J Am Podiatry Assoc* 73:70–74, 1983.

Vogler H: Ankle arthrodesis. *Clin Podiatry* 2:59–80, 1985.

Walter J, Pressman M: External fixation in the treatment of metatarsal non-unions. *J Am Podiatry Assoc* 71:297–301, 1981.

CHAPTER 9

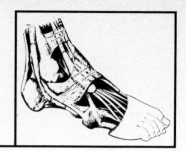

Postoperative Management

Stephen J. Miller, D.P.M.

THE IMMEDIATE POSTOPERATIVE PHASE

During the first three to five days following surgical intervention the body becomes engaged in a clean-up process at the operative site to remove debris, increase oxygen tension, and establish an environmental homeostasis amenable to tissue repair. The principle process is inflammation (Fig. 9.1). Hence this preparatory period is known as the inflammatory, substrate, or lag phase of healing. Whatever the surgeon does to assist the wound through this process will indeed optimize healing and minimize complications.

Management is aimed primarily at avoiding hematoma formation, excess edema, and infection while attempting to keep the patient comfortable and protect the surgical site. There must be an awareness of signs of impending complications so that a high index of suspicion will trigger prompt and decisive action appropriate to the situation.

Postoperative management begins with an organized set of considerations. In the hospital setting these are written as orders. They must be tailored to the individual patient but a good way to remember the major points is by using the acronym, SPADE (signs, sleep, pain, ambulation, diet, drainage, elevation, emesis, elimination).

These considerations regarding patient care are usually written as orders in the hospital, but the acronym can be used to cover the office setting as well.

S—Signs. Vital signs should be monitored immediately postoperatively, then every 15 minutes until the patient is stable.
S—Sleep. There should be a standby medication ordered for sleep.
P—Pain. Two types of pain medication should be ordered: a parenteral drug or cocktail for severe pain and an oral medication for moderate pain.
A—Ambulation. The surgeon must make very clear to the patient or in the hospital orders the limitations of activity. "Absolute bed rest" means no weight-bearing or bathroom privileges.
D—Diet. Gradual resumption to regular eating habits starts with clear fluids. Special diets as for diabetics should be ordered specifically.
D—Drainage. If drains are used, orders should be clear as to the removal of fluids and the change of suction devices.
E—Elevation. Immediate elevation of the extremity postoperatively is essential to prevent increased hemodynamic pressure and edema.
E—Emesis. Orders for antiemetic medication are important, especially following general anesthesia.
E—Elimination. Methods for waste removal should be clear. Catheterization, bathroom privileges, or bedside commode are examples.

Whether in the office or the hospital, management should be conducted by means of systematic patient evaluation. This is best done using the problem-oriented record (POR) approach that keeps the physician organized with the challenge to assess the findings and implement a plan. The progress note is first identified by number of the postoperative day to keep in perspective the time lapse since surgery.

Subjective findings are those described by the patient. They should be described in the patient's own words.

Objective findings are the observations of the surgeon.

Especially important are digital edema (indicating congestion caused by proximal swelling), color, temperature, sensation, and drainage. Also important are systemic indicators such as vital signs. Results of laboratory tests and radiographs should be noted, as well as the heart and lung status and any other pertinent information. The *assessment* is a statement or diagnosis based on the findings. It is a critical analysis that will help direct a course of action. Finally, the *plan* consists of any immediate treatment or investigation plus proposed future actions for patient care.

Postoperative Dressing

Surgery is never complete at final wound closure. The foot is a dependent end organ of an extremity with a rather awkward shape that requires very special dressing considerations.

A wound dressing has several functions, the goals

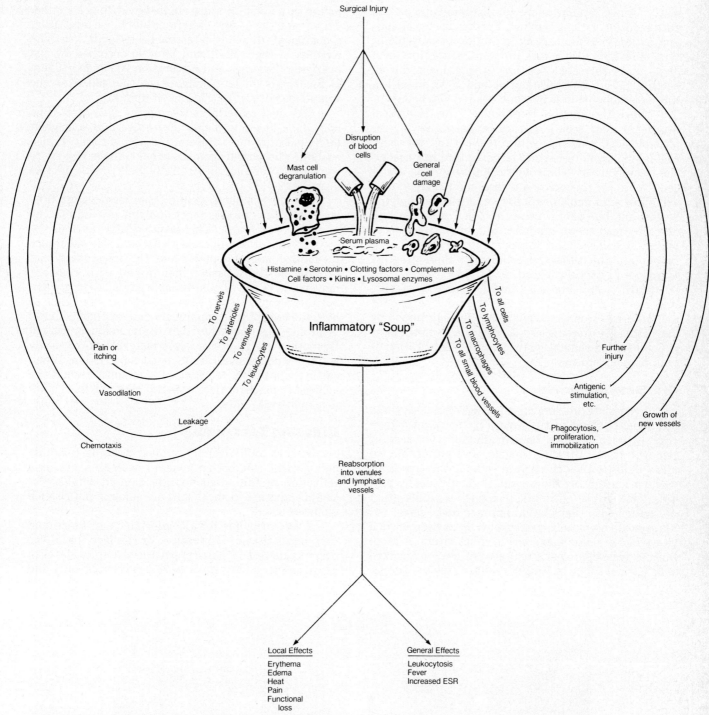

Surgical Injury

Disruption of blood cells

Mast cell degranulation

General cell damage

Serum plasma

Histamine • Serotonin • Clotting factors • Complement
Cell factors • Kinins • Lysosomal enzymes

Inflammatory "Soup"

To nerves
To arterioles
To venules
To leukocytes

To all cells
To lymphocytes
To macrophages
To small blood vessels

Pain or itching

Vasodilation

Leakage

Chemotaxis

Further injury

Antigenic stimulation, etc.

Growth of new vessels

Phagocytosis, proliferation, immobilization

Reabsorption into venules and lymphatic vessels

Local Effects

Erythema
Edema
Heat
Pain
Functional loss

General Effects

Leukocytosis
Fever
Increased ESR

Figure 9.1. Summary diagram of principle mechanisms involved in inflammatory reaction (Modified from Ryan GB, Majno G: *Inflamma-* *tion*. Kalamazoo, MI, The Upjohn Company, 1977, p 77.)

of which are to provide an optimum environment for healing and to maximize the body's ability to complete the task. It must first protect the wound from contamination and trauma. If possible it should provide antisepsis to prevent overgrowth or penetrance of pathogens. The second function is absorption. The dressing thus serves as a passageway to draw the fluids away from the wound and thereby prevent their accumulation, as well as tissue maceration, both of which

inhibit healing. It must avoid occlusion of the wound and leave a physiological environment for healing. By the combination of its capillary action and the entwining of protein and necrotic debris within its mesh, a dressing will provide a third function, that of wound debridement at the time of dressing change.

A dressing must provide temporary immobilization. This simply places a wound at rest allowing healing to take place without interference. Clots and newly formed capillaries are not disrupted and pain is decreased for patient comfort. Further bacterial contamination is minimized by limitation of movement. Immobilization also serves to maintain the foot or a digit in its corrected position or alignment during healing. Scar tissue can then be laid down in such a way as to support that new and desired alignment.

The fifth function is pressure. This is critical because it must seek a balance between allowing for physiological swelling while preventing excessive edema and avoiding further bleeding into the tissues. The technique of "controlled compression" is applicable here. By this method a dressing is applied that will allow a limited amount of swelling while applying a constant but gentle pressure. Such pressure will decrease dead space, minimize fluid and debris accumulation, and slow the transudation and exudation of fluids into the tissues. Healing can then progress unimpeded by local congestion.

Sixth, a dressing is a valuable source of specific information about the underlying wound. The amount and nature of wound secretions can be determined by inspecting the dressing as it is removed. Even the odor is important, a valuable clue for early identification of an infectious process.

Dressing Materials

A complete dressing must consist of at least three components. Next to the wound is the *contact layer* (Fig. 9.2) which must be nonadherent, for ease of removal at the dressing change, and permeable, to allow fluids to pass through into the absorptive layer without macerating the wound. It should ideally provide some sort of antiseptic to limit the proliferation of pathogens. Petrolatum-impregnated gauze or moistened Owen's silk soaked with an antiseptic such as povidone-iodine make nice contact layers. A more physiological approach is to use a gauze sponge soaked with normal saline or Ringer's solution and povidone-

iodine in a 50:50 mixture applied next to the wound. This draws the oozing secretions and blood away from the surgical site while deterring bacterial growth. The wetness is then dissipated as it is absorbed by the overlying dressings and maceration is avoided. There is amazingly little adherence of the gauze to the wound, as noticed at the time of removal.

The next material is the *intermediate layer* (Fig. 9.3). This must be highly absorptive and somewhat bulky material for storage of the wound fluids. It also cushions the wound against further trauma. Dry gauze sponges in lamination or fluffy bulk make up this layer.

Finally, the outer wrap or *compressive layer* (Fig. 9.4) binds the dressing together while providing some measure of pressure. This layer requires various degrees of conformability, elasticity, and self-adherence to control swelling and avoid the telescoping and slipping of the dressing that occurs with constant movement. A roll of conformable gauze, with or without interwoven elastic fibers, should be used first to hold the assembled components and anatomical parts in proper position. If further compression is desired then other layers of elasticized material can be gently applied, with special care to avoid constriction. When casting, however, elasticized materals should be avoided and appropriate pressure obtained from comformable gauze only.

Dressing Techniques

A neat and carefully applied dressing not only aids patient comfort and wound healing; it also is a reflection of the surgeon's attention to details. Patients and other medical staff are quick to notice such qualities.

A key principle for a comfortable and functional dressing is that of lamination, or the layering of the dressing materials, particularly the absorptive layer of gauze sponges. This must be done systematically and

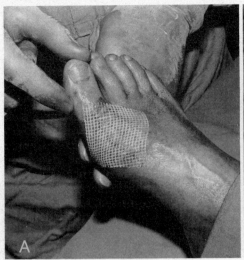 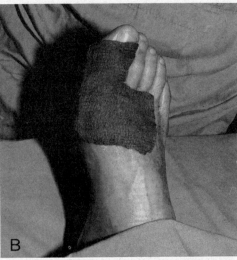

Figure 9.2.   Contact layer of dressing. (A) Petrolatum gauze with wide mesh impregnated with chlorhexidine gluconate. (B) Gauze sponge soak with 50:50 mixture of povidone-iodine solution and normal saline.

smoothly to avoid lumps or wrinkles that will concentrate pressure points causing pain and tissue ischemia.

Fluffed-up gauze can be applied in a bulky wad and then compressed over a wound where much swelling is anticipated. Another bulky dressing consists of wrapping the foot and leg in a roll of sterile cotton wadding and then compressing it with elastic bandages.

Dressing toes after nail surgery requires the all

important contact layer of impregnated gauze to prevent adherence balanced delicately with circumferential material that must provide elastic compression without constriction. The greatest danger is pressure ischemia. This is more noticeable in young people whose arteries are not firm enough to resist compression.

Dressing toes following corrective digital or hallux valgus surgery requires both technical skill and manual dexterity. Part of the absorptive layer may be used as a splint, either plain or, with the Hill modification, soaked in povidone-iodine solution. As the latter dries, a firm splint is formed. These splints may lay along the length of the dorsum of the toe or may encompass it so the tails are anchored plantarly (Fig. 9.5). Wrapping and anchoring digits with rolls of conforming gauze must serve not only to secure the dressing but also to hold each toe in its corrected alignment. The hallux should be rotated in a varus direction to counter the opposite deformity after hallux valgus surgery. The bandage should also plantarflex the great toe slightly. The fifth toe is usually wrapped so as to rotate it out of the varus position in most procedures, whereas the central three toes are especially secured about the proximal phalanx to draw the toe down into rectus alignment following most hammertoe surgery.

Circumferential dressings are difficult but important because they must supply digital compression to control swelling and hemorrhage without causing prolonged compression. A few practice wraps on one's own digits will provide a good guide to the appropriate amount of compression to use with various elastic materials.

The forefoot itself must be carefully wrapped and must be encircled to do so. The same principles apply

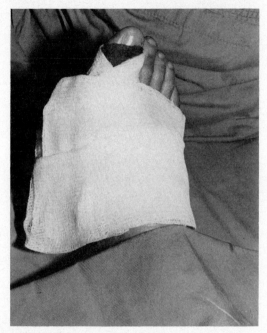

Figure 9.3. Contact layer of dressing. Sponges are applied smoothly for absorption and protection.

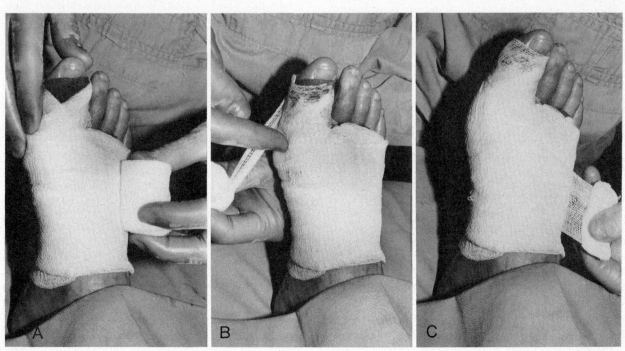

Figure 9.4. Compressive layers following hallux valgus correction. (A) Direction of application is important for derotating hallux. (B) Derotational wraps are anchored below axis of first metatarsophalangeal joint. (C) Dressing is anchored proximally.

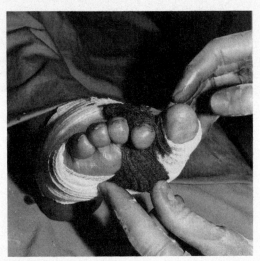

Figure 9.5. Povidone-iodine dressing of toe. As dressing dries it forms firm cast to immobilize toe in desired position.

in this area where layering is especially important to apply compression in all the dells between bony prominences. Keeping the dressing anchored in place so the patient can move about can be challenging. Tape can be quite irritating to the skin when used for many days at a time. Wrapping a nonadherent dressing in a figure-of-eight configuration about the ankle will solve this problem and will keep a forefoot dressing securely in place through much activity. Bony prominences and the Achilles tendon should be padded and the foot must be kept at right angles to the leg during application. If applied with the foot plantarflexed the dressing will surely bind at the anterior ankle flexure during ambulation. This can lead to pressure necrosis especially when hidden under a cast (Fig. 9.6).

Rearfoot and ankle dressings require special considerations in addition to the ankle flexure. Extensive and intense edema is a common feature of this area following trauma or surgical intervention. The larger anatomy allows for more extensive dead spaces and hence more devastating hematomata formation. With these problems in mind, the principle of "controlled compression" must be instituted.

The softer dressing materials, less apt to constrict, must be used for the initial wraps. Kerlix rolls are very useful here. Then a special compression dressing is applied.

Starting with Cast Padding and alternating with elastic bandages for two to three layers of each constitutes Ruch's modified Jones compression dressing. When plaster stirrup splints are added for further immobilization it becomes a relatively safe "compression cast" (Fig. 9.7). The area is thereby allowed to swell to some degree while constant, even compression resists further expansion and begins to milk the extracellular fluids from the local tissues. Immediate rigid

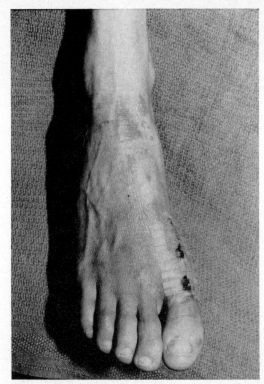

Figure 9.6. Pressure necrosis at anterior ankle flexure caused by binding of dressing during ambulation.

cast application is sometimes dangerous and may cause the patient unnecessary pain, even if cast splitting is anticipated.

Dressings should also protect pins and drains where they exit the skin. There must always be a protective layer between the device and the skin. The exit site should be painted with antiseptic solution at the conclusion of the surgery to minimize bacterial penetration.

Dressing Complications

An ominous sign when managing the postsurgical or posttrauma patient is pain unresponsive to even the strongest of analgesic agents. The most common causes are swelling whose expansion is being restricted, hematoma formation, and early infection. All three are relieved to some degree by releasing the pressure of the dressing and/or the cast.

Dressings should be split on the side opposite the wound. Casts should be split or bivalved to relieve pressure but usually the dressing must be released at the same time to provide relief.

Pressure ischemia is the end result of excess pressure (Fig. 9.8). Lumps or wrinkles in the dressings will cause localized ischemia whereas circumferential constriction results in diminished or absent distal blood supply. Prolonged ischemia will lead to necrosis

Figure 9.7. Compression cast application requires skill and care. (A) Materials required include cotton cast padding tension bandages and plaster splints. (B) First layer is cast padding. (C) Second layer is tension bandage. (D) Third layer is more cotton cast padding. (E) Fourth layer is another tension bandage. Notice criss-cross technique. (F) Fifth layer is cotton padding. (G) Sixth layer is plaster splints. (H) Plaster splints form stirrup. (I) Last layer is tension bandage.

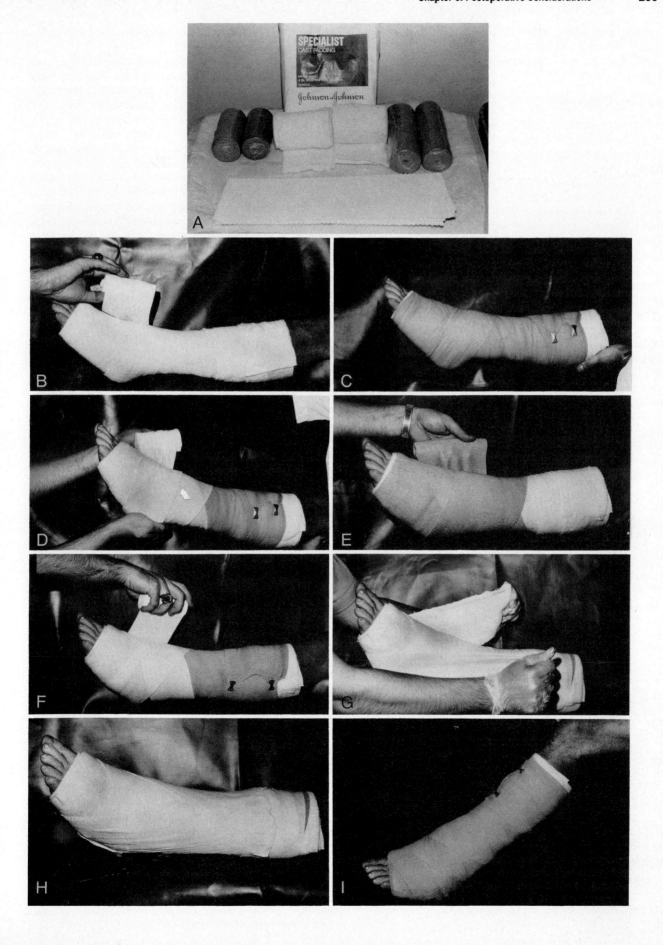

and frank gangrene unless sufficient circulation is promptly restored. Ulcers caused by pressure ischemia are very slow to heal and frustratingly resistant to treatment.

Dressing Change

Timing, technique, and wound evaluation are the key features of the postoperative dressing change. The first redressing for clean surgical cases without complications should usually take place no sooner than three days and no later than one week following the operative procedures, unless a long-term cast is applied at the time of surgery. The inflammatory phase of healing is seldom complete before 72 hours, making an early dressing change painful and biologically disruptive. For more extensive cases, particularly those involving the rearfoot and ankle, three to four days are necessary to allow the resolution of edema. The dressing, which has usually absorbed much blood and other secretions, should be changed before a cast is applied. If such manipulation is too painful for the patient, then a combination of analgesic and anxiolytic can be given before the procedures to make them more tolerable.

Removing the dressing should not be terribly uncomfortable for the patient. Only small, thin dressings should be cut off. The most logical and least disruptive method of removing a dressing is by unwinding it and taking off one layer at a time, simply reversing the method of application. If the contact layer does not come off freely then it should be soaked with hydrogen peroxide or normal saline or a mixture of both and allowed to soften.

Evaluation of the wound is a valuable exercise (Fig. 9.9). It should be done by the surgeon who understands the nature of the procedure performed and the course of events during the surgery. First, the dressing itself should be inspected to observe the character of the secretions and even the odor. Then the wound and surrounding tissues must be examined. Are the wound margins coapted for their entire length? Is there any drainage? In early dressing changes blood and serosanguinous fluids are common. Any drainage after 72 hours should usually be cultured. Are the surrounding tissues erythematous? The majority of inflammation should subside in the first three to five days. After that, redness and warmth may be early signs of infection or unusual tissue damage. How much swelling is present, close to the wound and generally? Localized swelling with unusual tenderness usually signifies the presence of a hematoma, whereas generalized swelling indicates extensive trauma and accompanying interstitial fluid congestion. Finally, the skin should be evaluated for signs of necrosis or dermatitis. Both should be treated promptly and aggressively to prevent further deterioration that would encourage infection.

The redressing consists usually of the same materials as the primary dressing except the contact layer that is needed only on moist or draining wounds. Besides wound protection, its primary functions are splintage for correct alignment and compression. The rules of application remain the same.

Finally, dressings are somewhat useless unless patients are instructed in how to look after them. The best method is to dispense to the patient written postoperative instructions that include information on dressing care (Fig. 9.10).

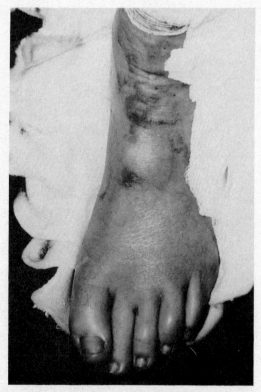

Figure 9.8. Pressure ischemia from overzealous compression bandaging.

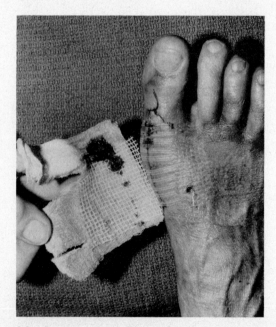

Figure 9.9. Dressing change. Evaluation of both wound and dressing can provide valuable information.

A surgical procedure has just been performed on your foot. The amount of discomfort will vary from one patient to another. The following instructions are for your benefit in order to help minimize swelling and pain and to insure good healing. Please follow them.

1. Go directly home and elevate feet on the way if possible. Do not sit with your feet down or crossed for any length of time. This causes the feet to swell and become painful.
2. A limited amount of swelling is expected. In some cases, the skin may take on a bruised appearance. This is no cause for alarm.
3. Elevate your feet about 6 inches above hip level by supporting feet and legs with pillows.
4. Keep your bandages clean and dry. Do not remove the bandages or inspect the wound. A small amount of blood on the bandage is normal.
5. Cover the foot with a plastic bag and hang outside the tub while bathing. NO SHOWERS!!! A standing sponge bath is acceptable.
6. Exercise your legs frequently by bending your knees and ankles to stimulate circulation and speed healing.
7. At night place a cradle made from a cardboard carton at the foot of the bed to protect your foot from the covers.
8. Take your medicine(s) as directed. If they cause stomach upset, headache, rash or other abnormal reactions, discontinue their use and call the doctor.
9. Crutches or walkers can be helpful at times to take the weight off the foot when walking or standing.
10. Curtail alcoholic beverages and smoking.
11. You should get plenty of rest with the foot elevated, drink plenty of fluids, and eat your regular well-balanced diet.
12. If your bandages become tight and/or your toes become numb, tingling or turn blue, call your doctor.
13. CALL YOUR DOCTOR IMMEDIATELY IF:
    * The bandages become overly stained.
    * Your medication does not stop the discomfort.
    * You should bump or injure your feet.
    * You develop a fever.
14. Your next appointment is _____.

Figure 9.10. Postoperative foot surgery instructions sample.

DRAIN MANAGEMENT

Evacuated fluids should be monitored for both quantity and quality. Samples may be cultured if so desired (Fig. 9.11). When a closed suction drain is no longer functional or no longer removing fluids, its purpose is complete and it should be removed. This usually occurs around the 48 to 72-hour mark (1).

Gravity drains may be left in for longer periods but any tube exiting the skin leaves a portal of entry for pathogens. Other complications include knotting or kinking of the tubing, which may require surgical extirpation (Fig. 9.12A), and pressure against the skin resulting in ischemia and pain (Fig. 9.12B). Under no circumstances should a drain be reinserted if it is accidentally pulled out, nor should any attempts be made to retrograde flush a drain with heparin or other

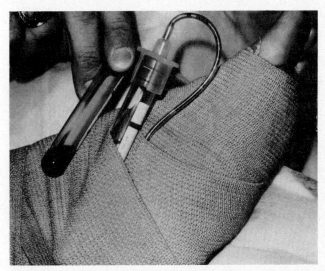

Figure 9.11. Closed suction drain. Evacuated fluids can be monitored for content and cultured if necessary.

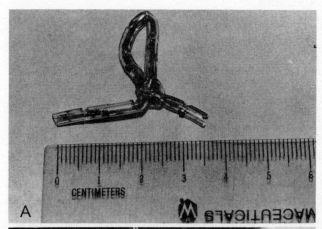

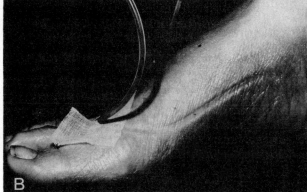

Figure 9.12. Complications of drains. (A) Knotted drain required surgical removal. (B) Pressure ischemia caused by direct pressure from unprotected drain.

fluids. The risk of contaminating a fresh surgical site is too high.

CASTS AND SPLINTS
Principles

The primary function of casts and splints is to provide immobilization so that healing can take place unhindered by motion. It usually applies to the healing of bone where there must be as close to zero motion as possible at the interface of cut bone for the osteons and budding capillaries successfully to bridge the gap.

A secondary function is protection of the wound site from outside trauma and some control of swelling although the latter must be done with caution.

Splinting

A splint is simply an orthosis that provides temporary support of a part. The greatest advantage is that it can be applied over a "controlled compression" dressing that will both allow and control postsurgical edema. It can also be easily removed if range of motion exercises or other physical therapy activities are required. Whether constructed of cast material or prefabricated they provide immobilization, with the biggest drawback being they are sometimes awkward and not always secure.

Casting

Casts provide long-term immobilization while maintaining the extremity and foot in very specific alignment. If a particular position is required, then the cast may be applied at the time of surgery at the risk of having to be split to accommodate swelling. However, it is better applied from three to five days following the surgery, after the wound has been inspected and redressed.

Casts that extend above the knee are necessary for the initial immobilization of some of the more complex foot and ankle surgeries. They are important when flexion and extension motion at the knee will adversely influence lower structures, such as after extensive multijoint surgeries or triceps surgery. Examples are triple arthrodesis, pantalar arthrodesis, and trimalleolar fracture reduction. The mechanism is one of torsional forces acting through the leg. When the knee flexes 15° the leg is unlocked and internally rotates. This force is transmitted along the tibia and fibula to the foot via the ankle, subtalar, and sometimes midtarsal joints. If the foot is locked in a cast and the knee is allowed to bend freely, the torque is taken up by the talus as it is "grasped" by the tibia and fibula. The result is motion interrupting the surrounding arthrodesis or fracture sites. When applying an above knee cast, it is important that the knee be flexed 25° to 35° to prevent rotation. A straight cast tends to use the foot as a lever when the cast rolls and the weight of the cast can thereby displace the ankle or subtalar joint that may have had surgery. With the cast applied above a bent knee the thigh absorbs any rotation that may be transmitted by the torque of cast weight, usually rolling externally. It is also the position of maximum comfort for that joint. At a later date an above knee cast can be reduced to a below knee cast for continuation of some restriction of motion.

Below knee casts are by far the best and most frequently used for immobilization of the foot and ankle. Above ankle casts are tempting but invite the danger of a boot-top leg fracture should the patient fall or stumble. Slipper casts provide only rigidity and limited local immobilization to the foot itself. They allow superstructural influences and are awkward for weight bearing. Casts may be bivalved and then can be reapplied as a removable device should physical therapy be required intermittently. Prefabricated removable below knee casts are also a valuable tool for immobilization interspersed with physical therapy or bathing (Fig. 9.13).

Casting materials range from plaster through resin-impregnated plasters to synthetic materials. Plaster, although distinctly heavier with about a 48-hour drying period, is ideal for positional molding to maintain a desired postsurgical configuration. Resin and plaster combinations are also satisfactory for positional molding (Table 9.1). They have the added advantage of lathering on for a smoother and harder finish providing added durability, which is helpful when casting active children. Finally, various types of synthetic materials are now available for casting (Table 9.2).

The newer synthetic casting materials have advantages and disadvantages that vary somewhat between manufacturers. They usually consist of knitted polyester and cotton substrates (roughly 65% and 35%) or fiberglass substrates impregnated with a unique wateractivated polyurethane resin. A cast made of this material will harden in seven minutes by way of an exothermic reaction once activated with water. Between 15 and 20 minutes later the cast will have achieved maximum strength. Such casts have the advantages of being lightweight, strong, porous, and relatively radiolucent. In addition to their rapid

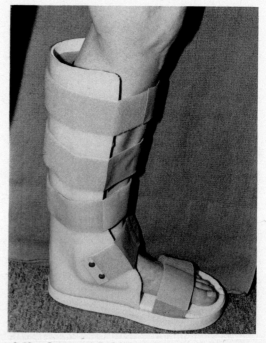

Figure 9.13. Commercially fabricated cast/splint may be removed for physical therapy and bathing.

setting time (once hardened, plaster takes about 48 hours to cure, depending on the ambient humidity) these synthetic materials are resistant to water damage. They are especially useful in treating children and active adults. Older patients appreciate the light weight.

There are disadvantages, however. Synthetic cast material may cost four to six times as much as plaster. The exothermic reaction is somewhat warmer, although less heat is given off if cool water is used for activation. Because the material can be activated simply by the ambient humidity, it has a limited shelf life, even in foil wrappers. The polyurethane resin will adhere strongly to skin when in direct contact so protection is necessary. Lastly, the synthetic tapes do not mold as well as plaster, although some brands are better than others.

The application of any cast requires adherence to several principles. First, the materials should be layered on smoothly without potentially irritating lumps or wrinkles. It should not be "pulled" on so as to cause constriction. Second, all bony prominences must be padded and protected, especially the heel, as well as the neck of the fibula where the common peroneal nerve can be impinged (Fig. 9.14). These two precautions will avoid the most common complications of casting: constriction and localized pressure, which can in turn lead to soft tissue ischemia and peripheral neuropathy. Third, attention must always be paid to the position of the foot in relation to the leg during casting. It should usually be at right angles so as not to cause future binding at the entire flexure. Finally, the toes should be protected, either by a plantar shelf

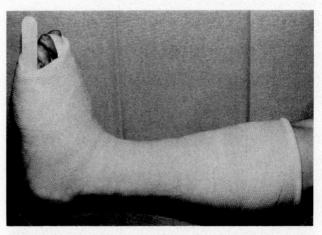

Figure 9.14. Potential cast irritation and compression sites. Care must be taken to pad and protect these areas. Tongue depressor allows room for fifth toe without cast binding.

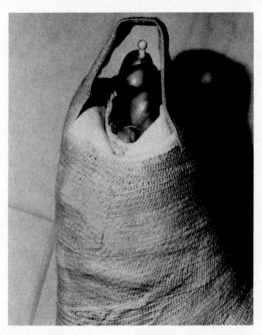

Figure 9.15. Cast of synthetic material with built-in toe protector to prevent pin damage.

extension or a distal toeshield, especially if pins are protruding from the digits (Fig. 9.15).

POSTOPERATIVE PROTECTIVE FOOTGEAR

When cast immobilization is not necessary, the postoperative foot can be protected by a variety of postsurgical shoes. These usually have firm wooden soles for protection and splinting, while slowing the patient's pace. They may be padded or altered as necessary (Fig. 9.16). If Kirschner wires are in place to immobilize the toes then the postoperative shoe should be long enough to protect them. To prevent digital bending at toe-off the shoe can be built up all the way forward from the heel to the sulcus.

Table 9.1
Resin/Plastic Cast Materials

Carapace	Carapace, Inc Tulsa, OK, 74145
Cellamin	Selomas, Inc Wilmington, DE 19899
Gypsona II	Smith & Nephew Chaston Medical & Surgical Products Dayville, CT 06241
Velroc	Johnson & Johnson Products, Inc New Brunswick, NJ 08903

Table 9.2
Synthetic Casting Materials

Delta-Lite	Johnson & Johnson Products Inc New Brunswick, NJ 08903
CutterCast	Cutter Biomedical Emeryville, CA 94608
TufStuf	DePuy Warsaw, IN
Scotchcast	Orthopedic Products Division/3M St. Paul, MN 55144
K-Cast	Kirschner Medical Timonium, MD 21093
Zimmer Cast	Zimmer Charlotte, NC 28212

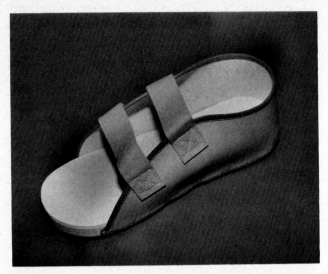

Figure 9.16. Postoperative shoe. Wooden sole protects foot while velcro straps encourage better patient compliance.

Cast boots are excellent for protecting the ambulatory cast. The soles are of a nonskid construction and give good support to the cast for full weight bearing.

In the best interest of economy, old shoes from the patient can be cut and altered for postsurgical use but their application is somewhat limited to toe and nail surgery.

Elevation and Position

Elevation is probably the single most important aspect in the management of the postsurgical foot and ankle. Dependency must be avoided to prevent excess swelling that occurs as a result of the tissue disruption. Noninflammatory transudates and inflammatory exudates must not be allowed to accumulate.

Overhead slings can be used following extensive surgery but the urethane foam cast elevator (e.g. Span aid) is an excellent re-usuable device for comfortably positioning and raising the extremity. The knee should be flexed and supported (usually with a pillow) at about 15° to 20°. The foot of the bed should be raised as well with the support strut in the highest position. Above the hips is the ideal height but above the heart is better (Fig. 9.17).

For further comfort the foot should be supported medially and laterally so it cannot roll and cause undue torque to the leg and foot. This is a powerful force that can be terribly disruptive at the surgical site, particularly if bone work is involved. A blanket cradle will keep the covers from irritating the surgical site. If the patient is recuperating at home a cardboard box can be cut out like a dog house for the same protection.

Postoperative Weight Bearing

A great deal of controversy surrounds the timing of weightbearing following foot surgery, particularly for the ambulatory patient, with and without bone work. My preference is to think of it as a progression tailored to the individual patient.

The progression takes the patient from rest and elevation and starts with range of motion exercises of the lower extremity joints while still in bed. This starts fluid drainage from the distal tissues, particularly when performed with the extremity still elevated. The next stage is to allow the patient to sit up and dangle the extremity over the edge of the bed for brief periods. This serves two functions: the first is to help restore the vestibular system to reorient the patient after anesthesia, surgery, and bed rest, and the second is to allow the distal vascular beds to become responsive again to the effects of gravity and thereby restore fluid

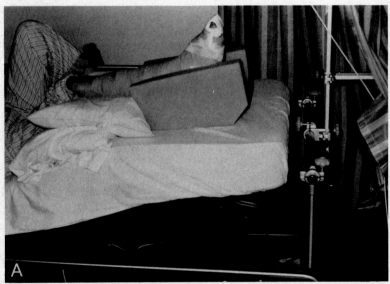

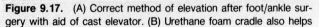

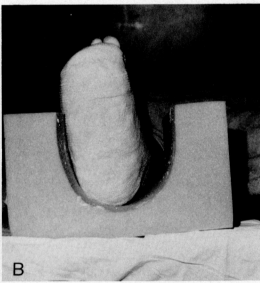

Figure 9.17. (A) Correct method of elevation after foot/ankle surgery with aid of cast elevator. (B) Urethane foam cradle also helps prevent gravitational torque caused by rolling of foot.

flow in a proximal direction during dependency. It is important to elevate the foot again after each dangle. Weight bearing is initiated after dangling or after cast removal, depending on the surgery and treatment program. In any event, it begins by placing the foot on the floor usually using a protective shoe. Just resting it there allows the proprioceptive system to equilibrate. Then *progressive weight bearing* is initiated. It begins by having patients weigh themselves and then apply foot pressure to the scale until they understand the force necessary to reach a desired approximate percentage of their weight. In this manner the surgeon can prescribe a progressive weight bearing program using simple percentages. For example, after a six-week cast removal following a base wedge osteotomy of the first metatarsal, the program might be 25% for three days, 50% for two days, 75% for one day, and then 100% weight bearing. The program must be simple and easy to follow.

This is not to say that early ambulation and movement are not encouraged. Indeed they are, but the physiological principles of healing must be followed. Imagine a foot where a neuroma was just removed in the office. Hemostasis looked good at the conclusion of the surgery, yet a void remained from the neurectomy and tissue disruption. Now the patient is told he or she can walk to the car because the foot is still numb. As the weight is imposed on those cells and blood vessels, it is easy to picture the extrusion of fragile platelet plugs, the destruction of other unprotected cells, and the forcing of extracellular fluid, blood, and serum into that dead space. The end result is an increased inflammatory response and additional unnecessary scar tissue because the body must clean up the extra extravastation.

Crutches and walkers are very helpful in assisting patients through non-weight-bearing to full weight bearing. Aside from the usual principles for using these devices one helpful measure is to have the patient obtain them and practice using them *before* the surgery. The familiarity will smooth the progression postoperatively.

Use of Ice

Pain Reduction

Cryotherapy has been shown to be very effective in reducing pain secondary to trauma, whether mechanical or surgical. It does so by the direct effect of cold on nerves, by reducing muscle spasticity and by reducing swelling through several mechanisms, including the diminution of inflammation.

Cold exerts its effect on nerves by elevating the excitation threshold of the pain receptors and afferent nerves, usually the delta fibers. Essentially, the conduction velocity is slowed considerably (2).

Reduction of muscle spasms, when they occur postoperatively, will tend to increase markedly patient comfort as well. The application of cold reduces the responsiveness of the muscle spindle to stretching (3) and affects the neuromuscular junction by blocking nerve conduction (4). Li (4) showed that, on cooling, neuromuscular transmission was impeded at 15° C and blocked at 5° C. Thus, cooling to appropriate levels will diminish unnecessary muscle irritation and activity.

The reduction of painful swelling and bleeding after trauma or surgery by cold application is the result of the principle mechanism of vasoconstriction (5). It is well known that cooling produces a reflex vasoconstriction via the sympathetic fibers; it also has a similar direct effect on the vessels themselves. Bazur and associates (6) demonstrated a more rapid recovery from ankle sprains when adding ice to compression bandages for therapy. Schaubel (7) examined the effects of cold on a large number of patients who underwent various orthopedic procedures requiring casting. He compared 207 patients treated with ice with 312 controls. Of those treated with ice, only 5.3% required cast splitting to relieve swelling, whereas 42.3% required splitting where ice was not used. Of equal importance, Schaubel found that the requirement for narcotics was markedly reduced when ice was applied (Table 9.3).

Swelling and pain are also reduced by using cold to diminish inflammation. Because the inflammatory reaction is itself temperature dependent, it is markedly slowed. Vasoconstriction also prevents the transudation of fluids. Finally, cold tends to retard the tissue destruction resulting from the inflammatory enzymes.

Disadvantages

When cold reduces skin temperatures to 2° C the vasoconstriction can be reversed, resulting in a marked increase in blood flow. This may lead to paradoxical swelling and hyperemia when the ice is discontinued. It is thought to be the result of the Hunting reaction that explains blood flow increase as an effort of the body to maintain sufficient temperature to prevent tissue damage (5).

It is also known that cooling wounds for too long tends to retard healing because of the prolonged vasoconstriction. Tensile strength can be reduced by as much as 20% (8).

Table 9.3
Average of Total Amount of Narcotics Required during first 72 hours after Operation, with and without Ice Treatment

Average Dosage	Cases with Ice			Cases without Ice		
	Codeine	Morphine	Demerol	Codeine	Morphine	Demerol
mg/Case	89.2	11.8	3.8	268.5	25.1	12.0

From Schaubel HJ: The local use of ice after orthopeadic procedures. *Am J Surg* 72:711–714, 1946.

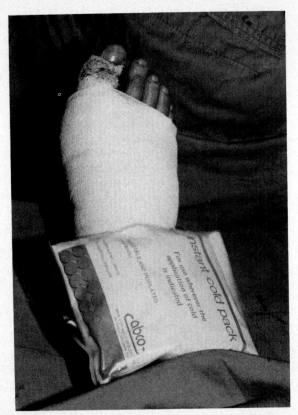

Figure 9.18. Correct application of ice at ankle flexure.

Techniques of Cold Application

Ice should rarely be applied directly to or over a wound. The ideal place is proximal to the wound where it can produce vasoconstriction and inhibit nerve conduction (Fig. 9.18). It should not be left in place for extended periods unless applied to a cast, where it can be surprisingly effective. The ice should be protected with waterproof material and covered with a cloth or towel before being located on the extremity. It is effective whether applied on skin, dressings, or casts (7).

Anxiety and Pain Management

The degree and severity of pain in the postoperative patient depends on three main factors: (*a*) the physiological and psychological makeup of the patient and his or her tolerance of pain; (*b*) the site and nature of the operation; and (*c*) the amount of surgical trauma (9) (Fig. 9.19). Thus, pain complaints reflect not only tissue injury, but many psychological dimensions of suffering as well (10). This psychological influence demands that the management of postoperative pain begin before the surgery itself.

Much unnecessary suffering can be avoided by reducing preoperative anxiety. Simple, clear, and honest communication with the patient should include an explanation of what will happen and when it will happen. Further, the patient's questions should be answered with care. It has been demonstrated that postoperative requirements of narcotics can be considerably reduced by proper preoperative instruction

(11). In fact, anxiety can be relieved with judicious use of a bedtime sedative-hypnotic agent. If surgery is performed on an outpatient basis with local or spinal anesthesia, a tranquilizer such as a benzodiazepine derivative can safely be given to allay fear and anxiety.

Pharmaceuticals for postoperative pain management should only be considered as supportive, in addition to protective dressings, elevation, rest, and ice. They should be used especially through the initial inflammatory phase of repair and diminished or discontinued as soon as possible.

A long-acting local anesthetic injected at the conclusion of the surgery will delay postoperative pain past the intense initial phases. This avoids the early use of narcotic analgesics that can depress respiration during the critical period of recovery from inhalation anesthesia. Use of a posterior tibial nerve block postoperatively is a two edged sword, besides prolonging

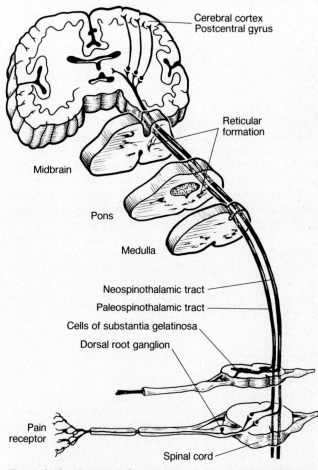

Figure 9.19. Anatomy of central nervous system pain pathways. From pain receptors, noxious stimuli are transmitted via sensory nerves to spinal nerves and into dorsal root ganglia. After entering spinal cord, impulse synapses and crosses cord. It then rises directly to either spinothalamic tract, which is on contralateral side, or to other component of spinothalamic tract, paleospinothalamic. Spinothalamic tract rises to medulla, where paleospinothalamic sends branch into reticular formation. This action is repeated in pons and midbrain. Neospinothalamic tract goes directly into cortex, synapsing in midbrain and sending impulses into postcentral gyrus, where pain is perceived.

Table 9.4
Inhibitors of Prostaglandin Biosynthesis Comparing the NSAIDs

Chemical Class	Drug	Usual oral Dose (mg)	Hours to Peak Serum Level	Serum Half-Life (Hours)	Anti-Inflam-matory	Approved as Simple Analgesic	Unique Side Effects Comments
Salicilates	Aspirin	650-975 q4h	¾–2	3–16	Yes	Yes	Increased bleeding time for life of the platelet (4–8 days); least expensive
	Diflunisal (Dolobid)	500 q12h	½–2	8	Yes	Yes	Good analgesic properties
Pyrazoles	Phenylbutazone (Butazolidin, Azolid)	100 q6h	2	84–96	Yes	No	Can cause bone marrow depression; highest incidence of fluid retention; safer if used for one week intervals
	Oxyphenbutazone (Tandearil, Ox-alid)	100 q6h	2–6	72–96	Yes	No	Metabolite of phenylbutazone; may cause bone marrow depression and hepatitis
Paraamino-phenol deriv-atives	Acetaminophen (Tylenol, etc.)	325–650 q4h	½–1	2–4	Very Weak	Yes	Active metabolite of phenacetin
Phenylalkanoic Acids	Ibuprofen (Motrin, Rufen)	400–600 q6h	1–2	2–3	Yes	Yes	Causes less gastric irritation than ASA. May cause fluid retention
Propionic Acids	Fenoprofen (Nal-fon)	300–600 q6h	1–2	3	Yes	Yes	Contraindicated in patients with impaired renal function. Similar to ibuprofen
	Naproxen (Napro-syn)	375–1200 q12h	2–4	13	Yes	Yes	GI intolerance is most common side effect
	Naproxen Sodium (Anaprox)	275–550 q12h	1–2	13	Yes	Yes	More rapidly absorbed than naproxen
Indole Acetic Acids	Indomethacin (In-docin)	25–50 q8h	2	3–4.5	Yes	No	Highest incidence of CNS side effects of all the NSAID's, eg. headaches, vertigo, confusion
	Sulindac (Clinoril)	200 q12h	2	13 (active metabolite)	Yes	No	Best choice for patients with renal impairments. Lower incidence of GI toxicity. Less effective than indomethacine
	Tolmetin (Tolectin)	400 q6–8h	½–1	1	Yes	No	Less CNS side effects than indomethacin
Fenamic Acids	Mefenamic acid (Ponstel)	250 q6h	2–4	2–5	No	Yes	Principally used for pain relief from primary dysmenorrhea
	Meclofenamic acid (Meclomen)	50–100 q6h	½–1	2–5	Yes	No	Relatively frequent diarrhea; effect may be dose related
Oxicams	Piroxicam (Feldene)	20 q24h	3–5	44–50	Yes	No	High GI upset potential

the local anesthesia. Distally it produces vasodilatation that immediately increases the blood supply to the operative site compromised by the hypoxia of tissue trauma, vasoconstrictive agents, and tourniquet ischemia when applied. This provides beneficial oxygen and nutrients while removing toxic wastes. However, the vasodilatation will also allow the transudation of serum and may even cause bleeding from severed vessels that had already retracted and occluded with a hemostatic plug. The result may well be added postoperative edema with possible hematoma formation. Therefore postoperative posterior tibial nerve blocks should be used judiciously. Local infiltration within the subcutaneous tissues with an anesthetic of long duration is very effective.

The injection of a short-acting soluble corticosteroid, such as dexamethasone phosphate, about the surgical site will diminish much of the initial painful swelling and inflammation associated with the intense lag phase of healing (12). It can be infiltrated before or after the first incision, mixed with a long-acting local anesthetic agent. Care should be taken to disperse the solution especially within the subcutaneous tissues where there is the greatest concentration of nerves and blood vessels affected by inflammation. Judicious application is important because steroids also weaken local tissue defenses against infection and have anabolic properties that might delay healing during their potency. As a result only a small amount should be used either alone or dispersed in the local anesthetic. Seldom is more than 1 cc of dexamethasone phosphate (4 mg/cc) necessary per foot. Many clinicians question the wisdom of using steroids in surgical sites as a routine practice.

Auxiolytics can be used alone or with analgesic medications to raise pain thresholds postsurgically. It must be remembered that supportive drugs for this period are given to control anxiety and not only to relieve pain (13).

Because inflammation is the hallmark of the initial and most painful postoperative phase, a logical approach is to incorporate antiinflammatory medications for the first 3 to 10 days. Aspirin is the prototype followed by the nonsteroid antiinflammatory drugs (NSAIDs) (Table 9.4). Most of these agents exert a variable amount of analgesia as well, making them attractive for mild to moderate pain control. All the NSAIDs, including aspirin, inhibit the enzyme cyclooxygenase of the prostaglandin cascade (Fig. 9.20), the end product of which is a prime mediator of acute inflammation. Prostaglandins may also augment pain perception and production (14). That the NSAIDs inhibit platelet aggregation and prolong bleeding time does not contraindicate their use postsurgically because the local clotting is already complete.

Factors to consider in selecting a NSAID for postoperative pain and inflammation control are the drug's half-life, hepatorenal toxicity, gastric irritation potential, and salt and water retention. Many studies have shown that the NSAIDs are effective in reducing postsurgical pain (14–20). Several of these studies even suggest that these agents can substitute for narcotic analgesia because their clinical efficacy may be equal or better. Once these factors are evaluated, final selection is a clinical decision based on experience and the patient profile.

The opiate or opiate-like drugs produce analgesia by entirely different mechanisms, so they can be used alone or in conjunction with aspirin, acetaminophen, or the NSAIDs. Combinations allow a greater amount of analgesia than when individual drugs are used alone (20). Codeine is the most popular adjunctive opiate because of its efficacy and wide margin of safety. It should only be used after mild analgesics such as aspirin, acetaminophen, or propoxyphene have been considered (21, 22). If codeine is insufficient then pentazocine or oxycodone compounds can be selected. Finally, a parenteral morphinelike analgesic may be used, usually on a prn basis (Table 9.5). It must be remembered that adverse reactions of opiate analge-

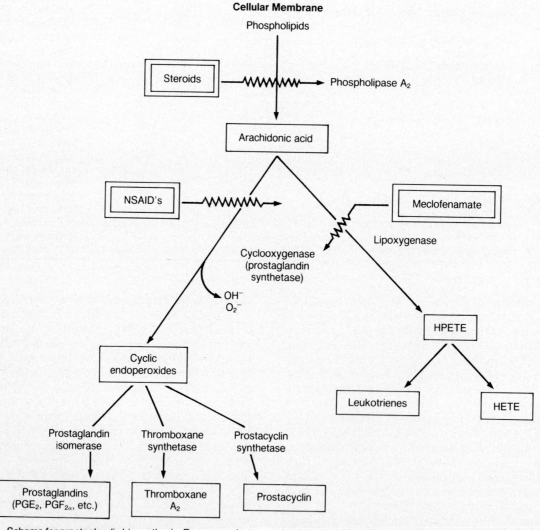

Figure 9.20.   Scheme for prostaglandin biosynthesis. Enzyme cyclooxygenase catalyzes reaction transforming arachidonic acid to endoperoxide compounds. Superoxide radicals OH and O2 are by-products of this reaction.

Table 9.5
Opiate Analgesics

Analgesic	Trade Name	IM Dose (mg)*	Peak (hr)	Duration (hr)
Morphine		10	¾–1	4–6
Hydromorphone	Dilaudid	1.5	½–¾	4–5
Oxymorphine	Numorphan	1–15	1	4–6
Oxycodone	Percodan	10–15 (oral)	2–4	4–6
Nalbuphine	Nubain	10	¾–1	3–6
Levorphanol	Levo-Dromaran	2–3	¾–1	4–6
Methadone	Dolophine	7.5–10	¾–1	3–5
Meperidine	Demerol	80–100	½–1	2–4
Pentazocine	Talwin	30–60	¾	4–5
Codeine		120	1–2	4–6
Propoxyphene	Darvon	60 (oral)	1–2	4–6

* Equivalent to 10 mg of morphine.

Modified from Marcus SA, Block BH (eds): *American College of Foot Surgeons—Complications in Foot Surgery. Prevention and Management.* Baltimore, Williams & Wilkins, 1984, p 79.

sics are dose-related. Thus the stronger the agent and the higher the dose, the greater the incidence of toxic reactions. Overdosage of the narcotic drugs is safely treated with 0.4 to 0.8 mg of naloxone, which has no specific narcotic actions of its own (23, 24).

Excessive anxiety will greatly reduce the pain threshold in the postoperative patient. It is important to identify the anxiety-prone patient, preferably preoperatively, and treat with sedatives or tranquilizers following the surgery. Caution is advised because these drugs can potentiate some of the effects of narcotics when used concurrently. Side effects of narcotics include hypotension, respiratory depression, urinary retention, nausea, and reduced peristalsis, which can lead to constipation or even ileus. These side effects are dose-dependent so the principle is to use as little narcotic as possible. Several studies and clinical experience have proved that the antihistamine, hydroxyzine is an excellent and safe adjunct when mixed with narcotic agents such as morphine and meperidine (25–30). Not only does it have its own analgesic properties but it also has attractive ataractic effects, so much so that narcotic doses can be reduced by one half or more when combined with hydroxyzine and still achieve the same analgesic result. It further exhibits other minor benefits, such as antiemetic, bronchodilatatory, and antiarrhythmic while producing minimal circulatory and respiratory depression (31).

Other antianxiety agents are mainly the relatively safe benzodiazepines, whether used as tranquilizers or sedative-hypnotics. Alternatives, especially for pediatric and elderly patients, include the barbiturates chloral hydrate, meprobamate, and diphenhydramine.

Vital Signs and Fever

Monitoring vital signs is critical both intraoperatively and postoperatively especially as the patient is emerging from anesthesia. From then on they should be monitored routinely until discharge.

Blood pressure tends to rise to presurgical levels once the anesthetic wears off. If the patient is known to be hypertensive then the same prescribed dose regimen of antihypertensive drugs should be resumed when the patient is stabilized.

The pulse is checked for rate, rhythm, and force. Anxiety is a prime cause of increased pulse, whether from apprehension or pain. It is a useful indicator of cardiac output.

The most critical times to monitor respirations are the initial period following anesthesia and when patients are receiving drugs such as narcotics, sedatives, or insulin.

Finally, the temperature is monitored regularly and, when elevated, is an important sign of potential complications. However, some ambiguity exists regarding the significance of postsurgical temperature changes (Fig. 9.21).

Body temperature is an important and vital indicator of body homeostasis. It is controlled about a reference "set point" thought to be seated in the hypothalamus by a complex thermoregulatory system. However, establishing a single numerical figure (i.e. 98.6° F) for normal "core" body temperature seldom fits the clinical situation. Rather, a "range of normal" of between 97.1° and 99.5° F has been established as more appropriate because it can be extended in either direction by a variety of benign conditions (30,32). For example, most people exhibit a diurnal flux in body temperature: lowest between 4 and 6 AM and highest between 8 and 11 PM, the variation ranging from 0.9° to 2.7° F (33–35).

Fever is the abnormal elevation in body temperature results from a disturbance of the thermoregulatory mechanism (36). When temperatures rise above the "normal range" it is important to take into account normal fluctuations such as those caused by diurnal variation, menstruation, or exercise, all of which can appreciably add to the core body temperature under nonpathological conditions. A better definition of fever then is an increase in temperature over what is normal for a given individual at that particular time of day and not merely an isolated temperature greater than 98.6° F (37).

It has been shown that temperature changes can occur postoperatively after extensive foot surgery, even when unassociated with pathological conditions (32). During the first few hours after general anesthesia it is usual to see a drop in body temperature of up to 2° F. If the body temperature were monitored during the anesthesia this "postoperative hypothermia" would probably be seen simply as the continuation of the "intraoperative hypothermia" caused by the interference with the hypothalamic thermoregulatory mechanism by general anesthesia (38). The body must then expend great effort to reduce this heat deficit in the immediate postoperative period. Although the most dramatic manifestation of this is in the form of intense shivering as the body regains control of its set point, it has been shown that even without shivering there is a considerable increase in oxygen consumption at this time (39). This is most likely indicative of

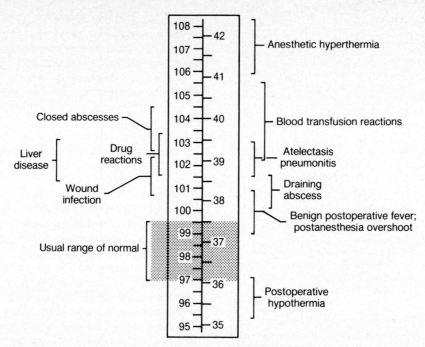

Figure 9.21. General guide to some approximate postoperative temperature elevations. (From Miller SJ: Body temperature following podiatric surgery: evaluation and management. *J Am Podiatry Assoc* 74:477–481, 1984.)

the nonshivering thermogenesis taking place in an attempt to restore body temperature.

In the absence of signs and symptoms of post-surgical complications a temperature rise of less than 2° F within the first 24 to 29 hours is probably a "postanesthesia overshoot" (32), which is a category of "benign postoperative fever" as described by Roe (40). He found in one group of patients that this phenomenon was not observed when the body temperature was successfully prevented from falling during the operation. It has been proven that the general anesthetic halothane by itself is not responsible for this phenomenon (41).

When mild postoperative temperature increases of less than 2° F are seen at approximately 48 to 54 and 72 to 78 hours postoperatively and there is an apparent absence of any signs of complications, then one can fairly make the diagnosis of true "benign postoperative fever." These temperature elevations are thought to be caused by the "leukocytic pyrogens" released during the inflammatory reaction following a threshold amount of tissue injury (32). Only observation and supportive therapy are required and further investigation is unnecessary.

For greater temperature elevations, evaluation of postoperative fever entails a lengthy differential diagnosis that must be narrowed by the interpretation of available data and the application of clinical experience. Important factors to consider are listed in Table 9.6.

Some common causes of postsurgical temperature changes to consider are presented chronologically in Table 9.7. Treatment is aimed at the associated pathological process. The use of antipyretic agents is dis-

Table 9.6
Key Factors to Review When Evaluating a Postoperative Fever

Age
General Health
Anesthesia used
Length of surgery
Amount of surgical trauma
Elapsed time since surgery
Drug therapy
Laboratory results
Postoperative status of patient
    Urinary retention
    Constipation
    Increased pain
    Signs of infection

From Miller SJ: Body temperature following podiatric surgery. *J Am Podiatry Assoc* 74:477–481, 1984.

couraged until the etiology of the fever has been determined or at least major pathology ruled out. Mild fevers of less than 2° F require no pharmaceutical therapy unless the patient is uncomfortable as a result of marked debilitation. Once the reason for the fever is realized antipyretic agents may be employed in cases where the temperature elevation is marked or persistent. Drugs of choice are aspirin and acetaminophen.

Chasing postoperative fevers can be frustrating and expensive. A knowledge of thermoregulation and fever pathogenesis, especially in relation to surgery, provides better clinical insight for judicious patient management. Each fever should be carefully examined and the more threatening and dangerous etiologies ruled out (42).

Table 9.7
Chronological Sequence of Postoperative Temperature Changes

Intraoperative	Heat pyrexia
	Malignant hyperthemia
	Hypothermia
First 12–24 hours	Postoperative hypothermia
Day 1	Postanesthesia overshoot
	Atelectasis/pneumonitis
Second 24 hours	Thrombophlebitis
Day 2	Pulmonary embolism
	Benign postoperative fever
Third 24 hours	Postsurgical infection
Day 3	Urinary tract infection
	Benign postoperative fever
	Constipation
Other causes appropriate to the situation:	Drug fever
	Catheter fever
	Blood transfusion reaction
	Intravenous fever

From Miller SJ: Body temperature following podiatric surgery. *J Am Podiatry Assoc* 74:477–481, 1984.

Table 9.8
Phenothiazines used in the Treatment of Nausea and Vomiting

Drug	Dosage	Suppository
Chlorpromazine (Thorazine)	10–50 mg q 2–4 h po or IM	25–100 mg q 6–8 hr
Perphenazine (Trilafon)	2–8 mg po or 5 mg IM (8–16 mg per day)	
Prochlorperazine (Compazine)	5–10 mg 3–4 times/ day po or IM (up to 40 mg/day)	25 mg twice a day
Promethazine (Phenergan)	12.5–25 mg q 4–6 hr po or IM	12.5–25 mg q 4–6 hr
Thiethylperazine (Torecan)	10 mg po or IM 1–3 times/day	10–30 mg/day
Triflupromazine (Vesprin)	15–30 mg/day po or IM in divided doses	

Modified from Gilman AG, Goodman LS, Gilman A: *The Pharmacological Basis of Therapeutics.* New York, Macmillan, 1980, p 417.

MANAGEMENT OF NAUSEA AND CONSTIPATION

Nausea

Because persistent vomiting is diminishing as a postanesthesia complication with the advent of newer agents, its occurrence should be observed and if necessary investigated for underlying causes. Prolonged vomiting can lead to dehydration and electrolyte disturbances, especially in children and in the elderly. Drug sensitivity, such as to morphine, meperidine, and codeine, may instigate severe nausea, and if so, these agents should be discontinued in favor of alternative analgesics.

Postoperative nausea responds well to small doses of phenothiazine antiemetics (Table 9.8), although some of the antihistamines such as diphenhydramine (Benadryl), dimenhydrinate (Dramamine), and hydroxyzine (Atarax) are effective alternatives. Other drugs that can be used include trimethobenzamide (Tigan), benzquinamide (Emete-con), and the butyrophenone derivative droperidol (Inapsine). Although an excellent antiemetic, caution is advised with the use of droperidol, which may cause hypotension, extrapyriamidal effects, and/or the potentiation of respiratory depression when narcotics are in use. Recommended initial dosages are 2.5 mg (1 ml) for the adult and 1.0 to 1.5 mg per 20 to 25 pounds for children over two years.

For mild, uncomplicated nausea, especially in children, an effective treatment is experienced with phosphorated carbohydrate solution (Emetrol), a pleasant, mint-flavored syrup containing levulose, dextrose, and orthophosphoric acid. For children the dosage is 5 to 10 ml at 15-minute intervals until nausea diminishes; in adults 15 to 30 ml are given in the same manner.

Finally, WANS antinausea suppositories may be used. These are a combination of an antihistamine (pyrilamine) and a sedative (pentobarbital). They are formulated in a pediatric size and two adult strengths. As with all of the antiemetic agents, precautions should be taken for adverse effects common to their drug family, as well as to the individual drug itself. Great care should be taken in administering centrally acting antiemetics to children. Also, the same precautions should be observed with the use of drugs for nausea and vomiting as with the use of potent analgesics in the treatment of pain, because they may mask diagnostic symptoms (43).

Constipation

Slowing of peristalsis begins as soon as the patient is immobilized for surgery. It is more evident in the elderly patients with less muscle tone. Fasting before surgery, diminished fluid intake, drugs such as narcotics, and inactivity can all lead to constipation postoperatively, and can ultimately cause fecal impaction if at least daily attention is not paid to the patient's bowel activity. Initial treatment should include increasing fluid intake, adding bulk and roughage to the diet, and encouraging activity.

Pharmaceutical treatment should begin with the mildest of laxative-cathartics, such as milk of magnesia or psyllium preparations (e.g. Metamucil). If unsuccessful, then a stool softener might be used; for example, dioctyl sodium sulfosuccinate (Colace) 50 to 250 mg. For resistant constipation other contact cathartics can be considered, such as biscodyl (Dulcolax) 5 to 10 mg po taken with a large glass of water. Saline enemas will also provide prompt evacuation of the bowel.

Caution must be advised when there is obstruction or other signs of gastrointestinal disorders. All laxatives and cathartics are contraindicated in a patient with cramps, colic, nausea, vomiting, and any undiagnosed abdominal pain (44).

FLUID MANAGEMENT

Blood loss is rarely sufficient to require replacement therapy in foot and ankle surgery, unless additional trauma has been involved. The encouragement of oral fluid intake postsurgically is usually sufficient to restore fluid homeostasis. There are, however, certain situations that require the maintenance of an intravenous line and fluid augmentation.

Postoperative fluid deficits (when present) have little reason to be large and will be more significant in children and elderly patients. Long periods of fasting, assisted ventilation, extended surgical cases, and prolonged vomiting are indications that usually require 8 to 24 hours of intravenous fluids, which may then be discontinued as long as the patient and vital signs are stable. The most important method of quickly assessing the patient's fluid status is to use the daily intake and output records. Serum electrolytes (Na+, K+, HCO_3 and pH) should be monitored if there is any question regarding the acid-base balance, and consultation requested as necessary.

The goal of fluid therapy following foot and ankle surgery is seldom more than normal maintenance requirements. Additional replacement for the previous 12 to 24 hours might be considered depending on the volume delivered intraoperatively and the status of the patient preoperatively. Normal maintenance requirements are composed of daily water and salt losses through normal urinary and feces output (sensible losses, usually 1000 to 1500 ml daily) plus evaporative losses through the skin and lungs (insensible losses, about 600 to 1000 ml daily). Thus daily fluid maintenance requirements for both sensible and insensible losses will approach 1500 to 2500 ml, depending on the patient's age, sex, weight, and body surface area (Table 9.9). Because electrolyte loss is negligible in these fluids, adequate replacement can be achieved in uncomplicated cases with a solution of 5% dextrose in water. In estimating these needs, a useful rule of thumb is to multiply the patient's weight (kg) times 30 ml/kg. For example, to meet normal maintenance requirements, a 70 kg male would need approximately 2100 ml of water using this formula (45, 46).

Other primary uses for intravenous infusion in the hospitalized podiatric patient include the administration of medications, particularly antibiotics. For patients requiring such therapy for periods longer than 48 to 72 hours, some considerations should be given to electrolyte maintenance. Exact calculation of ion needs is impractical and not really necessary on a daily basis; determination can be made generally. Daily sodium requirements are about 50 to 125 mEq whereas potassium and chloride approach 40 to 100 mEq. The usual replacement requirements for each of these ions, in practical terms, is roughly 60 to 70 mEq

Table 9.9
Daily Water Losses and Water Requirements for Normal Individuals Who Are Not Working or Sweating

	Losses				Requirements	
	Urine (ml)	Stool (ml)	Insensible (ml)	Total (ml)	ml/person	ml/Kg
Infant (2–10 Kg)	200–500	25–40	75–300 (1.3 ml/ Kg/hr)	300–840	330–1000	165–100
Child (10–40 kg)	500–800	40–100	300–600	840–1500	1000–1800	100–45
Adolescent or Adult (60 Kg)	800–1000	100	600–1000 (0.5 ml/Kg/hr)	1500–2100	1800–2500	45–30

Modified from Wilson JL: *Handbook of Surgery*, ed 5. Los Altos, CA, Lange Medical Publications, 1973, p 151.

Table 9.10
Composition of Intravenous Solutions

Solutions	Glucose (gm/l)	Na	Cl	HCO₃	K (mEq/1)	Ca	Mg	HPO₄	NH₄
Extracellular fluid	1000	140	102	27	4.2	5	3	3	0.3
5% dextrose and water	50								
10% dextrose and water	100								
0.9% sodium chloride (normal saline)		154	154						
0.45% sodium chloride (half-normal saline)		77	77						
0.21% sodium chloride (¼ normal saline)		34	34						
3% sodium chloride (hypertonic saline)		513	513						
Lactated Ringer's solution	130	109		28*	4	2.7			
0.9% ammonium chloride		168							168

* Present in solution as lactate but is metabolized to bicarbonate.
From American College of Surgeons: *Manual of Preoperative and Postoperative Care*, ed 3. Philadelphia, WB Saunders Co, 1983, p 47.

daily. To fulfill these needs, a second rule of thumb can be used by giving 1 mEq per kg of body weight of each of these electrolytes daily (45).

Unless the patient is on diuretic therapy or is mildly hypokalemic preoperatively, postassium is usually unnecessary during the first 24 hours postoperatively. Also, because there is some degree of fluid retention as a result of the release of aldosterone and antidiuretic hormone caused by the stress induced by surgery, only about two thirds of the maintenance fluid requirements are necessary during the first 72 hours postoperatively as a precaution to prevent volume overload (45).

Selecting an appropriate intravenous solution can be confusing, because many types are available in the hospital (Table 9.10). For most postoperative maintenance the following solutions or combinations are satisfactory: 5% dextrose in water (D5W), normal saline (NS), half-normal saline (½ NS), or lactated Ringer's solution (LR), which is a balanced salt solution. Useful combinations are D5NS, D5 ½NS, and D5LR. Orders for administration can be given as volume per time period. For example, for a patient requiring 1500 ml to meet normal maintenance requirements the order might be "500 ml D5LR IV q 8 hrs" or "60 ml per hour." Orders can also be given for infusion rates including KVO for "keep vein open" by maintaining drip only. The latter might be used when the patient is not fully stabilized and the IV line is available for the rapid administration of medication if necessary.

Cardinal Signs of Local Complications

The institution of prompt and decisive therapy for postoperative localized wound complications requires the early recognition of such problems. Acute pain usually aggravated by anxiety, and unresponsive to even the most potent narcotic analgesic agents, is a common denominator of postsurgical complications. The three most frequent causes are excessive swelling within a restrictive dressing or cast, hematoma formation, and infection later than 48 to 72 hours.

Fever may occur at various times following surgery but is not generally indicative of local infection until 72 hours or longer. Infection can also be present without fever because a threshold amount of leukocytic pyrogen is necessary to instigate a temperature rise.

Critical evaluation of the surgical site will provide definite clues to impending complications. Erythema, swelling, warmth, and tenderness are signs of intense inflammation. This is a normal tissue response if dissection was extensive. However, when it is excessive or prolonged, it may also be the result of hematoma.

Drainage is an ominous sign when present after 48 to 72 hours. Mild hemorrhage along the wound edges at the dressing change during this time is normal. However, the exudation or transudation of clear or serosanguinous fluid, especially in the presence of

other local danger signs such as erythema, swelling, and tenderness, means a relatively high probability of a developing infection. An abnormal amount of postoperative pain increases such a possibility. The drainage should always be gram stained and cultured and judicious antibiotic prophylaxis instituted at once. The first choice is a penicillinase-resistant penicillin with erythromycin as primary backup in the face of penicillin allergy, unless the gram stain indicates otherwise. For broader coverage, including some gram-negative bacteria, cephalosporin antibiotics are indicated.

Discharging the Patient

Whether the surgery is done in the office or in the hospital, the patient should be in possession of three important items at the time of discharge. First, and more importantly, is *written* postoperative instructions. These may be typewritten in standard format from the surgeon's office, even if the hospital dispenses instructions of its own (Fig. 9.10).

Second, prescriptions for antiinflammatory, analgesic, and, if necessary, antibiotics or other drugs, should be provided. Finally, ambulatory assistance to the transportation vehicle is essential. A wheelchair is ideal, especially for elderly or unsteady patients, but crutches can be provided instead. A health care person should accompany the patient to the home-bound vehicle.

Detailed management of edema, hematoma, and infection are thoroughly reviewed elsewhere in this text.

References

1. Miller SJ: Surgical wound drainage system using silicone tubing. *J AmPodiatry Assoc* 71:287–296, 1981.
2. DeJong PH, Hershey WN, Wagman IH: Nerve conduction velocity during hypothermia in man. *Anesthesiology* 27:805–810, 1966.
3. Ottoson D: The effects of temperature on the isolated muscle spindle. *J Physiol* 180:636–648, 1965.
4. Li CL: Effect of cooling on the neuromuscular transmission in the rat. *Am J Physiol* 194:200–206, 1958.
5. Lehmann JF, DeLateur BJ: Cryotherapy. In Lehmann JF (ed): *Therapeutic Heat and Cold*, ed 3. Baltimore, Williams & Wilkins, 1982, pp 563–602.
6. Bazur RL, Shephard E, Mouzag GL: A cooling method in the treatment of ankle sprains. *Pract* 216:708–722, 1976.
7. Schaubel HJ: The local use of ice after orthopedic procedures. *Am J Surg* 72:711–714, 1946.
8. Lundgren C, Maren A, Zederfeldt B: Effect of cold vasoconstriction on wound healing in the rabbit. *Acta Chir Scand* 118:1–4, 1959.
9. Pflug AE, Bonica JJ: Physiopathology and control of postoperative pain. *Arch Surg* 112:773–778, 1977.
10. Chapman CR: Psychological aspects of pain patient treatment. *Arch Surg* 112:767–772, 1977.
11. Egbert LD, Battit GE, Welch CE, Bartlett, MK: Reduction of postoperative pain by encouragement and instruction of patients: a study of doctor-patient rapport. *N Engl J Med* 270:825–827, 1964.
12. Curda GA: Postoperative analgesic effects of dexamethasone phosphate in bunion surgery. *J Foot Surg* 22:187–191, 1983.
13. Drew FL, Moriarty RW, Shapiro AP: An approach to the measurement of the pain and anxiety responses of surgical patients. *Psychosom Med* 30:826, 1968.

14. Borovoy M, Holtz P, Kaczander BI: Postoperative analgesia with naproxen in foot surgery. *J Am Podiatry Assoc* 74:125–128, 1984.
15. Naproxen: *AMA Drug Evaluations*, ed 4. Chicago, American Medical Association, 1980, p 80.
16. Stetson JB, Robinson K: Analgesic activity of oral naproxen in patients with postoperative pain. *Scand J Rheumatol* (Suppl) 2:50, 1973.
17. Ruedy J: A comparison of the analgesic efficacy of naproxen and acetylsalicylic acid-codeine in patients with pain after dental surgery. *Scand J Rheumatol* 2:50, 1973.
18. Simon LS, Mills JA: Non-steroidal anti-inflammatory drugs (part 1). *N Engl J Med* 302:1170–1185, 1980.
19. Van Pelt WL: Postoperative management of pain by the use of ponstel (mefenamic acid), a nonsteroidal, anti-inflammatory agent. *J Foot Surg* 22:78–79, 1983.
20. Inturrise CE: Targeting narcotic action to patients' needs. *Drug Ther* 10:49–55, 1980.
21. Beaver WT: Mild analgesics, a review of their clinical pharmacology. Part I. *Am J Med Sci* 250:577–604, 1965.
22. Beaver WT: Mild analgesics, a review of their clinical pharmacology. Part II. *Am J Med Sci* 251:576–599, 1966.
23. Marcus SA, Block BH: *American College of Foot Surgeons, Complications in Foot Surgery, Prevention and Management*, ed 2. Baltimore, Williams & Wilkins, 1984, pp 76–77.
24. Gilman AG, Goodman LS, Gilman A: *The Pharmacological Basis of Therapeutics*, ed 6. New York, Macmillan, 1980, pp 494–534.
25. Beaver WT: Analgesic combinations. In Lasagna L(ed): *Combination Drugs: Their Use and Regulation*. New York, Stratton Intercontinental Medical Book Corp, 1975.
26. Halpern LM: Analgesic drugs in the management of pain. *Arch Surg* 112:861–869, 1977.
27. Beaver WT: Comparison of morphine, hydroxyzine, and morphine plus hydroxyzine in postoperative pain. In *Proceedings, Recent Studies on the Nature and Management of Acute Pain. Hosp Prac*, Special Report, 11:23–25, January 1976.
28. Kantor TG: Studies of orally administered narcotics, ataractics, and combinations of the two. In *Proceedings, Recent Studies on the Nature and Management of Acute Pain. Hosp Prac* 11:29–32, January 1976.
29. Stambaugh JE Jr: Pharmacokinetic studies of the interactions between meperidine and other drugs. In *Proceedings, Recent Studies on the Nature and Management of Acute Pain. Hosp Prac*, 11:33–39, January 1976.
30. Beaver WT, Feise G: Comparison of the analgesic effects of morphine, hydroxyzine and their combination in patients with postoperative pain. In Bonica J, Albe-Fessard D (eds): *Advances in Pain Research and Therapy*. New York, Raven Press, 1976, pp 553–557.
31. Anderson TW, Gravenstein JS: Cardiovascular effects of sedative doses of pentobarbital and hydroxyzine. *Anesthesiology*, 27:272–278, 1966.
32. Miller SJ: Temperature regulation and postoperative fever: a preliminary study. *J Am Podiatry Assoc* 74:373, 1984.
33. Blake MJF: Relationship between circadian rhythm of body temperature and introversion-extraversion. *Nature* 215:896–897, 1967.
34. Kleitman N: Biological rhythms and cycles. *Physiol Rev* 29:1, 1949.
35. Mellette HC, Hutt BK, Askovitz SI, Horvath SM: Diurnal variations in body temperatures. *J Appl Physiol* 3:665, 1951.
36. Atkins E: Pathogenesis of fever. *Physiol Rev* 40:580–646, 1960.
37. Wolff SM, Fauci AS, Dale DC: Unusual etiologies of fever and their evaluation. *Ann Rev Med* 26:277, 1975.
38. Goldberg MJ, Roe CF: Temperature changes during anesthesia and operations. *Arch Surg* 93(2):365–369, 1966.
39. Roe CF, Goldberg MJ, Blair CS, Kinney JM: The influence of body temperature on early postoperative oxygen consumption. *Surgery* 120:85, 1966.
40. Roe CF: Surgical aspects of fever. *Curr Probl Surg* 1:43, 1968.
41. Sadove MS, Redlin TA, Katz D: Postoperative fever and the halothane controversy. *Compr Ther* 1(1):69–72, May 1975.
42. Miller SJ: Body temperature following podiatric surgery: evaluation and management. *J Am Podiatry Assoc* 74:477–481, 1984.
43. Gilman AG, Goodman LS, Gilman A: *The Pharmacological Basis of Therapeutics*, ed 6. New York, MacMillan, 1980, p 418.
44. Gilman AG, Goodman LS, Gilman A: *The Pharmacological Basis of Therapeutics*, ed 6. New York, MacMillan, 1980, pp 1010–1011.
45. American College of Surgeons: *Manual of Preoperative and Postoperative Care*, ed 3. Philadelphia, WB Saunders Co, 1983, pp 38–67.
46. Wilson JL: *Handbook of Surgery*, ed 5. Los Altos, CA, Lange Medical Publications, 1973, pp 150–174.

Additional References

Arrigoni-Martelli E: *Inflammation and Antiinflammatories*. New York, Spectrum Publications, 1977.

Bonica JJ, Benedetti J: Postoperative pain. In Condon RE, DeCosse JJ (eds): *Surgical Care. A Physiologic Approach to Clinical Management*, Philadelphia, Lea & Febiger, 1980, pp 394–414.

Braenden OJ, Eddy NB, Halbach H: Synthetic substances with morphine-like effect. Relationship between chemical structure and analgesic action. *Bull WHO* 13:937–998, 1955.

deStevans G (ed): *Analgesics, Medicinal Chemistry*, vol 5. New York, Academic Press, 1965.

Drago JJ, Jacobs AJ, Oloff LM: Elevated temperature in the postoperative patient. *J Foot Surg* 21(4):269–277, 1982.

Eddy NB, Halbach H, Braenden OJ: Synthetic substances with morphine-like effect. Clinical experience: potency, side effects, addiction liability. *Bull WHO* 17:569–863, 1957.

Fields HL, Levine JD: Pain—mechanisms and managements (medical progress). *West J Med* 141:347–357, 1984.

Gildea J: The relief of postoperative pain. *Med Clin North Am* 52:81–90, 1968.

Goforth P, Gudas CJ: Effects of steroids on wound healing: a review of the literature. *J Foot Surg* 19:22–23, 1980.

Haller JA: Analgesia in children. In Wilson RE(ed): *The Management of Pain in Surgical Practice*. New York, Appleton-Century-Crofts, 1979, p 75.

Hurley JV: *Acute Inflammation*, ed 2. New York, Churchill-Livingstone, 1983.

Kantor TG: Selecting the appropriate NSAID. *Drug Ther* 14:59–66, February 1984.

Lasagna L: The clinical evaluation of morphine and its substitutes as analgesics. *Pharmacol Rev* 16:47–83, 1964.

Roe BB: Are postoperative narcotics necessary? *Arch Surg* 87:912–915, 1963.

Sabiston DC (ed): *Davis-Christopher Textbook of Surgery*, ed 12. Philadelphia, WB Saunders Co, 1981.

Salib PI: *Plaster Casting*. New York, Appleton-Century-Crofts, 1975.

Simon LS, Mills JA: Non-steroidal anti-inflammatory drugs (part 2). *N Engl J Med* 302:1237–1243, 1980.

Spragg J: The plasma kinin-forming system. In Weissman G (ed): *Mediators of Inflammation*. New York, Plenum Press, 1974.

Van Pelt WL: Postoperative management of pain by the use of Ponstel (mefenamic acid), a nonsteroidal anti-inflammatory agent. *J Foot Surg* 22:78–79, 1983.

Wilson RE (ed): *The Management of Pain in Surgical Practice*. New York, Appleton-Century-Crofts, 1979.

Wittenberg M, Kinney KW, Black JR: Comparison of ibuprofen and acetaminophen-codeine in postoperative foot pain. *J Am Podiatry Assoc* 74:233–237, 1984.

Wolf DS, Ross WR: The foot. In Hill GJ (ed): *Outpatient Surgery*. Philadelphia, WB Saunders Co, 1980, pp 1158–1184.

Zweifach BW, Grant L, McCluskey RT (eds): *The Inflammatory Process*, ed 2, vol 5. New York, Academic Press, 1974.

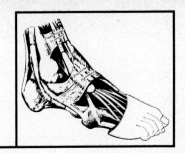

CHAPTER 10

Anesthesia

Raymond G. Cavaliere, D.P.M. and **Robert E. Bergman, D.O.**

Preoperative Testing

Approximately 15 million surgical procedures are performed annually with about one half of these operations being performed on persons classified as "normal and healthy." The surgical mortality among this group of patients is very low. The debate concerning what constitutes proper preoperative screening for routine surgery on healthy individuals continues today. It involves screening for disease before it is apparent, cost-benefit analysis, and medicolegal considerations.

The complete history and physical examination remain today as the best preoperative screening examination. From this the physician requests appropriate additional testing. The following recommendations are presented for healthy asymptomatic patients undergoing foot surgery.

Complete Blood Count

Anemia, unless severe, is usually asymptomatic and hence a preoperative hemotocrit or hemoglobin is worthwhile. The hematocrit should be above 30% (hemoglobin greater than or equal to 10 gm) for men and 27% for women or surgery should be delayed. Remember that polycythemia (hematocrit above 57% for men and 54% for women) carries with it additional risks of bleeding and thrombosis. White blood cell counts are rarely indicated. Values less than 2400/mm^3 with less than 900 to 1000 polymorphonuclear cells or above 16,000/mm^3 for both men and women are values deserving further study before elective surgery.

Electrocardiogram

The resting electrocardiogram EKG is unreliable for diagnosing ischemic heart disease but can recognize recent myocardial infarctions, frequent premature ventricular contractions (PVCs), and rhythms other than sinus. It is recommended for those over 40 years of age or with a positive medical history.

Chest X-Ray

Chest x-ray films are notoriously poor for diagnosing obstructive lung disease and very rarely pick up primary carcinoma in preoperative patients. Their use is recommended for those over 60 years of age unless otherwise warranted by the history and physical examination. Pulmonary function tests and arterial blood gases are rarely needed.

Blood Chemistry

An occasional abnormality may be found by blood chemistry and liver function tests, but in most cases these are false positives. Within this vast array of tests, three of them have good prognostic value. These include the SGOT, blood glucose, and BUN or creatinine. An elevated SGOT may signify hepatitis and therefore be important to both the anesthesiologist and all other health care members coming in contact with the patient. Although it is unusual for a patient with chronic renal disease to remain asymptomatic, a BUN or creatinine is valuable preoperatively to rule out renal insufficiency and to alert personnel to modify drug dosages. An elevated blood glucose could represent early type II diabetes and at least dictate an alteration of perioperative IV fluids with limited dextrose.

Urinalysis

A urinalysis is required to rule out infection, renal disease (proteinuria), and unsuspected diabetes mellitus. The test is cost effective and therefore worthy of use. Remember that urine sterility is recommended in patients undergoing implant arthroplasty or urinary catherization.

Coagulation Studies

Routine coagulation studies appear to have limited prognostic values except when a positive history for bleeding tendency is ascertained, the patient is undergoing surgery that carries the possibility of substantial hemorrhage, or if the patient will be severely compromised by bleeding at the operative site.

Preoperative Testing and Malignant Hyperthermia

Malignant hyperthermia is a potentially life-threatening disorder characterized by muscle rigidity, cardiac arrhythmias, fever, and acidosis. It can be precipitated by inhaled anesthetics, both depolarizing and nondepolarizing neuromuscular blocking agents, amide local anesthetics, and by other means. It can occur even after a previous uneventful anesthetic course. The incidence has been reported to be from 1 in 15,000 children to 1 in 100,000 adults with the overall incidence approximately 1 in 50,000 (1). Among those not properly treated, mortality is about 70%.

Proper identification of the person susceptible to malignant hyperthermia is complicated by the lack of any clearly associated diagnostic characteristics other than a possible family or personal history of complications with anesthesia. Some myopathies have been associated with susceptibility to malignant hyperthermia. The first is characterized by wasting of the lower ends of the vastus muscles with hypertrophy of the proximal quadriceps, usually without functional impairment. Inheritance is thought to be mendelian dominant. Another myopathy, recessively inherited in male patients, reveals cryptorchism, kyphosis or lordosis, webbed neck, and serratus weakness. In addition, elevated serum creatinine phosphokinase (CPK) or electromyogram or EKG abnormalities may be evident in patients susceptible to malignant hyperthermia. Other characteristics may be common to susceptible individuals such as muscular cramping, joint hypermobility, and dislocation and squint (2).

Remember that all of these indicators are nonspecific and frequently no signs are present to point to persons susceptible to malignant hyperthermia. Currently the only reliable diagnostic test for malignant hyperthermia susceptibility involves the use of a skeletal muscle biopsy specimen that has been exposed to halothane or caffeine in vitro. This test is expensive and only performed at specialized centers.

There is no simple noninvasive screening test for malignant hyperthermia before surgery. Susceptible patients as mentioned can demonstrate an elevated CPK preoperatively; about 80% of hyperthermia patients and some of their relatives reveal a higher than normal value (1). A good anesthetic and family history is the best preventive measure along with a high clinical suspicion and knowledge of management of the condition in case of its occurrence. Intravenous dantrolene sodium (Dantrium) is today the most effective drug for preventing and treating this clinical syndrome. Quick cooling of the body and reversal of the acidosis are also important in overall management.

Elective Surgery and Hypertension

In general, hypertension may contribute to coronary heart disease, intermittant claudication, stroke, and congestive heart failure. Obesity may be associated with hypertension. In the surgical patient uncontrolled hypertension indicates an increased risk for developing intraoperative or postoperative strokes and/or myocardial infarctions.

Most patients' antihypertensive medications should be continued without disruption during and after surgery. Diuretics may induce electrolyte abnormalities and therefore increase the risk of intraoperative cardiac arrhythmias. Hypertensive patients should ideally be seen by an internist preoperatively for assessment of blood pressure control, electrolyte assessment, and appropriate weight reduction. An EKG is suggested. Also, the anesthesiologist must be made aware of the patient's medications, some of which may interact with anesthetic agents.

Diabetes Mellitus and Elective Surgery

Microangiopathy is a lesion unique to diabetes that affects capillaries and is responsible for diabetic nephropathy and retinopathy, as well as cardiovascular disease. Peripheral vascular assessment, as well as examination for the presence of peripheral neuropathy should be considered preoperatively by the surgeon. Before surgery the patient's blood sugar should be well controlled (preferably less than 150 mg/dl) and the patient should be seen by a physician for a general assessment of diabetic control, state of the cardiovascular system, presence of neuropathy, retinopathy, glomerulopathy, and hidden infections.

Patients on oral hypoglycemic agents may or may not require insulin coverage perioperatively. Insulin dependent diabetics may receive one third to one half the daily dose of intermediate-acting insulin the morning of surgery and an intravenous solution of 5% dextrose in water is started and maintained throughout the perioperative period as long as the patient is taking nothing by mouth. Additional regular insulin should be administered according to a sliding scale based on plasma glucose levels versus urinary sugar.

Modest hyperglycemia will not interfere with leukocytic functions or wound healing.

Sickle Cell Disorders

Variants of sickle cell disease are types of hemolytic anemias caused by the substitution of valine for glutamic acid in the B-globin chains of HbA, the normal adult hemoglobin. Three principle variants exist. The homozygous state (SS) hemoglobinopathy is true sickle cell anemia. The heterozygous state (AS) hemoglofinopathy is the condition referred to as sickle cell trait. Lastly, the double heterozygous state (SC) disease consists of two abnormal hemoglobin chains.

Patients affected with the SS and SC hemoglobinopathies usually are aware of their disorders because of previous crises. Those affected with the AS hemoglobinopathy are usually asymptomatic and may not be aware of their underlying disorder. Most of the AS variant patients, under normal conditions, have no increase in morbidity or mortality as compared with the healthy population.

Three major factors contribute to red blood cell sickling: the HbS concentration, the partial pressure of oxygen, and the pH. Intraoperative use of tourniquets during extremity surgery certainly increases stasis, local acidosis, and hypoxia. Intravascular sickling during tourniquet use in sickle cell patients therefore affords a theoretical possibility of sickling in the patient with sickle cell disease. A review of the literature finds no increased risk of complications when using tourniquets in patients with sickle cell trait. Tourniquets should, however, be avoided (if possible) in those patients with sickle cell disease (homozygous or double heterozygous) because of their increased amounts of abnormal hemoglobin.

Preoperative patient evaluation should aim to identify those with sickle cell disorders. In addition to a sickle cell prep, those with uncertain hemoglobinopathies should undergo a hemoglobin electrophoresis. Intraoperatively and postoperatively, hypoxia, dehydration, and acidosis must be prevented in those with known sickle cell disease and caution should be used when using tourniquets on patients with sickle cell trait. With these precautions sickle cell crises with possible anemia, thrombosis, and infection can be avoided.

Emergency Surgery

Although podiatric surgery is usually considered an elective surgical specialty there are several instances where emergency surgery is indicated. These include acute fractures with neurovascular compromise, compartment syndromes, uncontrollable traumatic bleeding, and infection with septic complications.

Stat blood work should obviously be performed along with an adequate history and physical examination before surgery. Intraoperative endotracheal intubation may be necessary to prevent aspiration throughout the procedure.

Tourniquets

The use of pneumatic tourniquets for hemostatis is quite a common practice in podiatric surgery today. Complications such as thrombosis, inflammation, paralysis, tissue necrosis, and circulatory volume overload have been reported.

Noncardiac circulatory overload, often called tourniquet induced hypertension, may become more clinically significant especially if bilateral thigh tourniquets are used simultaneously (3–5). Significant decreases in patient's blood pressure following tourniquet release has also been reported (6). This has been attributed to a drop in peripheral resistance compounded by a postischemic reactive hyperemia.

Many studies have centered on systemic and local effects of tourniquet ischemia especially as related to acid-base changes, serum potassium, blood pressure rises and falls, and changes in PaO^2. Conclusions today are that no significant myocardial or pulmonary disturbances are produced after two or three hours of tourniquet ischemia and that the changes produced are only moderate and reversible provided that the blood pressure and acid-base status of the patient is stable. Note that these "changes" affect the myocardium to some degree and although tolerated well by the young and healthy patient, may be detrimental to other patients with foot deformities such as the rheumatoid arthritis patient and patients with other similar conditions.

Thigh tourniquets are usually preferred over ankle tourniquets because the thigh is the area of greatest circumference in the lower extremity and therefore provides maximum protection to nerves and blood vessels from pressure against bone. The use of the thigh tourniquet usually necessitates the use of either a general or spinal anesthetic to control ischemic pain although patients can usually tolerate an ankle tourniquet for one hour after inflation without the benefit of general anesthesia. Proper inflation pressure depends on the patient's blood pressure (systolic), local placement of the cuff, and the patient's size. Most physicians feel that thigh tourniquets should be inflated approximately 100 mm Hg above the preoperative systolic blood pressure with minor adjustments for the patient's size (7, 8). No correlation between thigh circumference and adequate tourniquet pressure has been established. Maximum ankle pressure is considered 250 mm Hg where pressures over 500 mm Hg at the thigh are considered unsafe. No tourniquet should be left inflated over two to three hours. Breathing periods of 5 to 15 minutes should be allowed before tourniquet reinflation. Note that no accepted safe duration of reinflation has been established after the breathing period.

The surgeon is urged to avoid tourniquets unless hemostasis is not achievable by anatomical dissection techniques and careful ligation and cautery of vessels.

Intubation

Endotracheal intubation may be considered for every elective surgical patient receiving general anesthesia. Specific indications include emergency surgery where one has to consider a full stomach on all patients. Intubation would prevent the dreaded complication of aspiration penumonitis. Other indications include: facilitation of tracheal suctioning, prolonged procedures, adverse operative position (i.e. sitting, prone, lateral, or head down); operative site near or involving the upper airway; or when airway maintenance is difficult by mask. Note that prolonged application of a mask on the face may result in tissue ischemia.

Although tracheal edema, croup, laceration, laryngeal trauma, and pneumothorax are potential complications of orotracheal intubation, most patients experience only a mild sore throat.

Positioning

The anesthesiologist and surgeon must prevent peripheral neuropathy and/or pressure necrosis in an anesthetized patient. In the supine position, the most common complication is that of brachial plexus injury, especially to the ulnar nerve. The anesthesiologist must prevent arm extension to avoid this.

The prone position carries danger from pressure to the orbit and dorsum of the foot. Proper padding can prevent these complications. Properly placed chest rolls will assist the patient in adequate ventilation.

For the patient in the lateral position the surgeon must be sure to place pillows between the knees and ankles and the anesthesiologist should provide padding to the patient's head and elbows.

As in any position, care should be taken to assure the viability of the IV line, endotracheal tube, and other measures used for monitoring.

GENERAL ANESTHETIC MANAGEMENT
Preoperative Medications

Preoperative medications, routinely used today, decrease the emotional and physical stress of surgery and thereby aid in the use of general anesthetic agents and lessen complications. They also make the patient more comfortable by decreasing the side effects of general anesthetic agents (i.e. salivation, nausea, vomiting, and brachycardia). Amnesia may be another benefit.

There are no set rules governing the choice of preoperative medications. Selection is usually based on the physician's experience and comfort with the agents, as well as the patient's age, sex, physical status, and contemplated procedure.

The agents commonly used include barbiturates, tranquilizers and sedative hypnotics, narcotics, anticholinergics (belladonna derivatives), plus histamine H2-receptor antagonists. Combinations of these agents often produce the best results, and they are seldom used alone.

Barbiturates

Pentobarbital (Nembutal) and secobarbital (Seconal) are the most commonly employed short-acting barbiturates. When used orally, they reach their desired maximum effect in one to one and a half hours and last for three to four hours versus one half hour and two to three hours, respectively, if given intramuscularly. They provide sedation and relieve apprehension in the preoperative patient. They produce minimal respiratory and circulatory depression, rare nausea and vomiting but do not produce analgesia. They do not have a specific antagonist.

Some evidence exists that these agents may hinder toxic effects of local anesthetic agents. Care should be taken not to give these agents to those with intermittent porphyria because to do so may precipitate an acute attack of this disease.

Tranquilizers and Sedative Hypnotics

Lorazepam (Ativan) and diazepam (Valium) are commonly used benzodiazepines employed to relieve anxiety and invoke amnesia preoperatively. Diazepam

is a specific anxiolytic agent and has greater blood levels after oral administration than after intramuscular injection. One should avoid IM administration because of slow and incomplete absorption. On the other hand, lorazepam is rapidly and almost completely absorbed after IM injection. Oral diazepam should be given one to two hours before the surgery in amounts of 5 to 10 mg. Lorazepam 2 to 4 mg orally is given in the same manner. In these doses diazepam rarely will incur significant cardiorespiratory depression; however, one must be careful because no specific antagonist exists for this drug.

Other popular agents include hydroxyzine (Vistaril), promethazine (Phenergan) and droperidol (Inapsine). Droperidol is also a potent antiemetic whereas hydoxyzine and promethazine possess antiemetic, sedative, and antihistaminic properties. Hydroxyzine and promethazine may also be used to augment the analgesic effects of narcotics without increasing respiratory depression.

Narcotics

The most frequently used premedication narcotics include morphine and meperidine (Demerol). Other agents include alphaprodine (Nisentil) and fentanyl (Sublimaze). Narcotics are credited with facilitating anesthetic induction and reducing anesthetic requirements while producing perioperative analgesia. Of significance is the reversibility of their effects by the direct narcotic antagonist naloxone (Narcan).

Adverse side effects include hypotension, respiratory depression, and nausea and vomiting. Current thinking reserves the use of preoperative narcotics to patients who will experience pain before or after surgery. Although these agents will allay patient apprehension, other agents such as barbiturates and tranquilizers are better and more effective for that desired effect.

Anticholinergics (Belladonna Derivatives)

Anticholinergics include atropine sulfate, scopolamine, and glycopyrrolate (Robinul). All agents are given intramuscularly about one half to one hour preoperatively and reduce respiratory tract secretions, protect against reflex bradycardia (an effect of general anesthesia), provide sedative and amnesic effects, as well as decrease gastric hydrogen ion secretion. Their side effects include dry mouth, poor visual accommodation, relaxation of the lower esophageal sphincter, heart rate changes, and body temperature elevation. Central nervous system toxicity includes restlessness, delirium, hallucinations, somnolence after anesthesia, and possible coma and convulsions. These central nervous system effects are seen mainly with scopolamine and atropine and rarely with glycopyrrolate because it does not cross the blood-brain barrier.

Glycopyrrolate has become increasingly more popular because it has no central nervous system effects, produces minimal cardiovascular and visual effects, and is more potent and longer lasting than atropine. Scopolamine causes many more central nervous system effects than atropine. Physostigmine is useful to reverse the effects of these agents.

Today, the antisialagogue effect of these medications is not as important as it was in years past when ether was a major anesthetic agent. In contrast, most inhalation agents today do little to stimulate upper airway secretions. In spite of this, the anticholinergic drugs remain popular and are used either alone or in combination.

Histamine H2-Receptor Antagonists

Cimetidine (Tagamet) given 300 mg orally, IM, or IV approximately one to two hours preoperatively appears to be useful in raising gastric fluid pH. Preoperative antacids provide the same benefit, however, with the addition of gastric fluid volume. The addition of this agent is not routine today, and its benefit in case of aspiration is not really known. One might consider its use in emergency surgery, patients with known gastroesophageal reflux, and in mask anesthesia especially with obese patients.

Remember that no medication alone or in combination can substitute for the patient-physician relationship. If performing outpatient surgery, one should consider the use of the oral barbituates, tranquilizers, and sedative-hypnotics. Other medications are better reserved for inpatient surgery where better patient monitoring is possible.

Induction

The induction of general anesthesia in the adult podiatric patient is usually accomplished by an intravenous short acting barbituate. Thiopental (Pentothal) is the most frequently used barbiturate for induction, the dosage being 3 to 5 mg/kg usually following a test dose of 50 mg intravenously. Induction with thiopental is usually rapid but smooth and with a brief duration of action. Thiopental is metabolized by the liver and excreted by the kidneys; however, its short duration of action is caused by redistribution of thiopental from the central nervous system to muscle, skin, bone, and fat tissue rather than to the metabolic action of the liver.

Methohexital (Brevital), another short-acting barbituate used for induction, is very similar to thiopental. Methohexital has a slightly shorter duration of action than thiopental; however, there is an increased incidence of coughing and singultus when methohexital is used for induction.

When an intravenous route is not available in a pediatric patient then rectal thiopental or methohexital in a 10% solution can be used as an induction agent. The patient is accompanied by a parent to a holding area where a maximum dose of thiopental (30 mg/kg) or methohexital is administered rectally. When administered this way sleep usually ensues within 10 to 15 minutes in 90% of the cases. This induction is frequently used in the nine months to four years of age group. It should be noted that this is considered an induction dose, not a preoperative med-

ication, and the anesthesiologist in charge should be available to treat any circulatory or respiratory problem that may occur.

Ketamine (Ketalar) can be used as an induction agent and for the maintenance of anesthesia. Ketamine produces a state referred to as dissociative anesthesia. The patient appears awake, with eyes open at times, and may continue to move; however, ketamine produces profound analgesia and the patient is unaware of his or her surroundings. Ketamine has certain advantages: it can be used intramuscularly in the uncooperative pediatric patient, the dose being 3 mg/kg; the child becomes quiet usually within 60 seconds.

Characteristics of ketamine are retained pharyngeal and laryngeal reflexes, stimulation of the circulatory system, increased salivation, and cerebrospinal fluid pressure. It can be used intravenously for induction and by repeated injections for the maintenance of anesthesia. Ketamine has been used in poor risk patients because of its circulatory stimulation and in patients who have eaten because of the retention of pharyngeal and laryngeal reflexes. Preoperative medication with a drying agent is important when using ketamine because of increased salivation. Vomiting with aspiration may occur with the use of ketamine and careful monitoring is essential.

Diazepam (Valium), a benzodiazepine derivative, has been used as an intravenous induction agent. It is reported to produce less circulatory and respiratory depression than thiopental. Diazepam is metabolized by the liver and its effect can be prolonged by hepatic cirrhosis. When diazepam is used prolonged somnolence may occur because of the metabolites produced. Another problem encountered with diazepam has been thrombophlebitis. A newer benzodiazepine (Midazolam) is expected to decrease these above problems.

Neuroleptanalgesia is a state of apathy and analgesia usually produced by a butyrophenone and a narcotic. Droperidol (Inapsine), a butyrophenone and major tranquilizer, can be given in high enough dosage with or without a narcotic to be used as an induction agent. Droperidol has a prolonged effect and potentiates the effects of narcotics. Droperidol is frequently used with fentanyl (Sublimaze) to produce neuroleptanesthesia.

Etomidate has been used as an intravenous induction agent in Europe for years and has recently been approved for use in the United States. The usual dosage is 3 to 5 mg/kg, which produces a rapid response, slightly slower than thiopental (Pentothal), and a rapid recovery in approximately three to five minutes. It is reported to cause fewer respiratory and circulatory changes and has been used in poor risk patients. One problem that has been seen frequently is severe pain in the extremity when administered intravenously. The pain can be reduced or eliminated by pretreatment with fentanyl (Sublimaze) to some extent.

Following the intravenous induction agent a mask is usually applied over the face and an anesthetic mixture of gases is administered to deepen and maintain anesthesia.

If an intravenous route is not available then induction by mask can be accomplished. When using a mask induction maximum gas flow at first is used, usually 6 to 8 liters of air per minute, for removal of nitrogen and to enable rapid uptake of anesthetic gases. The agents most frequently used for inhalation anesthesia are oxygen, nitrous oxide, and a potent volatile anesthetic agent.

Inhalation Agents

Nitrous oxide when used with oxygen as a sole analgesic in a 75% to 80% concentration usually will not produce adequate anesthesia in the healthy patient. Nitrous oxide is often combined with muscle relaxants and narcotics following an intravenous induction agent to provide good analgesia. One of the most useful administrations for nitrous oxide is in combination with a volatile anesthetic agent such as halothane, enflurane, or isoflurane. The use of nitrous oxide enables these agents to be used in lower concentrations, and as a result there is less circulatory and respiratory depression and a more rapid emergence.

Halothane (Fluothane) usually produces a rapid and smooth induction because of its low irritability to the respiratory tract. Halothane decreases blood pressure by decreasing cardiac contractility and causing peripheral vasodilation. Halothane also sensitizes the myocardium to catecholamines, which appears to be more of a problem when acidosis is present. If ventilation is adequate then infiltration of 0.15 ml/kg of 1:100,000 epinephrine in 10 minutes is considered safe by most authorities. A maximal dose of 0.45 ml/kg should not be used within one hour. Halothane is partially metabolized by the liver; the metabolites produced have been blamed for the reported cases of hepatic necrosis following halothane anesthesia.

Enflurane (Ethrane) first became available for general use in 1972. Enflurane, like halothane, produces rapid and smooth induction. When metabolized it produces free fluoride ions and for this reason the possibility of renal damage should be taken into consideration when used in a patient with existing renal disease. During the induction with enflurane motor hyperactivity has been noted; however, EEG studies and postanesthesia neurological examinations revealed no permanent changes. Because of the motor activity enflurane is not recommended for the patient with a history of a seizure disorder. Enflurane depresses myocardial contractibility and causes peripheral vasodilation; however, this appears to be less of a problem than with halothane. Enflurane does not appear to sensitize the heart to epinephrine to the same degree as halothane.

Isoflurane (Forane) was synthesized about the same time as enflurane but has just recently been approved for clinical practice. Isoflurane is a nonflammable fluorinated hydrocarbon like halothane and enflurane. Isoflurane has a pungent odor and when a mask induction is attempted breath holding, coughing, and laryngeal spasm can occur. The use of an intravenous agent allows isoflurane to be used for smooth and rapid anesthesia. Isoflurane is becoming very popular. It is metabolized only 0.2%, the rest being recovered unchanged through respiration. Cardiac contractibility is decreased during deep anesthesia; however, the cardiac output remains elevated because of an increase in the pulse rate. Isoflurane does not appear to sensitize the heart to catecholamines. The halogenated agents (isoflurane, enflurane, and halothane) can cause respiratory depression. When general anesthesia is used a patent airway with adequate ventilation must be assured.

Emergence

Emergence from these commonly used volatile agents is usually smooth and rapid. Halothane can produce prolonged emergence because of fat absorption of the agent. Isoflurane has the lowest blood solubility of the three agents and therefore the patient will usually respond more rapidly.

Problems that may be seen on emergence, which also may be seen during induction, include retching and vomiting, airway obstruction, and laryngeal spasm.

Postoperative pain is usually controlled with infiltration or nerve block anesthesia using long-acting local anesthetic agents. If any further pain medication is needed an intravenous or intramuscular narcotic is usually used. Shivering sometimes occurs postoperatively. This can be both uncomfortable and dangerous because of the increase in oxygen demand. The best way to treat this is by prevention using warm intravenous fluids and warm humidified gases. Small doses of intravenous narcotics have been used successfully to control shivering.

Nausea and vomiting can be very major problems. Many antiemetics are available and usually work with some success. The authors have recently used metoclopramide (Reglan) 10 mg IV over a 15-minute period with excellent results. It may cause an increase in sedation and it has been reported to cause extrapyramidal symptoms in about 1 patient in 500. Droperidol (Inapsine) in small doses, 0.25 ml to 0.5 ml, has been used intraoperatively to prevent postoperative nausea and vomiting with good results.

Adequate communication between the surgeon and the anesthesiologist should occur before the surgery. In this manner the anesthesiologist is informed as to the nature of the surgery, the time and positioning involved, as well as the health of the patient. In this way the best anesthetic agent and route is chosen that directly benefit the patient, surgeon, and anesthesiologist. The patient is consulted and informed about the nature of the surgical procedure and the anesthetic.

LOCAL ANESTHETIC AGENTS
Introduction

Local anesthesia can be traced back to the Peruvian nations who chewed erythroxylon coca plant leaves for pleasant stimulation and who also experienced reversible perioral numbness. Nieman, in 1860, identified cocaine as the active ingredient responsible for these effects. From that day forward research progressed, leading to the synthesis of the ester procaine in 1905 and the amide lidocaine in 1943. These advances heralded the beginning of modern local anesthesia. These two drugs remain today the prototype of each of their class. In podiatric practice these agents are used not only for minor surgical procedures but also for the diagnosis and treatment of many painful conditions. In surgery these agents are used to reduce general anesthetic requirements during lengthy procedures.

Chemical Aspects

All local anesthetics today contain three basic structural molecular components: an amine end, an aromatic end, and either an ester or an amide linkage connecting the two. Differences among these amide and aromatic components dictate the differences in drug potency, duration of action, and toxicity. Generally, larger components mean greater duration of action and potency. The addition of more complicated side chains renders the local anesthetic agent more "bindable" to tissue proteins, as well as more fat soluble. These additive features also make the drugs more "toxic" with additional potential to produce central nervous system and cardiac side effects.

The amide or ester linkage forms the basis of the two different classes of local anesthetic agents—the amides or esters (Table 10.1).

Pharmacodynamic Aspects of Local Anesthetic Agents

Local anesthetics act on the neuronal cell membrane to slow and eventually stop nerve conduction by somehow stabilizing the nerve cell membrane. Presently many theories exist as to how that occurs, all eventually leading to a decrease in the membrane permeability to ions, the final result being no nerve conduction.

Although many local anesthetics exist with different uses and properties, all fall into one of two major groupings as discussed earlier (Table 10.2). These two classes of drugs are metabolized in entirely different ways. The esther local anesthetics are broken down by plasma pseudocholinesterases, yielding amino alcohol and derivatives of para-aminobenzoic acid (PABA). Although true allergic reactions to local anesthetics in general are rare, they are more common in the esther group because of PABA. PABA is a common constituent found in sunscreens. Therefore esther-type local anesthetics should be avoided in any patient who has shown sensitivity to sunscreens or to PABA.

The amide-type local anesthetics, are metabolized by the liver and then excreted by the kidney. True "amide-type" allergic reactions are rare and one can use these agents cautiously in any patient reporting a history of sensitivity to local anesthetics (9). Diphen-

Table 10.1
Commonly used local anesthetics

Amides:	Esters:
Lidocaine	Cocaine
Mepivacaine	Procaine
Bupivacaine	Chloroprocaine
Etidocaine	Tetracaine
Prilocaine	

The basic structure of local anesthetics (4):

$$Ar - COO - (Ch2)n - N \begin{smallmatrix} R \\ R \end{smallmatrix} \quad HX \text{ (Hydrophilic)} \quad \text{(Salt)}$$

(Aromatic)   (Ester)

$$Ar - CO - (Ch2)n - N \begin{smallmatrix} R \\ R \end{smallmatrix} \quad HX \text{ (Hydrophilic)} \quad \text{(Salt)}$$

Aromatic   (Amide)

(From Rieglehaupt R, French S, Reinherz R: Properties of local narcotics. Pharmacologic Review. *J Foot Surg* 21:234–236, 1982.)

hydramine hydrochloride (Benadryl), 25 mg, locally has been reported to be substituted for local anesthetics in the patient with a history of true hypersensitivity (9). Its use has been widely reported in the general surgical and dental literature with minimal use within the podiatric profession. Hypersensitivity to Benadryl as a local anesthetic within the foot has been reported (10). It should be used cautiously and only when absolutely necessary until further documentation of its safe use within the foot is reported.

It is prudent to avoid large amounts of amide-type local anesthetics in patients with hepatic disease. One must also be careful with patients with significant renal disease to avoid local anesthetic toxicity.

All local anesthetics are weak bases and act on the nerve only after they cross the nerve's lipid barrier. Because diffusion is facilitated in the uncharged form one can now understand why local acidosis (i.e. infection) may slow down the anesthetic processs. In areas of local infection one may prefer to block proximally for optimal results.

Prevention and Management of Toxicity

When using a local anesthetic agent one must be aware of its maximum dose (Table 10.2) and this calculation should be performed for each individual. Preparations containing epinephrine permit a higher recommended maximum dose because of the local vasoconstrictive properties of epinephrine. Epinephrine will also increase the drug's duration of action for the same reason.

Toxic reactions may also be reduced by avoiding inadvertent intravascular injection. Frequent aspiration during injection is therefore advised. Using proper dosages of the right drug in the right patient is paramount.

Toxic effects may involve the cardiovascular and central nervous systems. Local anesthetics initially produce central nervous system and cardiovascular excitation followed by depressive effects eventually leading to coma, respiratory arrest, and cardiovascular arrest. The first essential treatment of any toxic seizure is establishment of an airway and oxygenation. If cardiovascular collapse has not occurred, intrave-

Table 10.2
Representative Local Anesthetic Agents in Common Clinical Use

Generic* and Common Proprietary Name	Approximate Year of Initial Clinical Use	Main Anesthetic Utility	Representative Commercial Preparation	Maximum Dose (mg)
Cocaine	1884	Topical	Bulk powder	200
Benzocaine	1900	Topical	20% ointment	—
Americaine		Topical	20% aerosol	
Procaine	1905	Infiltration	10 & 20 mg/ml solutions	1000
Novocain		Spinal	100 mg/ml solution	
Dibucaine	1929	Spinal	0.667, 2.5, & 5 mg/ml solutions	100
Nupercaine				
Tetracaine	1930	Spinal	Niphanoid crystals—20 mg/ml	200
Pontocaine		Spinal	10 mg/ml solutions	
Lidocaine	1944	Infiltration	5 & 10 mg/ml solutions	500
Xylocaine		Peripheral nerve blocks	10, 15, & 20 mg/ml solutions	
		Epidural	10, 15, & 20 mg/ml solutions	
		Spinal	50 mg/ml solution	
		Topical	2.0% jelly, viscous	
		Topical	2.5%, 5.0% ointment	
Chloroprocaine	1955	Infiltration	10 mg/ml solution	1000
Nesacaine		Peripheral nerve blockade	10 & 20 mg/ml solutions	
		Epidural	20 & 30 mg/ml solutions	
Mepivacaine	1957	Infiltration	10 mg/ml solution	500
Carbocaine		Peripheral nerve blockade	10 & 20 mg/ml solutions	
		Epidural	10, 15, & 20 mg/ml solutions	
Prilocaine	1960	Infiltration	10 & 20 mg/ml solutions	900
Citanest		Peripheral nerve blockade	10, 20, & 30 mg/ml solutions	
		Epidural	10, 20, & 30 mg/ml solutions	
Bupivacaine	1963	Infiltration	2.5 mg/ml solutions	200
Marcaine		Peripheral nerve blockade	2.5 & 5 mg/ml solutions	
		Epidural	2.5, 5, & 7.5 mg/ml solutions	
Etidocaine	1972	Infiltration	2.5 & 5 mg/ml solutions	300
Duranest		Peripheral nerve blockade	5 & 10 mg/ml solutions	
		Epidural	5 & 10 mg/ml solutions	

* USP nomenclature
(Modified from Miller, Ronald D. Anesthesia: New York Churchill-Livingstone, Inc., 1981. pg. 565.

nous injection of a barbituate or benzodiazepine will terminate a seizure. Vasoconstrictors and cardiac pacing can control cardiovascular depression.

An anaphylactic response to local anesthetics should be treated with vasopressors, antihistamines, corticosteroids, and supportive measures.

It is hoped that no practitioner will take local anesthetics for granted. They have widespread use within the professions; however, their potential for serious unpleasant results truly exists. Knowledge of their proper dosage and usage, as well as treatment of the patient who has a complication, will greatly reward the practitioner.

CLINICAL LOCAL ANESTHESIA
Intravenous Sedation and Nitrous Oxide

When one refers to intravenous analgesia, one usually refers to the use of a hypnotic, tranquilizer, or sedative with a narcotic analgesic and with or without the addition of nitrous oxide. This combination is based on the belief that many of these drugs reduce the concentration of inhaled anesthetics required for anesthesia and cause less depression of the cardiovascular system or other organ systems than do the inhaled anesthetic agents alone.

Many variations of the "nitrous oxide-narcotic" technique have become popular such as the use of innovar, thiopental, diazepam, and the nonnarcotic intravenous anesthetics, ketamine and procaine.

Harris and associates (11) have described the use of nitrous oxide and Valium to produce "conscious sedation" whereby the patient can respond but has total amnesia of the surgical procedure performed. This means of analgesia together with local anesthesia has proved safe even during office surgery with proper patient monitoring. Others have attested to the safe use of intravenous sedation during foot surgery (12–15). Donick and associates (16) have provided an excellent review of the concept of intravenous sedation and the agents employed for such analgesia.

Intravenous sedation can reduce operative anesthetic risks in properly chosen patients during most podiatric procedures while at the same time relieving patient anxiety and pain.

Nitrous Oxide

As mentioned earlier nitrous oxide is used in conjunction with other intravenous agents for the production of conscious sedation. It is the weakest of all anesthetic bases with a weak analgesic effect that is directly proportional to its inhaled concentration. Its effects, primarily on the central nervous system, range from somnolence to general anesthesia in increased doses. A 35% concentration has been proven to be the optimal concentration for sedation and analgesia. It is common for its concentration to vary from 15% to 50% depending on the particular patient. The drug has rapid onset and recovery. The gas, in addition, is not explosive or flammable. Mention must be made concerning the potential for possible irreversible myelopathy and neuropathy in those who chronically misuse this inhalation agent (17).

Epidural

Epidural anesthesia is a form of regional anesthesia in which the spinal nerves are blocked as they pass through the epidural space of the vertebral canal (Fig. 10.1). Peridural and extradural anesthesia are synonymous terms.

Epidural anesthesia is produced by passing a needle between the vertebral spines, at the desired level, just short of the dura and then depositing a local anesthetic agent. Important anatomical considerations include: (a) the epidural space extends from the foramen magnum to the coccyx, (b) the spinal cord ends at L2, and (c) the dural sac ends at S2. The preferred position for administration is the lateral prone position (Fig. 10.2). The use of epidural anesthesia includes operations on the lower extremities, use as a sympathetic block, and for the relief of intractable pain. It is often used when spinal anesthesia is required but where the anesthesiologist has reser-

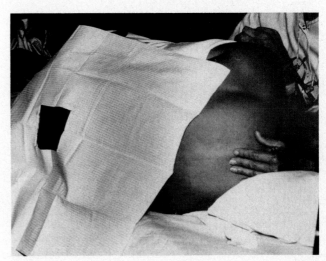

Figure 10.2. Patient shown in lateral prone position before epidural anesthesia.

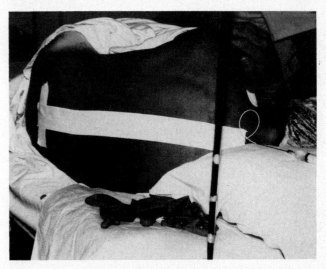

Figure 10.3. Continuous epidural block with indwelling catheter shown before bilateral ankle surgery.

vations about introducing the spinal anesthetic drug into the subarachnoid space. If properly performed no postspinal headache should result. Its onset is, however, somewhat delayed as compared to the onset of spinal anesthesia.

Epidural anesthesia is a viable anesthetic alternative in podiatric surgery patients who need complete anesthesia and where local anesthesia is difficult and general anesthesia prohibited. In prolonged procedures a continuous epidural block is possible with the use of an indwelling catheter (Fig. 10.3).

Spinal Anesthesia

Synonymous terms for spinal anesthesia include spinal analgesia and subarachnoid block. Here local anesthesia is introduced into the subarachnoid space by puncturing the dura and arachnoid in the lumbar area. Sensory, motor, and autonomic anesthesia result in the anterior and posterior roots in the area of the block. The procedure can be performed singly or as a continuous catheter drip.

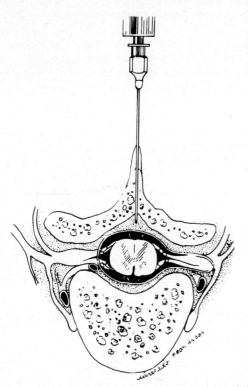

Figure 10.1. Diagram showing epidural space and its relationship to dura, periosteum, and arachnoid. (From Andriani J: *Labat's Regional Anesthesia: Technique and Clinical Application.* 1967, p. 381.)

The levels of anesthesia can be high, medium, low, or saddle. Podiatric surgery would employ a low block whereas high blocks should be avoided except in special circumstances because of their possible undesirable effects. An assortment of different local anesthetic agents are available for use. Proper positioning of the patient and use of strict asepsis are needed for this procedure.

Complications include hypotension, headache, possible palsies, cauda equina syndromes, and infection.

Infiltrative Block

Infiltrative block is a type of field block accomplished by injecting a wall of anesthetic solution across the path of nerves supplying an operative field. Knowledge of the location of nerves that cross the operative field and of their sensory distribution allow one to predict the distribution of anesthesia, as well as selectively perform specific nerve blocks. The field block is not an exact block per se and is usually used when surgery involves a small local area especially when dissection is in the superficial layers. In some cases the infiltration will involve all the layers of soft tissues including the subcutaneous layer, deep fascia, and muscle (as in the case of the Mayo block).

This block allows one to operate in a field undistorted by the effect of the injection and is a simple procedure to perform. More bleeding may be encountered because of the vasodilating action of the anesthetic fluid on the sympathetic nerves accompanying the blood vessels. This is especially noticeable with lidocaine. This increased bleeding is usually short-lived and should not affect the surgical procedure.

Intravenous Regional Anesthesia (Bier Block)

Intravenous regional anesthesia was first described by Bier (18) in 1908. The technique can be delivered by the operating surgeon; however, it is prudent to have an anesthesiologist present to monitor the patient and to treat any toxic reaction if one should occur.

An intravenous line as a route for drug administration is started in the upper extremity. Two pneumatic tourniquets are placed just below the knee and below the common peroneal nerve at the fibular neck. The tourniquets are checked for proper function. A suitable vein is cannulated with a small-gauge needle near the operative area and the limb is elevated to 45° for three minutes or exsanguinated with a Martin or Ace bandage (Fig. 10.4). The proximal tourniquet is then inflated to 275 to 300 mm Hg and lidocaine (Xylocaine) 0.5% or 1% at an amount of 3 mg/kg body weight is then injected. Anesthesia onset is rapid as lidocaine perfuses the tissues and prepping and draping of the operative area can now begin.

The distal tourniquet is inflated when the patient complains of tourniquet pain. Then the proximal tourniquet is released.

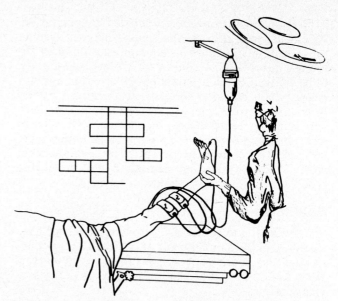

Figure 10.4. Technique shown for proper use of Bier block. (From Sanner F, Lawton J: Intravenous regional anesthesia in the lower leg and foot. *J Am Podiatry Assoc* 64:386, 1976.)

Lidocaine is the preferred intravenous local anesthetic because others have been associated with methemoglobinemia and thrombophlebitis. Lidocaine without epinephrine has been shown to be safer. Approximately 20 to 30 minutes of tourniquet use are needed to employ this technique. Earlier release of the tourniquet may trigger a toxic reaction caused by nondiffused local anesthetic in the central circulation. It is recommended that the tourniquet be deflated in intervals at the end of the procedure. Some indications for the use of this anesthesia include: a high risk patient for general anesthesia, a patient with a history of spinal arthritis or laminectomy in whom spinal anesthesia is less desirable, and a patient in whom specific nerve block techniques are for some reason impossible. Contraindications include a history of anaphylaxis to local anesthetic agents, previous phlebitis, history of vein stripping, and local infection. Intravenous sedation has been found to be a desirable adjunct to allay patient anxiety and fears.

Minor toxic reactions may occur and include ringing in the ears or a feeling of faintness. Of greater concern are major toxic effects, including decreased blood pressure, convulsions, or respiratory depression. With lidocaine at a dosage of 3 mg/kg body weight, serious toxic reactions are unlikely to occur.

Intravenous regional anesthesia can be safely used in surgery of the lower extremity. Its use, however, should not preclude concurrent use of specific nerve block anesthesia when applicable.

SPECIFIC NERVE BLOCK ANESTHESIA
Introduction

Regional anesthesia using specific peripheral nerve block technique should be widely used in surgery of the foot and ankle today. Infiltrative local anesthetic technique (field block) involves multiple injections, is painful, requires large volumes of local anesthetic, and frequently produces inadequate analgesia. Peripheral nerve blocks use precisely placed injections to anesthetize relatively large body areas with small amounts of local anesthesia. Knowledge of anatomy and sensory and motor nerve innervations are essential for proper use of this technique (Fig. 10.5).

Regional anesthesia does not interfere with body physiology as a whole, therefore making it an excellent method of anesthesia for most patients, as well as for poor risk and emergency patients. These patients should not eat or drink for at least four hours before surgery to minimize the danger of aspiration should a systemic reaction occur.

At Doctors Hospital the authors use local anesthesia even when the patient is under general anesthesia. This technique allows the anesthesiologist to carry the patient in a "light" plane of anesthesia and also aids us in anatomical dissection technique if epinephrine is added to the local anesthetic agent. Tourniquets are therefore usually unnecessary. We find 25 to 27 gauge needles most appropriate for the administration of the anesthetic.

Peripheral nerve block anesthesia should be considered the ultimate in foot and ankle surgery analgesia. Its use is gratifying to both physcian and patient while providing the patient with excellent postoperative pain relief for many hours depending on the choice of local anesthetic.

Tibial Nerve Block

Block of the sciatic nerve at its termination in the popliteal fossa should not be used routinely for surgical procedures involving the lower extremities. Its use is mainly reserved for procedures when anesthesia of the posterior aspects of the leg is desired (e.g. tendo achillis rupture, popliteal cyst, gastrocnemius recession, or tendo achillis lengthening).

Anatomy

The popliteal fossa is diamond shaped and is bounded inferiorly by the medial and lateral heads of m. gastrocnemius and superiorly by the long head of m. biceps femoris on the lateral side and the tendons of the semitendinosus and semimembranosus on the medial side (Fig. 10.6). The sciatic nerve separates into the larger tibial nerve and smaller common peroneal nerve about the middle of the back of the thigh. The common peroneal nerve diverges laterally gradually while the tibial nerve continues in the same direction as the sciatic and is parallel and 0.5 to 1 cm lateral to the midline of the popliteal fossa. Note that the sciatic nerve and its terminal branches are superficial to the popliteal vessels approximately 1.5 to 2 cm deep to the skin.

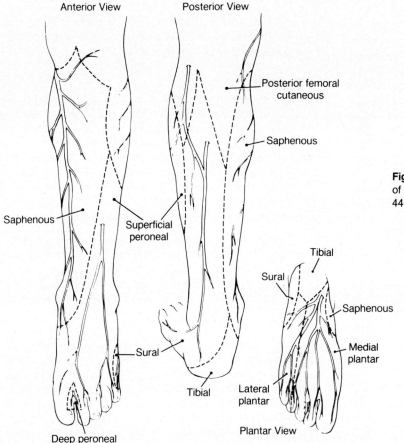

Figure 10.5. Cutaneous innervation of superficial nerves of foot and leg. (From Schurman DJ: *Anesthesiology*, vol 44. Philadelphia, JB Lippincott, 1976, pp 350–352.)

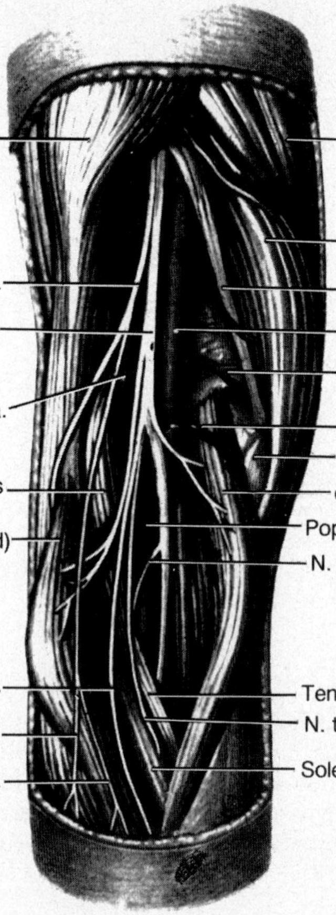

Figure 10.6. Dissection of left popliteal fossa. Upper boundaries have been pulled apart and aponeurosis to which two heads of gastrocnemius are attached has been split and heads separated. (From Romanes GJ: *Cunningham's Manual of Practical Anatomy. Upper and Lower Limbs*, vol 1. New York, Oxford University Press, p 129.)

Technique

The block should be performed with the patient prone and with the leg flexed 30° so that the popliteal fossa is easily outlined and structures easily palpated. An intradermal wheal of local anesthetic is then raised approximately 5 cm superior to the skin crease behind the knee in the location just described. Because of the large amount of fat within the popliteal fossa the needle is advanced until paresthesia is obtained. The needle is then withdrawn 1 to 2 mm to minimize the possibility of intraneural injection.

If difficulty is encountered in blocking the tibial nerve one may use a peripheral nerve stimulator for tibial nerve location.

Common Peroneal Nerve Block

The common peroneal nerve block is useful in a number of situations that include: (*a*) relaxation of the muscles about the ankle during an ankle stress radiograph following acute trauma, (*b*) for a diagnostic measure in peroneal spastic flatfoot, and (*c*) when other more distal blocks are prohibited because of trauma or infection.

Anatomy

The common peroneal nerve, after leaving the popliteal fossa, winds around the neck of the fibula and divides into deep and superficial peroneal nerves. This division occurs about the fibula neck and the upper fibers of the peroneal longus muscle. The nerve is very superficial at this level and can be palpated best posterior to the fibular neck.

Technique

An intradermal wheal is raised approximately 2 to 3 cm distal to the fibular head at the point where the nerve crosses the fibula. The needle is advanced slowly; the nerve should be no more than 1 to 1.5 cm deep to the skin. Once distal paresthesia is obtained, one aspirates to assure that the needle is not within a vessel and then deposits 3 to 5 cc of local anesthetic.

Superficial Peroneal Nerve Block

Ankle block anesthesia describes a process whereby six nerves, all innervating the foot, are anesthetized at the ankle. This nerve compromises of two of the nerves that transverse the ankle. These nerves, as well as the others, will be discussed separately.

Anatomy

The superficial peroneal nerve descends through the peroneal muscles after arising off the common peroneal nerve. It enters the superficial fascia at the junction of the middle and distal third of the leg and then branches into the medial and intermediate dorsal cutaneous nerves. Both nerves pass deep to the dorsal venous arch as they each divide and terminate into dorsal digital nerves of the foot (Fig. 10.7).

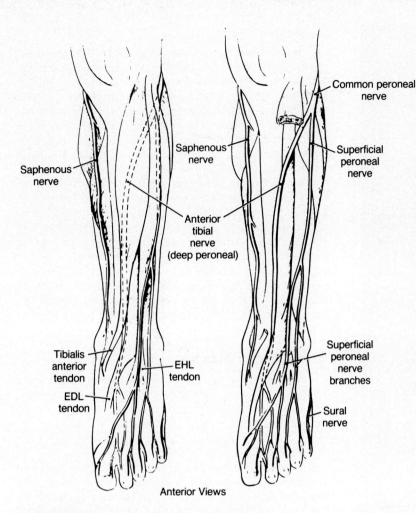

Figure 10.7. Anterior views of deep and superficial nerves of foot and leg. (From Schurman DJ: *Anesthesiology*, vol 44. Philadelphia, JB Lippincott, 1976, p 352.)

Anterior Views

Technique

Both nerves are located approximately 1 cm above the base of the medial malleolus on the anterior ankle. The medial dorsal cutaneous nerve lies lateral to the tendon of m. extensor hallucis longus and is felt as a strong cordlike structure that can be gently rolled under an index finger within the subcutaneous tissues. The intermediate dorsal cutaneous nerve can be palpated in the same manner running approximaely 1 to 1.5 cm anterior to the lateral malleolus. Lemont (19) has described a simple technique actually to visualize the nerve at this location by simply plantarflexing and inverting the foot (Fig. 10.8). Once the specific nerves are identified, approximately 0.5 to 1 cc of local anesthetic is infiltrated directly adjacent to or under them. Eliciting of paresthesia is not necessary.

Deep Peroneal Nerve Block

The deep peroneal nerve must be anesthetized when performing surgery about the first metatarsal interspace dorsally.

Anatomy

The deep peroneal nerve arises from the common peroneal nerve as it divides about the fibular neck. It pierces the anterior intermuscular septum and continues inferiorly as the anterior tibial nerve with the anterior tibial artery while lying on the interosseous membrane. It crosses the anterior ankle approximately midway between the malleoli usually between the tendons of m. extensor hallucis longus and m. extensor digitorum longus. At this point it is called the deep peroneal nerve (Fig. 10.7). It usually lies just lateral to the anterior tibial artery beneath the deep fascia.

Technique

A fine-gauge needle is advanced through the deep fascia just lateral to the pulse of the anterior tibial artery between the two long extensor tendons. Advancement is stopped when paresthesia occurs or when the needle touches the tibia. At this point 1 to 2 cc of local anesthesia is introduced for a complete block.

Of interest is that the anterior tibial nerve may vary in its relation to the tendon of m. extensor hallucis longus and its muscle, passing either laterally or medially to that structure (20).

Posterior Tibial Nerve Block

There is probably no single nerve block used in foot surgery as much as that of the posterior tibial nerve. It is blocked for tarsal tunnel surgery and surgery for soft tissue masses and foreign bodies about

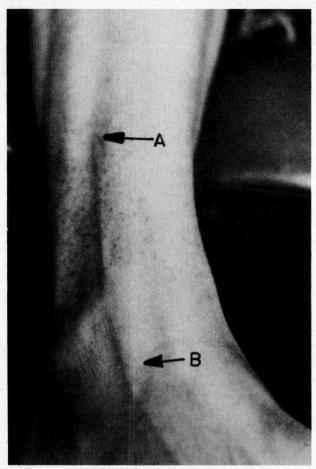

Figure 10.8. (A) Superficial peroneal nerve after exiting deep fascia and before its division. (B) Intermediate dorsal cutaneous nerve. Foot is plantarflexed and inverted. (From Lemont H: A simplified nerve block to control postoperative foot pain. *J Am Podiatry Assoc* 68:193, 1978.)

the plantar aspect of the foot. It is also used before injection therapy for painful heel conditions and as a therapeutic modality in the treatment of Sudeck's dystrophy.

Anatomy

The posterior tibial nerve is a continuation of the tibial nerve and passes through the posterior compartment of the leg, deep to the superficial calf muscles just beside the posterior tibial artery. In the lower leg it rests next to the posterior tibial surface and passes deep to the flexor retinaculum at the ankle as it enters the foot to divide into the lateral and medial plantar nerves between the first and second layer of plantar muscles (Fig. 10.9). The medial calcaneal branch divides higher about the malleolus and then pierces the deep fascia to supply the medial and posterior surfaces of the heel.

A cross section at the ankle will reveal these structures from anterior to posterior: the tendon of m. tibialis posterior, the tendon of m. flexor digitorum longus, the posterior tibial vein, the posterior tibial artery, the posterior tibial nerve, and the tendon of m. flexor hallucis longus (Fig. 10.10).

Technique

It has been the authors' experience that the most useful landmark is the pulsation of the posterior tibial artery just posterior and medial to the medial malleolus. One should inject slowly approximately 0.5 to 1 cm superior to this landmark so as to obtain anesthesia of all three branches before the trifurcation. Slow injection technique will allow one to feel the needle pass through the subcutaneous layer, pierce the deep fascia, and subsequently lie within the tarsal canal. Contact with the nerve should be at a depth of 1.5 to 2 cm. Paresthesias are occasionally elicited but do not have to be. Aspiration is essential here to avoid intravascular injection. If this occurs one redirects the needle more posteriorly. Approximately 3 to 5 cc of local anesthesia are adequate for this block.

Failure to achieve a complete block may be secondary to being within the wrong tissue layer or secondary to early nerve trifurcation. One should attempt a more proximal injection should this situation occur.

Sural Nerve Block

The sural nerve block represents another useful nerve block when performing foot or ankle surgery. Injury to or surgical entrapment of this nerve may be very disabling.

Anatomy

The sural nerve is a branch of the tibial nerve in the popliteal fossa and descends deeply between the heads of m. gastrocnemius to exit the deep fascia about the middle of the back of the leg. In its then superficial course it is joined by the peroneal communicating nerve and continues to travel with the short saphenous vein posterior to the lateral malleolus, superficial to the deep fascia. It courses approximately 1 to 1.5 cm inferior to the lateral malleolus and then has a variable distribution as it courses to the fifth toe (Fig. 10.9).

Technique

The nerve can be blocked just inferior to the lateral malleolus or just superior to it by fanning out approximately 3 to 5 cc of local anesthetic within the subcutaneous tissue. No paresthesias should be elicited. Many times one can palpate the nerve avoiding the fanning technique and using 0.5 to 1 cc of anesthetic. Anatomical variations of this nerve are rare about the malleolus.

Saphenous Nerve Block

The saphenous nerve must be anesthetized before surgery about the longitudinal arch because of diamond-shaped cutaneous innervation about the navicular region. Occasionally its innervation will extend to the metatarsophalangeal joint (21).

Anatomy

The saphenous nerve is the longest branch of the femoral nerve and arises in the femoral triangle and

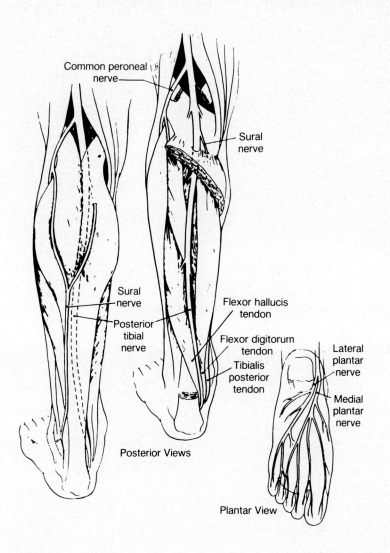

Posterior Views

Plantar View

Figure 10.9. Course of posterior tibial and sural nerves as they pass from leg into foot. (From Schurman DJ: *Anesthesiology*, vol 44, no 4, 1976, p 351.)

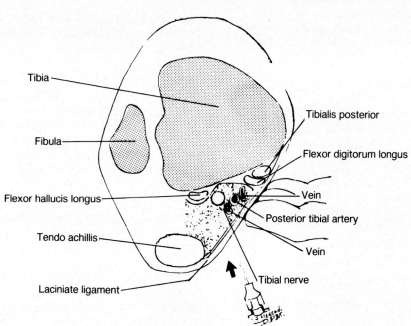

Figure 10.10. Cross section of left ankle. (From Mercado AO: *An Atlas of Foot Surgery. Forefoot Surgery*. Carolando Press, Oak Park, IL, 1979, pp 10, 11, 14.)

then pursues a complicated course before exiting the deep fascia just inferior to the medial epicondyle of the knee beside the greater saphenous vein. It then continues to travel with the greater saphenous vein within the superficial fascia and crosses the ankle just lateral to the vein. The nerve is palpable at that point (Fig. 10.7).

Technique

To anesthetize the saphenous nerve one may palpate it (if possible) and then inject approximately 0.5 to 1 cc of local anesthetic just lateral to the great saphenous vein. Aspiration here is most critical to avoid intravascular injection. Complete anesthesia is obtained quickly.

Digital Block

Not one previous nerve block thus far reviewed demands the finesse required by the digital block. Digital blocks may be avoided in the elderly or those with peripheral vascular disease by performing a proximal nerve block, thereby reducing more distal tissue insult.

Anatomy

Each digit is supplied by four nerves, two dorsally and two plantarly, running on the medial and lateral aspects of the toe within the subcutaneous tissues.

Technique

The authors have found that the two-point digital block (hallux or lesser toe) as described by Forman (22) has resulted in profound anesthesia in almost all cases (Fig. 10.11). Two wheals are raised on the dorsomedial and dorsolateral aspects of the proximal digit. The needle is then advanced within the subcutaneous layer until it is palpated plantarly. Approximately 0.25 to 0.5 cc of local anesthetic is deposited evenly along both the medial and lateral aspects of

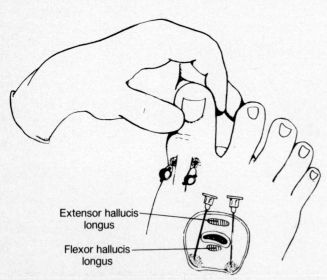

Figure 10.11. Digital block technique used for hallux or lesser digit anesthesia. (From Mercado AO: *An Atlas of Foot Surgery. Forefoot Surgery.* Carolando Press, Oak Park, IL, 1979, pp 10, 11, 14.)

Extensor hallucis longus

Flexor hallucis longus

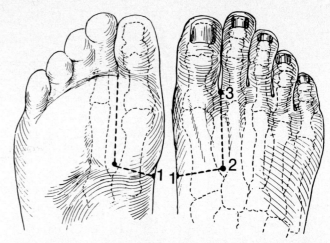

Figure 10.12. Field block for disarticulation of great toe, hallux valgus correction, or amputation. For base wedge osteotomy block is performed more proximal. (From Andriani J: *Labat's Regional Anesthesia: Technique and Clinical Application*, 1967, p 526.)

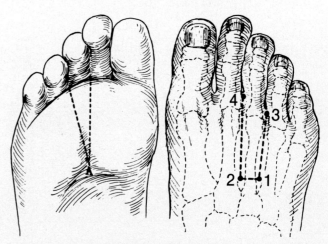

Figure 10.13. Field block for resection of third toe or third ray. (From Andriani J: *Labat's Regional Anesthesia: Technique and Clinical Application*, 1967, p 526.)

the toe. The anesthetic agent should be deposited just as close to skin as possible for rapid anesthesia. Anesthesia is usually profound except in rare cases.

Ring block technique (four point digital block about the base of the toe) should always be avoided for fear of creating a fluid tourniquet. Besides, this procedure is much more painful.

Mayo Block

The Mayo block is a type of field block that involves infiltration of local anesthetic through all tissues proximal to the surgical site in a ring block fashion (Fig. 10.12) It is an intermediate procedure between specific nerve block anesthesia and pure local infiltration. The procedure allows use of less local anesthesia than would be needed if one were to infiltrate the surgical field directly. Surgical tissue planes are therefore preserved in addition.

Field block anesthesia is useful when excising soft tissue tumors, correcting hallux valgus, or performing ray resections (Fig. 10.13). The Mayo block describes a proximal block about the first metatarsal (or lesser metatarsal) base. A wheal is raised proximally in the first interspace and then the needle is advanced plantarly. Approximately 1.5 cc of local anesthetic is infiltrated evenly along the course of the injection. The needle is then withdrawn partially and redirected medially and a subsequent wheal is raised along this course. The needle is now re-entered medially and advanced plantarly, again depositing approximately 1.5 cc evenly. The final injection is performed from medial to lateral at the plantar proximal aspect of the first metatarsal. No more than 5 cc of local anesthetic is needed for a complete block. Hallux valgus correction along with any first metatarsal osteotomy can then be comfortably performed.

EPINEPHRINE AND FOOT SURGERY

The medical literature abounds with concepts denouncing the use of epinephrine-containing local anesthetics in digital surgery.

Excellent studies and surveys have been performed within the podiatric profession documenting both the safe and effective use of 1:100,000 and 1:200,000 concentrations of epinephrine used for injection into the toes. In an experimental study performed by Tipton and Gudas (23) at the University of Chicago using skin temperature as a method for obtaining information about circulation in a toe they concluded that lidocaine had a substantial vasodilatory effect whereas epinephrine caused dose-dependant vasoconstriction that not only counteracted the vasodilatory effect of lidocaine but also lost its effect in 15 to 20 minutes. They did not observe any compartment syndromes after injection of 3 cc of local anesthetic per digital block.

Another study performed by Green and associates (24) at the Pennsylvania College of Podiatric Medicine used light-sensitive plethysmography as an indicator of digital perfusion while comparing bupivicaine and lidocaine with and without epinephrine as local anesthetics. They found that blood perfusion levels returned to baseline values by approximately one hour post injection. This concurred with the study of Scarlet and associates (25). This study also documented that even during the maximum time of vasoconstriction, circulation to the digits was never completely occluded.

Roth (26) in 1981 reported on complications of epinephrine-containing local anesthetic solutions in the toes in over 2,100,000 injections. This study again documented an acceptable therapeutic level of safety for 1:100,000 and 1:200,000 concentrations of epinephrine. Furthermore, Kaplan and Kashuk (27) and Steinberg and Block (28) have documented their lack of complications using digital injections of lidocaine with epinephrine 1:100,000 in over 65,000 and 200,000 injections, respectively.

Discussion

There appears to be a very large difference of opinion regarding the use of epinephrine in the digits in the current medical literature. More correctly stated, the morbidity attributed to the use of epinephrine in local anesthetic agents has probably been as a result of several other factors. These factors include poor patient selection, inadequate medical and peripheral vascular assessment, improper preparation of injectable solutions, improper injection technique, improper tissue handling, excessive operative dissection, and, especially, injection of excessive volumes. Of particular importance is that denervated blood vessels (i.e. decreased sympathetic tone) are hypersensitive to the vasoconstrictive effects of epinephrine. Therefore if careful neurological evaluation reveals a neurotrophic foot, one should be especially conservative in the use of epinephrine. This may well provide the answer to age-related increased sensitivity to epinephrine injections in the toes. Such sensitivity may be secondary to age-related partial denervation.

Contraindications to epinephrine-containing solutions include known sensitivity and thyrotoxicosis. Epinephrine may be used prudently in patients with coronary artery disease or hypertensive cardiovascular disease. A relative caution to the use of epinephrine in the digits is found in patients taking amitriptyline HCL (Elavil) and other tricyclic antidepressants. This class of drugs appears to react with both anticholinergics and epinephrine centrally and peripherally augmenting their effects. Careful dose adjustment or avoiding epinephrine entirely is suggested (29). Epinephrine also sensitizes the myocardium when used concomitantly with inhalation agents such as halothane (Fluothane) and cyclopropane. Because of the potential for causing cardiac arrhythmias, its use here should be avoided or carefully controlled after consultation with the anesthesiologist. Vasoconstrictors should also be avoided or used very conservatively in patients taking other antidepressant medication and monoamine oxidase (MAO) inhibitors (30, 31).

Epinephrine added to local anesthetics does have definite advantages such as prolonging anesthesia, permitting the use of a smaller volume of injectable, thereby reducing the incidence of toxic reactions, and providing excellent control of capillary bleeding within the operative field. Such hemostasis provides good visualization and allows the use of anatomic dissection techniques without the use of a tourniquet.

Conclusion

Although adverse effects such as cerebral hemorrhage and local tissue necrosis have been reported with the use of epinephrine, these all appear to be dose related and associated with other cumulative variables. The group at Doctors Hospital has used epinephrine in concentrations of 1:100,000 and 1:200,000 with minimal complications in over 50,000 foot surgery procedures. They advocate the use of 1:200,000 to 1:100,000 concentration of epinephrine to be an effective and safe means of local vasoconstriction used to facilitate anatomical dissection. The technique the authors reference has been used in over 2000 procedures per year for 27 years. Complications have been extremely rare and when present have appeared to relate more to the volume of the anesthetic than to epinephrine. The authors do not consider a tourniquet as a viable alternative unless absolutely necessary.

COMPLICATIONS OF LOCAL ANESTHESIA

Adverse reactions to the use of local anesthetics for peripheral nerve blocks are either local effects or systemic reactions.

Systemic toxic reactions result from inadvertent intra-arterial or intravenous injection, administration of an excessive dose, or from rapid absorption of the drug from a highly vascular area. The use of the smallest effective volume of the weakest effective concentration is therefore suggested. Signs, symptoms, and treatment have been discussed earlier. Another systemic reaction is the true allergic reaction seen almost exclusively with the ester-type local anesthetic agents. These reactions are extremely rare.

Local adverse reactions may be of a toxic nature secondary to preservatives and solvents. Other local reactions include hematoma, infections, inflammation, neuritis (rare), edema, and possible slough.

Intelligent use of local anesthetic agents with a knowledge of emergency treatment make the use of local anesthesia safe and rewarding.

NONSURGICAL USE OF REGIONAL ANESTHESIA

Sympathetic Dystrophy and Related Disorders

Nerve blocks can be performed to establish a diagnosis, to differentiate one entity from another, or to establish whether surgical intervention or chemical neurolysis would be helpful.

Among the syndromes affecting the lower extremity amenable to nerve block are reflex sympathetic dystrophy (Sudeck's atrophy) (32–36, 40), peripheral vascular disease, chronic vasospastic disorders, hyperhydrosis, bursitis, capsulitis, tendinitis, myofascial pain syndromes (37–39), tenosynovitis (41), metatarsalgia, causalgia (36, 42), and entrapment syndromes.

All of the peripheral vessels except the capillaries are innervated by the sympathetic nervous system. These nerves are the first affected by local anesthetic agents and are followed by the nerves mediating the sensations of cold, pain, touch, deep pressure and heat. Motor nerves are affected last. The relief of pain and discomfort following the block often outlasts the sensory blockade by many hours (32, 38). Sympathetic interruption has also been found to be present for up to 48 hours after the return of normal motor and sensory function (34). The reason for this phenomenon is unknown. Repeated peripheral chemical sympathectomy (posterior tibial nerve blocks) or repeated infiltration of painful areas with local anesthetics may permanently relieve or at least reduce pain in many of these entities (36).

Regional intravenous block with local anesthetics

and soluble corticosteroid has been described in the treatment of posttraumatic dystrophy of the extremities with good results (32). Mobilization of the extremity followed by physiotherapy is an important addition to therapy. Early recognition and treatment of this disorder is recommended (33, 36).

Obviously nerve block anesthesia represents a most useful tool both diagnostically and therapeutically, besides its established role in surgical anesthesia. Timely application of its use can relieve many clinical syndromes just described; its therapeutic value outlasts its immediate effects. Its use can also prevent the development of the chronic pain syndrome and alleviate anxiety that may have great psychological value (42). The relief of pain allows for decreased muscle spasm, facilitates motion, and therefore prevents the complication of disuse.

CONCLUSION

Nothing is of greater concern than the safe and uncomplicated journey of our surgical patients. Their safety begins with a thorough understanding of the preoperative patient evaluation, as well as with our knowledge of anesthetic principles and guidelines. Complications and their treatment are another area deserving of concern. Although major complications are rare, one should be prepared to be confronted with one at any time.

Anesthetic principles and techniques encompass a vast amount of material. Individual excellence in local anesthesia with its various medical and surgical uses requires an in-depth understanding of anatomical principles and relationships. Through continued study, research, practice, and a desire for "perfection," the practitioner can offer superior quality care for those he or she treats.

References

1. Byrd JP: Malignant hyperthermia. *South Med J* 76:890–893, 1983.
2. Murphy AL, Conlay L, Ryan JF, Roberts JT: Malignant hyperthermia during a prolonged anesthetic for reattachment of a limb. *Anesthesiology* 60:149–150, 1984.
3. Maurer NH, Voegeli PT, Sorkin BS: Non-cardiac circulatory overload secondary to penumatic thigh tourniquets. *J Am Podiatry Assoc* 73:589–592, 1983.
4. Bradford E: Haemodynamic changes associated with the application of lower limb tourniquets. *Anaesthesia* 24:191–197, 1969.
5. Kaufman RD, Walts LF: Tourniquet induced hypertension. *Br J Anaesth* 54:333–336, 1982.
6. Modig J, Kolstad K, Wigren A: Systemic reactions to tourniquet ischemia. *Acta Anaesthesiol Scand* 22:609–614, 1978.
7. Estersohn H, Sourifman H: The minimum effective midthigh tourniquet pressure. *J Foot Surg* 21:281–284, 1982.
8. Reid H, Camp RA, Jacob WH: Tourniquet hemostasis. A clinical study. *Clin Orthop* 177:230–234, 1983.
9. Stein JM, Warfield CA: The pain clinic. Local anesthetics: principles of safe use. *Hosp Pract* 21:73–78, 1983.
10. Howard K, Conrad T, Heiger J, Manzi J: Diphenhydramine hydrochloride as a local anesthetic. A case report. *J Am Podiatry Assoc* 74:240–242, 1984.
11. Harris WC Jr, Alpert WJ, Giu JJ, Marcinko D: Nitrous oxide and valium use in podiatric surgery for production of conscious sedation. *J Am Podiatry Assoc* 72:505–510, 1982.
12. Choi GW, Donick II: Blood gas analysis with intravenous

sedation and local anesthesia. *J Am Podiatry Assoc* 67:231–232, 1977.
13. Gilman EA, Borovoy M: Lorazepam (ativan). An intravenous sedative in podiatric surgery. *J Am Podiatry Assoc* 73:307–310, 1983.
14. Alafriz E:Intravenous sedation with valium and sublimase with the addition of nitrous oxide. *J Am Podiatry Assoc* 67:187, 1977.
15. Grayson RJ, Laine W: Intravenous sedation with diazepam. *J Am Podiatry Assoc* 72:347–357, 1982.
16. Donick II, Choi G, Block L, Berlin S, Costa A: Intravenous sedation combined with anesthesia in foot surgery. *J Am Podiatry Assoc* 67:177–185, 1977.
17. Lunsford MJ, Wynn M, Kwan WH: Nitrous oxide induced myeloneuropathy. *J Foot Surg* 22:222–225, 1983.
18. Bier A: A new method for local anesthesia in the extremities. *Ann Surg* 48:780, 1908.
19. Lemont H: A simplified nerve block to control postoperative foot pain. *J Am Podiatry Assoc* 68:193, 1978.
20. Locke RK, Lock SE: Nerve blocks of the foot. *J Am Coll Emerg Phys* 5:698–702, 1976.
21. McCutcheon, R: Regional anesthesia for the foot. *Can Anaesth Soc J* 12:465–474, 1965.
22. Forman WM: A two-point hallux block. *J Am Podiatry Assoc* 70:253–254, 1980.
23. Tipton PE, Gudas CJ: The effects of a local anesthetic on digital circulation. *J Am Podiatry Assoc* 70:142–146, 1980.
24. Green D, Walter J, Heden R, Menacker L: The effects of local anesthetics containing epinephrine on digital blood perfusion. *J Am Podiatry Assoc* 69:397–409, 1979.
25. Scarlet JJ, Water JH, Bachman RJ: Digital blood perfusion following injection of plain lidocaine and lidocaine with epinephrine. A comparison. *J Am Podiatry Assoc* 68:339–346, 1978.
26. Roth RD: Utilization of epinephrine-containing anesthetic solution in the toes. *J Am Podiatry Assoc* 71:189–199, 1981.
27. Kaplan EG, Kashuk K: Disclaiming the myth of use of epinephrine local anesthesia in feet. *J Am Podiatry Assoc* 61:335, 1971.
28. Steinberg MV, Block P: The use and abuse of epinephrine in local anesthetics. *J Am Podiatry Assoc* 61:341, 1971.
29. *Physicians Desk Reference*, ed 37. Oradell NJ, Medical Economics Co, 1983, p 1293.
30. Hara B, Lock RK, Lowe W(eds): *Complications in Foot Surgery*. Baltimore, Williams & Wilkins, 1976, pp 18–28.
31. Goodman LS, Gilman A(eds): *The Pharmacological Basis of Therapeutics*. New York, MacMillan, 1975, pp 379–400.
32. Andriani J: Non-surgical uses of regional anesthesia: diagnostic and therapeutic nerve blocking. In *Labat's Regional Anesthesia*. Philadelphia, WB Saunders Co, 1967, pp 529–533.
33. Poplawski J, Wiley AM, Murray JF: Post-traumatic dystrophy of the extremities. *J Bone Joint Surg* 65A:642–655, 1983.
34. Louis J, McNamara G, Weinstein A: Local sympathectomy of the foot. *J Am Podiatry Assoc* 70:604–608, 1980.
35. Steinberg MD, Steinberg LB, Fields GS, Fields LS: Gout and Sudeck's atrophy, a simplified office approach to treatment. *J Am Podiatry Assoc* 65:379–383, 1975.
36. Stephen E, Abram MD: Causalgia and reflex sympathetic dystrophy. *Current Concepts in Pain* 2:10–16, 1984.
37. Mandel LM, Berlin SJ: Myofascial pain syndromes and their effect on the lower extremities. *J Foot Surg* 21:74–79, 1982.
38. Louis JM, Naftolin NH: Myofascial pain syndromes in the foot. *J Am Podiatry Assoc* 70:89–93, 1980.
39. Bruno D, Bartoli V, Grisius D, Beconi D: Fibrositic myofascial pain in intermittent claudication. Effect of anesthetic block of trigger points on exercise tolerance. *Pain* 6:183–190, 1979.
40. Hodgson RM: Reflex sympathetic dystrophy syndrome. *Lancet* 1:1419, 1976.
41. Scranton Jr PE: Metatarsalgia: diagnosis and treatment. *J Bone Joint Surg* 62-A:723–732, 1980.
42. Carron H, Giorgio AR, Kepes ER: Nerve Block. *Aches Pains* 4:41–46, 1983.

Additional References

Andriani J: Epidural anesthesia. In *Labat's Regional Anesthesia*. Philadelphia, WB Saunders Co, 1967, pp 380–388.
Andriani J: Spinal anesthesia. In *Labat's Regional Anesthesia*. Phil-
adelphia, WB Saunders Co, 1967, pp 326–379.
Cangialosi CP: Podiatric anesthesia revisited. *J Am Podiatry Assoc* 72:448–452, 1982.
Corman LC: Medical evaluation of the preoperative patient. *Med Clin North Am* 63:1131, 1979.
Costley DO, Lorlan PH: Intravenous regional ansthesia. *Arch Surg* 103:34–35, 1971.
Covino BG: Local anesthesia. *N Eng J Med* 286:1035–1042, 1972.
Covino BG, Vassalls HG: *Local Anesthetics. Mechanisms of Action and Clinical Use.* New York, Grune & Stratton, 1976.
Covino BG: Local anesthesia. *N Eng J Med* 286:975–983, 1972.
Ecker RI: More on local anesthetics of digits. *J Dermatol Surg Oncol* 6:165, 1980.
Finsterbush A, Stein H, Robin GC, Geller R, Cotev S: Recent experience with intravenous regional anesthesia in limbs. *J Trauma* 12:81–84, 1972.
Gallant EM, Ahern CP: Malignant hyperthermia: responses of skeletal muscles to general anesthetics. *Mayo Clin Proc* 58:758–763, 1983.
Goldman L: Which tests are necessary for "healthy" patients? *Consultant* 24:331, 1984.
Haber J, Hammer DJ, Butler B: Malignant hyperthermia—a review of case report. *J Am Podiatry Assoc* 73:422–426, 1983.
Humphrey MJ, Thomas JJ, Blanck MD. Malignant hyperthermia: rapid treatment and problematic prevention. *Consultant* 7:61–66, 1984.
Jassen MR: Proper use of the tourniquet. In *Doctors Hospital Eleventh Annual Surgical Seminar. Reconstructive Surgery of the Foot and Leg.* Atlanta, Doctors Hospital Podiatry Institute, 1982.
Keller DL, Benson DE: Sickle cell disease: preoperative and postoperative management. A case report. *J Am Podiatry Assoc* 73:11, 1983.
Klenerman L, Biswas M, Hulands G, Rhodes AM: Systemic and local effects of the application of a tourniquet. *J Bone Joint Surg* 62B:385–388,1980.
Kofoed H: Peripheral nerve blocks at the knee and ankle in operations for common foot disorders. *Clin Orthop* 168:97–101, 1982.
Lucas GL. Intravenous regional anesthesia in peripheral extremity surgery. *Clin Orthop* 65:138–142, 1969.
Martin WJ, Green DR, Dougherty N, Morgan D, O'Heir D, Zarro M: Tourniquet use in sickle cell disease patients. *J Am Podiatry Assoc* 74:291–294, 1984.
Mercado OA: *An Atlas of Foot Surgery-Forefoot Surgery*, vol 1. Chicago, Carolando Press, 1979.
Miller RD: *Anesthesia*. New York, Churchill-Livingstone, 1981.
Podolsky J: Management of diabetes in the surgical patient. *Med Clin North Am* 66:1361, 1982.
Poulton TJ, Mims GR: Peripheral nerve blocks. *Am Fam Phys* 16:100–109, 1977.
Riegelhaupt R, French S, Reinherz R: Properties of local narcotics. Pharmacologic Review. *J Foot Surg* 21:234–236, 1982.
Romanes GJ: The lower limb. In *Cunningham's Manual of Practical Anatomy. Vol I. Upper and Lower Limbs.* New York, Oxford University Press, 1976, pp 97–183.
Rorie DK, Byer DE, Nelson DO, Sittipong R, Johnson KA: Assessment of block of the sciatic nerve in the popliteal fossa. *Anesth Analg* 59:371–376, 1980.
Sanner F, Lawton JH: Intravenous regional anesthesia in the lower leg and foot. *J Am Podiatry Assoc* 64:383–391, 1974.
Schad RF: Pre and postoperative medications. *Therapeutics* 39:3–13, 1981.
Schuman DJ: Ankle-block anesthesia for foot surgery. *Anesthesiology* 44:348–352, 1976.
Schwartz PS, Newman A, Green AL: Intravenous regional anesthesia. *J Am Podiatry Assoc* 73:201–204, 1983.
Shaw J, Murray D: The relationship between tourniquet pressure and underlying soft-tissue pressure in the thigh. *J Bone Joint Surg* 64-A:1148–1152, 1982.
Thorn-Alquist AM: Intravenous regional anaesthesia—a seven year survey. *Acta Anaesthiol Scand* 15:23–32, 1971.
Tzagournis M: A deadly duo: hypertension and diabetes mellitus. *Consultant* 21:247, 1981.
Willinsky JS, Lepow R: Sickle cell trait and the use of the penumatic tourniquet. *J Am Podiatry Assoc* 74:38–41, 1984.
Zier BG: Clinical considerations for the hypertensive patient in podiatric practice. *J Am Podiatry Assoc* 73:573, 1983.

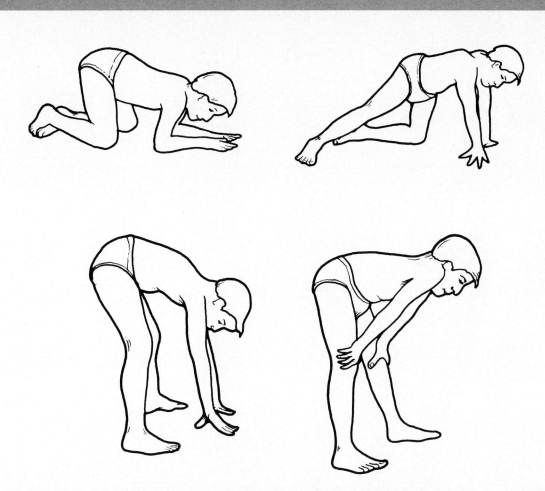

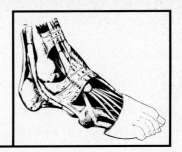

CHAPTER 11

Peroneal Spastic Flatfoot

John M. Buckholz, D.P.M.

In contradistinction to the kinematic origins of flatfoot there exists a clinical condition referred to as peroneal spastic flatfoot. Alternative terms used for this condition include spasmodic flatfoot, spastic flatfoot, peroneal extensor spasm, spasmodic peroneals, rigid flatfoot, spasmodic clubfoot, spasmodic valgus, inflammatory flatfoot, and toxic tonsil foot.

Peroneal spastic flatfoot (PSFF) is an infrequent, yet striking clinical state of pronatory splinting by the evertor muscles of the foot. Any number of noxious stimuli to the tarsus can provoke this reflex action. Identification of the initiating source is the first assignment for the clinician attempting to manage its course.

HISTORICAL RECOGNITION

The earliest citing of PSFF was described by the French surgeon Nelaton (1) in 1852. Nelaton treated an adolescent girl for peroneal spasm of the left foot by tenotomizing the peroneals below the ankle. At this early account he theorized the cause to be in the bones of the foot. Sayre (2) attributed the etiology of PSFF to tarsal inflammation. He employed injections of strychnia into the tibialis anterior muscle and tenotomized the peroneals before 1872. Shaffer (3) termed the condition "inflammatory flatfoot" and related it to tarsal osteitis secondary to an advanced flatfoot. Lorenz (4) advocated midtarsal joint injections of cocaine. The first description of tarsal coalition inducing PSFF was made by Goldthwaite and Painter (5) in 1909, although Slomann (6) has been consistently credited. Goldthwaite and Painter were apparently the first surgeons of many who failed to relieve PSFF by the simple excision of osseous coalition. Additional causes of PSFF became evident with advances in diagnostic techniques.

ETIOLOGY

PSFF can be attributed to a variety of factors. Occupational strain was the etiological consideration of the physicians first concerned with this problem.

The identity of tarsal coalition as a specific cause gained the attention of clinicians in the first half of the twentieth century and the general concept of strain fell into disfavor. In spite of the development of precise radiographic projections to reveal various tarsal coalitions, there remains a significant number of cases reported without a definitive diagnosis. Circumstantial evidence supports the likelihood of strain-inducing PSFF in at least some patients. Increased numbers of patients with PSFF treated at the turn of the century indicates many of these appeared related to the demand of prolonged labor (7). Males experience PSFF by at least a 2:1 frequency compared to females yet the incidence of tarsal coalition is equally distributed between the sexes. Many of the symptomatic patients are overweight. Finally, although no physeal plates are present in the tarsus during adolescence, there appears to this author the possibility of a load-stress osteochondrosis existing in the tarsal interfaces of this age group. This may occur when adult demands are made without the benefit of full maturity of the tarsal bones.

Fracture in the tarsal area, including the ankle joint, may produce PSFF. Reported sites initiating spasm include osteochondral lesions of the talar dome, the head of the talus (8, 9), the subtalar joint (10), the calcaneocuboid joint (11), and the talonavicular joint (8, 12). Ankle sprain has also been cited as a cause. However, the possibility of a coexisting coalition aggravated by the injury should be considered. Arthropathies most likely to produce PSFF are rheumatoid, osteo-, and bacterial arthritis. Tuberculous arthritis is the most commonly reported in the latter category. Additional etiologies for PSFF include fibrosarcoma of the sinus tarsi as reported by Richards (13) and Johnson (14). This author has observed a single case of peroneal extensor spasm throughout the second and third stages of reflex sympathetic dystrophy.

The complex motions of the subtalar and midtarsal joints are easily thwarted by various structures including those produced by surgical operations. Subtalar arthrodesis or the Green-Grice extra-articular subtalar arthrodesis can provoke PSFF. The most common cause of PSFF is the congenital anatomical anomaly. The balance of this chapter will focus on such anomalies specific to tarsal function.

PATHOPHYSIOLOGY

The mystery of how the crurotarsal joints trigger the evertor reflex has not been solved. Lapidus (15) attributed the initiation to stretch of the talocalcaneal interosseous ligament during inversion. Kyne and Mankin (16) studied the intra-articular pressure of the subtalar joints during supination and pronation and found increased pressure values in supination. They subsequently suggested that the splinting is a response to proprioceptive receptors. This answer fails to explain PSFF resulting from "extrasubtalar" sites such as the ankle, talonavicular, calcaneocuboid, or naviculocuboid joints. In addition, splinting sometimes occurs with maximum supination in response to subtalar lesions that trigger the invertor muscles (17, 18). Outland and Murphy's (19) attempt to trace the tarsal nerves anatomically has offered no new answers to the question.

In the typical case the responding muscles are m. peroneus brevis and m. extensor digitorum longus. These are the most powerful evertor muscles of the foot. M. peroneus longus does not appear to participate in PSFF. This is evidenced by the lack of plantarflexion of the first ray and has been recognized by Blockney (20) during EMG studies.

Jayakumar and Cowell (21) have argued that the peroneals are not spastic and prefer that the condition be called rigid flatfoot. Their contention is a return to Harris and Beath's interpretation that adaptive shortening of the peroneals takes place as a result of limited subtalar joint motion. Unfortunately, this view can undermine the clinician's understanding and appropriate efforts to treat the deformity. When tarsal coalition maintains a fixed valgus position of the foot, the everting muscles will undergo shortening by dynamic contracture. During examination the unwary clinician may note the tightened peroneals and misinterpret the muscles to be reflexly splinting the tarsus. This circumstance rarely exists and would be the only case where the term "rigid flatfoot" could apply. The singular concept of adaptive shortening ignores several anatomically remote clinical examples of persistent muscular contracture by reflex (neurogenic) pathways. Such examples include hamstring splinting following knee injury or spastic pes varus of the foot secondary to specific tarsal lesions such as calcaneal fracture or coalition (18). An additional argument is provided by the fact that in many cases PSFF responds to nerve blocks, releasing the tarsus to complete reinstatement of subtalar and midtarsal joint motion. The term PSFF does not include the spastic deformity produced by upper motor neuron lesions.

CONGENITAL TARSAL COALITION AND CONGENITAL ARTHROEREISIS

The once clinically obscure tarsal coalition has surfaced in recent years to gain recognition as a pathoanatomical variant imposing a serious deterrent to tarsal function. So much so that the once unheeded accounts of tarsal anomalies described by nineteenth century anatomists are now portrayed as pathological anomalies by clinicians (22–26). This is especially true for interpretation of the clinical influence of the calcaneonavicular bar. This discussion will seek to evaluate the clinical implications of tarsal coalition, as well as review the diagnostic and surgical course of its management.

Classification and Definitions

In the following classification, two categories of tarsal anomalies are treated: congenital tarsal coalition and congenital tarsal arthroereisis. The blending of tarsal arthroereisis with coalition as etiology for PSFF is a compatible concept when these anomalies are examined from a clinical perspective. Essentially these anatomical variations may inflict limited or abnormal motion to the tarsal joints. This eventuates in pain, deformity, and disability of the PSFF. Limitation of motion may occur by actual coalition of two or more tarsals or by premature abutment of one tarsal to another by an intervening accessory ossicle or by a "fender" of bone projecting from the anatomical bone. The latter two possibilities do not directly adjoin one tarsal to another, as in coalition, and can best be interpreted as a biological arthroereisis. A classification would then develop as follows.

I. Coalitions
  A. Types
    1. Synarthrosis—fusion occuring within an anatomical joint
    2. Synostosis—tissue extensions joining one bone to another from outside the anatomical joints
    3. Synarthrostosis—coexisting synarthrosis and synostosis
  B. Histological Structure
    1. Fibrous
    2. Cartilaginous
    3. Osseous
II. Arthroereisis
  A. Accessory ossicles—inconstant sesamoids that may block motion
  B. Accessory processes—apparently remnants of incomplete morphological bone formation; the process is continuous with the parent tarsal bone
  C. Conglomerants—accessory ossicles that are fused to an anatomical parent bone

It should be noted that these above variations are congenital and are not the result of disease. The term "synostosis" indicates that two bones are abnormally united and does not identify a tissue type in coalition.

Anatomical Features

In view of the total tarsal structure, the distribution of tarsal anomalies has a limited range of possible sites for appearance. Typical locations for tarsal coalition and arthroereisis are given in the following description of their morphology.

Calcaneonavicular Anomalies

Two forms of coalition and five forms of biological arthroereisis exist as possible deterrents to tarsal motion. The well-known calcaneonavicular bar is an isthmus of tissue passing from the distal dorsomedial aspect of the calcaneus to the lateral plantar corner of the navicular. In the adult the isthmus is usually fully ossified, whereas in the juvenile it can be totally cartilaginous, making it difficult or impossible to demonstrate on x-ray studies. As the bridge becomes ossified by converging osteogenesis from the calcaneus and navicular, a level, usually in early adolescence, is reached where only a thin plate remains cartilaginous. This plate is often irregular and on x-ray studies suggests fracture of the bar to the clinician, especially if the patient is experiencing concomitant pain in the area. Caution should precede the conclusion of a fractured calcaneonavicular bar. The fact that calcaneonavicular coalition in the isthmus form is frequently discovered incidentally on x-ray should underline the possibility that no significant clinical or pathomechanical effect exists with some bars. Standard evaluation for tarsal range of motion can surprisingly reveal a full and functional freedom of motion with coalesence by this bar, though the direction of the motion may be quite aberrant.

The second form of calcaneonavicular coalition is far more rare than the isthmus, but produces serious effects on the function of the tarsus. This coalition, the platysmal bridge, extends across the complete field of the plantar calcaneonavicular ligament. Cruveilhier's (22) original plate of this coalition nicely illustrates its form. The deep location and breadth of its size magnifies the problematical considerations inherrent for its surgical removal.

Congenital arthroereisis of the calcaneonavicular area produces variable degrees of tarsal restraint. The size and location of the bony block determines the extent of obstruction that will take place.

Two accessory bones can act as a congenital arthroereisis. The os calcis secundus (secondary calcaneus) is the most important of these because of its strategical position between the calcaneus and navicular (27, 28). The bone is most often pyramidal in shape, with the apex directed plantarly and medially. It is positioned at the "four corners" interval of the midtarsal joint, which explains its ability to block tarsal motion. If the bone is sufficiently large it may be mistaken as the calcaneonavicular isthmus or as a fractured calcaneonavicular bar. The os calcis secundus is not rare in occurrence. Pfitzner (29) discovered its presence 16 times in 840 dissections, a 2% incidence in that study.

The second accessory ossicle that may block tarsal movement is a type of accessory navicular that projects posteriorly and plantarly (11). The bone abuts against the anterior sustentaculum tali during supination or may force the forefoot to abduct if bone to bone contact is continuous.

A third accessory bone, the secondary cuboid, exists as a possible rare form of arthroereisis (11).

Three processes occur that may produce arthroereisis. First is an anterior dorsal projection of the calcaneus that is directed toward the navicular. This process has been proposed as a conglomerant of the os calcis secundus with the calcaneus and as an incomplete calcaneonavicular bar (30). The second process occurs frequently yet is not often recognized. The navicular can demonstrate a plantar bone bud that jams against the anterior dorsal aspect of the calcaneus during supination. Ordinarily it has no detrimental effect other than being misinterpreted as a calcaneonavicular bar on an oblique x-ray study (31). A third anomaly is the posterior lateral projection of the navicular that may be interpreted as a complete calcaneonavicular bar (i.e. isthmus) (32).

Talocalcaneal Anomalies

The description of talocalcaneal anomalies is complicated by a wide range of irregularities. Synarthrosis may exist in massive forms (33–35) or by narrow inconspicuous fusion in a portion of the anterior talocalcaneal articulation (36). The medial face of the sustentaculum tali is disposed to anatomical distortion that defies classification (37). For this reason a complete description of the variants is prohibitive, but the following should suffice for clinical application.

Arthroereisis of the talocalcaneal articulations most often occurs medially. Bony protuberances along the margin of the sustentaculum tali or bony stalactites directed at the sustentaculum tali from the medial surface of the talus may individually or in combination produce discordant subtalar motion. An accessory bone, the os sustentaculum proprium (os sustentaculare) has been credited with limiting motion as well (10, 30, 37). Anatomists have also considered the variations of the sustentaculum tali to be a conglomerant with the os sustentaculum proprium (30).

When these rough, irregular bony processes are united, the term "medial talocalcaneal bridge" (synostosis) (10) has been used to describe the coalition. In addition to the os sustentaculum proprium, two additional accessory ossicles can create a talocalcaneal arthroereisis. Both are unusual but probably occur more often than is appreciated. The first is arthroereisis by way of the os trigonum (11, 30). This common accessory bone may be a conglomerant with the calcaneus reducing motion, or may exist as a conglomerant adjoined to both the talus and calcaneus establishing a coalition (38, 39). The third accessory bone producing arthroereisis is the os talocalcaneale, which lies in the sinus tarsi. When of sufficient size this bone will limit eversion (40). Massive talocalcaneal coalition by synarthrosis has been sporadically described throughout the past two centuries, more often as a teratological curiosity or as an associated deformity with meromelia (30, 33, 41, 42).

Talonavicular Anomalies

Talonavicular coalition is a rare anomaly of the tarsus (43–45). Complete synarthrosis of the talonavicular articulation is the classic description of this coalition, which is often discovered incidentally (46). This condition alone may not produce clinical symptoms. However, talonavicular synarthrosis often exists with other congenital anomalies, such as ball and socket ankle joint, meromelia, additional coalitions, symphalangism and congenital bowing of the tibia (47, 48). Thus talonavicular coalition may find its clinical significance as a sign of the presence of coexisting malformations. Arthroereisis of this joint has not been described but has been suggested as a possibility by way of the dorsal accessory bone, os pirie (11, 49).

Other Anomalies

Calcaneocuboid, naviculocuboid, naviculocuneiform, and intercuneiform coalition may all be categorized in the most rare of tarsal anomalies (50 – 52). It is therefore difficult to assess their clinical importance with the sparse reportings available. One case of PSFF has been attributed to arthroereisis of the naviculo-cuboid interval by the rare accessory ossicle, the os cuboidum secundum (11).

Etiology

Correlated embryonic studies, as well as case reports, suggest a genetic dominant autosomal mechanism for tarsal coalition and arthroereisis. The primitive synovial joints are formed early in morphogenesis, between the fifth and seventh postovulatory week by the vacuolization of chondral inner zones (53, 54). A genetically induced synarthrosis is produced by failure of the primitive synovial joint to form and should therefore be observable embryologically. Such observations have been confirmed (55, 56). Both fetal observation and familial accounts of calcaneonavicular coalition have been made (57–60). Hereditary talonavicular synarthrosis (42, 44, 61, 62) and talocalcaneal synarthrosis (33), as well as medial talocalcaneal bridging, have been reported (31). The Pfitzner (30) theory explaining accessory ossicles as evolutionary anlage is without support.

Clinical Findings

As previously cited, tarsal coalition and tarsal arthroereisis can produce abnormal or limited motion of the tarsus. It is from this effect that the clinical picture emerges. When limitation is primary, i.e. directly resultant from the anomaly, a fixed pronated foot is to be found (63, 64). Pain associated with this deformity is more likely to be produced by fatigue and strain secondary to the pathomechanical positioning of the pronated foot. When the anomaly provokes tarsal pain, reflex splintage of the tarsal components is induced. In the absence of this deformity tarsal coalition may be suggested by range of motion examination where limited inversion is the usual circumstance.

Tarsal pain alone may be the first indication of tarsal coalition or arthroereisis. This tarsalgia usually occurs about the sinus tarsi or over the sustentaculum tali especially during supination maneuvers (31). It is not unusual then for supination injuries to initiate pain and/or reflex splintage especially in adolescence when osseous maturity is near completion. More extensive synarthroses are not as likely to present with

this picture and are more likely to show functional adaptation of the tarsal joints with growth. Late maturing osseous obstacles are likely to cause pain and splintage as these anomalies impose their presence late—near full development of the foot (65). On survey of the historical background for PSFF (7, 66–69), it is apparent that musculoskeletal activity and load will instigate tarsalgia, as well as enforce peroneal extensor spasm. The incidence of tarsal coalition and tarsal arthroereisis is greater than is generally appreciated. The results of several random studies indicate a 2% incidence in the general population (10, 29, 70).

Roentgenographical Signs and Techniques

For the purposes of screening, the standard dorsoplantar and lateral weight-bearing x-ray studies of the foot provide suitable exposures for signaling the presence of tarsal coalition or arthroereisis. Because calcaneonavicular and talocalocaneal coalition and/or arthroereisis are less obvious, and yet more likely to occur, roentgenographical signs and techniques for their detection will be emphasized in this section.

Calcaneonavicular coalition may be suggested on dorsoplantar projection by the "comma sign" (31) of the navicular. This sign is to be noted by a narrowing in the width, anterior to posterior of the lateral end of the navicular, as well as an elongated lateral horn that curves abruptly in a hooked fashion to meet the anterior of the calcaneus. A second indicator is visualized on a lateral projection when the anterior dorsal aspect of the calcaneus is projected dorsodistally in what may be termed a "bow spar" configuration. If either or both of these indicators are noted, the 45° oblique projection as described by Slomann (71) may be used to confirm coalition (72). In making this projection the central ray must not be posterior to the midtarsal joint. If the suspected foot is a pronated type in stance, the central ray is projected vertically to the midtarsal interval with the foot non-weight-bearing and positioned at a 45° angle to the weight-bearing surface. If the foot presents with fixed cavus deformity, the exposure is taken at 45° to the weight-bearing surface with the foot fully weight-bearing. Coalition should not be diagnosed by mere overlap of the navicular with the os calcis as occurs in a more laterally projected central ray. Also, the central posterior bony process of the navicular should be ruled out as masquerading a genuine coalition (31).

Projections for demonstrating the presence of os calcis secundus have been described by Voyers (73). The foot is non-weight-bearing and the plantar surface is everted 10° to the plantigrade position. The central ray is directed vertically at the midtarsal joint.

Talocalcaneal coalition and/or arthroereisis is suggested by lateral views. On close examination of a normal subtalar joint the middle articular facet immediately above the sustentaculum tali can be visualized through its full extent. When coalition or arthroereisis is present, irregularity, obliteration, or eburnation of this facet may be noted. Coalition may then be revealed by posterior sustentacular tangential projection (10, 74). These exposures were originally presented by Korvin; however, Harris and Beath have received credit for their discovery. Exposures should be taken at 30°, 35°, 40°, and 45° to the weight-bearing plane as suggested by Conway and Cowell (36). Attempts to measure the inclination of the sustentaculum tali on lateral weight-bearing view may meet with unsatisfactory imaging. Tomograms of the subtalar joint will produce unnecessary radiation exposure and are not usually required for x-ray diagnosis.

The anterior and posterior talocalcaneal facets are nicely demonstrated on projections as demonstrated by Isherwood (75). The lateral/oblique projection of this set is useful in demonstrating coalition by an os trigonum conglomerant. The os sustentaculum proprium is visualized by posterior tangential projections of the os calcis or suroplantar projections. The os talocalcaneale is revealed on anteroposterior x-ray studies of the ankle with inclusion of the tarsus (40). The presence of accessory ossicles about the talocalcaneal articulation does not affirm coalition or arthroereisis, but rather implies its possibility. Additional roentgenographical indicators of tarsal coalition represent secondary alterations that occur as a result of the functional effect of the anomaly. Approximately 50% of all coalitions produce talar breaking (36). This saddlehorn exostosis is noted at the dorsal-distal-lateral aspect of the talus on lateral projection. To a lesser extent it may be viewed in a dorsoplantar projection at the lateral rim of the talar head facet. Late stages may reveal other sites of spurring such as the calcaneocuboid joint (76). Swirling and bizarre patterns of trabeculation may be viewed on lateral projections that represent the deviation of stress force flow coursing through the tarsus.

Decrease of the calcaneal tuber angle, as well as increased width of the talofibular facet, will occur less frequently as a result of coalition (36, 77). The decrease of the tuber angle results from the extended anterior process of the calcaneus in calcaneonavicular arthroereisis or coalition. The higher reference point for forming the angle gives a false indication of a depressed subtalar joint. Subtalar joint motion usually includes measurements confirming subtalar valgus.

Differential Diagnosis

The frequency of tarsal anomalies deserves consideration during evaluation of the painful tarsus presenting with limited motion with or without PSFF or spastic pes varus (78). Obviously there must be consideration for other causes that may induce these clinical symptoms. Talar beaking does not confirm tarsal coalition or arthroereisis. Rheumatoid arthritis, compensatory equinus, acromegaly, forced casting, or arthrodesis of the subtalar joint (36, 79, 80) commonly create plowing of the navicular into the talar head causing this exostosis (37). A fair assessment of these possibilities is justified before the diagnosis of tarsal coalition and/or arthroereisis is formed.

Treatment

Depending on the clinical circumstance, the treatment aim may be pursued by three possible pathways: conservative, surgical, and preventive.

Conservative

Immediate conservative measures should be instituted to mitigate the tarsal irritation and splintage (31, 81, 82). This may be accomplished by injections in the sinus tarsi with long acting local anesthetics and corticosteroids, tibial and peroneal nerve blocks, restive immobilization, soothing physiotherapy, and such antiinflammatory drugs as phenylbutazone and salicylates (67, 83, 84). Muscle relaxants have proven to be of no value in this author's experience.

Efforts to overcome peroneal extensor spasms or limited motion by forced inversion are to be discouraged, because these attempts will meet with exacerbation of the symptoms and reflex splinting. This includes manipulation of the tarsal articulations using general anesthesia (5, 67). The clinician should rather support the direction of splintage to quiet the tarsalgia. Usually this is in the pronatory direction and is best accomplished by a non-weight-bearing below-knee cast for three to six weeks. Once the symptoms of tarsal irritation are relieved, functional motion of the tarsus should be discouraged by use of an orthosis that accommodates the foot in its pronated position (31, 85).

Surgical

If symptoms recur or persist, surgical intervention may be considered. The exception to this rule is the resistant juvenile cases that should be casted for extended periods of time, unless the calcaneonavicular bar is proven to be the culprit. In these younger age groups the calcaneonavicular bar may be excised (86–89). As a generalization, the operative procedures designed to overcome the effects of tarsal coalition have been conceived for symptomatic improvement.

From the first recorded case of PSFF where Nelaton (1) performed peroneal tenotomy, to the recent Dwyer's calcaneal osteotomy, the attempt has been to relieve symptoms (90). Only in the circumstances of calcaneonavicular bar resection or arthroereisis excision is function restored to the tarsus. As early as 1909, Goldthwaite and Painter (5) identified and reported removing bony spurs from about the talocalcaneal articulation in an effort to restore function and relieve peroneal extensor spasm. Dunn and Simpson (7) employed crushing of the superficial peroneal nerve and transfer of the tenton of m. peroneus longus to the navicular in 1912. Slomann (6) suggested excision of the calcaneonavicular bar, which was later achieved by Carl Badgley (86) in 1927. Ryerson's (91) triple arthrodesis has held the attention of most surgeons to the present with good reason. Triple arthrodesis permits relief of pain and revisional alignment of the foot to the leg and forefoot to rearfoot. This procedure should be awarded as a thoroughly tested operation for tarsal coalition (92–94). Resection of the calcaneonavicular bar is likewise a time tested procedure. On review of the literature this latter procedure is confined to patients younger than 14 years of age, when there is no evidence of arthritic insult or chronic tarsalgia (72, 83, 86–89); however, this author has had successful results following bar excision for patients of 20 to 30 years of age.

The calcaneonavicular bar is approached by Ollier's incision with identification and preservation of the intermediate dorsal cutaneous nerve. M. extensor digitorum brevis is freed from a posterolateral to a dorsodistal direction. The bar can then be removed by a transverse proximal osteotomy at the juncture with the calcaneus, as well as a vertical oblique osteotomy directed plantar medially at the navicular end of the isthmus. The direction of this osteotomy is crucial to avoid leaving the plantar lateral corner of the navicular. Once the bar is excised the surgical void is filled with the m. extensor digitorum brevis. Providing the surgical void is made sufficiently wide, interpositional arthroplasty is important to prevent recurrence of the bar, but should not require a foreign implant such as a silicone insert. When the calcaneonavicular bar is symptomatic in older patients, or patients with arthritic changes, triple arthrodesis should be performed (82, 88, 89). Although the author can find no record of, and have had no experience in, removing the platysmal bridge, it would seem that its excision is too extensive to permit consistent satisfactory results.

When considering calcaneonavicular bar excision, coexisting talocalcaneal coalition must be ruled out by sustentacular x-ray views. Postoperative care following resection of the calcaneonavicular bar should be aimed at early motion to the ankle with casting no longer than three weeks. The author disagrees with the belief that excision of a completed osseous coalition is contraindicated (95).

A second coalition, which may be excised with satisfactory results, is the os trigonum conglomerant (39). Attempts to excise medial talocalcaneal synostoses have met with consistent failure and in this anomaly triple arthrodesis is indicated (5, 10, 96, 97). Dwyer's varus osteotomy of the calcaneus, which reduces the valgus heel to neutral, suggests a possible alternative to triple arthrodesis (90); however, the procedure should be considered in the observational phase at this time.

If the juvenile foot requires arthrodesis the extra-articular subtalar arthrodesis of Green and Grice will permit continued growth and maturity of the foot while stabilizing the tarsal joints (98). This operation must be viewed as a holding procedure until sufficient maturity of the tarsus is reached for triple arthrodesis. In most cases of biological arthroereisis, excision of the accessory ossicle or bony process is indicated with the exception of os sustentaculum proprium (28, 31, 40, 99–101). Asher and Mosier (102) have reported successful results with three cases of subtalar middle facet by synarthrosis by fat interposition arthroplasty.

Preventive

If objective evaluation reveals pronatory function, orthoses can be employed to prevent stress propagation within the limb by control of the pronatory syndrome. Close observation of this treatment mode should be maintained to assure that the tarsal joints are not antagonized to splintage and subjective symptoms. If tarsal coalition or arthroereisis is clinically silent and without deformity, observation alone may be the best choice. A few surgeons consider excision of the calcaneonavicular bar at an early age as a preventative form of treatment, even though symptoms are nonexistent. In view of the number of incidental discoveries of the calcaneonavicular bar, the argument for this supposition seems questionable.

Adjunctive treatment may be required when tarsal coalition or tarsal arthroereisis coexists with other pronatory forces acting on the foot (e.g. short tendo achillis). When tarsal coalition exists and tendo achillis lengthening is to be performed to alleviate pronation during equinus, the surgeon is obligated to consider the effect of tarsal coalition after heel cord lengthening. Postoperative increase of subtalar joint motion may now induce stress forces within the coalition provoking what previously may have been an asymptomatic anomaly. A second example would include the effect of a coalition after bunionectomy where pronation caused by the coalition is influential on the first metatarsophalangeal joint. Thus wherever deformities are present secondary to pronation caused by tarsal coalition or arthroereisis, adjunctive treatment of the latter must be considered.

References

1. Atlee, WF: *Lectures on Surgery by M Nelaton*. Philadelphia, JB Lippincott Co, 1855.
2. Sayre L: *Lectures on Orthopedic Surgery*, ed 2. New York, Appleton & Co, 1883.
3. Shaffer NM: *Selected Essays on Orthopedic Surgery*. New York, GP Putnam's Sons, 1923.
4. Lorenz A: *Wien Klin Wochenschr* 11:189, 1889.
5. Goldthwaite J, Painter C, Osgood R: *Diseases of the Bones and Joints*. Boston, Heath & Co, 1909.
6. Slomann HC: On coalition—calcaneonavicularis. *J Orthop Surg* 3: 586–602, 1921.
7. Simpson GCE, Dunn N: On spasmodic contraction of the peronei in flatfoot. *Br Med J* 2:1369–1371, 1912.
8. Merryweather R: Spastic valgus of the foot. *Proc R Soc Lond* 48:103–106, 1955.
9. Cowell HR: Talocalcaneal coalition and new causes of peroneal spastic flatfoot. *Clin Orthop* 85: 16–22, 1972.
10. Harris RI, Beath T: Etiology of peroneal spastic flatfoot. *J Bone Joint Surg* 30B:624–634, 1948.
11. Outland T, Murphy ID: Relation of tarsal anomalies to spastic and rigid flatfeet. *Clin Orthop* 1:217–224, 1953.
12. Sanghi JK, Roby HR: Bilateral peroneal spastic flatfeet associated with congenital fusion of the navicular and talus. *J Bone Joint Surg* 43A:1237–1240, 1961.
13. Richards JF: Peroneal spastic flatfoot syndrome due to fibrosarcoma. *Inter-Clin Inform Bull* 11:9, 1971.
14. Johnson EE: Peroneal spastic flatfoot syndrome. *South Med J* 69:6, 807K–809, 1976.
15. Lapidus PW: Spastic flatfoot. *J Bone Joint Surg* 28A:126–136, 1946.
16. Kyne PJ, Mankin HJ: Changes in intra-articular pressure with subtalar joint motion with special reference to the etiology

of peroneal spastic flatfoot. *Bull Hosp Joint Dis* 26:181, 1965.

17. Maudsley RS: Spastic pes varus. *Proc R Soc Lond* 49:181, 1956.
18. Simmons EH: Tibialis spastic varus foot with tarsal coalition. *J Bone Joint Surg* 47B:533–536, 1965.
19. Outland T, Murphy ID: The pathomechanics of peroneal spastic flatfoot. *Clin Orthop* 16:64–73, 1960.
20. Blockney NJ: Peroneal spastic flatfoot. *J Bone Joint Surg* 37B:191–202, 1955.
21. Jayakumur S, Cowell HR: Rigid flatfoot. *Clin Orthop* 122:77–84, 1977.
22. Cruveilhier J: *Anatomie pathologique du corps humain.* Tome I: 1829–1835.
23. Zuckerkandl E: Ueber einen fall von Synostose zwischen Talus und Calcaneus. *Allegen Wein Mediz Zeit* 22:293–294, 1877.
24. Anderson RJ: The presence of an astragalo-schapoid bone in man. *J Anat* 14:452–455, 1879–1880.
25. Chaput H: Etude anatomo-pathologique de deux pieces depeid plat valgus (tarsalgie des adolescents), queris par ankylose, suivie de quilques considerations sur la pathogenie et le mecanisme de ces lesions. *Prog Med* 14:857–860, 1886.
26. Holl M: Beitrage zur chirurgischen Osteologis des fusses. *Archir fur Klinisch Chirurgie* 25:211–223, 1880.
27. Mercer J: The secondary os calcis. *J Anat* 66:84–97, 1931.
28. Krida A: Secondary os calcis. *JAMA* 80:752–753, 1953.
29. Pfitzner W: Beitrage zur kenntniss des menschliehen exlremitatenshelets: VII die variationen in aufboss des fusshelets. In Schwalbe G: *Morphologische Arbeiten, Band 6,* Jena, Fischer, 1896.
30. O'Rahilly R: A survey of carpal and tarsal anomalies. *J Bone Joint Surg* 35-A:626–642, 1953.
31. Buckholz J: Peroneal spastic flatfoot. *Surgical Management of Pes Cavus, Clubfoot and Flatfoot.* Northlake Hospital Surgical Syllabus. Chicago 1972.
32. Chambers CH: Congenital anomalies of the tarsal navicular with particular reference to calcaneo-navicular coalition. *Br J Radiol* 23: 480–586, October 1956.
33. Buffon GLL, Comte de: *Histoire Naturell avec les Description de Cabinet de Roy.* Tome 3:47, 1750.
34. Austin FH: Symphalangism and related fusions of tarsal bones. *Radiology* 56:882–885, June 1951.
35. Miller E: Congenital ankylosis of joints of hands and feet. *J Bone Joint Surg* 22A:560, 1922.
36. Conway JJ, Cowell HR: Tarsal coalition: clinical significance and roentgengraphic demonstration. *Radiology* 92:799–811, March 1969.
37. Harris RI: Rigid valgus foot, due to talocalcaneal bridge. *J Bone Joint Surg* 37-A:169–183, 1955.
38. Bentzon PGK: Bilateral congenital deformity of the astragalocalcanean joint. Boney coalescence between os trigonum and the calcaneus. *Acta Orthop Scand* 1:359–364, 1930.
39. Galinski A, Crovo R, Ditmars J: Ostrigonum as a cause of tarsal coalition. *J Am Podiatry Assoc* 69:3, 191–197, 1979.
40. Hirschtick A: An anomalous tarsal bone. *J Bone Joint Surg* 33A:907–910, 1951.
41. Bloom A: Hereditary multiple ankylosing arthropathy. *Radiology* 29:166–171, 1937.
42. Bersani FA, Samilson RL: Massive familial tarsal synostosis. *J Bone Joint Surg* 39-A: 1187–1190, October 1957.
43. Boyd HB: Congenital talonavicular synostosis. *J Bone Joint Surg* 26A: 682–686, October 1944.
44. Rothberg A, Feldman J, Schuster O: Congenital fusion of astragalus and schapoid: bilateral; inherited. *New York State Journal Medicine* 35:29–31, 1935.
45. Lapidus PW: Congenital fusion of the bones of the foot; with a report of a case of congenital astragaloschopoid fusion. *J Bone Joint Surg* 14A:888–894, 1932.
46. Bullett JB: Variations of the bones of the foot. Fusion of the talus and navicular, bilateral and congenital. *American Journal Roentgenology* 20:548–549, 1928.
47. Schreiber R: Talonavicular synostosis. *J Bone Joint Surg* 45-A:170–172, 1963.
48. Shands A, Wentz I: Congenital anomalies, accessory bones, and osteochondritis in the feet of 850 children. *Surg Clin North Am* 33:1643–1666, 1953.
49. Pirie AH: Extra bones in the wrist and ankle found by roentgen rays. *American Journal Roentgenology* 8:569–573, 1921.
50. Basu SS: Naviculo-cuneo-metatarso-phalangeal synostoses. *Indian Journal Surgery* 25: 750–751, 1963.
51. Del Sel JM, Grand NE: Cubo-navicular synostosis: a rare tarsal synostosis. *J Bone Joint Surg* 41-B:149, 1959.
52. Waugh W: Partial cubonavicular coalition as a cause of peroneal spastic flatfoot. *J Bone Joint Surg* 39-B:520–523, 1957.
53. O'Rahilly R, Gardner E, Gray D: The skeletal development of the foot. *Clin Orthop* 16:7–14, 1960.
54. Whillis J: The development of synovial joints. *J Anat* 74:277–283, 1940.
55. Solger B: Ueber abnorme versch melzung knorpeliger skelettheile beim fotus. *Zentrale fur Allgeminc Pathologie und pathologisch Anatomie* 1:124, 1890.
56. Harris BA: Anomalous structures in the developing human foot. *Anat Rec* 121:399, 1955.
57. Leboucq H: De la soudure congenitale de certains os du tarse et du metatarse. *Bulletin Academy Royal Medicine Belgique* IV:103, 1890.
58. Glessner JR Jr, Davis GL: Bilateral calcaneonavicular coalition occurring in twin boys. A case report. *Clin Orthop* 47:173–176, 1966.
59. Leonard MA: The inheritance of tarsal coalition and its relationship to spastic flatfoot. *J Bone Joint Surg* 56-B:520–526, 1974.
60. Wray J, Herndon C: Hereditary transmission of congenital coalition of the calcaneus to navicular. *J Bone Joint Surg* 45-A:365–371, 1963.
61. Harle TS, Stevenson JR: Hereditary symphalangism associated with carpal and tarsal fusions. *Radiology* 89:91–94, 1967.
62. Geelhoed G, Neel J, Davidson R: Symphalangism and tarsal coalitions: a hereditary syndrome. *J Bone Joint Surg* 51B:278, 1969.
63. Harris RI: Retrospect - peroneal spastic flatfoot (rigid valgus foot). *J Bone Joint Surg* 47-A:1657–1667, 1965.
64. Rankin EA, Baker GI: Rigid flatfoot in the young adult. *Clin Orthop* 104:244–248, 1974.
65. Hark FW: Congenital anomalies of the tarsal bones. *Clin Orthop* 16: 21–25, 1960.
66. Armour TR, Dunn N: Spasmodic clubfoot. *Br Med J* 2:1371–1372, 1912.
67. Todd AH: Etiology and treatment of spasmodic flatfoot. *Br Med J* 2: 602–604, 1939.
68. Malkin SAS: Discussion on spasmodic flatfoot. *Proc R Soc Lond* 23:973–981, 1930.
69. Braddock GTF: A prolonged follow-up of peroneal spastic flatfoot. *J Bone Joint Surg* 43-B: 732–737, Nov 1961.
70. Vaughan W, Segal G: Tarsal coalition with special reference to roentgenographic interpretation. *Radiology* 60:855, 1953.
71. Slomann HC: On the demonstration and analysis of calcaneo-navicular coalition by Roentgen examination. *Acta Radiol* 5:304–312, 1926.
72. Heikel HVA: Coalition calcaneo-navicularis and calcaneus secundus, a clinical and radiological study of twenty-three patients. *Acta Orthop Scand* 32:72–84, 1962.
73. Holland T: The accessory bones of the foot with notes on a few other conditions. In *Robert Jones Birthday Volume. A Collection of Surgical Essays.* London, Oxford University Press, 1928, pp 157–182.
74. Korvin H: Coalitio talocalcanea. *Z Orthop* 60:105–110, 1934.
75. Isherwood I: A radiological approach to the subtalar joint. *J Bone Joint Surg* 43B:566–574, 1961.
76. Jack EA: Bone anomalies of the tarsus in relation to peroneal spastic flatfoot. *J Bone Joint Surg* 11B:831–837, 1929.
77. Gold GS: Tarsal coalitions: clinical significance, diagnosis and treatment. *J Am Podiatry Assoc* 61:1, 409–422, 1971.
78. Webster RS, Roberts UM: Tarsal anomalies and peroneal spastic flatfoot. *JAMA* 146:1099–1104, 1951.
79. Cowell HR: Diagnosis and management of peroneal spastic flatfoot. In *American Academy of Orthopaedic Surgeons Instructional Course Lecture,* Vol 24, St Louis, The CV Mosby Co, 1975, p 94.
80. Herschel H, Von Ronnen J: The occurrence of calcaneonavi-

cular synostosis in pes valgus contractures. *J Bone Joint Surg* 32A:280–282, 1950.

81. Stoller M: Tarsal coalition: study of surgical results. *J Am Podiatry Assoc* 64:1004–1015, 1974.

82. Coventry MB: Flatfoot with special consideration of tarsal coalition. *Minn Med* 33:1091–1097, 1103, 1950.

83. Musgrave RE, Goldner JL: Results of triple arthrodesis for (spastic) flatfeet. *South Med J* 49:32, 1966.

84. Magee RK, Benson RA: Calcaneo-scaphoid bar. *Can Med Assoc J* 55:287, 1946.

85. Buckholz J: The diagnosis and surgical management of tarsal coalition. Grand Community Hospital Syllabus of Surgery, Detroit, 1973.

86. Badgley CE: Coalition of the calcaneus and the navicular. *Arch Surg* 15:75–88, 1927.

87. Bentzon RGK: Coalitia calcaneo-navicularis, mit vesonderer bezungnahme auf die operative behandlunge des durch diese anomalie vedinten plattfusses. *Verhand Deutsch Orthop Gesel* 23:269–274, 1929.

88. Kendrick JI: Treatment of calcaneonavicular bar. *JAMA* 172:1241–1244, 1960.

89. Mitchell GP, Gibson JMC: Excision of calcaneonavicular bar for painful spasmodic flatfoot. *J Bone Joint Surg* 49B:281–287, 1967.

90. Cain T, Hyman S: Peroneal spastic flatfoot. Its treatment by osteotomy of the os calcis. *J Bone Joint Surg* 60B:527–529, 1978.

91. Ryerson EW: Arthrodesing operations on the feet. *Am J Orthop Surg* 5:453, 1923.

92. McCarroll R, Musgrave R, Goldner J: Results of triple arthrodesis for rigid (spastic) flatfoot. *South Med J* 49:32, 1966.

93. Crego CH, Ford LT: An end result study of various operative procedures for correcting flatfeet in children. *J Bone Joint Surg* 34A:183, 1952.

94. Patterson RL: Various factors involved in triple arthrodesis. *Clin Orthop* 85:59–61, 1972.

95. Mosier K, Asher M: Tarsal coalitions and peroneal spastic flatfoot. *J Bone Joint Surg* 66A:983, 1984.

96. Sutro C: Anomalous talocalcaneal articulation. A cause for limited subtalar movements. *Am J Surg* 74:64–65, 1947.

97. Kaplan E, Kaplan G, Vaccari O: Tarsal coalition: review and preliminary conclusions. *J Foot Surg* 16:4, 136–143, 1977.

98. Grice DS: An extra-articular arthrodesis of the subastragalar joint for correction of paralytic flatfeet in children. *J Bone Joint Surg* 34A:927, 1952.

99. Kidner FC: Prehallux (accessory scaphoid) in its relation to flatfoot. *J Bone Joint Surg* 11A:831, 1929.

100. Krida A: Secondary os calcis. *JAMA* 80:752–753, 1923.

101. Contomposis J: Common adolescent dance injuries. *Clin Podiatry* 1:638, 1984.

102. Asher M, Mosier K: Coalition of the talocalcaneal middle facet: treatment by surgical excision and fat graft interposition. *Orthop Trans* 7:149–150, 1983.

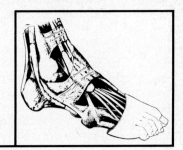

CHAPTER 12

Neuromuscular Deformities

Clinical Evaluation and Treatment of Dropfoot Deformity

Marla Jassen, D.P.M.

Paralysis of muscles acting on the foot and ankle can result in many deformities depending on the muscle imbalance that is created. One such condition is dropfoot, which can be caused by a variety of neurological and muscular disorders (1).

TWO MAIN TYPES

Dropfoot can be divided into two main types (2). The first type presents as a flail foot caused by loss of motor power and resulting in loss of stability of the ankle and foot. There is partial or complete paralysis of the anterior and possibly lateral compartment muscles of the lower leg making it difficult for the patient to dorsiflex during gait. Gait becomes awkward because the patient's hip and knee must be raised high enough for the plantarflexed foot to clear the ground.

The second type develops as adaptive bony structural changes occur creating a fixed deformity. One then sees the fixed equinus with a marked imbalance between dorsiflexors and plantarflexors and a varus deformity caused by the unopposed action of the tendon of m. tibialis posterior.

Unfortunately there is only a fine line between these two categories. Many conditions and degrees of muscular weakness and adaptive changes exist making thorough and complete clinical evaluation imperative before rendering treatment.

CLINICAL EVALUATION

The first step in evaluating the deformity is to determine the cause. This often requires a team approach because the patient may present with a confusing spectrum of symptoms involving many organ systems. Very often a definitive diagnosis can only be reached after a thorough clinical history, physical examination, laboratory, and electrophysiological investigation (1, 3, 4).

The extremity is evaluated to determine the severity of the disease, the extent of the paralysis, and the presence and nature of the deformity. One must determine if the deformity is caused by structural blockage, muscle contracture, muscular weakness, excessive muscle tone, or combinations of them all (5).

The examination begins with gait analysis (1, 3, 4). In certain neurological conditions muscle tone varies according to the patient's body position and it is therefore important to reproduce physiological postures (5). The examiner must have a thorough understanding of normal muscle function in the gait cycle, as well as isolated muscle action. The patient as a whole must be considered with functional improvement being the primary goal of treatment that should be kept in mind during the entire examination. When surgical planning is undertaken, it is dependent on accurate visual gait analysis to determine which muscles are responsible for the abnormalities noted (6). Also the functional disability must be shown to be structural or muscular in origin and not caused by sensory, perceptual, or cognitive abnormalities.

Dropfoot gait shows a distinctive pattern (1). It is an awkward high steppage gait with the ankle maintained in plantarflexion during the swing phase. If any function of the long extensors is present, an attempt is made to dorsiflex the foot and this manifests as extensor substitution or digital contractures. If there is no function of the digital extensors toe curling occurs, which decreases stability during stance and makes the wearing of shoes difficult. Varus deformity secondary to the unopposed pull of the tendon of m. tibialis posterior is noted during stance and swing. The degree of this effect is dependent on the degree of function of m. peroneus brevis. Spasticity or contractures of the posterior muscle group will modify the gait pattern and the use of a local anesthetic nerve block to achieve relaxation can reduce these effects, making evaluation easier.

Manual Muscle Testing

Manual muscle testing is performed to determine the degree and distribution of muscular weakness and strength. The testing is based on the use of gravity and resistance and is outlined as follows (1, 3, 4):

0—No contraction
1—Trace contraction
2—Muscle contraction and range of motion with gravity eliminated
3—Muscle contraction and range of motion against gravity with no resistance
4—Muscle contraction and range of motion against gravity and some resistance
5—Normal power

A plus and minus can also be used for those muscles that fall between these categories. Quantifying the patient's response both to range of motion and strength can be done with a goniometer and a strain gauge, respectively. The accuracy and reproducibility of the results is sometimes limited by the examiner's technique, instrumentation, and/or patient compliance.

Testing of muscles demands precise anatomical and functional knowledge (4). The relaxed muscles and joints of the extremity are first palpated and placed through a passive range of motion to determine if any abnormalities or painful areas could limit the test results. Mobility and position in relationships of the rearfoot, forefoot, and toes are noted. Ideally the part is then placed in the position of maximum contracture of the muscle and resistance is applied until the muscle yields. The examiner also palpates the contracting muscle at the same time.

The test results are limited by a number of factors. Any pain can alter the patient's response. The use of a local anesthetic to relieve the discomfort may produce a more accurate representation of function. Local anesthetics can also be used to block competing innervation temporarily eliminating spasticity of antagonistic muscles. It must also be remembered that the dependability of testing is affected by both the patient's understanding and compliance.

Following manual muscle examination, nerve conduction velocity measurements and electromyographical studies are obtained and correlated with the examination (4). They are helpful in evaluating the appropriateness of proposed tendon balancing procedures.

X-ray evaluation is used to determine the degree of structural adaptations and arthritic involvement. Standard views including lateral, oblique, dorsoplantar, and calcaneal axial are used. Stress laterals are often helpful in separating structural from functional

involvement. Again the use of a local anesthetic to relieve spasticity should be considered.

CONSERVATIVE TREATMENT
Orthotic Management

Some authorities believe that most deformities of the foot and ankle can be improved with an appropriate orthosis (1). In a dropfoot condition, an ankle/foot orthosis can provide adequate toe clearance and maintain a functional position during the swing phase of gait (Fig. 12.1). It can also control excessive movement and prevent contractures. Functional improvement is the primary goal with minimal restriction.

The ideal brace must be simple to apply and remove. Strength and durability are important to provide the best mechanical advantages, although the device must be lightweight enough to be functional. Its cosmetic appearance is extremely important because if it is not acceptable there will be poor patient compliance (7).

When inadeqaute dorsiflexion alone is the problem, a lightweight posterior insert ankle/foot orthosis will control the patient's foot (8–10) (Figs. 12.2, 12.3). This device is rigid enough to provide adequate toe clearance during the swing phase of gait, and at the same time produces flexibility to allow mild plantarflexion and dorsiflexion during stance. This versatility is achieved by narrowing the posterior portion of the orthosis to permit mild bending, secondary to weight bearing (Fig. 12.4). If there is overactivity of the posterior muscle group, a more rigid orthosis is needed (8–10).

Lateral instability and/or varus deformity is another condition that is often found associated with dropfoot deformity because of the unopposed function of m. tibialis posterior. Frontal plane, as well as sag-

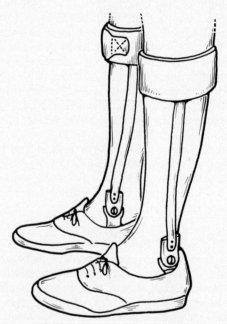

Figure 12.1. Ankle foot arthosis.

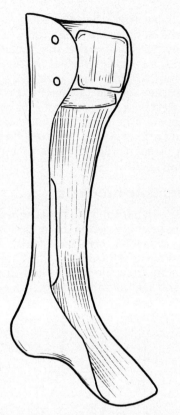

Figure 12.2. Plastic posterior orthosis.

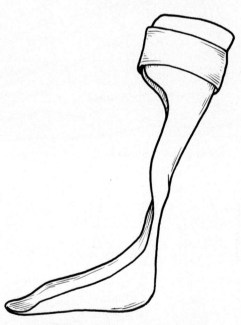

Figure 12.3. Plastic posterior orthosis.

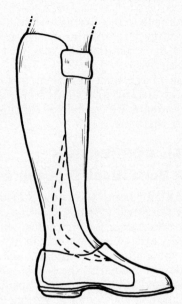

Figure 12.4. Plastic posterior orthosis illustrating trim lines to allow for increased ankle joint flexibility.

of the orthosis while maintaining a narrowed posterior support (8–10).

There are many other types of orthoses to control dropfoot that are not mentioned here and are beyond the scope of this chapter. Consultation with an orthotist is highly recommended before final prescription.

Peroneal Nerve Stimulator

Experimental correction of dropfoot has been achieved by electrical stimulation of the peroneal nerve (11–13). Both improvement of gait and dorsiflexion have been reported.

The stimulator device consists of essentially three parts. A stimulator that generates and transmits an electrical signal, a switch box that synchronizes the electrical activity with the swing phase of gait, and an electrode that stimulates the peroneal nerve to produce dorsiflexion. The switch box can be placed either on the heel of the affected side or the insole of the opposite foot. Once activated during the gait cycle, an electrical impulse is sent to stimulate the ankle dorsiflexion muscles to provide a more normal gait.

This method of treatment, although sometimes successful, does offer problems and has several limitations. Direct stimulation of the dorsiflexion muscles is not usually possible because the amount of current necessary to produce an adequate effect often produces pain. The peroneal nerve must therefore be stimulated directly either by skin electrodes or surgically implanted ones. The apparatus must therefore be functioning normally and because of individual sensitivity still has been shown to produce discomfort, limiting its use. If surface electrodes are used, it is sometimes difficult to locate the correct stimulation site and skin irritation has been noted. For the stimulator to be effective sufficient ankle joint range of motion and muscle strength of the dorsiflexors needs to be present.

ittal plane, stability is needed for the patient to function securely on uneven surfaces. Dynamic inversion control can be provided in several ways. The posterior portion of the orthosis can be extended anteriorly, although this will not allow any dorsiflexion or plantarflexion to occur during stance. If flexibility is desirable, a T-strap can be applied to the lateral aspect

For this approach to be effective the dropfoot must be caused by an inactive anterior muscle group and not complicated by structural blockage or by posterior muscle spasticity.

Because of the many problems associated with the use of the electrical stimulator, only a small percentage of patients are candidates for this method of treatment at this time.

SURGICAL CORRECTION

Posterior Bone Block Procedures

The posterior bone block procedure was initially reported by Campbell (14) in 1923 (Fig. 12.5). It was indicated for the correction of dropfoot when no other foot deformity existed except the inability to dorsiflex the foot at the ankle (15). A linear longitudinal incision is made just medial to the tendon and posterior to the ankle and subtalar joints. Capsular tissue is reflected, exposing the posterior surface of the talus and calcaneus. Care is taken not to injure either the tendo achillis or the tendon of m. flexor hallucis longus. With the foot held in dorsiflexion the posterior surface of the talus is resected and bone is reflected superiorly and anteriorly from the superior surface of the calcaneus, forming a peak of bone posterior to the ankle joint and preventing plantarflexion (16) (Fig. 12.6). Care is taken to avoid roughening the posterior surface of the tibia to prevent the occurrence of a fusion site between the bone block and the ankle joint.

The procedure has since been modified by several authorities (17, 18). It is sometimes done in conjunction with a tendo achillis lengthening and/or a triple arthrodesis. If done in conjunction with a triple ar-

throdesis, bone from that procedure can be used in creating the bone block (Fig. 12.7). The Gill bone block is another modification that removes a wedge of bone from the posterior surface of the calcaneus and places it into an osteotomy created in the posterior superior surface of the talus (19) (Figs. 12.8, 12.9). Unfortunately over time the posterior bone block procedures have shown a high incidence of recurrence of the deformity, resorption or fracture of the bone block, as well as osteoarthritic changes with resulting pain and disability (20).

Lambrinudi Arthrodesis

In 1927 Lambrinudi (21) described a procedure for the surgical correction of dropfoot. Indications were later expanded to include equino varus, equino valgus, and cavus deformities. The surgeon excises a wedge of bone from the plantar and distal portion of the talus so that the talus remains in equinus at the

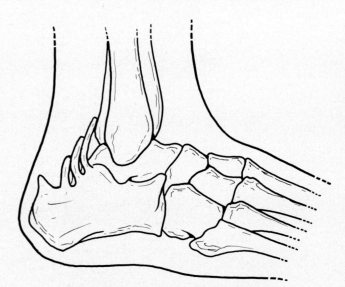

Figure 12.6. Posterior bone block procedure.

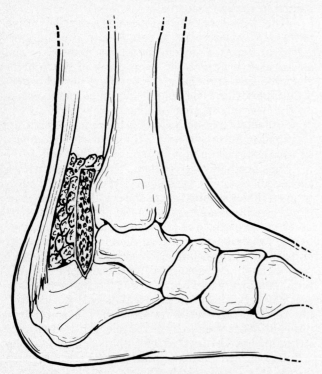

Figure 12.5. Campbell's posterior bone block procedure.

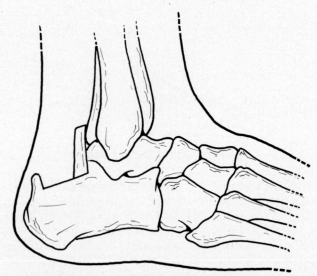

Figure 12.7. Posterior bone block procedure.

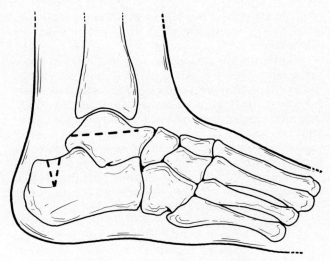

Figure 12.8. Gill posterior bone block.

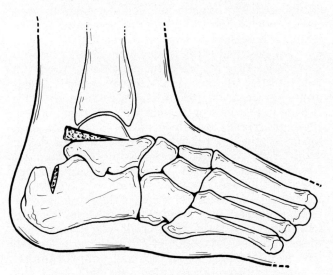

Figure 12.9. Gill posterior bone block.

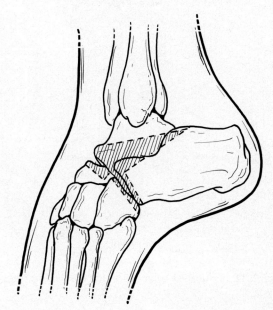

Figure 12.10. Bone wedge to be resected for Lambrinudi arthrodesis.

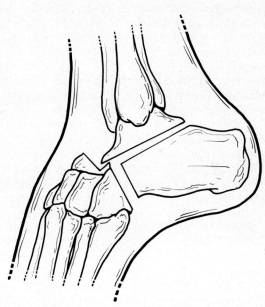

Figure 12.11. Bone resected for Lambrinudi arthrodesis.

ankle joint, while the forefoot is repositioned in dorsiflexion and fused to the rearfoot (Figs. 12.10, 12.11). Similar to the bone block procedures, further plantarflexion of the foot is prevented by the posterior process of the talus jamming against the posterior distal tibia.

The procedure is similar to the traditional triple arthrodesis with the exception of the position of the fusion site. Before surgery a template is made from a lateral radiograph taken in maximum plantarflexion to determine the size and angulation of bone wedges necessary for correction of the deformity. A wedge of bone is first removed from the plantar and distal portions of the neck and head of the talus. The plane of the osteotomy should be parallel to the transverse axis of the ankle joint. A corresponding osteotomy is made through the superior surface of the calcaneus parallel to the longitudinal axis of the foot. A wedge of bone is removed from the calcaneocuboid joint, being careful not to invert the forefoot, and an osteotomy is created in the proximal plantar navicular (2, 15, 18, 21, 22) (Figs. 12.10, 12.11).

With the osteotomy sites held in the reduced positions the forefoot should be in mild abduction and the rearfoot in mild valgus. Slight equinus of the forefoot is acceptable because of the shortening of the extremity that is created by the removal of bone (Fig. 12.12).

There are many reported complications secondary to the procedure. The most common technical areas include painful nonunions, removing too small a wedge from the subtalar joint, leaving excessive equinus, and a residual forefoot varus or supination deformity caused by the angulation of the wedge of bone removed from the calcaneocuboid joint (20, 23). The procedure demands that a sizeable wedge of bone be removed from the talus and subtalar joints to

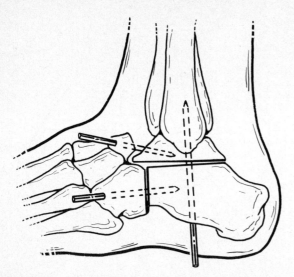

Figure 12.12. Lambrinudi arthrodesis—final position with fixation.

achieve a plantargrade position of the forefoot. Shortening of the extremity, although commonly reported, does not usually present a problem. The occurrence of avascular necrosis of the talus was rarely reported although flattening of the head of the talus either secondary to avascular necrosis or postoperative arthritis is sometimes found on lateral radiographic examination.

Severe painful osteoarthritis of the ankle joint was reported in a number of studies and can be secondary to many factors (20, 23). Inherent in the surgical procedure and original deformity the narrow posterior articular surface of the talus is made to articulate in the ankle joint in place of the wider anterior segment. This increasing joint incongruity, as well as laxity of the anterior and lateral ligaments of the ankle joint, secondary to either stretching or the surgical procedure itself, can lead to instability predisposing the patient to arthritic changes (24).

Muscle power has also been shown to have an effect on the surgical results. Even with stabilization and realignment of the foot secondary changes occur with time (24). Dislocation of the ankle joint caused by an imbalance between dorsiflexors and plantarflexors and varus deformity of the ankle joint caused by the overpowering influence of the tendon of m. tibialis posterior have been reported. The highest incidences of failures occurred in the flail foot type and the best results were seen when the dorsiflexors and plantarflexors were balanced or there was a fixed equinus (22, 23).

Anterior Transfer of the Tendon Of M. Tibialis Posterior

Anterior transfer of the tendon of m. tibialis posterior provides a replacement for the nonfunctioning anterior group muscles, restoring balance to the foot and ankle (25–28). The surgical procedure removes a varus deforming force and provides active dorsiflexion and tenodesis, as well as improved stability, by producing better muscle balance. Successful

treatment depends on complete evaluation that covers all aspects of the patient's disability and potential for rehabilitation.

Certain basic principles must be followed before the tendon transfer. All fixed deformities must be reduced. The tendon transfer itself provides a dynamic force for correction of movement that can only function after contractures are released and osseous stability is achieved (18, 29–32). Fixed varus and/or equinus necessitates performing such procedures as triple arthrodesis, Dwyer's osteotomy, tendo achillis lengthening, posterior capsulotomy, plantar fascial stripping, m. flexor hallucis longus, and/or m. flexor digitorum longus lengthening (20, 24, 33).

Strength and range of motion of the muscle-tendon unit to be transferred must be adequate to perform the intended function (18, 24, 29). A loss of power of at least one grade is expected postoperatively and therefore any muscle below a grade four should not be used. The original function of the muscle must be expendable and its effects postoperatively on remaining muscular balance considered (32, 34).

The insertion of the tendon of m. tibialis posterior is variable. After it is split it is possible to insert each half into the tendons of m. extensor hallucis longus and m. extensor digitorum longus, respectively. This is done in the hope of providing a stabilizing force to the digits and is usually done in conjunction with flexor lengthening procedures and/or osseous digital stabilizing procedures. M. tibialis posterior does not have to be split and can be inserted directly into one of the tarsal bones. Its final position is dependent on the remaining muscular strength of the extremity (32). Primary concern is to avoid creating a varus or valgus foot. The tendon is therefore usually placed fairly close to the midline. The tendon of m. tibialis posterior will have a greater force across the ankle joint the further it is inserted from the axis of motion. However, it will require a smaller excursion to produce ankle joint range of motion if the insertion is closer to the axis (30). The final position of insertion is not as critical when the procedure is performed in conjunction with bony stabilization such as triple arthrodesis (1).

The tendon of m. tibialis posterior can also be transferred around the medial side of the ankle (20, 30). Although this method is less likely to damage the tibial nerve, it does have certain disadvantages. The pull of the muscle tendon complex is now in a long spiral direction, rather than in a direct line of pull, decreasing both force and range of motion on the ankle. The tendon is also more likely to come in direct contact with the bone, increasing the possibility of adhesions. Also, such transfer is performed subcutaneously rather than within an existing tendon sheath and gliding motion seen postoperatively will be restricted.

Regardless of the method of transfer the patient is kept non-weight-bearing with the foot and leg immobilized in a cast in mild dorsiflexion for approximately four to six weeks. The cast should extend to the distal aspect of the digits supporting the toes in a neutral position. The cast is then bivalved and passive range of motion exercises are begun. These are followed by active assisted range of motion exercises and finally gait training. It is recommended that a night splint be used for approximately six months following the surgical procedure to protect the transfer and to aid in the stretching of accommodative contractures that may be present (27, 32).

M. tibialis posterior is primarily a stance phase muscle and when it is transferred anteriorly to act as a dorsiflexor it must change its pattern of firing to the swing phase to function properly during the gait cycle. Voluntary dorsiflexion is usually fairly easy to accomplish postoperatively; however, true phasic conversion is much more difficult and in some patients, as shown by dynamic electromyographical studies, never occurs (35, 36). In these cases one should not presume a failure. A tenodesis effect can often be seen that is sufficient to resist dropfoot and allow a more normal gait. In more than 300 tendon transfers performed at Doctors Hospital in the past 25 years only 2 could be termed as failures. Yet even those two failures were sufficiently improved to permit the patients to discontinue the use of double upright braces.

Much of the success of the procedure is dependent on reeducation of the muscle, which can take an extended period of time (35–38). A team effort among the patient, physiotherapist, and surgeon is helpful. Reeducation can be made easier by teaching the patient preoperatively to isolate and maximally contract m. tibialis posterior. Its action must be isolated from the flexors and other posterior group muscles with which it is synergistic. Postoperatively muscle training can be assisted by direct electrical stimulation. This helps the patient to isolate and feel the muscle's new function, as well as to reduce atrophy and increase strength. Electrical stimulation can also reproduce the normal muscular firing sequence during gait assisting in muscle reeducation and phasic transfer (1).

Other tendon balancing procedures used have been reported for the correction of dropfoot deformity. Dual transfer of the tendons of m. tibialis posterior and m. flexor digitorum longus is believed to have the advantage of increased dorsiflexion strength (27, 39). Transfer of m. peroneus longus to the dorsum of the foot along with the tendon of m. tibialis posterior increases the strength of dorsiflexion, as well as applies additional transverse plane stability to the foot (1). The use of either m. flexor hallucis longus and/or m. flexor digitorum longus provides an active dorsiflexory range of motion that does not disrupt the function of m. tibialis posterior (40). This can be an important consideration so as not to create a valgus foot if m. peroneus brevis is functioning strongly (1, 27).

As mentioned earlier, digital deformities are commonly associated with dropfoot. Correction of these is necessary to allow the patient to wear normal shoes and function adequately. The procedure chosen is dependent on the muscular imbalance present, as well as the other surgical procedures to be performed. It must be determined whether extensor substitution or simple curling of the digits are present. In either case osseous stabilizing procedures are recommended over simple arthroplasties. These are performed in conjunction with digital muscle tendon balancing procedures.

SUMMARY

The main goal of treatment when dealing with dropfoot deformity is functional improvement whether it be by conservative or surgical measures. A proper course of treatment can only be decided on after careful patient evaluation and must be considered in relation to the total functional capacity of the patient.

Achieving successful surgical results is dependent on proper patient selection, a thorough preoperative evaluation to determine the best surgical procedure, and a complete postoperative program. As with all reconstructive procedures, patient motivation is essential to achieve the best possible results.

Unfortunately there is no one best surgical procedure for the correction of dropfoot deformity. There are many variations of muscle and/or structural abnormalities that can produce the condition and for this reason each surgical approach must be individualized to the patient's needs.

Paralytic Flatfoot

Stephen Silvani, D.P.M. and Barry L. Scurran, D.P.M.

Flatfoot is a general term used to describe any condition of the foot that results in an abnormally low longitudinal arch as assessed clinically and radiographically. This section describes those neuromuscular conditions that produce the so-called flatfoot, or paralytic pes valgo planus. Table 12.1 lists the common etiological factors. An overview of the conservative and surgical management of this group of conditions is presented here.

CLINICAL FEATURES

Although the presenting complaint may be that of a flatfoot, a thorough and complete physical examination must be performed. The systemic disorders that produce a neuromuscular pes valgo planus deformity may be identified by complex diagnostic evaluations that are beyond the scope of this section (41). Thorough examination of the skin, head, back, extremities, motor and sensory systems, the cranial nerves, and reflexes contributes to an accurate diagnosis. A detailed lower extremity biomechanical analysis is necessary. Laboratory, electromyographical, eletrodynographical, muscle, and nerve biopsies may be indicated to complete the diagnostic evaluation.

Clinically the neuromuscular pes valgus foot tires easily and is often associated with discomfort under minimal stress (42–44). The patient may report pain in the arch, calf, and low back after minimal periods of standing or walking. Examination of the foot, non-weight-bearing, may or may not reveal a well-formed arch; however, the foot appears totally flat with weight bearing (Fig. 12.13 A, B). Eversion of the calcaneus may be present during stance.

Standard weight-bearing radiographs are taken in the angle and base of gait for further evaluation and documentation of the flatfoot deformity, as well as to rule out local osseous etiologies (e.g. tarsal coalition) (Fig. 12.14 A, B). A decreased calcaneal inclination angle is observed on the lateral view (Fig. 12.15). An increase in the normal talocalcaneal angle is noted on

the dorsoplantar (anteroposterior view). Because of incomplete ossification these measurements cannot be identified with accuracy until age six. However, radiographic measurements will serve as an indicator of the severity of the deformity.

ETIOLOGICAL CONDITIONS AND THEIR TREATMENT

Cerebral Palsy

Cerebral palsy is a complex of symptoms that are caused by fixed, nonprogressive brain lesion(s) occurring prenatally, at parturition, or in the immediate postnatal period. In most affected patients the primary disorder affects the musculoskeletal system; in others, mental retardation, speech, hearing, or sensory disturbances may be present (45). Because multiple types of cerebral palsy exist diagnostic differentiation must be undertaken before surgical procedures are planned. These types include extrapyramidal-athe-

Table 12.1
Etiology of the Paralytic Flat Foot

Cerebral Palsy
Poliomyelitis
Progressive Muscular Dystrophy
Myelomeningocele
Diastematomyelia
Posttraumatic
Ischemia
Compartment Syndrome
Cerebral Vascular Accident
CNS Neoplasms
Amaurotic Familial Idiocy

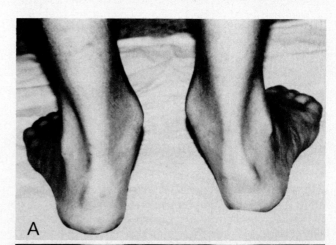
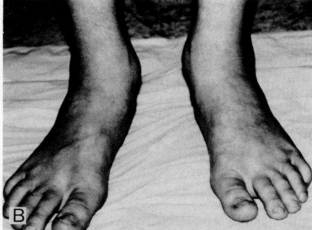

Figure 12.13. (A, B) Clinical appearance of paralytic flat foot secondary to mild poliomyelitis.

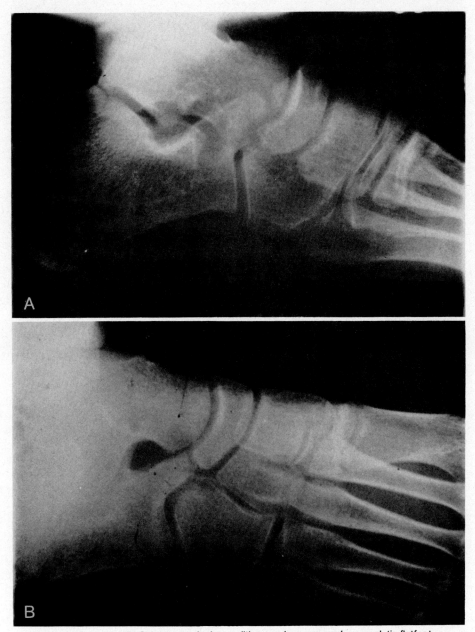

Figure 12.14.   (A, B) Calcaneonavicular coalition produces secondary paralytic flatfoot.

toid, mixed, ataxic, rigid or tremor, and pyramidal-spastic. The differential diagnosis is beyond the scope of this discussion (46–49).

The management of the patient with cerebral palsy is a multidisciplinary problem requiring a team approach to treatment that may extend over many years (50–52). The goal of podiatric surgery is to improve structrual stability and motor function. This must be integrated into the dynamics of growth, development, and maturation of the central nervous system. The interaction and relation of the hip, knee, and ankle joints to local foot deformities must be closely evaluated (53).

Spastic pes valgus deformity seen in the patient with cerebral palsy is usually associated with a triceps surae equinus (41). This can be secondary to foot biomechanics or to a dynamic muscular imbalance between evertors and invertors. Passive stretching exercises should be initiated first functionally to lengthen the triceps surae and peroneal tendons (54). Night splints that hold the ankle neutral or slightly dorsiflexed may help control further contracture. Stretching or a wedged plaster cast does not seem to be well tolerated by children with cerebral palsy.

Operative correction of the equinus deformity is indicated if toe-toe or toe-heel gait persists up to 4 to 6 years, or earlier if especially severe. Lengthening of the Achilles tendon is usually done to correct myostatic contracture, to alter the point at which the stretch reflex is elicited, and to develop control over a weak m. tibialis anterior thus establishing a dynamic muscle balance between ankle dorsiflexors and plan-

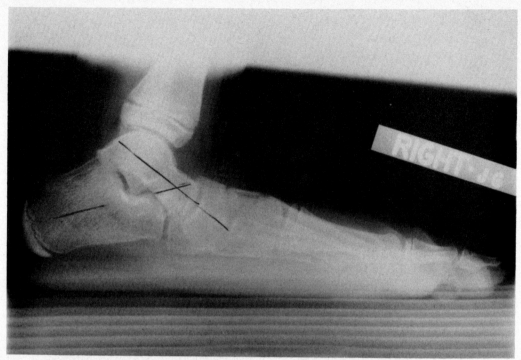

Figure 12.15.   Radiograph of paralytic flatfoot secondary to brain trauma (auto accident).

tarflexors. Many types of lengthening procedures have been reported in the literature (54–59), each with its own advantages and disadvantages. The results usually are more closely related to patient selection and follow-up care than to the type of procedure selected.

The White sliding lengthening, as advocated by Banks and Green, is widely favored because there is little disruption of the anatomical continuity of the tendo achillis and relatively early mobilization is permitted. Subcutaneous and Z-type lengthenings have shown poor long-term results, with frequent overlengthening or scarring down of the tendon often with recurrent equinus. The Vulpius procedure maintains the continuity of m. soleus fibers by transecting only the aponeurotic tendon portions of m. gastrocnemius and m. soleus (56). It has been noted, however, that this procedure may produce a genu recurvatum by eliminating the posterior dynamic support for the knee. The Strayer (56, 57) method divides the tendon of m. gastrocnemius transversely at the conjoined junction and with the foot dorsiflexed to neutral the tendon is sutured to the underlying m. soleus. Neurectomy of the motor branches of the tibial nerve to m. gastrocnemius has also been advocated (59) but only in cases where severe clonus hinders weight bearing or bracing.

Pierrot and Murphy (60) in 1959 proposed an anterior advancement of the insertion of the tendo achillis on the calcaneus to shorten its lever arm and decrease its strength without changing its resting length. Throop (61) and associates demonstrated 89.9% satisfactory results with this advancement.

If by one year after tendo achillis lengthening the patient cannot overcome a cerebral zero tibialis anterior, Tachdjian (62) recommends shortening m. tibi-

alis anterior and transferring m. extensor hallucis longus to the first metatarsal base through the tibialis anterior sheath.

With correction of the equinus component of the neuromuscular pes valgus deformity associated with cerebral palsy the child is followed until age 8 to 10 years. If pes valgus persists an extra-articular subtalar arthrodesis is recommended (Grice procedure). The results are reported as satisfactory in approximately 65% of the cases (45), provided overcorrection is not effected, other muscular contractures are alleviated, and pseudarthrosis is avoided. Subtalar arthroereisis peg or peglike procedures (lateral subtalar joint arthroereisis) may also be used once the equinus component has been eliminated (Fig. 12.16).

Dwyer's opening lateral calcaneal osteotomy, and displacement osteotomies are also used to reduce or correct valgus deformity of the rearfoot. These procedures tend to offer a more anatomical weight-bearing alignment of the foot while preserving subtalar joint range of motion. It appears that Baker and Hill's (63) medial displacement osteotomy may be superior because bone grafting is not required.

Triple arthrodesis may be indicated in the skeletally mature patient with painful valgus feet or where a fixed osseous deformity prevents appropriate bracing.

POLIOMYELITIS

The poliomyelitis virus destroys the anterior horn cells of the spinal cord and denervates the associated motor units. The resultant flaccid muscle paralysis may cause a pes valgo planus deformity, and the transferring of active muscles to replace those para-

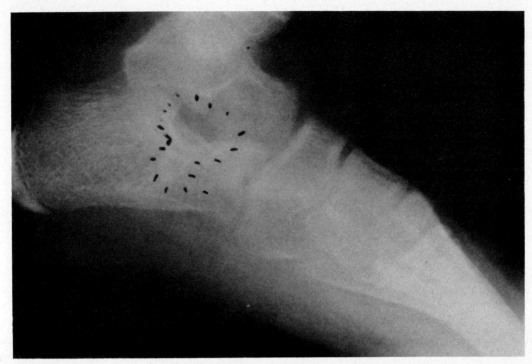

Figure 12.16. Radiograph of postoperative lateral subtalar joint arthroereisis (STA peg) in same patient as in Figure 12.15.

lyzed may be indicated to reestablish dynamic muscle balance. Basic concepts of tendon transfer are beyond the scope of this chapter and may be found in the chapters on tendon surgery and pes valgus deformity.

Muscle imbalance will produce an initial deformity that is flexible in nature. With skeletal growth fixed soft tissue and osseous deformity may occur; therefore tendon transfers are most effective when performed on younger patients.

Paralysis of m. tibialis anterior will cause an equinovalgus foot to develop. The digital extensors become overactive in an attempt to replace ankle dorsiflexors and cock-up toes often result. Passive gastrosoleus stretching with protective night splinting is encouraged. If severe fixed equinus is present a posterior surgical release of the ankle and subtalar joints is recommended and the Achilles tendon is stretched with plaster casting if feasible rather than being surgically lengthened. A plantigrade, stable foot for ambulation can thus be achieved.

PROGRESSIVE MUSCULAR DYSTROPHY

Progressive muscular dystrophy, a hereditary primary disease of skeletal muscle, generally has a poor prognosis. The initial symptoms of delayed motor development, difficulty in rising from the floor (Gower's sign), and a tendency to fall frequently present within the first three years of life. The gait is waddling. Pes valgo planus deformity occurs because of the unopposed gastrosoleus contracture secondary to a weak anterior muscle group. The diagnosis is confirmed by muscle biopsy and an elevated serum creatinine phosphokinase (41).

The clinical course is rapid and progressive with the patient wheelchair bound by the second decade. The muscle weakness, contractures, and inactivity are problems that must be considered along with their emotional sequelae. Passive stretching and appropriate splinting can relieve some equinus. When fixed equinus is noted slide tendo achillis lengthening is recommended, along with postoperative knee-ankle-foot orthosis to allow ambulation.

MYELOMENINGOCELE

Myelomeningocele is an intrauterine defect with failure of fusion of the vertebral arches and dysplasia of the spinal cord with cystic protrusion of the meninges. With nerve tissue present in the sac, distal neurological defects are seen below the level of the lesion. This complex congenital problem requires a team therapeutic approach because many organ systems are usually involved. Flaccid paralysis is seen with lesions of the lumbosacral region; spastic paralysis is seen with lesions at the cervicothoracic level. A thorough pediatric neurological examination is necessary to relate the musculoskeletal deformity to a specific neural level. Modern techniques of neonatal surgery are decreasing the mortality rate for these affected infants and are preserving lower extremity neurological function. This, however, creates an increase in the number of patients with associated musculoskeletal deformities. These patients are best cared for by a multidisciplinary approach.

The goal of lower extremity surgery should be to have the patient ambulatory with orthotic assistance by 18 months. Pedal problems are common because of muscle imbalance, spasticity, fibrous contracture of denervated muscles, intrauterine malposition, and teratogenic and repetitive malpositioning of the limb after birth (42).

The type of paralytic pedal deformity can be correlated to the neural level of the lesion. When the lesion is at or above the third lumbar vertebral segment, equinovalgus may result that will persist with weight bearing. Stretching and orthotic support may adequately control the problem. A paralytic vertical talus is seen with talar plantarflexion and subluxation of the talonavicular joint when the lesion is at the fourth lumbar segment. Early pantalar release (six months) is advocated for this serious deformity.

The goal should be the provision of a plantigrade foot that will avoid the common neuropathic pressure lesions. Therapy includes soft tissue release, orthotic management, and well-padded custom-made shoes.

DIASTEMATOMYELIA

Diastematomyelia is a congenital sagittal division of the spinal cord by protrusion of an osseous or fibrocartilaginous mass coursing from the anterior vertebral body to the posterior dura. Various skin deformities (dimpling, tufts of hair, vascular and fatty tumors) are usually found over the level of the lesion.

Delayed ambulation and spastic or flaccid paralysis may occur depending on the level of the lesion. Radiographic or myelographic studies with CT scanning visualizes the pathological lesion. Neurosurgery may be indicated to prevent the progression of the neurological defect. The treatment of the paralytic pedal disorder is similar to that described for the deformities of poliomyelitis.

POSTTRAUMATIC, ISCHEMIC, AND COMPARTMENT SYNDROMES

Peripheral nerve disorders can produce paresis or paralysis of intrinsic or extrinsic muscles, neuropathies, painful states, and contractures. The resultant foot deformities may be treated by stabilization with arthrodesis and tendon transfers when indicated. Orthotic devices may be useful to protect and stabilize the paralyzed foot. The advances in microvascular surgery and improved limb salvage procedures have decreased the late sequelae of neural ischemia.

The careful and detailed neurological examination to determine the level, extent, and distribution of the paralysis is indicated but is beyond the scope of this section. The types of traumatic and ischemic neuropathies are listed in Table 12.2. Many injuries are mixed, a combination of contusion, stretch, and ischemia. Compressive or ischemic lesions are often associated with a fracture or with subsequent fracture treatment. The primary etiological factor must be identified and treated or eliminated to the extent possible. The residual effects of a paralytic pes valgus foot are then managed with the aforementioned prin-

Table 12.2
Eiology of Neuropathies

Direct Injury
1. Laceration
2. Traction Injury
3. Crush and Contusion
4. Gunshot Injuries
5. Thermal Injury
6. Intraneural Injection of Toxic Substances
7. Radiation Injuries

Compression Injury
1. Tourniquet
2. Internal Compression

Ischemic Neuropathies
1. Arterial Embolism
2. Arterial Nervorum Occlusion
3. Vascular Spasm
4. Traumatic

Entrapment Neuropathies
1. Tarsal Tunnel Syndrome.

ciples of stabilization, contracture releases, and tendon transfers as indicated.

CENTRAL NERVOUS SYSTEM ORIGIN

Hemiplegia is the most common neurological deficit following a cerebrovascular accident with the majority of the spontaneously resolving neurological deficits occurring in the first six to eight months (43). If spasticity or flaccidity persists, bracing of the ankle joint to prevent footdrop may be necessary to enable ambulation. Intensive physical therapy must be instituted early in the treatment program with increased motivation of the patient.

Surgical correction is indicated if equinus persists after six to eight months of appropriate rigid ankle foot orthotics and stretching. The White sliding tendo achilles lengthening is commonly performed. The ankle is dorsiflexed to neutral and a below knee cast is applied with weight bearing for six weeks. Postcasting the tendon is protected for six weeks with a posterior splint.

MISCELLANEOUS

Many strategically located CNS space-occupying tumors or metastases can cause upper motor neuron spasticity with potential lower extremity muscular spasticity or paralysis. Once the lesion is stabilized and no further neurological changes are seen in the periphery, the paralytic pes valgus deformity can be stabilized through arthrodesing procedures as described previously. Amaurotic familial idiocy, a hereditary disorder with diminished eyesight, mental retardation, and in many instances a paralytic flatfoot, is best stabilized through arthrodesing procedures.

Digital Deformity and Neuromuscular Disease

Edwin W. Wolf, D.P.M.

Orthopedic and surgical literature report techniques of corrective surgery for pedal deformities secondary to neurological dysfunction as early as 1881 (64). During this same time period authors such as D'Angers (1827, syringomyelia) and Smith (1849, neurofibromatosis) (65–67) described neurological syndromes not previously published. Although the exact etiology, pathophysiology, progression, and residual effects of the neuromuscular disorders were not fully understood, attempts were made to stabilize and restore function to the lower extremities of afflicted individuals.

Today with diagnostic aids such as computerized axial tomography, myelography, electromyography, and nerve conduction velocity studies, the medical community has arrived at a better understanding of the etiology, diagnosis, and prognosis of neurological and neuromuscular disorders described over a century ago. It is with these advances in technology, as well as the greater sophistication of surgical techniques, that we attempt to obtain the same objectives as early surgeons: diminution of discomfort, restoration of function and stability, and improved cosmetic restoration of those with a pedal manifestation of neurological and neuromuscular disease.

Although it is virtually impossible to attribute a pedal deformity to a specific neurological or neuromuscular disorder, lesions or aberrations in specified areas of the central nervous sytem or neural pathway, or abnormalities of peripheral nerves may affect musculature influencing the foot itself and thus have a propensity to manifest a specific pedal deformity. In this manner pedal deformity can be attributed to one or several possible disorders.

Lower extremity musculature receives innervation from spinal cord segments L1 through S2. Numerous texts list specific innervations of muscle groups of the lower extremity. Aberration in the innervation, nerve root, spinal cord, or nerve tract will be manifested in corresponding muscular deficits. These aberrations may be congenital as in cerebral palsy or spina bifida or acquired as in poliomyelitis.

Generally speaking the more proximal the location of nervous disfunction the greater the variation of pedal deformity manifested.

For example, Allan (68) cites the development of pes cavus deformity with lesions occurring at the L4 level and pes calcaneus with those occuring at L5. Tachjian (66) relates development of pes calcaneus, pes valgus, or equinovarus with spina bifida cystica occurring at or proximal to L3. It is with lesions at this level that a flail foot and ankle occur. However, in response to intrauterine forces any of the three described deformities may ensue.

With a defect at L4, m. tibialis anterior will be powerful in dorsiflexing and inverting the forefoot while the hindfoot is in calcaneovalgus or equinus producing a paralytic vertical talus (66).

Lesions occurring at L5 may manifest through progressive calcaneus deformity (67), because the peroneal, anterior tibial, and long digital extensor muscles are strong and the triceps surae and long flexors are inactive.

Pes cavus deformity results from overpowering by the long and short digital extensors with diminution of flexor and intrinsic muscle function (67). Lesions at S1, S2, or nerve damage of the superficial peroneal nerve or tibial nerve can result in this extensor prevalence with subsequent hammering of the digits.

An equinus deformity may be the result of spasticity and overpowering of the anterior crural musculature by the triceps surae. Equinovarus deformity is caused by relative overactivity of m. tibialis posterior and the long digital flexor muscles causing a varus attitude of the rearfoot.

An equinovalgus presentation may represent a compensatory morphology in an individual with initial equinus. Inability to dorsiflex the ankle causes extreme pronation and hence a valgus attitude of the rearfoot is assumed (69).

In the assessment of foot deformity in every individual and, more importantly, those with cerebral palsy it is essential to examine the more proximal elements both osseous and muscular and appreciate the influence these factors exert on the morphology and function of the foot.

Spastic hemiplegia results in hip and knee flexion, internal rotation, and adduction of the entire limb. The foot in this case may be in equinus. The presence of soft tissue contracture also complicates presentation because one must distinguish the primary deformity from the resultant contracture.

Individuals with Down's syndrome frequently exhibit ligamentous laxity and subsequently a pes planovalgus deformity (70). Spasticity of ankle dorsiflexion, if and when present, can exacerbate the deformity by compensatory pronation and hence predispose to the development of hallux valgus.

ANATOMICAL AND BIOMECHANICAL DIGITAL PATHOLOGY

A determination of the etiology of digital deformity secondary to neuromuscular disease is facilitated by a thorough understanding of "normal" digital structure and function.

The function of the digits arises from the integrated and alternated activity of extensors, flexors, and intrinsic musculature in the stance, toe-off, swing,

357

and heel contact phases of gait. Deviation from "ideal" functioning of flexors, extensors, and intrinsic muscles results in digital deformity.

Essential to the assessment of these digital deformities is the consideration of the following four factors. Digital function is an expression of both structure and function of more proximal segments (i.e. midtarsal, subtalar, rearfoot, and talocrural segments). Digital pathology may be inherent in the forefoot or may be the result of compensation activity for proximal segments (i.e. forefoot deformity caused by spastic equinus with calcaneovarus). Longstanding deformity is increased by adaptive osseous and soft tissue contracture in accordance to Wolff's and Davis' laws, respectively. Assessment of the deformity's fixed (rigid) or flexible (reducible) nature.

Hammertoe Deformity

A hammertoe deformity occurs with dorsiflexion of the proximal phalanx at the metatarsophalangeal joint and either neutral or planterflexed attitude of the proximal interphalangeal joint (71, 72).

Clawtoe Deformity

A clawtoe deformity is one in which there is dorsiflexion of the proximal phalanx at the metatarsophalangeal joint and either plantarflexion or neutral position of the middle phalanx with the distal phalanx plantarflexed (72). Several authors including Young (72) have considered the incidence of multiple hammerdigits as clawtoe deformity.

Mallet Toe Deformity

A mallet toe deformity is described as the deformity in which both the proximal and middle phalanges are stable but the distal phalanx is plantarflexed.

Digital deformity has been attributed to three basic biomechanical phenomena and occurs in both those with neuromuscular disease and in unaffected individuals as a result of structure and function. These are extensor substitution, flexor substitution, and flexor stabilization (D.R. Green, unpublished observations). The events precipitating these mechanisms of compensations will be described.

Extensor Substitution

Extensor substitution occurs in the swing and heel contact phases of gait when the anterior muscle group functions to dorsiflex the foot at the ankle. This can occur in anterior or combined equinus deformities (71, 73, 74), muscular weakness of the lumbricales, tight heel cord, or rigid cavus deformities. Several authors believe this extensor substitution is a major influence in the development of clawtoes (75, 76).

Flexor Substitution

Flexor substitution is seen in the stance phase of gait and occurs when there is a weakness of the triceps surae. The flexors and m. tibialis posterior attempt to substitute for the triceps surae. Extreme supination

and external rotation of the leg may also occur as a result in the late stance phase (D.R. Green, unpublished observations).

Flexor Stabilization

Flexor stabilization results from interosseous muscle weakness as in neuromuscular disease, in the hypermobile pes valgus deformity, and the pronated foot. The mechanism is noted in the stance phase of gait with increased force of pull of the long flexors over the interossei (D.R. Green, unpublished observations).

In addition, the loss of intrinsic muscle power is noted in abnormal pronation (77, 78).

Determination of the presence of one of these three phenomena can be made during gait analysis of the individual who is ambulatory. This information is then corroborated with static testing of specific muscle groups.

Testing of muscle function should include active and passive ranges of motion and muscle power against resistance. Spasticity should be noted.

Selected myoneural blocks as described by Kasser (71) consisting of 0.25% Marcaine administered within the muscle belly will temporarily eliminate muscle action selectively and enhance assessment of remaining musculature.

Electromyographical studies have also been performed to demonstrate muscle power deficits (79). These studies conducted before tendon transfer procedures assist in prognosis and postoperatively are invaluable in the retraining and physiotherapy of patients with neuromuscular disease.

Conservative Treatment. The treatment of digital deformity secondary to neuromuscular disease, whether surgical or conservative, is directed toward six objectives: (*a*) providing greater stability, (*b*) increasing ambulatory capacity, (*c*) decreasing severity of progression, (*d*) minimizing soft tissue contracture, (*e*) diminution of discomfort, and (*f*) improved cosmetic appearance.

Shoe therapy with orthotic control is recommended to control rearfoot and subtalar joint motion (70). Stretching, splinting, dynamic bracing, and strength enhancement are also recommended (69). Forcible manipulation is discouraged vehemently because of the potential of ligamentous or tendinous damage (80).

Surgical Correction of Digital Deformities Secondary to Neuromuscular Disease

The goals of surgical therapy of the digital deformities, as in conservative treatment, are to: (*a*) restore and/or maintain ambulatory ability, (*b*) provide greater stability, (*c*) delay rapidity of progression and severity of deformity, (*d*) diminish discomfort, (*e*) prevent complications such as trophic ulcerations over osseous prominences in the individual with sensory deficit, and (*f*) improve cosmetic appearance.

In surgical correction of these deformities the

following are important considerations: (a) presence of rearfoot deformity, (b) severity of the digital deformity, (c) flexibility (reducibility) or rigidity (nonreducibility) of the digits, (d) responsiveness to conservative therapy, (e) age of the patient, and (f) ambulatory potential of the patient.

Because digital deformities in the presence of neuromuscular disease afflicting the lower extremity are rarely encountered without rearfoot, talocrural, or forefoot aberrations, the surgical treatment entails intervention or at least investigation of each segment. For this reason surgical correction is sometimes staged and is often directed at more proximal segments that may consititute the etiology.

In staging of surgical procedures tendon transfers that attempt to restore muscle balance and delay the progression and severity of digital deformity have been suggested before skeletal maturity (82). Additional soft tissue procedures have been recommended before the patient's ambulation as an infant (69).

Osseous procedures such as Dwyer's calcaneal osteotomy have proven to be most effective before skeletal maturity (80).

Soft Tissue Procedures

Soft tissue procedures for digital deformities will relieve contracture and prove corrective only if the deformity expressed in the digits is flexible in nature and not a result of rearfoot deformity as caused by neuromuscular pathology.

The transfer of the tendons of m. extensor digitorum longus to corresponding metatarsal bases as described by Hibbs (82) has been noted to correct digital deformity and restore muscle balance.

Extensor tenotomy and capsulotomy have failed to provide more than temporary relief of dorsal lesions (83).

Other soft tissue procedures noted to decrease digital deformity are tendon transfers such as split tibialis anterior tendon transfer (STATT), tendo achillis lengthening (TAL), peroneus longus transfer, and tibialis posterior transfer in that they restore muscle balance and minimize rearfoot influence, depending on the muscle group involved.

The modified Jones forefoot suspension has also been cited as correcting forefoot equinus and related hammerdigits (84).

Osseous Procedures

Surgical correction of more severe deformity of the digits entails osseous resection combined with soft tissue procedures. The procedure most frequently cited consists of interphalangeal fusion at the proximal interphalangeal joint plus extensor transfer (77, 80, 81, 85, 86). Interphalangeal fusion plus flexor transfer was also reported (87).

Certainly the exact biomechanical etiology of the deformity should be identified and addressed in the attempt at surgical correction.

Green in his symposium on the etiology and treatment of hammerdigits describes the stepwise approach in the surgical treatment of digital deformity (D.R.

Green, unpublished observations). Although he does not differentiate between pathomechanics secondary to structural deformities and those arising from neuromuscular affliction, one can extrapolate and base surgical therapy on his observations.

In instances where formation of hammerdigits is caused by *extensor* substitution, proximal interphalangeal arthroplasty, extensor hood recession, extensor digitorum longus lengthening, and dorsal, medial, and lateral capsulotomy of the metatarsophalangeal joint can be attempted with intraoperative manipulation of the stump of the proximal phalanx at each step before continuation. The Hibbs procedure is effective in these cases because extensor pathology is in part responsible for deformity.

Neuromuscular disease frequently causes the demonstration of extensor substitution concomitant with flexor stabilization. In such cases interphalangeal joint arthrodesis is advisable.

Digital deformity resulting from flexor substitution can be ameliorated by proximal interphalangeal joint arthrodesis. In these cases arthroplasty alone is not effective. Muscle transfer to increase triceps surae strength is also frequently advisable (D.R. Green, unpublished observations).

Discussion

The vast majority of the literature reviewed concerns neuromuscular disease with resultant rearfoot deformity with little or no mention of subsequent digital abnormality. Those sources addressing the surgical correction of digital deformity fail to specify neuromuscular disease as an etiological factor.

Several authors suggest that correction of the rearfoot deformity may eliminate digital deformity if it is flexible (80).

Beyond a reasonable doubt the correction of rearfoot deformities secondary to neuromuscular deformities will reduce digital deformity or minimize its progress, the earlier the diagnosis of neuromuscular disease the better the prognosis with treatment, and corrective soft tissue procedures reduce the severity of the progression.

References

1. Jordan C: Adult neurologic diseases. In Cruess RL, Rennie WRJ (eds): *Adult Orthopedics*. New York, Churchill-Livingstone, 1984, pp 513–546.
2. Tang SC, Leong JCY, Hsu LCS, Lambrinudi C: Triple arthrodesis for correction of severe rigid drop-foot. *J Bone Joint Surg* 66B:66–70, 1984.
3. Omer GE Jr: Physical diagnosis of peripheral nerve injuries. *Orthop Clin North Am* 12:207–227, 1981.
4. Walton JN: Clinical examination of the neuromuscular system. *Disorders of Voluntary Muscle*, ed 4. New York, Churchill-Livingstone, 1981, pp 448–467.
5. Mooney V, Goodman F: Surgical approaches to lower extremity disability secondary to strokes. *Clin Orthop* 63:142–152, 1969.
6. Waters RL, Perry J, Garland D: Surgical correction of gait abnormalities following stroke. *Clin Orthop* 131:54–63, 1978.
7. Hutchison J: Present orthotic practice in the lower extremity. In Murdock G (ed): *Prosthetic and Orthotic Practice*. London, Edward Arnold, 1970, pp 461–469.
8. McCollough NC: Orthotic management in adult hemiplegia. *Clin Orthop* 131:38–46, 1978.

9. Meyer PR: Lower limb orthotics. *Clin Orthop* 102:58–70, 1974.

10. Waters R, Montgomery J: Lower extremity management of hemiparesis. *Clin Orthop* 102:133–143, 1971.

11. Waters RL, McNeal D, Perry J: Experimental correction of foot-drop by electrical stimulation of the peroneal nerve. *J Bone Joint Surg* 57A:1047–1054, 1975.

12. Takebe K, Kakulka C, Narayan MG, Milner M, Basmajian JV: Peroneal nerve stimulator in rehabilitation of hemiplegic patients. *Arch Phys Med Rehabil* 56:237–239, 1975.

13. Takebe K, Basmajian JV: Gait analysis in stroke patients to assess treatment of foot-drop. *Arch Phys Med Rehabil* 57:305–310, 1976.

14. Campbell WC: An operation for correction of "drop-foot." *J Bone Joint Surg* 5:815, 1923.

15. Patterson RL Jr, Parrish FF, Hathaway EN: Stabilizing operations of the foot. A study of indications, techniques used and end results. *J Bone Joint Surg* 32A:1–26, 1950.

16. Suppan RJ: Bone block procedures for dropfoot. *J Foot Surg* 16:133–135, 1977.

17. Ingram AJ, Hundley JM: Posterior bone block of the ankle for paralytic equinus; an end result study. *J Bone Joint Surg* 33A:679–691, 1951.

18. Ingram AJ: Anterior poliomyelitis. In Edmonson AS, Crenshaw AH (eds): *Campbell's Operative Orthopedics*, vol II. St Louis, The CV Mosby Co, 1980, p 1418.

19. Gill AB: An operation to make a posterior bone block at the ankle to limit foot-drop. *J Bone Joint Surg* 15:166, 1933.

20. Omer GE: Tendon transfers as reconstructive procedures in the leg and foot. In Omer GE, Spinner M (eds): *Management of Peripheral Nerve Problems*. Philadelphia, WB Saunders Co, 1980, p 873.

21. Lambrinudi C: New operation of dropfoot. *Br J Surg* 15:193–200, 1927.

22. MacKenzie IG: Lambrinudi's arthrodesis. *J Bone Joint Surg* 413B:738–742, 1959.

23. Bernau A: Long term results following Lambrinudi's arthrodesis. *J Bone Joint Surg* 59A:473–479, 1977.

24. Omer GE: Reconstructive procedures for extremities with peripheral nerve defects. *Clin Orthop* 163:80–90, 1982.

25. Turner JW, Cooper RR: Anterior transfer of tibialis posterior through the interosseous membrane. *Clin Orthop* 83:241–244, 1972.

26. Williams PF: Restoration of muscle balance of the foot by transfer of the tibialis posterior. *J Bone Joint Surg* 58B:217–219, 1976.

27. Wiesseman GJ: Tendon transfers for peripheral nerve injuries of the lower extremity. *Orthop Clin North Am* 12:459–467, 1981.

28. Eyring EJ, Earl WC, Brockmeyer JF: Post tibial tendon transfers in neuromuscular conditions other than arterio-poliomyelitis. *Arch Phys Med Rehabil* 55:124–126, 1974.

29. Turek SL: *Orthopedics—Principles and Their Application*, ed 4, vol I. Philadelphia, JB Lippincott Co, 1984, pp 545–552.

30. Lipscomb PR, Sanchez JJ: Anterior transplantation of posterior tibial tendon for persistent palsy of common peroneal nerve. *J Bone Joint Surg* 43A:60–66, 1961.

31. Spector EE, Todd WF, Wilson F: A review of selected posterior tibial tendon transfer procedures. *J Am Podiatry Assoc* 69:325–328, 1979.

32. Westin GW: Tendon transfers about the foot, ankle and hip in the paralyzed lower extremity. *J Bone Joint Surg* 47A:1430–1445, 1965.

33. Sorell DA, Hinterbuchner C, Green RF, Kalisky Z: Traumatic common peroneal nerve palsy: a retrospective study. *Arch Phys Med Rehabil* 57:360–365, 1976.

34. Schneider M, Balon K: Deformity of the foot following anterior transfer of the posterior tibial tendon and lengthening of the Achilles tendon for spastic equino-varus. *Clin Orthop* 125:113–118, 1977.

35. Close JR, Todd FN: The phasic activity of the muscles of the lower extremity and the effect of tendon transfer. *J Bone Joint Surg* 41A:189–208, 1959.

36. Verghese M, Radhakrishnan M, Chandrapal H, Jacob MV: Phasic conversion after tibial posterior transfer. *Arch Phys Med Rehabil* 56:83–85, 1975.

37. Takebe K, Hirohata K: EMG biofeedback in tendon transplantation for foot drop. *Arch Orthop Trauma Surg* 97:77–79, 1980.

38. Basmajian JV, Kukulka GG, Narayan MG, Takebe K: Biofeedback treatment of foot drop after stroke compared with standard rehabilitation technique: effects of voluntary control and strength. *Arch Phys Med Rehabil* 56:231–236, 1975.

39. Garayon A, Bourrell P, Bourges M, Touze M: Dual transfer of posterior tibial and flexor digitorum longus tendons for drop foot. *J Bone Joint Surg* 49A:144–148, 1967.

40. Tracy HW: Operative treatment of plantar-flexed inverted foot in adult hemiplegia. *J Bone Joint Surg* 58A:1142–1145, 1976.

41. Mayo Clinic. *Clinical Examinations in Neurology*, ed 4. Philadelphia, WB Saunders Co, 1976.

42. Harris RJ, Beath T: *Army Foot Surgey—An Investigation of Foot Ailments in Canadian Soliders*. Ottawa, National Research Council of Canada, 1947.

43. Basmajian JV, Steco G: The roles of muscles in arch support of the foot. *J Bone Joint Surg* 45A:1184, 1963.

44. Morton D: *The Human Foot*. New York, Columbia University Press, 1935.

45. Jones MH: Differential diagnosis and natural history of the cerebral palsied child. In Samilson RL (ed): *Orthopedic Aspects of Cerebral Palsy*. Philadelphia, JB Lippincott Co, 1975, p 5.

46. Banks H: The foot and ankle in cerebral palsy. In Samilson RL (ed): *Orthopedic Aspects of Cerebral Palsy*. Philadelphia, JB Lippincott Co, 1975, p 195.

47. Banks HH, Paragakos P: Orthopedic evaluation of the lower extremity in cerebral palsy. *Clin Orthop* 47:117, 1966.

48. Bleck EE: *Orthopedic Management of Cerebral Palsy*. Philadelphia, WB Saunders Co, 1979.

49. Goldner JL: Cerebral palsy. Part I: general principles. *AAOS Instructional Course Lectures* 20:20, 1971.

50. Phelps WM: Treatment of cerebral palsies. *Clinics* 2:981, 1943.

51. Phelps WM: Complications of the orthopedic surgery in the treatment of cerebral palsy. *J Bone Joint Surg* 41A:440, 1959.

52. Phelps WM: Complications of orthopedic surgery in the treatment of cerebral palsy. *Clin Orthop* 53:39, 1967.

53. Mullaferozi P, Vora PH: Surgery on the lower limbs in cerebral palsy. *Dev Med Child Neurol* 14:45, 1972.

54. Banks HH, Green WT: The correction of equinus deformity in cerebral palsy. *J Bone Joint Surg* 40A:1359, 1958.

55. Craig JJ, Van Vuren J: The importance of gastrocnemius recession in the correction of equinus deformity in cerebral palsy. *J Bone Joint Surg* 58B:84, 1976.

56. Silver CM, Simon SD: Gastrocnemius—muscle recession (Silfverskiold) for spastic equinus deformity in cerebral palsy. *J Bone Joint Surg* 41A:1021, 1959.

57. Strayer LM Jr: Recession of the gastrocnemius, an operation to relieve spastic contracture of the calf muscles. *J Bone Joint Surg* 32A:674, 1950.

58. Strayer LM Jr: Gastrocnemius recession—five year report of cases. *J Bone Joint Surg* 40A:1019, 1958.

59. Stoffel A: The treatment of spastic contractures. *Am J Orthop Surg* 10:611, 1913.

60. Pierrot AH, Murphy OB: Heel cord advancement. A new approach to spastic equinus deformity. *Orthop Clin North Am* 5:117, 1974.

61. Throop FB, DeRosa GP, Reeck C, Waterman S: Correction of equinus in cerebral palsy by the Murphy procedure of tendon calcaneus advancement: a preliminary communication. *Dev Med Child Neurol* 17:182, 1976.

62. Tachdjian MO: *The Child's Foot*. Philadelphia, WB Saunders Co, 1985, p 389.

63. Baker LK, Hill LM: Foot alignment in the cerebral palsy patient. *J Bone Joint Surg* 46A:1, 1964

64. Mann RA: Tendon transfer and electromyography. *Clin Orthop* 85:64–66, 1972.

65. Adams RD, Victor M: *Principles of Neurology*. New York, McGraw-Hill, 1977, p 486.

66. Tachjian M: *Pediatric Orthopedics*, vol II. Philadelphia, WB Saunders Co, 1972, p 896.

67. Tachjian M: *Pediatric Orthopedics*, vol II. Philadelphia, WB Saunders Co, 1972, p 902.

68. Allan HJ, Adams JP (eds): *Current Practice in Orthopedic Surgery.* St Louis, The CV Mosby Co, 1963.

69. Waskins MR, Frost JP, Hatalowich GS: Cerebral palsy: a podiatric overview. *J Foot Surg* 22:362–365, 1983.

70. Lindsay R, Drennan J: Management of foot and knee deformities in the mentally retarded. *Orthop Clin North Am* 12:107–112, 1981.

71. Kasser JR: Examination of the cerebral palsy patient with foot and ankle problems. *Foot Ankle* 4:135–144, 1983.

72. Young CS: An operation for the correction of hammer-toe and clawtoe. *J Bone Jt Surg* 20:715, 1938.

73. Schlefman BS, McGlamry ED, Bodamer PE: Severe pes valgus in spastic diplegia. *J Am Podiatry Assoc* 73:133–140, 1983.

74. McGlamry ED, Kitting RW: Equinus foot. *J Am Podiatry Assoc* 63:165–184, 1973.

75. Subotnick S: Digital deformities: etiology and treatment. *J Am Podiatry Assoc* 65:542–549, 1975.

76. Fenton CF III, Schlefman BS, McGlamry ED: Surgical considerations in the presence of Charcot-Marie-Tooth Disease. *J Am Podiatry Assoc* 74:490–498, 1984.

77. Schlefman BS, Fenton CF III, McGlamry ED: Peg in hole arthrodesis. *J Am Podiatry Assoc* 73:187–195, 1983.

78. Sabir M: Pathogenesis of pes cavus in Charcot-Marie-Tooth disease. *Clin Orthop* 175:173–178, 1983.

79. Waters RL, Frazier J, Garland DE, Jordan C, Perry J: Electromyographic gait analysis before and after operative treatment for hemiplegic equinus and equinovarus deformity. *J Bone Joint Surg* 64A:284–288, 1982.

80. Dwyer FC: The present status of problem of pes cavus. *Clin Orthop* 106:254–274, 1975.

81. Levitt R, Canale ST, Garltand J: The role of foot surgery in progressive neuromuscular disorders in children. *J Bone Joint Surg* 55A:1396–1409, 1973.

82. Hibbs RA: An operation for "claw-foot". *JAMA* 73:1583, 1919.

83. Sgarlatto T: Transplantation of the flexor digitorum longus muscle tendon in hammertoes. *J Am Podiatry Assoc* 60:383–388, 1970.

84. Macken O: Procedure for distal digital contracture. *J Foot Surg* 11:64–66, 1972.

85. Shapiro F, Bresnan M: Orthopedic management of childhood neuromuscular disease. *J Bone Joint Surg* 64A:949–953, 1982.

86. Chuinard E: Claw-foot deformity. *J Bone Joint Surg* 55A:357–362, 1973.

87. Knecht J: Pathomechanical deformities of the lesser toes. *J Am Podiatry Assoc* 64:941–954, 1974.

Additional References

Adams RD, Victor M: *Principles of Neurology.* New York, McGraw-Hill, 1977.

Aho C: Some considerations for total excision of the middle phalanx. *J Foot Surg* 5:137–138, 1966.

Asher M, Olson A: Factors affecting the ambulatory status of patients with spina bifida cystica. *J Bone Joint Surg* 65A:350–356, 1983.

Bannister R: *Brian's Clinical Neurology.* New York, Oxford University Press, 1973.

Barenfield P, Weseley MS, Shea JS: The congenital cavus foot. *Clin Orthop* 79:119–126, 1971.

Basmajian JV: Functional and anatomical considerations of major muscle tendon imbalance. *J Am Podiatry Assoc* 65:723–729, 1975.

Bowlus T, Dobas DC: Congenital vertical talus. *J Am Podiatry Assoc* 67:609–612, 1979.

Cahill BR, Connor DE: A long-term follow-up on proximal phalangectomy for hammertoes. *Clin Orthop* 86:191–192, 1972.

Chusid J: *Correlative Neuroanatomy and Functional Neurology,* ed 14. Los Altos, CA, Lange Medical Publications, 1970.

Crenshaw AH (ed): *Campbell's Operative Orthopedics,* ed 5, vol II. St Louis, The CV Mosby Co, 1971, p 1368.

DeKel S, Weissman SL: Osteotomy of the calcaneus with concomitant plantar stripping in children with talipes cavo-varus. *J Bone Joint Surg* 55B:802–808, 1973.

Dennyson WG, Fulfond GE: Subtalar arthrodesis by calcaneal graft and metallic internal fixation. *J Bone Joint Surg* 55B:507–510, 1976.

Duckworth T, Smith TWD: The treatment of paralytic convex pes valgus. *J Bone Joint Surg* 56B:305–313, 1974.

Dwyer FC: Osteotomy of the calcaneus for pes cavus. *J Bone Joint Surg* 41B:80–86, 1959.

Fenton CF III, Gilman RD, Jassen M, Dollar DM, Smith GA: Criteria for selected major tendon transfers in podiatric surgery. *J Am Podiatry Assoc* 73:561–568, 1983.

Fenton CF III, McGlamry ED, Perrone M: Severe pes cavus deformity secondary to Charcot-Marie Tooth disease. *J Am Podiatry Assoc* 72:171–175, 1982.

Ferciot CF: The etiology of developmental flatfoot. *Clin Orthop* 85:7–10, 1972.

Fields L: The limping child. *J Am Podiatry Assoc* 71:60–64, 1981.

Fine W: Hammer and mallet toes. *J Foot Surg* 6:154–155, 1967.

Gerber A: Corrective procedures for disorder of the foot. *J Am Osteop Assoc* 74:992–996, 1975.

Green DR: Overview of hammerdigit syndrome. Class notes presented at Pennsylvania College Podiatric Medicine, 1982.

Green N, Griffin P, Shiavi R: Split posterior tibial-tendon transfer in spastic cerebral palsy. *J Bone Joint Surg* 65A:748–754, 1983.

Hoffer M, Reiswig JA, Garrett AM, Perry J: The split anterior tibial tendon transfer in treatment of spastic varus hindfoot of childhood. *Orthop Clin North Am* 5:31–37, 1974.

Jacobs A, Oloff L, Visser HJ: Calcaneal osteotomy in management of flexible and nonflexible flatfoot deformity. *J Foot Surg* 20:57–66, 1981.

Jahss M: Tarsometatarsal truncate-wedge arthrodesis for pes cavus and equinovarus deformity of the forepart of the foot. *J Bone Joint Surg* 55A:1385–1395, 1973.

Jay R, Schoenhaus HD: Further insights in the anterior advancement of tendo achillis. *J Foot Surg* 7:73–75, 1981.

Kasser JR, MacEwen GD: Examination of the cerebral palsy patient with foot and ankle problems. *Foot Ankle* 4:135–144, 1983.

Koutsogiannis A: Treatment of mobile flat foot by displacement osteotomy of the calcaneus. *J Bone Joint Surg* 53B:96–100, 1971.

Leonard M, Gonzales S, Breck L, Bascom C, Palafox M, Kosicki Z: Lateral transfer of posterior tibial tendon in certain selected cases of pes plano valgus (Kidner operation). *Clin Orthop* 40:139–144, 1965.

Lichtblau S: A medial and lateral release operation for club foot. *J Bone Joint Surg* 55A:1377–1384, 1973.

Menks J: *Textbook of Child Neurology,* ed 2. Philadelphia, Lea & Febiger, 1975.

McGlamry ED, Ruch JA, Green DR: Simplified technique for split tibialis anterior tendon transposition (STATT procedure). *J Am Podiatry Assoc* 65:927–937, 1975.

Mitchell GP: Posterior displacement osteotomy of the calcaneus. *J Bone Joint Surg* 59B:233–235, 1977.

Neale D (ed): *Common Foot Disorders—Diagnosis and Management.* New York, Churchill-Livingstone, 1981.

Parker AW, Bronks R: Gait of children with Down syndrome. *Arch Phys Med Rehabil* 61:345–350, 1980.

Patterson RL: Various factors involved in triple arthrodesis. *Clin Orthop* 85:59–61, 1972.

Paul F: Fifth toe arthroplasty of the middle phalanx. *J Foot Surg* 12:14, 1973.

Scheck M: Etiology of acquired hammertoe deformity. *Clin Orthop* 123:63–69, 1977.

Schleffman BS, McGlamry ED, Bodamer PE: Severe pes valgus in spastic diplegia. *J Am Podiatry Assoc* 73:133–140, 1983.

Ruda R, Frost HM: Cerebral palsy. *Clin Orthop* 79:61–70, 1971.

Silver J: Repair of underlapping fifth toes by middle phalangectomy. *J Foot Surg* 7:24, 1975.

Sgarlato T, Sharpe DA: Triple arthrodesis: a new approach. *J Am Podiatry Assoc* 65:41–49, 1975.

Sharpe DA: A comprehensive look at triple fusion of tarsal bones of human foot. Master's thesis, California College of Podiatric Medicine, San Francisco, CA, 1974, p 1–22.

Sharrard WJW, Grosfield I: The management of deformity and paralysis of the foot in myelomeningocele. *J Bone Joint Surg* 50B:456, 1968.

Silver CM, Simon SD, Lichtman HM: Calcaneal osteotomy. *Clin Orthop* 99:181–187, 1974.

Sorto LA: Surgical correction of hammertoes. *J Am Podiatry Assoc* 64:930–940, 1974.

Spector E, Todd WF, Wilson F: Review of selected posterior tibial tendon transfer procedures. *J Am Podiatry Assoc* 69:325–328, 1979.

Tachjian M: *Pediatric Orthopedics*, vol II. Philadelphia, WB Saunders Co, 1974.

Tax H: *Podopediatrics*. Baltimore, Williams & Wilkins, 1980.

Tax H, Person V, Tuccio M: A podiatric presentation of diastematomyelia. *J Am Podiatry Assoc* 72:337–341, 1982.

Turco V: Surgical correction of resistant club foot. *J Bone Joint Surg* 53A:447–496, 1971.

Turner J, Cooper RR: Anterior transfer of tibialis posterior through interosseous membrane. *Clin Orthop* 83:241–244, 1972.

Vignos PJ Jr: Diagnosis of progressive muscular dystrophy. *J Bone Joint Surg* 49A:1212, 1967.

CHAPTER 13

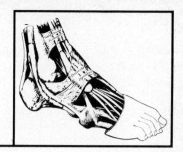

Neurological Disorders

Charles F. Fenton III, D.P.M.

Patients presenting with the signs and symptoms of neuromuscular disease require special consideration. It is not sufficient to have the surgical and technical skills to perform foot surgery. The surgeon must be thoroughly familiar with the neuromuscular disease encountered. Some procedures that may be indicated in one disease entity may be doomed to failure in another disease.

It is the surgeon's responsibility to see that a thorough history and physical examination is performed in these patients. The findings will determine the proper treatment. The prognosis of treatment is dependent on a number of factors. Among these are the particular disease entity, the age of onset, the age of the patient, the family history, the severity of the disease, and the history of previous treatment.

Following the history and physical examination the surgeon will have a knowledge of the assets and liabilities of the particular patient. The surgeon should determine if the disease is in a stage of progression or stability. If surgery is undertaken during a period of stability, better results may be obtained (1). However, if the disease is in a stage of progression more aggressive procedures may be necessary if an acceptable long-term result is to be expected. In fact patients with some neuromuscular diseases such as poliomyelitis are better off having surgery only during stages of stability.

Three guidelines should be followed when treating a patient with a neuromuscular disease. First, all fixed deformities must be reduced. Second, proper muscle and tendon balance must be obtained. Third, the goal of any surgery should be to limit the likelihood of the recurrence of the deformity. However, the surgeon's responsibility to these patients does not end following surgery. Preoperative and postoperative counseling will permit the patient and family to understand the disease process. In some cases genetic counseling may be desirable.

Following examination the surgeon will have objective information concerning the patient. The patient's disease can then be classified as either a my-opathy such as muscular dystrophy or a neurogenic disorder such as cerebral palsy or poliomyelitis. Neurogenic disorders can further be classified as upper motor neuron diseases (e.g. cerebral palsy) or lower motor neuron diseases (e.g. poliomyelitis).

In lower motor neuron syndromes the neurological deficit lies at or below the level of the anterior horn cells of the spinal cord. Whereas in upper motor neuron lesions the deficit will lie above this level. Differentiation is important because each condition will give rise to a different set of signs and symptoms. In lower motor neuron diseases muscle weakness and wasting will be seen along with areflexia and flaccid paralysis. In upper motor neuron lesions muscle rigidity, spastic paralysis, and hyperreflexia will be present. A positive Babinski reflex and ankle clonus will be present in upper motor neuron lesions and reflexes will be absent in lower motor neuron lesions.

EVALUATION

Before examination the physician must obtain a complete history. Obtaining a history in a neuromuscular disease is no different than in any other disease. Many neuromuscular diseases present in childhood and therefore the physician must rely on the parents' observation of the child's development. A child's history must include data concerning the prenatal period. Information as to whether the pregnancy was carried to term or any history of complications such as rubella must be documented. A history of any delay in developmental skills should likewise be documented.

In general the symptom of neuromuscular disease will be weakness. Such weakness may be manifested as a gait disturbance such as waddling, tripping, or clumsiness. A history of the disease process should be noted. Most neuromuscular diseases have an insidious onset, but a disease such as Guillain-Barré syndrome will have a rapid onset (2). The age of onset is also important. A disease such as Duchenne's muscular dystrophy will have an onset in childhood, usually age three to five (3), whereas Charcot-Marie-Tooth disease may first present in childhood, adolescence, or early adulthood. The age of onset in Charcot-Marie-Tooth disease will provide a prognosis as to the expected severity of the disease. Some neuromuscular diseases such as poliomyelitis may present following a febrile illness. Then there are diseases such as Refsum's syndrome that will have a history of remissions and relapses.

An attempt should be made to determine the history of prior treatment or prior surgery. Old medical records or roentgenograms should be examined if available. The success or failure of prior surgery is important. In illnesses such as cerebral palsy an equinus deformity may recur following a tendo achillis lengthening.

The family history should be ascertained. In diseases such as poliomyelitis there will usually be no other family members affected. However, in diseases such as Charcot-Marie-Tooth disease or Friederich's ataxia a positive family history is usually present. Once a diagnosis is established other family members should be examined. Such examination may reveal other family members who are only slightly affected or who have only minor signs such as cavus foot deformity.

EXAMINATION

The examination of any patient with a neurological disease must be thorough in nature. In most cases the disease will be progressive. This progression will manifest as increased weakness and muscle imbalance. With increasing muscular imbalance the static and dynamic position of the foot will be in a state of flux. The initial careful clinical and radiographic examination and documentation will be subsequently used as a baseline on which to measure the progression of the disease.

Evaluation of the patient with a neuromuscular disease will more often than not demonstrate a pes cavus deformity. However, merely documenting that pes cavus is present is not enough; the examiner must note the nature of the cavus deformity. Is the cavus mild or severe? Is the condition rigid, semirigid, or flexible? Is the cavus condition caused by a rearfoot condition such as calcaneal varus, or a forefoot condition such as a plantarflexed first ray? Are clawtoes or dropfoot deformities also present? The examiner must carefully evaluate the foot biomechanically both weight bearing and non-weight-bearing and note any difference.

Gait examination is invaluable in these patients to evaluate the dynamic deficits present. During the gait examination of a patient with neurological disease it is less important to evaluate the pronatory capabilities of the subtalar and midtarsal joints as it is to evaluate the patient as a whole.

A patient with Charcot-Marie-Tooth disease will present with a high steppage gait. Because of weakness of m. tibialis anterior the patient is unable to dorsiflex the foot to clear the ground. Therefore the patient will flex the pelvis in an attempt to shorten the limb. The patient will actually appear to be stepping over tiny invisible fences. The patient raises the knees high in the air to avoid dragging the foot on the ground. A patient with Friederich's ataxia will demonstrate similar gait patterns and will be very unstable on standing. The patient may actually have to hold onto the wall for stability while walking.

A cerebral vascular accident patient may show a broadly based gait. This is done in an attempt to gain added stability. If the cerebral vascular accident was severe and muscle weakness was advanced the patient may drag the forefoot of the affected side when walking.

A poliomyelitic patient will often demonstrate a short limb syndrome. Weakness of the affected knee will manifest as hyperextension or genu recurvatum in gait. A dropfoot condition may or may not be present. Circumduction of the limb will help the affected side to clear the ground.

A patient with Parkinson's disease will demonstrate a shuffling gait. There is a typical "pill rolling" motion of the hands. Additionally there is difficulty in starting and stopping gait.

Patients suffering from cerebral palsy will demonstrate a scissors gait or severe knock-knee gait because of spasticity of the adductor group. This spasticity causes adduction and internal rotation of the hips, which causes the knees to be in a position of internal rotation. These patients often demonstrate gross instability and lack of coordination in gait. There will be a wide base of gait and the arms and hands will swing wide to create balance (Fig. 13.1).

Patients suffering from muscular dystrophy will demonstrate a Trendelenburg gait. Because of weakness of m. gluteus medius the torso will shift over the contralateral side during the swing phase of gait. This minimizes the falling of the pelvis on the ipsilateral side.

Muscle examination and evaluation is the cornerstone in evaluating patients with neuromuscular disease. A complete muscle inventory is required before any tendon transfer procedure.

Each individual muscle should be inspected and palpated. Note should be made of the consistency (firm or flabby), enlargement or atrophy, and presence of tenderness or spasticity. The deep tendon reflexes should then be evaluated. The strength of each muscle should be evaluated on a scale of 0 to 5 as follows:

Grade 0: No contraction
Grade 1: Trace contraction
Grade 2: Motion with gravity eliminated
Grade 3: Motion against gravity
Grade 4: Motion against mild resistance
Grade 5: Normal strength

Each muscle in the leg and foot should be evaluated separately and documented as such. Evaluation of each limb should be performed separately because there may be more weakness of one limb. For example, a patient with Charcot-Marie-Tooth disease may have

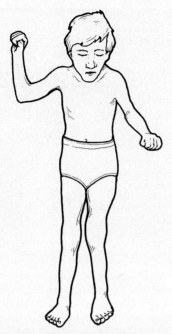

Figure 13.1. Patient with cerebral palsy will demonstrate incoordination during gait. Arms swing wide to help with balance. Additionally, adductor spasticity will result in scissors gait.

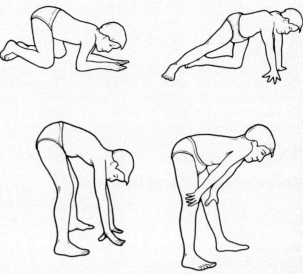

Figure 13.2. Gower's sign is typical of patient suffering from Duchenne's muscular dystrophy. Patient is unable to rise normally from floor. Patient must first rise up onto hands and knees and next rise to feet. Finally patient uses hands to climb up legs until body is upright.

a weak m. peroneus longus on one side and a weak m. tibialis posterior on the other. Therefore each leg will require a different tendon transfer for treatment. The muscle inventory will provide a baseline by which to assess the progress of the disease and will also be used as a guide when planning tendon transfer surgery. The muscle inventory is a record of the assets and liabilities of the patient.

Several special examinations may shed light on the neuromuscular disease. The Romberg test and the test for rapid alternating movement will be abnormal in patients with cerebellar diseases such as Friedreich's ataxia. Such patients will be unable to heel or toe walk, to tandem walk, or to touch their fingers to their nose. Abnormalities seen in patients with cerebellar disease are similar to those seen in patients suffering from acute alcoholic intoxication.

Patients with muscular dystrophy will have difficulty climbing stairs. The classical sign of Duchenne's muscular dystrophy is Gowers' sign, which is also called tripoding. The patient is unable to arise normally from a seated position on the floor. The patient first rises up to the hands and knees, then the hands are used to climb up the leg until the patient is finally standing (Fig. 13.2).

The serum creatinine phosphokinase (CPK) assay is the most sensitive laboratory test in patients with neuromuscular disease. The CPK acts as an enzyme to break down phosphocreatinine into phosphoric acid and creatinine. It also serves to transform adenosine diphosphate (ADP) into adenosine triphosphate (4). This enzyme is found in high concentrations in the sarcolemma of striated muscle. Damage to the sarcolemmal membrane will cause leakage of the en-

zyme into the bloodstream. Even the damage caused by an electromyographical needle will cause a rise in the CPK (2, 5).

Increased CPK levels are noted in conditions other than neuromuscular diseases. These include trauma, acute myocardial infarction, acute alcoholic intoxication, and extensive exercise or exertion. Marked elevation (levels greater than 10 times normal) is indicative of a myopathic disorder such as myositis, myasthenia gravis, spinal muscular atrophy, dermatomyositis, and limb-girdle muscular dystrophy. In early Duchenne's muscular dystrophy the CPK may be 200 to 300 times normal (5). Neuromuscular disorders of neurogenic origin such as Charcot-Marie-Tooth disease may show little if any elevation of the CPK.

In a neuromuscular disease it is usually prudent to request a neurological consultation before surgery. Following such a consultation an electromyogram, nerve conduction study, or muscle biopsy may be requested.

HEREDITARY PERIPHERAL NEUROPATHIES

The hereditary peripheral neuropathies encompass a group of disorders that are clinically similar. However, they all differ in certain respects. The category includes Charcot-Marie-Tooth disease, Dejerine-Sottas disease, Roussy-Lévy disease, Refsum's disease, and Friedreich's ataxia. The student and uninformed clinician may ask what is the difference in these diseases. The answer eludes even the researchers. There is debate as to whether these syndromes represent different disease entities or represent "forme frustes" or abortive cases of each other. In fact, in any particular family, hereditary conditions could vary and therefore may not accord with classical descriptions of these diseases. Such cases could give rise to a seemingly "new" disease entity.

There is no known treatment for these diseases. Foot surgery will allow the patient to continue a somewhat normal ambulatory function in life. In stable cases surgery may be of permanent value. In progressive cases surgery will not arrest the disease process but will provide the patient with a longer period of near normal mobility.

Charcot-Marie-Tooth Disease*

Charcot-Marie-Tooth disease or progressive peroneal atrophy was described simultaneously by Tooth (6) in England and Charcot and Marie (7) in France. The disease involves peripheral distal muscular atrophy that begins in the feet and legs and later involves the hands and distal aspects of the arms. Foot involvement is commonly manifested as a pes cavus deformity.

The incidence of this disease has not been established (8, 9). The disease affects males five times more frequently than females (9). All races are affected except blacks (10).

Allan (11) has described three patterns of inheritance. These are dominant, sex-linked recessive, and simple recessive. The dominant form is usually the mildest in severity and manifests itself around the age of 30. The sex-linked recessive form is more disabling and affects teenaged males. In the simple recessive form manifestation before the age of eight is common with rapid progression of symptoms such that the victim soon becomes incapacitated. Allan's theory allows one to extrapolate valuable clinical information. The pattern of inheritance determines the age of onset and the degree of severity of the disease, which gives one insight into the prognosis of the disease.

Examination of these patients will reveal weakness and wasting of the lower extremities and often of the upper extremities. Classically the peroneals, tibialis anterior, long extensors, gastrocnemius, and intrinsic muscles are involved (10). In actuality Fenton and associates (12) have shown that m. peroneus longus is normal in 59% of the cases of Charcot-Marie-Tooth disease (Fig. 13.3). The wasting of the muscles leads to atrophy of the lower legs, which results in plump thighs and slender calves. This has been referred to as an "ostrich," "stork leg," or "inverted champagne bottle" appearance (Fig. 13.4). The musculature of the face and trunk is usually spared.

This atrophy usually leads to a pes cavus deformity. The cavus deformity may be either rigid or flexible depending on the degree of muscular atrophy. The strength of m. peroneus longus may determine if the foot is rigid or flexible. With normal strength there will be rigid plantarflexion of the first ray. In advanced

*Taken in part from Fenton C, Schlefman B, McGlamry ED: Surgical considerations in Charcot-Marie-Tooth Disease. *J Am Podiatry Assoc* 74:490–498, 1984. by permission)

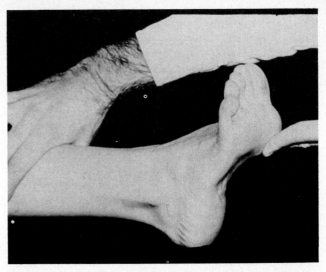

Figure 13.3. Proper method of testing strength of m. peroneus longus involves measuring strength of plantarflexion of first ray. Assessing strength of m. peroneus longus by testing eversion power of foot is erroneous and will often result in false weakness of m. peroneus longus. Improper manual muscle testing of m. peroneus longus has led to the myth that the muscle is weak in all cases of Charcot-Marie-Tooth disease.

weakness m. peroneus longus will be weak and a flexible deformity may ensue.

Hand deformity, which indicates severe progression of the disease, is as impressive as the foot deformity. There is often wasting of the thenar muscle mass. As such, opposition of the thumb is lost and the hand assumes a "monkey fist" appearance (8) (Fig. 13.5).

Gait examination will reveal a steppage-type gait. As atrophy of the anterior muscles progresses a dropfoot deformity will develop (Fig. 13.6). In later stages the weakness of the legs will lead to an inability to heel or toe walk. In extremely severe cases the patient may require a wheelchair.

Neurological examination may include nerve conduction studies, electromyographical (EMG) studies, or muscle biopsy. The conduction velocities of the peripheral nerves will be markedly slower than normal. The EMG will show abnormal activity and the muscle biopsy will show muscular atrophy (13). The achilles reflex is often lost and the patellar reflex may or may not be absent. Sensory examination will reveal decreased vibratory and position sensation. This is often in a glove and stocking distribution. Pain sensation may likewise be diminished. Therefore the use of narcotic analgesics may be reduced postoperatively.

Because of the various progressions and degrees of deformity associated with this neuromuscular disease many surgical procedures have been used in the past. Miller (14) in 1924 first recommended subtalar arthrodesis for the treatment of foot deformities associated with Charcot-Marie-Tooth disease. Later Jacobs and Carr (10) in 1950 recommended triple arthrodesis along with appropriate soft tissue procedures and tendon transfers. They noted an increased varus deformity in patients in whom the force of the tendon

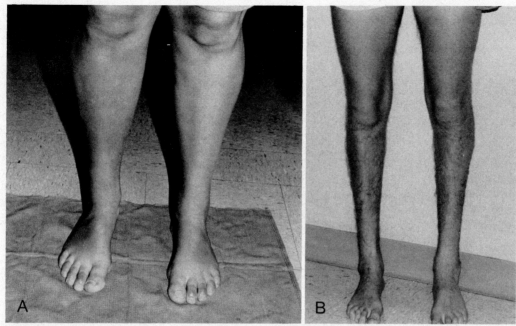

Figure 13.4. (A) Classical "inverted champagne bottle" appearance of legs in young female with Charcot-Marie-Tooth disease. Note plumpness of proximal calf and atrophy of distal lateral calf. (B) Brother of young female in A. The disease in this teenaged male was more advanced. Therefore there was more extensive wasting of calf muscles (From Fenton CF, Schlefman BS, McGlamry ED: Surgical considerations in the presence of Charcot-Marie-Tooth disease. *J Am Podiatry Assoc* 74:490–498, 1984, by permission.)

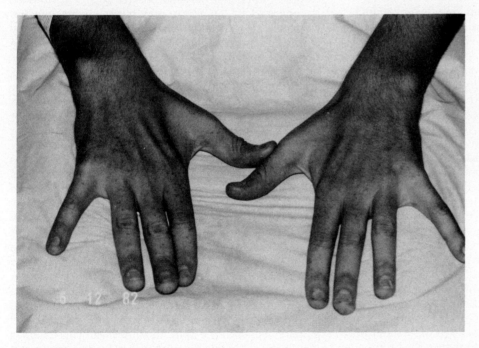

Figure 13.5. Hand deformity in Charcot-Marie-Tooth disease is as impressive as foot deformity. Because atrophy of thenar eminence hand assumes appearance of "monkey fist." Shaking hands with this patient is like "shaking hands with a skeleton." (From Fenton CF, Schlefman BS, McGlamry ED: Surgical considerations in the presence of Charcot-Marie-Tooth disease. *J Am Podiatry Assoc* 74:490–498, 1984, by permission.)

of m. tibialis posterior was not removed, either by sectioning or by transposition. Because the ankle joint is usually weak laterally the intact tendon of m. tibialis posterior can pull the ankle into a position of ankle varus even though the subtalar joint is fused.

Karlholm and Nilsonne (15) in 1968 desired to avoid osseous procedures and recommended soft tissue procedures consisting of plantar fasciotomy, tendo achillis lengthening, and tibialis posterior transfer to the dorsum of the foot via a subcutaneous tunnel anterior to the ankle. They concluded that posterior tibial tendon transfer was the most important step in the correction of the deformity. Levitt and associates (16) concurred with Jacobs and Carr and recommended triple arthrodesis as the procedure of choice in this disease. They further noted that soft tissue procedures performed on patients undergoing surgery before skeletal maturity allowed the patients more time before the necessity of triple arthrodesis.

Cavuoto (17) reported excellent to good results following peroneus longus tendon transfer to the dorsum of the foot. Gould (18) in 1984 recommended a

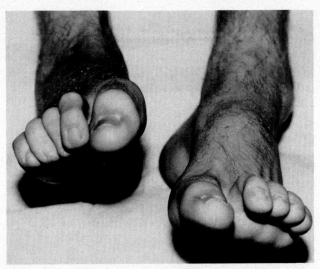

Figure 13.6. Dropfoot deformity is demonstrated on left foot. Patient seated on bed is attempting to dorsiflex foot. Right foot is able to dorsiflex only to right angle despite previous posterior tibial tendon transfer. Left foot is unable to dorsiflex at all. Note clawing of digits as long extensor tendons attempt to assist dorsiflexion of foot.

protocol to avoid triple arthrodesis as follows: double plantar fasciotomies, dorsal closing wedge proximal greenstick osteotomies of all of the metatarsals, the Jones procedure, tenotomy of the long flexor tendons to the lesser digits, and occasionally Dwyer's calcaneal osteotomy. Although he reported good results in 10 patients, several fallacies are apparent with this approach. First, Charcot-Marie-Tooth disease is a progressive disease and therefore patients with severe or progressive disease will require the stability that only a triple arthrodesis can afford. Second, it is technically difficult if not impossible to perform five metatarsal dorsiflexion osteotomies and have them all heal on the same transverse plane. Third, in Charcot-Marie-Tooth disease the long extensors become weak very early in the disease and therefore a Jones transfer will be ineffective. The Jones transfer is an unnecessary step and accomplishes nothing that the dorsiflexion osteotomy did not already accomplish. Fourth, tenotomy of the long flexor tendon will not provide long-term correction of clawtoe deformity. In fact preservation of long flexor function via peg-in-hole arthrodesis or flexor tendon transfer will combat the extensor substitution phenomenon that often contributes to clawtoe deformity (19, 20). Finally, a great omission in Gould's protocol is that there is no recommendation for a tendon transfer procedure to reduce the dropfoot deformity that is so common in these patients. Even Jahss (21) rebukes this study and recommends triple arthrodesis for long-term stability.

Fenton and associates (12) in 1984 published an exhaustive study on the surgical considerations in Charcot-Marie-Tooth disease. No strict criteria can be established because of the various presentations of patients with this disease. Surgery must therefore be individualized. Fenton and associates advocate an aggressive surgical approach consisting of three steps.

First, an osseous rearfoot procedure will be required to reduce the rearfoot varus and provide long-term stability. In mild cases Dwyer's calcaneal osteotomy may be adequate. However, additional procedures such as a Steindler stripping or a dorsiflexion first metatarsal osteotomy may be necessary. In moderate cases that appear progressive or in severe cases a triple arthrodesis will provide the best long-term stability. Second, a tendon transfer will be necessary to reduce the dropfoot deformity. A split tibialis posterior tendon transfer routed through the interosseous membrane is preferable. However, a split peroneus longus tendon transfer may be adequate in mild cases and a combination of both may be necessary in severe cases. The Jones, Hibbs, or split tibialis anterior tendon transfers are not adequate because of the weakness of m. extensor hallucis longus, m. extensor digitorum longus, and m. tibialis anterior. Finally, most cases will require digital stabilization to reduce the clawtoe deformity. Fenton and associates' approach is very aggressive but is required for an adequate long-term result (Fig. 13.7).

Dejerine-Sottas Disease

Dejerine-Sottas disease is also known as hypertrophic interstitial polyneuropathy (22). This disease is inherited by an autosomal recessive mechanism. Clinically there is distal muscular weakness especially of the lower extremity. This will manifest with pes cavus and dropfoot deformities. Loss of tendon reflexes, distal sensory disturbances, and kyphoscoliosis are often present. This disease first appears in later childhood or early adult life and is progressive in nature. This condition appears clinically similar to Charcot-Marie-Tooth disease; however, at present it remains a distinct clinical entity.

The distinctive clinical feature of Dejerine-Sottas disease is enlargment of the peripheral nerves. This most frequently affects the internal cutaneous nerve of the forearm, the ulnar nerve, the saphenous nerve, the peroneal nerve, and the superficial cervical nerve (23). The enlargement of these nerves is the result of an increase in volume of the interstitial connective tissue elements of the nerves. Classically there is "onion bulb" formation manifested as concentric proliferation of Schwann's cells around a central core with segmental demyelination of Schwann's cells (24). This hypertrophy causes the nerves to be firm and palpable beneath the skin. In some cases these nerves may even be visible beneath the skin. Diagnosis can be obtained by biopsy of the sural nerve.

Roussy-Lévy Syndrome

Roussy-Lévy syndrome is a dominantly inherited peripheral neuropathy similar to Charcot-Marie-Tooth disease (25). Clinically the patient will present with clumsy gait, abnormal equilibrium, absent tendon reflexes, acquired cavus deformity, and atrophy of the hand, foot, and leg. Additionally there is a superim-

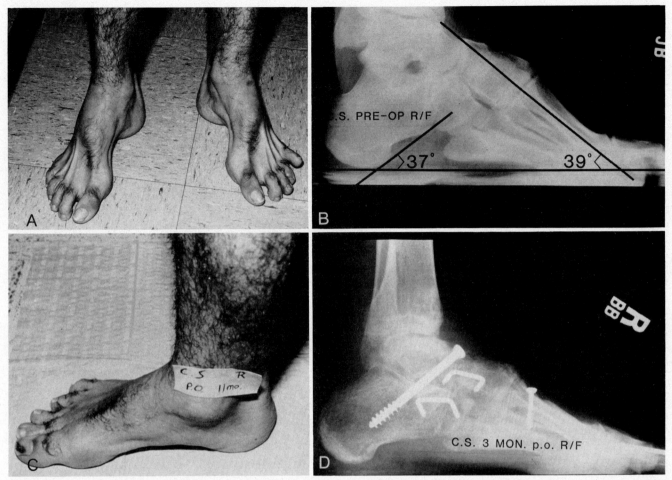

Figure 13.7. (A) Preoperative clinical appearance of severe pes cavus deformity in patient with Charcot-Marie-Tooth disease. Note high arch, plantarflexed first ray, inversion of rearfoot, clawing of digits, bowstringing of extensor tendons, and taut plantar fascia. (From Fenton CF, McGlamry ED, Perrone M: Severe pes cavus deformity in a patient with Charcot-Marie-Tooth disease—a case report. *J Am Podiatry Assoc* 72:171–175, 1982, by permission.) (B) Preoperative radiographs demonstrate pes cavus deformity. Note high calcaneal inclination angle, high first metatarsal declination angle, and prominent sinus tarsi. Rearfoot supination is so severe that anterior trochlear surface of talus is demonstrated on this lateral radiograph. (C) Clinical appearance of foot 11 months following surgery demonstrating reduction of multiple foot deformities and stabilization of foot. (D) Postoperative radiographs three months following surgery. Procedures involved triple arthrodesis, dorsiflexion osteotomy of first metatarsal, arthrodesis of hallux interphalangeal joint, peg-in-hole arthrodesis of second, third, and fourth digits, arthroplasty of fifth digit, and split posterior tibial tendon transfer to dorsum of foot. (From Fenton CF, McGlamry ED, Perrone M: Severe pes cavus deformity in a patient with Charcot-Marie-Tooth disease. *J Am Podiatry Assoc* 72:171–175, 1982, by permission.)

posed essential tremor. The tremor occurs while tensing the hand muscles and is absent while at rest (26).

Roussy-Lévy syndrome is a slowly progressive disease with limited disability. It has been referred to as a "forme fruste" of Charcot-Marie-Tooth disease (26, 27). It presents similar to Charcot-Marie-Tooth disease but with a superimposed essential tremor.

Refsum's Disease

Refsum's disease was first described as "heredopathia atactia polyneuritiformis" by Refsum (28) in 1946. The patient will present with progressive paresis of the distal aspects of the extremities, dropfoot, pes cavus, decreased knee and ankle reflexes, cerebral ataxia, nerve deafness, ichthyosis, and night blindness. In fact the night blindness is often the first symptom of the disease. This disease is autosomal recessive. There have been no cases reported where the parents of the offspring were affected with the disease (29). Males and females are affected equally.

The disease first appears following a febrile illness. The course of the disease is highly unpredictable. There will be acute exacerbations followed by periods of stability. The acute exacerbations often follow stresses such as a viral infection or pregnancy (30).

Refsum's disease is more appropriately classified as a lipoidosis, similar to Gaucher's disease. The primary etiology of the disease is a disturbance in lipid metabolism. In particular phytanic acid accumulates in all of the tissues at least 50 times the normal levels. The diet is the sole source of phytanic acid because there is little or no endogenous production of this fatty acid. There is a genetic defect in the capacity to oxidize phytanic acid. It therefore accumulates in the tissues and this accumulation results in a neurological deficit.

The diagnosis of Refsum's disease is by the presence of phytanic acid in the serum at least 50 times normal (29). Preliminary studies indicate reducing from the diet foodstuffs that contain phytol or phytanic acid. This will reduce subjective and objective symptoms of the disease.

Friedreich's Ataxia

Patients with Friedreich's ataxia will usually present with a pes cavus deformity similar to that seen in Charcot-Marie-Tooth patients (31). However, Friedreich's ataxia is a more severe and disabling disease. It will begin in childhood or adolescence. Progression is slow yet steady, such that by the age of 30 most victims are incapacitated.

The disease is equally common in both sexes. The etiology of the disease is degeneration of the posterior and caudal regions of the spinal cord of unknown cause (32). The condition is commonly inherited by a recessive mechanism. Yet dominant and partially sex-linked transmission have also been reported (32).

The patient's main symptoms will often be ataxia and instability of the lower extremities. On examination there will be a pes cavus deformity with a dropfoot often present. Spinal deformities such as scoliosis and kyphoscoliosis are common. Weakness of the lower extremity, especially those muscles supplied by the peroneal nerve, will be seen. Later weakness of those muscles of the hand supplied by the ulnar nerve will occur. Decreased sensation, especially proprioception, vibratory, and pain sensations will occur in a glove and stocking distribution. Gait examination will reveal a lurching or Trendelenburg gait because of weakness of m. gluteus medius.

Friedreich's ataxia is more severe than the other peripheral neuropathies. This is because of the degree of cerebellar involvement. Such cerebellar involvement will produce incoordination, nystagmus, speech disorders, absence of reflexes, and positive Babinski response (32).

CEREBRAL VASCULAR ACCIDENTS

Although cerebral vascular accidents occur most frequently in older persons they can occur in any age group (Fig 13.8). In the older population strokes will account for most of the damage to the brain. In younger people head trauma from car accidents or gunshot wounds can produce cerebral trauma. A female of childbearing age is at risk of a cerebral vascular accident if she smokes and takes birth control pills. Therefore one may see the side effects of cerebral vascular disease in any age group.

A cerebral vascular accident patient's presenting signs and symptoms will vary. This is because of the variable sites and degree of damage that can occur. Although the sites of damage may vary the condition of the illness is static and nonprogressive. Therefore surgical repair is likely to be of more permanent value

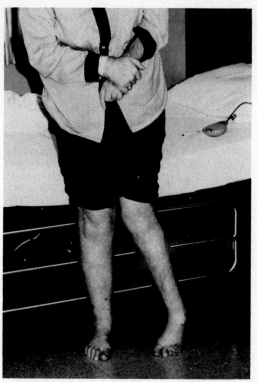

Figure 13.8. Hemiplegia secondary to cerebral vascular accident. Paralysis of left arm and leg is apparent. Equinovarus deformity is present in foot secondary to dynamic muscular imbalance.

than in patients suffering from a progressive illness such as Charcot-Marie-Tooth disease.

Eventually spastic contractures will develop because of the unbalanced position of the joints. Spastic contracture of an agonist with inhibition of the tone of the antagonist will result in joint contractures (33). For example, if the triceps become spastic and the extensors are weak then an equinus deformity will ensue. Such contractures may manifest themselves as conditions such as equinovarus deformity, clawtoe deformity, spastic equinus deformity, and dropfoot deformity.

The goal of treatment is to stabilize a poorly controlled joint. Conservative care will take the form of bracing and physical therapy. Bracing may be as involved as a double upright dropfoot brace or as simple as a cotton roll toe crest device. Some patients find braces too cumbersome. Surgery should aim to allow the patient to be free from bracing and to ambulate as well as possible. In cases where there is a poorly controlled joint because of spastic contracture arthrodesis is preferred over arthroplasty procedures. Arthrodesis will stabilize the joint in the position that is functionally optimal and will prevent recurrence of the deformity.

Many patients who have had a cerebral vascular accident are on anticoagulant therapy to prevent a recurrence of the cerebral vascular accident. A carefully performed history will reveal this fact. When performing surgery on a patient receiving blood thinners a close liaison between the surgeon and the internist is advisable. Interruption of therapy before surgery places the patient at risk of developing a thromboembolism, whereas not interrupting therapy poses the risk that the patient may hemorrhage profusely during surgery. If surgery is undertaken while the patient is taking anticoagulants, then the prothrombin time should be adjusted to 1½ to 2½ times the control level (34). During surgery absorbable hemostatic agents, ligatures, and pressure dressings will reduce bleeding. Finally, the physician must be aware of the unfavorable reaction these drugs have with concurrent medications. In particular the surgeon must avoid prescribing the oral nonsteroidal anti-inflammatory agents postoperatively because of their potentiation of the anticoagulants.

MUSCULAR DYSTROPHY

The muscular dystrophies cover a group of disorders in which the muscle tissue dies off or becomes dystrophic. These diseases are classified as myopathies (i.e. as a primary disease of the muscle fibers). Clinically there will be weakness, atrophy, loss of reflexes, secondary contractures, deformities, and mental impairment. Because the muscle weakness is not uniform, contractures and deformity develop.

The three common types of muscular dystrophy are Duchenne's pseudohypertrophic, faciscapulohumeral, and limb-girdle dystrophy. Duchenne's muscular dystrophy is the most common. This is referred to as pseudohypertrophic because fat is deposited within the interstitial spaces of the muscle. This causes them to be unusually large and firm, even though they are actually weak. Duchenne's muscular dystrophy affects only male children because it is sex-linked. The onset is between age one and three with rapid progression thereafter until the patient is wheelchair-bound.

Because there is no definitive treatment for the muscular dystrophies care is directed toward management of secondary problems. The goal of treatment is to maintain the patient in an ambulatory status for as long as is possible (35). Surgery should be tailored towards releasing contractures and reducing deformities to serve this purpose. Surgery should be undertaken before the patient is wheelchair-bound. However, surgery may be necessary on occasion even in patients confined to a wheelchair. Surgery may be needed to relieve pain or to reduce a deformity that inhibits the use of adequate footgear.

Ankle equinus and equinovarus deformity are common foot conditions seen in patients with muscular dystrophy. Physical therapy, surgery, and bracing are advocated for treatment. Physical therapy should be employed continuously. Such therapy should include stretching to reduce contractures and water exercises to build strength and confidence. Patients with muscular dystrophy are able to exercise in water much easier than on hard surfaces. Additionally, actual swimming helps to exercise the muscles of respiration (36).

Common surgical procedures performed for patients with muscular dystrophy include sectioning of a tight iliotibial band. A tibialis anterior tendon transfer may be necessary to reduce an equinovarus deformity. Tendo achillis lengthening or tenotomy may be necessary to reduce ankle equinus. A tibialis posterior tendon transfer may be combined with a tendo achillis lengthening to prevent redevelopment of equinus contracture. Following surgery bracing can be used to maintain position and prevent recurrent contracture. A night splint will maintain the foot at 90° to the leg to delay contracture of the triceps muscle group (35). Surgery has been shown to prolong ambulation one to three years (37).

Any period of inactivity results in a rapid progression of muscle weakness (38). Therefore cast immobilization must be kept to a minimum and physical therapy must be ongoing.

MYELODYSPLASIA

Myelodysplasia refers to a group of developmental deformities of the spinal cord. Most often the lumbar and sacral areas are involved. Included in this category is spina bifida with meningocele, myelomeningocele, myelocele, and spina bifida occulta. The developmental deformity involves failure of the neural arch to close during development. Subsequently the neural elements protrude through the defect. This results in motor and sensory deficits with resultant foot deformity.

Meningocele refers to the condition where a meningeal sac containing the dura and arachnoid tissues protrudes through the defect and a visible sac develops beneath the skin (Fig. 13.9). Myelomeningocele refers to the condition where additionally elements of the spinal cord and nerve roots have protruded through the defect and are contained within the sac. Myelocele, the most severe form of spina bifida, occurs when the skin has failed to close over the neural elements. The neural elements are completely exposed and menengitis often results. These three forms of spina bifida result in varying degrees of neurological deficit of the lower extremity.

On the other hand, spina bifida occulta refers to the condition whereby the neural arch has not closed, yet all of the neural elements remain in the spinal canal. Spina bifida occulta results in mild if any neurological deficit. This form of spina bifida may be revealed as a secondary finding on spinal radiographic

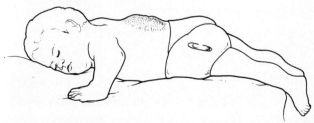

Figure 13.9. Classical "sac" located over lumbrosacral region in infant with meningocele.

examination or may be suggested by a dimple or hair growth over the lumbosacral region (Fig. 13.10).

In 1918 Frazier (39) reported that the mortality rate was 90% for patients afflicted with myelodysplasia. Because of surgical techniques to repair the neural arch and to control the accompanying hydrocephalus the survival rate today is much greater (40). Therefore more patients with spina bifida are able to lead prolonged lives and will therefore develop problems with their lower extremities.

Because this disease affects the lumbosacral region of the spinal cord, the upper extremities and torso are spared. Lower extremity involvement is often manifested by foot deformity. The foot deformity may be mild or severe. The degree of deformity will be dependent on two factors. First, the level of the defect will determine the extent of involvement. The higher the defect the more involvement of the lower extremity. Second, the type of condition will determine the severity of the disease. Myelomeningocele will present more severely than spina bifida occulta.

Spina bifida results in a dynamic imbalance of the muscles of the lower extremities. Therefore the deformities get gradually worse as the disease progresses. Commonly a pes cavus deformity will develop (Fig. 13.11). However, equinus, equinovarus, and valgus deformities are common (41).

Two factors are of importance when performing surgery on these patients. First, most spina bifida patients suffer with paralysis of the bladder. Therefore they should be catheterized during surgery. Following surgery the physician must be on the alert for bladder infection. Second, there is often insensitivity to pain. Such insensitivity leads to trophic ulceration on the plantar aspect of the foot. In a pes cavus deformity trophic ulceration may occur under the first or fifth metatarsophalangeal joint (42). Such ulceration may easily lead to osteomyelitis if left untreated. Also, because of the insensitive nature of the foot, fractures occur secondary to undue stress on the foot. Such fractures occur without pain and may not be noticed by the patient except as prolonged swelling of the foot.

The goal of treatment is to produce a plantigrade foot that can be placed in a shoe and also one must aim to prevent redeformity (41). There must not be any undue pressure on any area of the foot that might cause future ulceration. Serial splinting and casting of young children should be avoided (41). Such casting has the potential of causing undue pressure on the foot and leg, which may, because of insensitivity to pain, produce ulceration with resultant infection. In young children soft tissue procedures consisting of tenotomies, tendon lengthenings, and tendon transfers are indicated. In older children additional osseous procedures such as metatarsal and calcaneal osteotomies and stabilization procedures such as the Grice extra-articular arthrodesis may be necessary. In severe cases definitive stabilization via triple arthrodesis will have to be deferred until after osseous maturation. Following surgical repair, care must be taken when applying casts because the possibility of ulceration is always present in these patients.

Sharrard and Grosfield (41) have reported that repair of the spinal defect and hydrocephalus should proceed as soon as possible after birth. They believe that soft tissue procedures on the foot and lower extremity are most beneficial when performed between the agees of one and two. The main drawback in performing surgery on young children is the difficulty in assessing the exact sensory and motor defects.

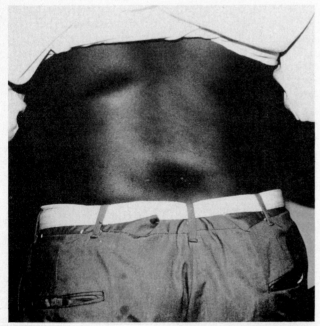

Figure 13.10. Classical "dimple" overlying lumbrosacral region suggestive of spina bifida occulta.

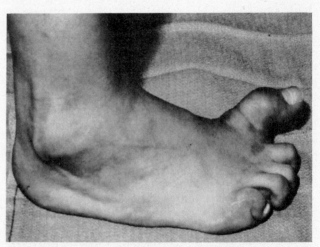

Figure 13.11. Pes cavus deformity in patient with spina bifida. This teenager had developed mal perforans beneath first metatarsal head. Subsequent destruction of intersesamoidal ligament resulted in dislocation of first metatarsophalangeal joint, as demonstrated here. (From Schlefman BS, McGlamry ED, Hilkeman RJ: First metatarsophalangeal joint dislocation in spina bifida: a case report. J Am Podiatry Assoc 74:147–152, 1984, by permission.)

POLIOMYELITIS

Poliomyelitis is a disease that is seen only sporadically today. The use of vaccines has all but eliminated acute cases of the disease. However, there remain over 300,000 people in the United States who are suffering from the sequellae of poliomyelitis that was contracted before the development of the vaccines. Therefore the practitioner must still understand the disease and be able to treat the resultant deformities.

Poliomyelitis is a viral infection of the anterior horn cells of the spinal cord. The virus enters via the nasopharangeal orifices and a febrile illness develops. The virus settles in the anterior horn cells of the spinal cord and subsequently destroys the cell. This results in paralysis of the innervated muscle. Most muscles are innervated by columns of anterior horn cells. Therefore, depending on the extent of viral infection, only a portion of muscle power may be lost. Those muscles such as m. tibialis anterior, which is innervated by a short column of anterior horn cells, are more vulnerable to complete paralysis (43). As a result paralysis will be spotty and asymmetrical.

The acute stage will last several days to a week and is characterized by fever, malaise, myositis, and paralysis. During the acute phase the muscles will be tender and painful. The patient will therefore contract and shorten the muscle to relieve the pain. If the muscle is left in that position for long then permanent contracture and resultant deformity will develop (44).

During the following days a variable degree of muscle strength will return. Muscles that remain completely paralysed after four weeks have little likelihood of recovery (45). During the subacute or convalescent stage, which lasts up to two years, improvement can be anticipated. During this stage aggressive physical therapy and bracing should be instituted. Surgery should be avoided except to correct gross deformities.

During the chronic stage most patients have made as much improvement as they are likely to make. Most patients seen today will have already reached this phase of the disease. This is a period of stability and surgical procedures will yield the best results in this stage. Operations during this phase should reduce fixed deformities and restore function to the limb, thereby allowing the patient to reduce bracing and ambulate better. Therefore stabilization procedures such as ankle arthrodesis or triple arthrodesis and tendon transfer procedures yield the best results (Figs. 13.12, 13.13). Chronic poliomyelitis is a nonprogressive disease; therefore surgery will yield a more lasting result than would be expected in diseases such as Duchenne's muscular dystrophy, Charcot-Marie-Tooth disease, or spina bifida, which are progressive diseases.

CEREBRAL PALSY

Cerebral palsy is a congenital neuromuscular disease caused by a brain lesion. The lesion may form

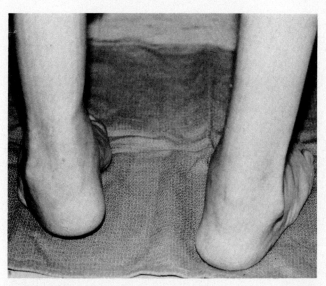

Figure 13.12. Fixed equinovarus deformity of left foot in patient with left limb shortage secondary to chronic poliomyelitis.

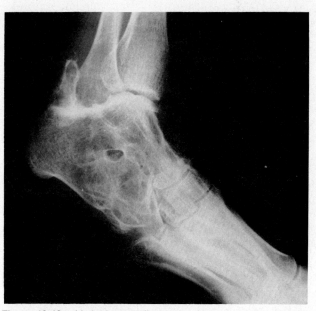

Figure 13.13. Limb shortage in patient with poliomyelitis. The patient had surgery 20 years previously consisting of triple arthrodesis and posterior ankle block. Patient now ambulates with ease in molded shoe with heel raise.

before, during, or immediately after birth. Common causes for the lesion developing include congenital maldevelopment of the brain, cerebral anoxia during the perinatal period, trauma during birth, erythroblastosis secondary to Rh incompatibility, neonatal encephalitis, and prematurity. Once formed the brain lesion is irreparable yet it is nonprogressive. Although the brain lesion is not progressive various deformities will gradually develop during growth because of the neurological imbalance produced by the lesion. The incidence of cerebral palsy has been estimated to be 6 per 100,000 births (46).

The location and extent of the brain lesion will

determine the type and severity of the cerebral palsy, as well as the degree of mental deficiency. Spastic cerebral palsy is the most common type and occurs in 65% of the cases. Athetoid cerebral palsy is the next common type and accounts for 20% of the cases. The other types, ataxic, rigidity, tremor, and atonia comprise the remaining 15%.

Of these types the spastic form of cerebral palsy responds well to the surgical repair of secondary deformities (46, 47). The other types do not respond well to surgery and will not be addressed. The spasticity is more pronounced in certain muscles. Those muscles that cross more than one joint, such as m. gastrocnemius, are often more spastic than muscles that cross only one joint. This accounts for the fact that spastic equinus is one of the most common findings in cerebral palsy. The muscles of flexion, adduction, and internal rotation tend to overpower those muscles of extension, abduction, and external rotation (46). This explains the common finding of lower extremity deformity consisting of flexion, adduction, and internal rotation of the hip, knee flexion and genu valgum, and ankle equinus (48). This spasticity produces the so-called scissors gait that is typical of a cerebral palsy patient. Secondary to the spastic equinus, talipes equinovalgus commonly develops. However, other foot deformities such as talipes calcaneus, pes cavus, hallux valgus, and hammertoe deformities are also seen.

Treatment in cerebral palsy should begin during the first year of life. Such treatment should consist of active physical therapy with splinting and bracing to resist contracture (48). Surgical correction should begin as early as possible to prevent bad locomotor habits from developing (49). Strayer (50) believes that a gastrocnemius recession will yield the best results in a child who has not yet walked. In that way the child will walk with the heels on the floor from the outset and will develop good walking habits.

The object of treatment is to facilitate training and rehabilitation. This is done by restoring muscle balance, realigning joints, and correcting posture (49). Surgery will be of the most benefit to the ambulatory patient. Yet it is also of benefit to the nonambulatory patient if it will facilitate physical therapy and nursing care (47). Surgery should be directed towards releasing contractures and correcting fixed deformities.

Treatment of spastic equinus can begin as stretching. Night splints can also be used in young children. Serial plaster of paris casts with wedging can facilitate the stretching of spastic muscles (47). Surgery for spastic equinus can take the form of a gastrocnemius recession or a tendo achillis lengthening. In cases where the triceps surae is shown to be spastic throughout the gait cycle, a Murphy tendo achillis advancement may be warranted (51). Such advancement weakens the effect of the triceps at the ankle by 50% yet only weakens toe-off ability by 15% (51).

Triceps surgery in spastic equinus is not without consequence. The surgeon must watch for overcorrection, which in a cerebral palsy patient will lead to the development of a devastating calcaneus deformity.

Recurrence can occur if the dorsiflexors are weak or if the triceps is in spasm (47). Recurrence may also occur during periods of rapid growth when the long bones grow fast and the soft tissue structures do not grow as fast. Such recurrence can be limited by adequate postoperative care including physical therapy and night splints (47).

Surgery for fixed deformities in cerebral palsy patients is best done by arthrodesis procedures such as the Grice extra-articular arthrodesis. In older patients the element of time has allowed more severe deformity to develop. Therefore more aggressive surgery will be required. Triple arthrodesis is often required to stabilize the foot and provide a stable base of support. Release of knee and hip contractures is often advisable if a satisfactory result is to be obtained.

CONCLUSION

The diseases presented here represent the most common neuromuscular diseases the foot surgeon is likely to encounter in an office setting. When performing surgery on a patient with a neuromuscular disease the surgeon must be totally familiar with the particular disease entity. Some procedures will yield miraculous results in patients with one neuromuscular disease yet have poor results in another disease entity. It is the surgeon's responsibility not only to perform the surgery but also to evaluate the patient preoperatively and to oversee rehabilitation postoperatively.

References

1. McCarroll HR: Discussion. *J Bone Joint Surg* 32B:38, 1950.
2. Swash M, Schwartz M: *Neuromuscular Disease: A Practical Approach to Diagnosis and Management*. New York, Springer-Verlag, 1981, p 4.
3. Siegel IM: *The Clinical Management of Muscle Disease*. Philadelphia, JB Lippincott Co, 1977, p 3.
4. Politz M: *Clinical Podiatric Laboratory Diagnosis*. Mt Kisco, NY, Futura Publishing Co, 1977, p 172.
5. Drennan J: *Orthopaedic Management of Neuromuscular Disorders*. Philadelphia, JB Lippincott Co, 1983, p 4.
6. Tooth HH: *The Peroneal Type of Progressive Muscular Atrophy*. London, HK Lewis Co Ltd, 1886.
7. Charcot JM, Marie P: Sur une forme particuliere d'atrophie musculaire progressive souvent familiale debutant par les pieds et les jambes et atteignant plus tard les mains. *Revue de Medecine Interne* (Paris) 6:97–138, 1886.
8. Tachdjian MO: *Pediatric Orthopaedics*. Philadelphia, WB Saunders Co, 1972, pp 1058–1067.
9. Louis JM, Giraudi CF: Charcot-Marie-Tooth disease: a case report. *J Am Podiatry Assoc* 70:43–46, 1980.
10. Jacobs JE, Carr C: Progressive muscular atrophy of the peroneal type (Charcot-Marie-Tooth disease). *J Bone Joint Surg* 32B:27–38, 1950.
11. Allan W: Relation of hereditary pattern to clinical severity as illustrated by peroneal atrophy. *Arch Intern Med* 62:1123–1131, 1939.
12. Fenton CF, Schlefman BS, McGlamry ED: Surgical considerations in the presence of Charcot-Marie-Tooth disease. *J Am Podiatry Assoc* 74:490–498, 1984.
13. Schwartz A: Charcot-Marie-Tooth disease. A 45 year follow-up. *Arch Neurol* 9:623–634, 1963.
14. Miller OL: Reporting cases of an infrequent type of foot deformity. *South Med Surg* 86:512–514, 1924.
15. Karlholm S, Nilsonne U: Operative treatment of the foot deformity in Charcot-Marie-Tooth disease. *Acta Orthop Scand* 39:101–106, 1968.

16. Levitt RL, Canale ST, Cooke AJ, Gartland JJ: The role of foot surgery in progressive neuromuscular disorders in children. *J Bone Joint Surg* 55A:1396–1410, 1973.

17. Cavuoto JW: Foot surgery in Charcot-Marie-Tooth disease. *J Foot Surg* 19:130–134, 1980.

18. Gould N: Surgery in advanced Charcot-Marie-Tooth disease. *Foot Ankle* 4:267–273, 1984.

19. Schlefman BS, Fenton CF, McGlamry, ED: Peg in hole arthrodesis. *J Am Podiatry Assoc* 73:187–195, 1983.

20. Marcinko DE, Lazerson A, Dollard MD, Schwartz N: Flexor digitorum longus tendon transfer: a simplified technique. *J Am Podiatry Assoc* 74:380–385, 1984.

21. Jahss M: Editorial. *Foot Ankle* 4:227, 1984.

22. Dejerine J, Sottas J: Sur la nevrite: interstitielle hypertrophique et progressive de l'enfance. *Competes Rendus Seances Societe Biologie Filiaks* (Paris) 45:63, 1893.

23. Sears WG: Progressive hypertrophic polyneuritis. *J Neurol Psychopathol* 12:137–147, 1931.

24. Anderson Rm, Dennett X, Hopkins IJ, Shield LK: Hypertrophic interstitial polyneuropathy in infancy. *J Pediatr* 82:619–624, 1973.

25. Roussy G, Levy G: Sept cas d'une maladie familiale particuliere: troubles de la marche, pieds bot et areflexie tendineuse generalisee, avec acessoirement legere maladresse des mains. *Rev Neurol* 1:427–450, 1926.

26. Yudell A, Dyck PJ, Lambert EH: A kinship with the Roussey-Lǘy syndrome. *Arch Neurol* 13:432–440, 1963.

27. Symonds CP, Shaw ME: Familial claw-foot with absent tendon jerks: a "forme-truste" of the Charcot-Marie-Tooth disease. *Brain* 49:387–403, 1926.

28. Refsum S: Heredopathia atactia polyneuritiformis. Familial syndrome not hitherto described, contribution to clinical study of hereditary diseases of nervous system. *Acta PsychiatrNeurol*, (suppl 38):1, 1946.

29. Steinberg D, Vroom FQ, Engel WK, Cammermeyer J, Mize CE, Auigan J: Refsum's disease—a recently characterized lipidosis involving the nervous system. *Ann Intern Med* 66:365–395, 1967.

30. Kolodry EH, Hass WK, Lane B, Drucker WD: Refsum's syndrome. *Arch Neurol* 12:583–596, 1963.

31. Makin M: The surgical management of Friedreich's ataxia. *J Bone Joint Surg* 35A:425–436, 1953.

32. Heck AF: A study of neural and extraneural findings in a large family with Friedreich's ataxia. *J Neurol Sci* 1:226–255, 1964.

33. Mooney V, Perry J, Nickel VL: Surgical and nonsurgical orthopaedic care of stroke. *J Bone Joint Surg* 49A:989–1000, 1967.

34. *Physician's Desk Reference*, ed 38. Oradell NJ, Medical Economics Co, 1984, pp 918–920.

35. Spencer G: Orthopedic care of progressive muscular dystrophy. *J Bone Joint Surg* 49A:1201–1203, 1967.

36. Reinherz R, Mann I: Lower extremity involvement in Duchenne's muscular dystrophy. *J Am Podiatry Assoc* 67:796–801, 1977.

37. Eyring EJ, Johnson EW, Burnett C: Surgery in muscular dystrophy. *JAMA* 222:1056–1057, 1972.

38. Zundel W, Tyler F: The muscular dystrophies. *N Engl J Med* 273:537–543, 1965.

39. Frazier CM: *Surgery of the Spine and Spinal Cord*. New York, Appleton-Century-Crofts Inc, 1918, p 272.

40. Hayes JT, Gross HP: Orthopedic implications of myelodysplasia. *JAMA* 184:762–767, 1963.

41. Sharrard WJW, Grosfield I: The management of deformity and paralysis of the foot in myelomeningocele. *J Bone Joint Surg* 50B:456–465, 1960.

42. Schelfman BS, McGlamry, ED, Hilkemann RJ. First metatarsophalangeal joint dislocation in spina bifida: a case report. *J Am Podiatry Assoc* 74:147–152, 1984.

43. Turek S: *Orthopaedics*, ed 4. Philadelphia, JB Lippincott Co, 1984, p 516.

44. Abbott LC: The orthopedic care in anterior poliomyelitis. *J Pediatr* 39:663–671, 1951.

45. Wickstrom JK, LaRocca HS: Management of the poliomyelitic foot. In Giannestras NJ (ed): *Foot Disorders. Medical and Surgical Management*. Philadelphia, Lea & Febiger, 1976, pp 302–330.

46. Salter RB: *Textbook of Disorders and Injuries of the Musculoskeletal System*. Baltimore, Williams & Wilkins, 1970, pp 233–267.

47. Pollock GA: Surgical treatment of cerebral palsy. *J Bone Joint Surg* 44B:68–81, 1962.

48. Evans EB: The status of surgery of the lower extremities in cerebral palsy. *Clin Orthop* 47:127–139, 1966.

49. Baker LD: A rational approach to the surgical needs of the cerebral palsy patient. *J Bone Joint Surg* 38A:313–323, 1956.

50. Strayer LM: Recession of the gastrocnemius, an operation to relieve spastic contracture of the calf muscles. *J Bone Joint Surg* 32A:671–676, 1950.

51. Jay RM, Schoenhaus HD: Further insights in the anterior advancement of tendo achilles. *J Am Podiatry Assoc* 7:73–76, 1981.

CHAPTER 14

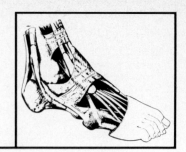

Medical and Surgical Considerations for the Patient with Diabetes Mellitus

Louis G. Pack, D.P.M. and **Grace M. Guastella, D.P.M.**

DIABETES MELLITUS

Introduction

The human foot is a mirror of systemic disease. Diabetes and a host of other diseases may show their first signs and symptoms in the foot. In the chronic disease state significant pedal changes may well be noted.

Diabetes mellitus and its complications are now the third leading cause of mortality in the United States. The estimated prevalence ranges between 3% and 6% of the population, and it is increasing rapidly (1). Approximately 80% of patients with diabetes are over 40 years of age and, interestingly, surgical intervention is highest in this population. Causative factors resulting in the increased incidence of morbidity in the diabetic patient include cardiovascular, renal, neuropathic, and ophthalomological complications of the disorder. Because of the extensive and serious pathology associated with the disease, diabetic patients require special considerations when surgery is contemplated. Thorough systemic and local evaluation combined with appropriate surgical measures and meticulous wound care will often permit successful surgery and limb salvage (2).

Definition

Diabetes can be defined as a group of metabolic derangements that share one feature in common: hyperglycemia. Diabetes is a disease complex characterized primarily by relative or absolute insufficiency of insulin secretion. In many patients there is a concomitant insensitivity or resistance to the metabolic action of insulin on target tissues. Type I, or insulin-dependent diabetes mellitus, is the form characterized by destruction of the insulin-producing beta cells and an absolute lack of insulin. It usually appears during childhood but may appear at any age, which is why the terms "juvenile" and "juvenile-onset" are no longer

recommended. Type II, or non-insulin-dependent diabetes mellitus, is characterized by a relative lack of insulin usually accompanied by some degree of peripheral insulin resistance creating a state of relative insulin deficiency despite circulating insulin levels that may be normal or increased (3).

Obesity is a major risk factor for the development of this type of diabetes mellitus, probably because of the decreased insulin receptor density and abnormal coupling of receptors to metabolic processes that occur in the obese state. Because insulin insensitivity is frequently the more dominant component of the pathological process, type II patients do not require injected insulin to survive. Nevertheless many patients who clearly are continuing to produce some endogenous insulin do require supplementation with injected insulin for control of symptoms and/or appropriate regulation of their blood glucose level.

Pathophysiology

Gluconeogenesis takes place primarily in the liver and kidneys and is controlled principally by insulin, glucagon, and adrenal steroids. In diabetic conditions with insulin deficiency the breakdown of natural fat to free fatty acids and glycerol is increased. Because of a lack of insulin, transport of glucose into muscle and adipose tissue is restricted and blood glucose therefore rises. Glucagon and adrenal steroids increase gluconeogenesis and both may contribute to an overproduction of glucose (4). In this hypercatabolic state increased amino acid and fat mobilization from adipose tissue and muscle produce further hyperglycemia, hyperlipidemia, and ketosis, in addition to the increased blood glucose reflecting accelerated gluconeogenesis. The situation is further complicated by secondary fluid and electrolyte imbalances from the osmotic diuresis that ensues (3). Thus the development of life-threatening dehydration, peripheral vascular collapse, and electrolyte abnormalities will result in the seriously insulin-deficient state (5).

DIABETIC PATIENT AS A SURGICAL CANDIDATE

Effects of Surgery on the Diabetic State

Because of the large number of individuals with diabetes in our population and the foot pathology associated with the disorder, these patients are frequently seen by the podiatrist (6). The podiatric physician is in a unique position to evaluate and maintain the status of the lower extremity. Often the decision to operate is made after conservative measures have failed to relieve a recurrent lesion that has the potential to threaten seriously the viability of the limb.

Surgery can be extremely stressful and therefore requires an optimal metabolic state to tolerate successfully anesthesia and prevent tissue injury. It is important to recognize that "good control" of the diabetic patient does not alter the pathological conditions present.

The patient with diabetes mellitus has an increased risk for morbidity and mortality as compared with the general population. In the general population stress stimulates the secretion of reactive anti-insulin hormones, resulting in the elevation of blood glucose levels and the mobilization of alternative fuels (3). Furthermore, reduction in peripheral insulin sensitivity triggered by the release of epinephrine diminishes glucose clearance. This elevated activity of epinephrine, norepinephrine, cortisol, growth hormone, and glucagon ultimately influence the hemodynamic and substance responses required for the physiological adaptation of the stressed individual (2). In the healthy person these changes are offset by an immediate increase in insulin release that enhances peripheral glucose use and inhibits alternative fuel mobilization (3). In the patient with poor insulin production the failure of this fine-tuned feedback loop can produce a wide range of metabolic complications.

In the type I diabetic patient the synergistic activity of the counterregulatory hormones results in a heightened catabolic response caused by insulin deficiency. This is characterized by increased glucose production and glycogenolysis leading to hyperglycemia and glycosuria. Hepatic ketogenesis is fueled by released triglycerides and protein breakdown occurs as amino acids are diverted to gluconeogenesis (2). Severe ketosis and shock may result from dehydration and peripheral vascular insufficiency in a patient with insulin-dependent diabetes mellitus not properly prepared for surgery. To preclude these complications fastidious management of insulin, fluids, and electrolytes is necessary (3). In addition an anesthetic itself may affect carbohydrate metabolism as does stress caused by the release of catecholomines. Chloroform and ether have the greatest effect on blood glucose and increases of 10 to 50 mg per 100 ml have been documented (7). Halothane is known to inhibit insulin release and nitrous oxide, tricholoroethylene, and cyclopropane promote sympathetic stimulation and catecholamine release. Barbituates can exhibit similar properties, as well as prevent normal circulatory clearance of glucose. The ultimate choice of anesthetic agent depends on the type of operation, the medical status, and surgical risks and should be based on the judgment of the anesthesiologist (2).

Effects of Diabetes on Surgery

The complications of diabetes frequently require surgical intervention. However, these patients are at a greater risk for perioperative and postoperative complications. The triad of vascular disease, neuropathy, and increased potential for infection enhance the surgical risk. Patients with uncontrolled diabetes are prone to thrombotic episodes and abnormalities of leukocyte and platelet function. Anemia, if present, will minimize oxygen delivery to the tissues. Furthermore it has been suggested that insulin is necessary to enhance the earliest stages of granulation and collagen formation. An insulin deficiency therefore would result in a decreased production of collagen and a reduction in strength of the surgical wound (8).

Faris (8) discusses three factors that ultimately lead to impaired wound healing: (a) the reduced blood supply to the affected area, (b) the decreased effectiveness of the inflammatory response, and (c) the alteration in the repair process that results in the formation of fibrous tissue. Because a successful surgical result depends on a sequence of closely related progressive changes, the metabolic derangements present in diabetes may reduce the body's ability to strengthen and heal a surgical wound.

Diabetes is one of the major diseases that predisposes patients to early development of atherosclerosis affecting coronary, cerebral, and peripheral arterial circulation (2, 9). Elevated free fatty acid levels accompanying poorly controlled diabetes are believed to contribute to this accelerated atherosclerosis. Because of this the patient with diabetes may frequently have "silent" coronary artery disease. Intraoperative and postoperative myocardial infarction is the most common cause of death in diabetic patients undergoing surgery (10, 11). Obesity, frequently associated with adult-onset diabetes mellitus, increases the risk of pulmonary, thromboembolic, and anesthetic complications. It is wise for the physician to recommend weight reduction in an effort to reduce blood glucose levels and enhance peripheral receptor function. In addition, excess weight and thick subcutaneous adipose can make for difficult surgical exposure and impede proper wound closure.

Lastly, diabetic nephropathy greatly predisposes the patient to septic complications. The presence of renal insufficiency influences not only the amount of intravenous fluids that can be given but also influences the excretion of various medications.

Development of Pedal Lesions

The same factors that may lead to complications in diabetic foot surgery also predispose the patient to ulceration (8). Diabetic neuropathy, combined with poor blood supply, and susceptibility to infection enhance the likelihood of skin ulceration in areas exposed to pressure. Such factors reduce the ability of the patient to cope with minor injuries that then progress to form major lesions.

Vascular Pathology

Vascular disease is a primary factor responsible for the pathogenesis of foot lesions. Typically patients with diabetes present with atherosclerosis (macroscopic lesion) identical to the nondiabetic population. Individuals with diabetes, however, develop these lesions earlier and to a greater degree than the nondiabetic (12, 13). The sequence of endothelial cell damage, platelet aggregation, vascular smooth muscle proliferation, deposition of lipid into places of intimal injury, and formation of atheromatous plaques results in occlusive disease (14).

Small vessel disease is the pathognomonic vascular lesion in the diabetic. Basement membrane thickening in these vessels leads to a diffusion defect that interferes with normal tissue nutrition (12, 13). Capillary disease may be the prime cause of inadequate vascular delivery, especially to the distal foot. Diabetic digital occlusive disease and autosympathectomy may make a pedal examination quite deceiving. This warm, pulsatile, apparently vascular foot may well become a gangrenous disaster. Tissue hypoxia and impedence of peripheral perfusion caused by microangiopathy may further contribute to the rapid progression of infection and the delayed response to treatment (14).

Infectious Process

Infection is an important contributing factor to the morbidity of diabetic patients with foot problems. Particular susceptability to infection results in forms of infection that are more common to this population (staphylococcal skin infections, fungal infections, and osteomyelitis) (8). Furthermore diabetes impairs the normal defense mechanisms against infection increasing the risk for the development of progressive deep infection and gangrene. Excellent studies exist to show that chemotaxis, engulfment, plagocytosis, and eventual lysozymal destruction of bacteria are all impaired for the hyperglycemic patient and that these metabolic abnormalities are reversed by adequate control of blood glucose. This disordered function of polymorphonuclear cells probably contributes to the well-recognized susceptibility of diabetics to infection, particularly in poorly vascularized tissues.

Primary infection occurs in areas of minor trauma, skin breakdown such as results from fungal infections, neuropathic ulcers, and ischemic lesions. It is critical, when treating a diabetic patient, to control minor skin impairments and to prevent them.

Neuropathic Abnormalities

Diabetic peripheral neuropathy is characterized by a slower nerve conduction time following a stimulus (13). The important neurological alterations in the diabetic foot are primarily the result of metabolic changes. Motor, sensory, and autonomic fibers can be affected with the characteristic histological feature in the peripheral nerves being segmental demyelination (8, 13). The pathology may reflect ischemia of the peripheral nerves secondary to disease of the vasonervorum and posterior column degeneration in the spinal cord. This is one theory. There are others that do not attribute this loss to microangiopathy (i.e. demyelination and loss of Schwann's cells). The slowly progressive deterioration of peripheral nervous system function seen in the symmetrical distal polyneuropathies is probably not attributable to an infarction process. It is currently believed that chronic hyperglycemia may lead to excess sorbitol formation in Schwann's cells of nerve trunks (15). Osmotic gradients cause swelling of Schwann's cells and disturbance of axonal integrity. With progressive deterioration axonal and nerve cell death may occur and this accounts for the sensory anesthesia observed in these patients (15).

Clinically this is manifested as a mild, distal polyneuropathy. There is a decreased sensation of pain, temperature, and touch, impaired proprioception, and sluggish or absent deep tendon reflexes (8, 13). Symptoms such as numbness, burning, or cold sensation of the feet and lower legs tend to be more severe at night. It is at this stage that the "unaware" foot is most susceptible to injury and insult. Early lesions such as blisters, callouses, and minor abrasions are overlooked. Footgear problems are common because diminished proprioception contributes to abnormal gait patterns. Gradual muscle weakness results from motor neuropathy and denervation of the small foot muscles. Motor changes in the lumbricales, interosseous, and extensor brevis muscles fix the metatarsophalangeal joint in a position of hyperextension and the interphalangeal joint in flexion. Shortening of the flexor tendons may occur, leading to hammertoe deformities. The metatarsal heads protrude plantarly, foot mechanics are altered, and pressure overload accelerates tissue breakdown (2, 8). In addition the loss of subcutaneous tissue, tissue moldability, and the anterior displacement of the protective metatarsal fat pad increase the risk of plantar metatarsal head ulceration. Therefore correction of maldistributed weight to prevent pressure areas and potential ulceration is important.

The aforementioned neurological changes produce the characteristic "mal perforans." Charcot joints develop insidiously with further denervation of other joints leading to degenerated joint spaces and damaged subchondral bone (8). The pathology of the early Charcot foot is felt to be repeated unappreciated microfractures (2, 13). In addition changes in the autonomic nervous system result in abnormalities in temperature regulation leading to dryness, scaling, and cracking of the skin. Interestingly, the normal vascular triple response (wheal formation, erythema, and inflammation) that occurs after a local injury is impeded in diabetics with autonomic neuropathy (8). This situation, coupled with diminished cutaneous defenses and arterial insufficiency is of great significance in a stressful situation. Vasoconstriction in response to catecholamines and stress causes a situation that enhances the susceptibility to septic complications.

MANAGEMENT OF THE DIABETIC SURGICAL PATIENT

Preoperative Assessment

Successful repair of an injury or deformity depends upon a sequence of closely related and progressive changes. Metabolic alterations in the patient with diabetes may reduce the effectiveness of the wound healing process. Therefore, it is wise to thoroughly evaluate those clinical signs that help predict healing potential. Local assessment is directed at determining the severity of existing infection, if any, and the degree of arterial disease and neuropathy (8).

Podiatric surgical intervention is aimed at the elimination of any deformities that may exist, as well as the correction of potential problems. Foot deformities such as hammertoes, bunions, and plantarflexed metatarsals are common causes of tissue breakdown. Neuropathic ulcers and ischemic lesions are common portals of entry for infecting organisms. Recurrence of these ulcerations despite conservative measures may be prevented by removal of the offending osseous structures. Early appreciation of these deformities and prophylactic surgery are aimed at the prevention of secondary morbidity in the diabetic population.

Once a decision to intervene surgically has been made it is the surgeon's responsibility to properly assess the state of the illness and appropriately handle the preoperative period. In a poorly controlled hyperglycemic patient it is advisable to admit the patient one to two days early. This time is needed to obtain numerous blood glucose measurements and adjust the insulin, diet, and electrolytes. When diabetes is seriously out of control or particularly unstable and difficult to manage it may be beneficial to seek consultation (or conjoint management) with an endocrinologist or diabetes specialist to optimize control of diabetes before, during, and after surgery. Successful tissue repair in the diabetic patient begins with a thorough preoperative assessment of the level of diabetic control. A history of metabolic instability may indicate a potential for associated imbalances postoperatively. The presence of retinopathy, obesity, chronic urinary tract infections and prominent pedal manifestations increase the surgical risk. Additionally, diabetic glomerulosclerosis with anemia, hypoproteinemia, and diminished glomerular filtration adversely affect wound healing and increase the risk of sepsis. Drug excretion is modified in this situation as well and careful assessment of renal function is crucial in selecting proper doses of drugs that may contribute to further nephrotoxicity (10, 14).

Besides those previously mentioned, pedal clinical signs may indicate a decreased healing potential. The presence of diabetic neuropathy is often a marker of undetected involvement of the autonomic nervous system which compromises vascular responses during and after surgery. Finally, a poorly controlled patient manifests delay in wound healing because of impaired nutritional status and protein depletion (2). With the above mentioned diabetic complications it can certainly be seen why thorough preoperative evaluation is imperative. The surgeon should be aware of advanced neurological indices such as decreased vibratory sensation and loss of reflexes that reflect advanced stages of the disease.

In the presence of infection diagnostic studies should include culture and sensitivity tests of open lesions and routine roentgenograms to rule out osseous involvement. When radiographs are inconclusive technetium scanning may be helpful. Gallium scanning can delineate the extent and location of soft tissue infection as it is concentrated in metabolizing white blood cells (13).

In vitro studies support a predominance of gram-positive bacterial growth in infected diabetic lesions (8). Multiple organisms are frequently exhibited; among the aerobes are Escherichia coli, Staphylococcus, Enterococcus, and Proteus. Of particular interest is the frequency of pseudomonal hospital infections, second only to staph infections in our experience. Anaerobes include Bacteroides and Peptococcus.

Infected areas require special attention. It is advantageous to obtain a culture of the ulcer before hospital admission. Administration of the antibiotic of choice should be keyed closely to anticipated or established flora. Usually treatment with an appropriate broad-spectrum antibiotic is instituted and then revised according to the culture results and clinical response. Preoperative antibiotic therapy has two goals: control of cellulitis and prophylaxis if no infection is present at the time of surgery. Obviously, in the case of cellulitis without an abcess, the treatment is aimed at curing the infection.

Where an abcess is present the authors recommend prompt incision and drainage as the cardinal treatment rather than relying on antibiotic therapy as a sole means of limiting the spread of the infection. There are a number of reasons the authors believe this mode of therapy is appropriate. First, incision of the abcess site permits culture of the wound and prevents the use of inappropriate antibiotics. Second, immediate drainage reduces the chance of ischemia and necrosis of the overlying skin. In addition, a closed, infected wound is a favorable environment that fosters bacterial growth. Finally, penetration and subsequent bacteriocidal activity of antibiotics may be impossible in abcess cavities of sufficient size.

Inspection of the wound can offer excellent clinical clues. For instance, a nonsuppurative cellulitis suggests a streptococcal infection and penicillin is the drug of choice. A local inflammatory reaction, on the other hand, may signal a staphylococcal infection and is adequately treated with a penicillinase-resistant antibiotic and surgical drainage (2).

In noninfected cases, giving preoperative antibiotics may have some value in reducing the incidence of wound infections postoperatively (8). The timing and administration of the drug should be tuned to achieve therapeutic blood levels at the start of the operative procedure. Antibiotic dosages must be carefully selected with regard to the patient's degree of renal function.

A thorough preoperative arterial evaluation should be conducted. Arterial disease can be assessed by palpation of lower extremity pulses and skin temperature gradients. It is generally assumed that if distal pulses (posterior tibial and dorsalis pedis) are present there is adequate blood supply to allow healing following local surgery (8, 12). The podiatrist facing a decision to perform surgery on the diabetic should be aware that this can be a misleading situation especially if the surgery is more distally oriented. In fact in marked counterdistinction to the former and generally held opinion, the authors believe that distal pulses can be present in a diabetic foot that has a high potential for ischemia. It is believed that neuropathy adversely affects the microcirculation in the distal small vessels through poorly functioning nerves controlling small vessel responsiveness. It follows that hemorrhage, infection, pressure, and possibly surgical stress can precipitate ischemia and delay wound healing.

In the infected foot it is strongly recommended that proper evaluation of the clinical signs of inflammation be accomplished before deciding to operate. This is much more informative and important than the results of a standard vascular examination. Such signs can suggest the individual's capability to handle tissue repair. For example, evidence of good local signs of inflammation around an ulcer is a promising clinical clue for satisfactory postoperative healing. If doubt remains about the degree of circulatory efficiency special vascular tests can be used.

Good preoperative management should always include recommendations to cease smoking, manage hypertension, and control diet and blood sugar levels.

Perioperative Management

The management of the patient's diabetes will depend on the extent of the operative procedure and the severity of the disease (2). The stress of surgery and the anesthetic agents contribute to the rise in blood sugar perioperatively (15). Hyperglycemia inhibits polymorphonuclear cell activity and can therefore lead to exacerbation of a septic process (5, 16). Ideally, then, patients undergoing surgical procedures should be in an anabolic state (16–19). The absence of increased gluconeogenesis is dependent on effective control of blood sugar. Good control also promotes a more favorable environment for protein synthesis and wound healing (5, 8).

Documentation of adequate blood glucose control and the insulin adjustments needed to attain the state is facilitated by frequent determination of the patient's blood glucose level. Capillary blood sugars (fingerstick) can be obtained and recorded by the nursing staff with results available in just a few minutes, a procedure that is efficient and obviates the need for multiple venipunctures. Blood sugars should be monitored at least twice a day and may need to be done four or more times daily in the type I patient with a history of metabolic instability. Bed rest, trauma, and active infection are all factors that contribute to blood glucose elevations and frequently require increased insulin doses in the diabetic patient being prepared for surgery.

In general obese type II patients have a higher requirement for insulin because they are relatively insensitive to the action of injected insulin just as they are to their own insulin. All type I patients have some degree of metabolic instability and one must anticipate some variability in blood glucose levels under the most optimum conditions. Long-duration type I patients and patients with endocrine deficiency states (adrenal insufficiency, hypothyroidism) tend to be very sensitive to insulin and need much greater caution when prescribing additional doses of insulin to correct hyperglycemia. Renal insufficiency inhibits insulin clearance and may require significant reduction in the insulin dosage to prevent hypoglycemia. Patients with advanced renal disease are usually difficult to regulate. This is thought to reflect binding and unbinding of insulin to circulating antibodies.

The most important principles of safe management are knowing the current plasma glucose values and intervening with sugar or insulin as needed. Generally a safe "surgical zone" is considered to be 150 to 250 mg/100 ml (3, 10, 20). Because during surgery a patient can exhibit extremes in blood glucose values, good control and safe management should include intraoperative measurements of the plasma glucose levels.

The following are suggested guidelines for intraoperative insulin management in the surgical diabetic patient.

Minor Procedures

Non-insulin-dependent diabetes mellitus

Patients taking oral agents can usually continue using them in minor surgical procedures. If a general anesthetic is used and surgery is in the morning, the oral agent should be discontinued (11, 20, 21). The patient can be successfully managed with good postoperative observation consisting of frequent blood glucose monitoring. In the type II patient previously under good control moderately high glucose values (less than 300 mg/100 ml) will usually fall to previous levels over the 24 to 48 hours postoperatively and do not require specific intervention. Successive blood glucose levels greater than 300 mg/100 ml are best treated with relatively small (6 to 16 units) doses of soluble (regular) insulin given at four to six hour intervals and with subsequent dose adjustments as determined by the patient's response to the previous dose (4). Patients treated with temporary insulin coverage should receive insulin of the highest purity (human insulin or highly purified porcine insulin) to minimize the antigenic exposure and the subsequent risk of insulin allergy should they become insulin-requiring at some future date. At all times it is wise to consult a diabetes specialist before intervention on the patient's diabetic control is made.

Insulin-dependent diabetes mellitus

A minor office procedure on an insulin-dependent individual can usually be done without an IV infusion. Surgery should be scheduled early in the morning and the preoperative insulin dose can be withheld. Afterwards, providing the patient can eat, the patient should receive approximately two thirds to all of the usual dosage depending on the time of day (4, 11). The lower dose is suggested if the patient's day is starting late and the customary dose given if breakfast and subsequent meals are to be taken at or about the usual times. When a reduced dose of insulin is given frequent monitoring is advised because "surgical stress" can elevate the blood glucose and require small supplementary "coverage" doses of soluble insulin later in the day.

Major Procedures

The literature reviews numerous protocols in an attempt to formulate a convenient and acceptable mode of insulin therapy for all diabetic patients in the perioperative period (16). It is the authors' opinion that no single protocol can adequately manage the degree of variability among diabetic patients. The evaluation of risk benefit ratios of each mode of insulin administration suggests that no single schedule of insulin administration will be uniformly effective in a situation where the stresses are variable (16). Therefore optimum control is obtained with frequent blood glucose analysis and appropriate therapy with intravenous insulin either as a continuous or intermittent infusion (15, 16). Of course patients receiving supplemental insulin should have an intravenous glucose infusion until adequate oral intake can be assured.

Before anesthesia is induced a plasma glucose value is obtained. If the patient is in control, a 5% dextrose infusion is given 2 ml/kg/hour. Capillary blood glucose determinations are often preferred for use in the operating room for periodic laboratory confirmation. In patients whose fasting serum glucose values are below 200 mg/dl perioperative insulin supplementation is generally not required. Intravenous insulin, 1 to 2 units per hour, can be given if the blood glucose is equal to or greater than 250 mg/dl. Extra glucose is given when the blood glucose is less than 150 mg/dl (14, 16).

Care of the Surgical Site

It is the authors' opinion that when recurrent pedal lesions and persistent tissue breakdown are chronic problems, prophylactic surgery should be considered. This may be far more beneficial than prolonged and constant treatment of ulcers. Such surgery attempts the restoration of normal foot architecture by correction of clawed or hammered digits, as well as by removal of bony prominences to eliminate sources of pressure and irritation.

Preoperative surgical care should consist of meticulous attention to the surgical site. Successful postoperative healing is best achieved when surgery is done through healthy tissue. Perioperative considerations are directed toward assuring good surgical technique that would result in prompt wound healing without infection. It is extremely important to provide the same level of care postoperatively to ensure a safe surgical result without complications.

Preoperative Care of the Surgical Site

Local preoperative care of the diabetic patient is aimed at reducing the risk of infection. When considering surgery for heloma molle, attention is drawn to the interspace hyperhydrosis that can lead to maceration, setting up an environment conducive to bacterial growth. The authors recommend home care for one week before surgery. This consists of cleansing the interspace with Betadine twice daily. The interspace should be dried thoroughly and a foam pad used to separate the toes. If excessively wet, gentian violet may be used periodically.

If hammertoe surgery is to be performed any underlying infection or ulceration should be healed before surgery if at all possible. Debridement and daily applications of wet to dry dressings are suggested. Foam padding behind the lesion to eliminate pressure is helpful. Any portal of entry must remain closed until the day of surgery.

Many diabetic patients will present with pedal fungal infections. Treatment is aimed at getting them out of the acute stage or controlling the chronic stage. Erythema, blisters, and scaling suggest an acute stage. Deep cracks and fissures suggest a chronic problem and should be healed before surgery is performed. Likewise, manifestations of dermatitis should be controlled before surgery.

The surgical prep (i.e. shaving) should be done carefully to prevent any nicks or scratches that may serve as portals of entry for bacteria. The authors do not recommend the use of a wrap after the surgical prep because it may increase the chance for hyperhydrosis. Instead, booties should be worn when ambulation is necessary, but removed for sleeping.

Perioperative Considerations

The most important consideration is excellent technique. The authors insist on good hemostasis without the use of a tourniquet. Prompt ligature and cauterization of vessels will reduce the postoperative edema, especially dangerous in the patient with small vessel disease. This will also decrease the incidence of postoperative hematomas and significantly decrease pain. Gentle tissue handling and removal of foreign material such as bone fragments that result from the use of drills and saws is important. Buried suture material may reduce the resistance to staphylococcal infection by 1000 to 10,000 times (22). Therefore fine sutures and accurate hemostasis should reduce the incidence of wound infection.

The authors do not recommend irrigation of subcutaneous tissue with povidone iodine solution because of the potential for tissue irritation. Instead the authors prefer irrigation with normal saline.

Postoperative Care of the Surgical Site

The diabetic patient requires special attention after surgery. It is of primary importance to ensure that the neurovascular status is not impaired. Loose bandaging with light gauze is recommended and the authors also try, when possible, to eliminate the use of a cast. When any kind of external support such as a cast, bandage, or splint is applied it is imperative that the circulation to the toes be observed. Care should be taken to prevent any constriction leading to interference with blood or nerve supply. When applying a cast, extra padding over bony prominences is suggested, as well as frequent cast changes. The surgeon has the option to bivalve the cast if this is more convenient. Bivalving is encouraged because the operative site can then often be examined and cast disease prevented. If the patient has a local fungal infection an antifungal medication may be applied before bandaging. Gentian violet is often used in the interspaces to prevent maceration. Although most postoperative visits are one week after surgery, the diabetic's wound should usually be inspected more frequently, especially when neuropathy is present. The patient should be advised to elevate the limb, remain nonambulatory, and watch for fever or excessive pain.

While the patient is resting in the hospital daily wound inspection for normal temperature and healthy color is mandatory. Excessive coolness of the skin, cyanosis, rubor, or paleness may indicate interference with proper blood flow and the cast or dressing should be examined.

CONCLUSION

In conclusion it is important to realize the complexity of the situations that require surgical intervention in the diabetic patient. This individual is consequently at a special disadvantage when facing surgery because of the disturbed metabolism. Therefore the podiatrist must secure competent medical consultation so that the patient be provided with complete care. The vascular and neurological status, as well as the diabetic control, must be considered before surgery. Judicious choice of procedure, surgical expertise, and sharply defined medical management will minimize complications and assist in rehabilitation.

Continued patient education programs after surgery are essential. Daily foot inspection and periodic podiatric evaluation will help to ensure a healthy patient. Prophylaxis against foot injury includes the use of appropriate orthotic devices and proper shoe gear.

If these measures are addressed the podiatrist can successfully manage a variety of surgical situations directed at preventing life-threatening ischemia and gangrene. It is extremely rare that the diabetic patient looses a limb from diabetes alone. It is diabetes and a minor foot problem such as an ingrown toenail, corn, or callus that is the precipitating factor. In most instances limbs can be salvaged if proper treatment is instituted. Most of these problems never need to become severe if minor surgical procedures and other modes of therapy are considered.

References

1. Molitch ME, Reichlin S: The care of the diabetic patient during emergency surgery and postoperatively. *Clin Orthop* 9:811–823, 1978.
2. Shuman CR: Surgery in the diabetic patient. *Compr Ther* 8:38–45, 1982.
3. Gallina DL, Mordes JP, Rossini AA: Surgery in the diabetic patient. *Compr Ther* 9:8–16, 1983.
4. Oakley WG, Pyke DA, Taylor KW: *Diabetes and its Management*, ed 3. London, Blackwell Scientific Publications, 1978, p 6.
5. Rossini AA: Why control blood glucose levels? *Arch Surg* 111:229, 1976.
6. Walts LF: Managing diabetics during surgery. *AORN J* 37:928–941, 1983.
7. Steinke J: Management of diabetes in the surgical patient. *Med Clin North Am* 55:939–945, 1971.
8. Faris I: *The Management of the Diabetic Foot*. London, Churchill-Livingstone, 1982.
9. Johnson DG, Bressler R: Preoperative management of the diabetic patient. *Contemp Anesth Pract* 3:39–44, 1980.
10. Byyny R: Management of diabetics during surgery. *Diabetes* 68:191–201, 1980.
11. Larkins RG: Perioperative problems in the diabetic. *Aust NZ J Surg* 48:238–241, 1978.
12. Mann RA: *DuVries Surgery of the Foot*, ed 4. St Louis, The CV Mosby Co, 1978.
13. Bessman AN: Foot problems in the diabetic. *Compr Ther* 8:32–37, 1982.
14. Winters B: Promoting wound healing in the diabetic patient. *AORN J* 35:426–451, 1982.
15. Bayless TM, Brain MC, Cherniack RM: *Current Therapy in Internal Medicine 1984–1985*. St Louis, The CV Mosby Co, 1984.
16. Taitelman V, Reece EA, Bessman AN: Insulin in the management of the diabetic surgical patient. *JAMA* 237:658–660, 1977.
17. Miller J, Walts LF: Perioperative management of diabetes mellitus. *Contemp Anesth Pract* 3:91–104, 1980.
18. Clarke RSJ: The hyperglycemic response to different types of surgery and anesthesia. *Br J Anaesth* 42:45, 1970.
19. Greene NM: Insulin and anesthesia. *Anesthesiology* 41:75, 1974.
20. Rossini AA, Hare JW: How to control the blood glucose level in the surgical diabetic patient. *Arch Surg* 111:945, 1976.
21. Stein JH: *Internal Medicine*, vol 2. Boston, Little, Brown & Co, 1983.
22. Crenshaw AH: *Campbell's Operative Orthopaedics*, ed 5. St Louis, The CV Mosby Co, 1971.

CHAPTER 15

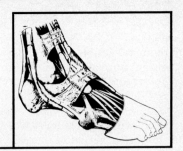

The Rheumatic Patient – Medical Considerations in Foot Surgery

Richard D. Roth, D.P.M.

Arthritic disorders affecting the foot produce extensive joint and soft tissue damage, deformity, pain, and disability. Conservative management with debridement of excrescences, padding, strapping, removable pressure relief devices, orthoses, shoe modifications, altered shoe styles, custom-molded shoes, and use of medications will provide satisfactory relief of pain and prevention of the progression of deformity for many afflicted patients. Others may require canes, braces, aluminum walkers, forearm crutches, or other assistive devices to achieve such relief and prevention of additional deformity. Surgical intervention becomes a consideration when these measures fail to provide satisfactory relief of pain and/or are insufficient to prevent progressive deformity. Surgery also becomes a consideration when these measures prove unduly burdensome for the patient.

Individual or multiple joint involvement with degenerative joint disease (osteoarthritis) represents the vast majority of pedal arthritic problems. Vascular, dermatological, neuromuscular, orthopedic (including biomechanical), radiographic, and general medical assessments should be undertaken when surgical care of these joints or related structures is contemplated. The patient's age, level of motivation, extent of pain and deformity, rate of progression, and potential for rehabilitation must also be considered. The presence of osteoarthritis in and of itself does not require related consideration of increased medical risks and associated conditions that could jeopardize surgical results.

Similar destructive joint changes are found in many other arthritides. Inherent differences in a number of those arthritides do, however, increase the hazards of surgical intervention. Some of these differences can jeopardize the results of such surgical procedures. Many of the arthritic disorders are systemic diseases that may affect numerous areas and organ systems throughout the body. Failure to adequately recognize and consider the overall manifestations of these diseases can prove dangerous and even lethal to the arthritic patient undergoing a surgical procedure.

TEAM APPROACH

Patients with rheumatic disorders will usually gain optimal benefit from required foot surgery if such care is integrated into the framework of an overall treatment plan. Formulation of a treatment plan for a patient with degenerative joint disease limited to a single pedal joint may be a relatively simple matter. The patient with extensive and progressive rheumatic disease involving multiple joints and organ systems will require a significantly more complex treatment plan. Such comprehensive treatment plans must consider extensive medical and psychosocial, as well as surgical, factors. They are best formulated by health care team approaches where the patient, surgeon, rheumatologist, internist, nursing staff, and physical therapist work closely together. The addition of a social worker, psychologist or psychiatrist, and occupational therapist to the team can be quite beneficial.

The team approach provides availability of health care professionals skilled in assessing extensive rheumatic involvement, simultaneously caring for the various manifestations of the disease processes and coordinating care so as to provide optimal benefit to the patient. The team not only provides valuable assistance to the foot surgeon; it also provides a route through which the surgeon can provide valuable input in achieving the best possible overall patient care. Many patients will require extensive physical therapy and multiple surgical procedures. Any patient's motivation to undergo such multiple procedures and to enter into lengthy and demanding follow-up therapy may be unnecessarily and substantially limited. This is often caused by fear of associated postoperative pain, temporary or potentially permanent increased disability, and limited overall benefit. Under such circumstances required foot surgery (e.g. forefoot reconstruction) with usually limited postoperative discomfort and rapid, dramatic relief of pain and disability should be scheduled initially. Limited postoperative pain and dramatically increased functional capacity following such surgery can substantially allay fears of future surgery and increase overall patient motivation. Some arthritic patients will require extensive pedal surgical procedures, the outcome of which will largely depend on the results of intensive and longterm physical therapy. Where a patient's motivational level makes cooperation in such therapy questionable, surgical procedures (e.g. first metatarsophalangeal joint or hip replacement) requiring little patient cooperation can often be initially scheduled. The patient's ability and desire to cooperate in postoperative care can then be better assessed.

Many patients requiring multiple joint replacements have numerous foot deformities. These deformities can often lead to skin necrosis, potential ulceration, and subsequent infection with seeding of proximal joint prostheses. Their surgical correction may result in wound dehiscence, necrosis, and ulceration with subsequent similar risk to proximal joint prostheses. Scheduling corrective or reconstructive foot surgery before proximal joint replacements can help to avoid such risks.

It is necessary to return a rheumatic patient to maximal functional capacity as soon as possible postoperatively if disability associated with foot surgery is to be minimized. Preoperative evaluation of the upper extremities should be performed when assistive devices will be required for early postoperative ambulation. Rheumatic involvement of the shoulder can prevent effective use of crutches or pose a significant danger to an already diseased shoulder joint should regular crutches be used. Similar involvement of the wrists or hands can make crutch use impossible or dangerous. When use of these assistive devices is anticipated, the physical therapist, physician, or physician's staff can familiarize the patient with the device, give instruction in its use, and monitor the patient's initial practice. Preoperative patient familiarity with these devices can prove quite beneficial in allaying patient fears and helping to ensure the earliest possible ambulatory efforts.

Many rheumatic patients will have unrealistic expectations with regard to the outcome of their surgery. The team can thoroughly assess each patient's overall capacity for rehabilitation. The foot surgeon can assess the anticipated benefits of specific surgeries within this framework. It is essential that each patient be guided to achieve realistic expectations with regard to any surgery performed. In those instances where the patient maintains unrealistic expectations with regard to a specific surgery, the failure of that surgery's outcome to meet his or her expectations may prove sufficient cause for the patient to abandon an overall treatment program and the benefits that can be derived from it.

Use of joint replacements is considered in many rheumatic patients' foot surgeries. The anticipated life span of these implants needs to be evaluated carefully with regard to each specific patient. Patients with rheumatoid arthritis require arthroplasties in which joint replacements may be used at an average of 10 years younger than would be done in similar patients with degenerative joint disease (1). Patients with systemic lupus erythematosus requiring similar surgery are generally young and on high doses of steroids. If these patients have no detectable renal involvement their life expectancy is near normal. Those with renal involvement have a significantly reduced life expectancy. The choice of when to use a joint replacement may therefore be more dependent on a given patient's manifestations of a disease than on the specific disease that the patient may have.

ANTIRHEUMATIC DRUGS

Inflammation with associated swelling, pain, and destructive changes is an inherent part of most rheumatic disorders. Antiinflammatory drugs are usually effective in relieving many of the symptoms of patients with arthritis. Autoimmune pathogenic processes are active in many rheumatic diseases. Immunoregulatory drugs can induce significant improvement and even remissions in patients with such diseases. Gold salts, antimalarial agents, and drugs altering collagen metabolism can provide similar benefits in many arthritic patients. These medications are recognized as antirheumatic drugs. Their efficacy, widespread use, potential side effects, and associated risks warrant thorough familiarization by any surgeon attending patients with rheumatic disorders.

SALICYLATES

Antiinflammatory agents include the salicylates, nonsteroidal antiinflammatory drugs (NSAIDs), and glucocorticoids (steroids). Although these agents are extensively used to treat the symptoms of rheumatic disease there is no substantial or conclusive evidence that they alter the overall course of rheumatic diseases. Aspirin (acetylated salicylate) is the most widely used antiinflammatory agent in rheumatic disorders. It is available under numerous brand names, in a variety of buffered compounds, and in considerable numbers of combination forms. A number of timed release preparations, generally marketed as "arthritis" relief drugs, are also widely available. Aspirin and salicylates are extensively used for control of pain noted in traumatic, degenerative, mechanical, and disease-associated arthropathies. They are used to control fevers associated with rheumatic fever, systemic lupus erythematosus, and juvenile polyarthritis, and less frequently with rheumatoid arthritis, spondyloarthropathies, and other rheumatic diseases.

Whereas single doses of salicylate-containing medication are sufficient to provide mild analgesic and antipyretic efficacy, antiinflammatory effects are only achieved with much higher doses. To obtain a serum salicylate level sufficiently high to provide antiinflammatory activity, 8 to 12 standard 325 mg tablets in divided doses will usually need to be taken daily. At such higher doses (4000 mg per day should not be exceeded) their antiinflammatory effects are used to treat arthritis, pleuritis, and pericarditis in patients with rheumatoid arthritis, systemic lupus erythematosus, and other connective tissue diseases. When salicylates have been effective in controlling these rheumatic symptoms, a preoperative decrease in dosage or abrupt withdrawal can cause recurrence or exacerbation of disease activity. Associated potentially life-threatening flares in disease activity may be noted under such circumstances.

Side effects associated with acute and chronic intake of aspirin can significantly increase the risks of surgery. Gastric upset and gastrointestinal ulceration with potential hemorrhage can be associated with aspirin use. Stress associated with surgery and rehabilitation may increase this risk. Testing of stool for occult blood preoperatively may prove beneficial in detecting gastrointestinal bleeding. The surgeon should be aware that patients taking vitamin C (ascorbate) supplementation may have a false positive guaiac test. In those patients with gastrointestinal problems potentially associated with aspirin use, if continued use of the drug is desirable it should be taken in a buffered form or with antacids. This is especially true in those patients concurrently taking steroids or with potential ethanol intake. The sodium content of buffering agents and antacids used in this manner should be carefully monitored in hypertensive patients.

Another potential side effect of aspirin is increased bleeding time during and after surgery. This is related to acetylation of platelet groups by the acetyl portion of the aspirin molecule. Acetylation of platelets decreases their adhesive properties required in the initial stages of normal clot formation. The acetyl portion of the aspirin molecule can, with prolonged use, induce a hepatitis. This hepatitis decreases the availability of vitamin K dependent clotting factors. It can also alter the rate of detoxification of drugs used in preoperative, intraoperative, and postoperative care. Chronic use of aspirin can also affect renal function. Subsequent decreased renal function can alter the rate of clearance of certain drugs and their metabolites from the body. Resultant buildup of these drugs and their metabolites can produce toxicity and complications. Assessments of prothrombin time, partial thromboplastin time, Ivy or Duke bleeding time, and serum transaminase, creatinine, and uric acid values should be a part of the preoperative assessment of any patient on long term aspirin therapy. This is true for both patients continuing to take the drug and those who have discontinued significant use of it within two weeks to a month before surgery.

Many believe that potential gastrointestinal, hematological, hepatic, and renal side effects warrant routine discontinuation of aspirin use preoperatively. The efficacy of this drug in controlling specific symptoms and disease activities can make such withdrawal unwise and even dangerous. Aspirin tends to be the most effective drug for controlling a number of potentially dangerous rheumatic complications, as with pleuritis in systemic lupus erythematosus. It should never be abruptly withdrawn unless the symptoms and disease activity it is being used to control are understood and a potential flare in those processes is acceptable or unless a safer alternative can be selected. In many of the instances where aspirin withdrawal is deemed advisable nonacetylated salicylates can be effectively used. These include sodium (Pabalate), potassium (Pabalate SF), magnesium (Magan, Mobigesic, Efficin), choline (Arthropan), salsalate- (Disalcid, Mono-Gesic), and choline magnesium (Trilisate) salts of salicylate. A newer nonacetylated salicylate derivative, recently marketed under the brand name of Dolobid, will be discussed later in this section.

Effective replacement can often be accomplished with one of the nonacetylated salicylate drugs. Because of the absence of the acetyl portion of the aspirin molecule, gastrointestinal, hematogenous, hepatic, and renal side effects associated with its presence can be avoided. The presence of salicylate in these compounds may, however, be associated with similar side effects in a limited number of patients, although this has yet to be clearly substantiated. If increased risks of surgery associated with aspirin use are to be avoided through withdrawal or replacement therapy, such action should be taken a minimum of one to two weeks preoperatively.

Aspirin and the nonacetylated salicylates in moderate to low doses can block the activity of the antihyperuricemic agents probenicid and sulfinpyrazone. This should be considered by any surgeon dealing with a hyperuricemic patient who needs to continue taking either of these medications perioperatively.

Inflammation plays an important role in the body's normal defenses against acute and chronic infections. Because aspirin, the salicylates, and the nonsteroidal antiinflammatory drugs exhibit antiinflammatory activity, it would seem that they should affect the course of these infections. In fact the inflammatory impetus of these infections in almost all instances far outweighs the antiinflammatory powers of these drugs. They will not affect the course of such infections (2).

NONSTEROIDAL ANTIINFLAMMATORY DRUGS

The nonsteroidal antiinflammatory drugs comprise a class of agents widely used in acute and long-term management of rheumatic disorders. Those nonsteroidal antiinflammatory agents currently available in the United States are outlined in Table 15.1. These drugs offer analgesic and antiinflammatory activity comparable to, or even greater than, that of salicylates. Their use is also associated with fewer gastrointestinal side effects. They offer more favorable dosing schedules with associated improved patient compliance. Whereas aspirin was historically considered the "first

Table 15.1

Class	Drug	Trade Name	Available Dosage	Usual Dose Frequency	Maximum Daily Dose	Relative Duration
Salicylate derivative	Diflunisal	Dolobid	250 mg, 500 mg	BID	1500 mg	Long
Pyrazole derivative	Phenylbutazone	Butazolidin	100 mg	QID	400 mg	Intermediate
		Butazolidin Alka	100 mg	QID	400 mg	Intermediate
		Azolid	100 mg	QID	400 mg	Intermediate
	Oxyphenbutazone	Tandearil	100 mg	QID	400 mg	Intermediate
		Oxalid	100 mg	QID	400 mg	Intermediate
Pyrole acetic acid derivatives	Indomethacin	Indocin	25 mg, 50 mg	TID	200 mg	Intermediate
		Indocin SR	75 mg	QID-BID	150 mg	Long
	Sulindac	Clinoril	150 mg, 200 mg	BID	400 mg	Long
	Tolmetin Sodium	Tolectin	200 mg	TID-QID	1600 mg	Intermediate
		Tolectin DS	400 mg	TID-QID	1600 mg	Intermediate
Propionic acid derivatives	Ibuprofen	Motrin	300 mg, 400 mg, 600 mg	TID-QID	2400 mg	Intermediate
		Rufen	400 mg	TID-QID	2400 mg	Intermediate
		Nuprin	200 mg	QID	1200 mg	Short
		Advil	200 mg	QID	1200 mg	Short
	Fenoprofen Calcium	Nalfon	200 mg, 300 mg, 600 mg	TID-QID	3200 mg	Intermediate
	Naproxen	Naprosyn	250 mg, 375 mg, 500 mg	BID	1000 mg	Long
	Naproxen Sodium	Anaprox	275 mg	TID-QID	1375 mg	Short
Fenemates	Meclofenamate Sodium	Meclomen	50 mg, 100 mg	QID	400 mg	Intermediate
	Mefenamid Acid	Ponstel	250 mg	QID	1000 mg	Intermediate
Oxicam	Piroxicam	Feldene	10 mg, 20 mg	QID	20 mg	Long

line" drug in the treatment of most rheumatic diseases, many of these drugs have now achieved that status (3). These drugs have become increasingly popular in recent years for reducing narcotic analgesic requirements after foot surgery in both rheumatic and nonrheumatic patients. Their widespread use and potential efficacy warrant foot surgeons' familiarity with their appropriate use, interactions, and side effects.

Many rheumatic candidates for foot surgery present with histories of brief or long-term aspirin, nonsteroidal antiinflammatory drug, and/or steroid use. Actual and potential side effects and interactions of these drugs can increase attendant risks of surgery. They can complicate postoperative care and rehabilitation. Preoperative withdrawal of any such medication must be carefully assessed for each individual patient. Considerations should include the effectiveness of each drug in suppressing or controlling local and systemic disease activity, what effect flares of such activity will have with regard to the intended surgery, and what the efficacy is of potentially comparable replacement drugs.

At first glance it would seem that the replacement of aspirin, another nonsteroidal antiinflammatory drug, or a steroid with a specific nonsteroidal antiinflammatory drug would provide comparable antirheumatic efficacy. Although the efficacy of a specific nonsteroidal antiinflammatory drug is generally comparable to aspirin (salicylates) or other drugs in its class, such efficacy cannot be assumed for any individual patient. Indocin and Butazolidin are usually the most effective agents for use in gout and ankylosing spondylitis. Other nonsteroidal antiinflammatory agents are in most instances far less effective in these diseases. Patients with other rheumatic disorders do, however, show remarkably individualized responses to specific nonsteroidal antiinflammatory drugs (4). Different patients with the same rheumatic disease, and even with similar presenting symptoms and levels of disease activity, will often respond remarkably differently to a given nonsteroidal antiinflammatory drug. Those responding well to one drug may show minimal if any response to a drug of quite similar chemical structure (5). Patient responses to a given drug are usually both individualized and dose-dependent (6). When reduction or replacement of one of the nonsteroidal antiinflammatory drugs is required, such action should be undertaken sufficiently before surgery to ensure the efficacy of the reduced dose or replacement medication.

Inadequate clinical response or untoward side effects may make perioperative replacement of a nonsteroidal antiinflammatory agent advisable. Probability of satisfactory clinical response and/or avoidance of specific side effects is improved when an agent from a different class (Table 15.1) is used.

Therapeutic and economic incentives have led to the marketing of many similar nonsteroidal antiinflammatory drugs during the past few years. This proliferation of available agents and the associated marketing efforts have induced many surgeons to cultivate extensive familiarity with one or a few members of this class of drugs and to limit their prescriptions of such agents to one or a few specific drugs. This may suffice for the needs of those using these drugs solely for the reduction of postoperative narcotic analgesic requirements in nonrheumatic patients. The widespread use, requirement for perioperative continuation, and characteristic efficacy of these drugs in rheumatic patients does, however, warrant that surgeons maintain familiarity with the proper dosing, specific efficacy, side effects, and drug interactions peculiar to each of these agents.

All of these drugs can produce gastrointestinal problems that are best avoided by taking each dose in the middle of a reasonably substantial meal. In patients using these drugs preoperative assessment should be made for potential gastrointestinal distress, anemia secondary to occult blood loss, and gastrointestinal ulceration. Dizziness, headaches, and other CNS-associated side effects can be noted with almost all of these drugs. They are more frequently seen in elderly patients. Patients should be advised to refrain from any potentially dangerous activity during initial use and until they can determine if these side effects are noted. All of these drugs can produce skin rashes and most are capable of producing exceedingly rare ocular side effects. Almost all such agents have produced kidney damage in animal studies, but no such findings have yet appeared in humans. Occasional urinalyses should be performed in patients on chronic use of these agents.

Most of these drugs can affect coagulation. This effect is generally much less prominent than that seen with aspirin use. Such drugs are contraindicated in patients who have nasal polyps and have demonstrated angioedema and bronchospastic reactivity to either aspirin or any other nonsteroidal antiinflammatory drug. Because these agents are mostly detoxified in the liver and eliminated through the kidneys, they should be prescribed with caution in patients with any known hepatic or renal impairment. With the exception of tolmetin sodium, these agents are not recommended for use in children. Nonsteroidal antiinflammatory drugs should be preferentially prescribed in place of hypnotic agents when rheumatic symptoms are the cause of insomnia. They all travel in plasma with some degree of binding to proteins, and can require reduction in use of anticoagulant and oral antihyperglycemic agents. Preoperative assessments of coagulation, bleeding time, and serum glucose should be performed in any patient with a history of recent use of these drugs. All cause a degree of fluid retention that can aggravate or even induce congestive heart failure.

Diflunisal (Dolobid)

Although maintaining antiinflammatory properties diflunisal (Dolobid) is primarily marketed as an analgesic for mild to moderate pain. Substantial postoperative analgesia can be obtained with initial doses of 500 to 1000 mg followed by 250 mg every 8 to 12 hours. Although structurally similar to aspirin diflunisal lacks an acetyl radical. Aberrations in platelet function and bleeding times associated with the acetyl radical are therefore avoided in its use. Concomitant use of antacids containing aluminum salts will decrease the absorption of diflunisal. This drug has a uricosuric effect, increasing renal excretion of uric acid and thereby lowering serum uric acid (7). If used concurrently with acetaminophen, diflunisal will increase that drug's plasma levels. Excessive acetaminophen plasma levels can be associated with hepatotoxicity. Side effects associated with use of this drug are similar to those of the safer members of the nonsteroidal group. Its gastrointestinal side effects are rarely sufficient to justify its discontinuation.

Phenylbutazone (Butazolidin, Butazolidin Alka, Azolid)

Phenylbutazone and its buffered (Alka) form represent one of the most potent, if not the most potent, antiinflammatory agents in this group. The recommended maximum daily dose can be exceeded in treating acute gout. Such a treatment regimen may include a 400 mg loading dose followed by 100 mg every four hours (1000 mg the first day, followed by 600 mg each additional day). Relatively rare but potentially fatal side effects associated with the use of this drug should prevent its use from usually exceeding seven days' duration. Younger patients receiving this drug can develop a non-dose-dependent agranulocytosis that is usually reversible on withdrawal of the drug. Patients over 60 years of age can develop irreversible aplastic anemia with prolonged use. The severity of side effects that may accompany the use of this drug makes its safety questionable in view of the availability of similarly efficacious drugs with far less devastating potential side effects. In those rare cases where long-term use of this drug is warranted, blood testing must be frequently performed. Fluid retention associated with use of this drug limits its safety in hypertensive patients and those with cardiac problems. Such fluid retention can aggravate or even induce congestive heart failure. Unless blood studies clearly document the absence of hematological side effects this drug should be immediately discontinued in any patient receiving it who develops an infection.

Oxyphenbutazone (Tandearil, Oxalid)

The efficacy, indications, and potential hazards associated with oxyphenbutazone's use are essentially the same as those noted for phenylbutazone. Although this drug has a lower incidence of gastrointestinal side effects than does phenylbutazone the potential severity of other similar side effects makes its use seldom warranted.

Indomethacin (Indocin, Indocin Sr)

Concurrent use of indomethacin and diflunisal has resulted in fatal gastrointestinal hemorrhage. This and the potential compounding of other side effects associated with salicylates and nonsteroidal antiinflammatory agents makes concurrent administration of this drug with other antiinflammatory agents inadvisable. Over 10% of those receiving this drug will develop headaches. Concurrent administration of probenecid (Benemid) will increase the plasma levels of indomethacin. This drug can also reduce the efficacy of concurrently administered thiazide diuretics and furosemide (Lasix). It should be used with caution and careful monitoring in hypertensive patients controlled with these medications. In acute gout a loading dose of 100 mg followed by 50 mg three times a day until symptoms subside can be given. A dose of 50 mg two times a day or 25 mg three times a day should then be continued for a few additional days. The incidence of side effects is higher when there is a failure to reduce the dosage of this medication as inflammatory findings decrease during its usage. Because of associated central nervous system side effects its use should be avoided in overtly depressed or unstable patients. It can rarely reduce host resistance to infection. A reversible peripheral neuropathy may also be associated with its use (8, 9). This drug and phenylbutazone are the most efficacious in the treatment of the seronegative arthropathies and gout.

Sulindac (Clinoril)

The structure, efficacy, and side effects associated with sulindac are quite similar to those of indomethacin. This drug does, however, appear to lack most of the central nervous system side effects noted with indomethacin. Prolonged plasma half-life associated with sulindac allows for effective twice daily dosing (10). This drug is a poor choice for postoperative analgesia because about one half of the patients receiving it take up to a week's time to show a beneficial response and others require an even more prolonged trial. Because sulindac travels fairly loosely bound to plasma proteins its use is associated with fewer problems in those patients receiving oral anticoagulants or antihyperglycemic medications than is use of similar nonsteroidal antiinflammatory agents. If a patient is using dimethylsulfoxide concurrently with sulindac a peripheral neuropathy may result (10, 11). This drug has less effect than aspirin on platelet function and has no uricosuric effect. Gastrointestinal side effects are fairly commonly noted with its use.

Tolmetin Sodium (Tolectin, Tolectin Ds)

Tolmetin sodium is the only nonsteroidal antiinflammatory agent currently approved for use in pediatric (over two years of age) patients. Although similar in chemical structure to indomethacin, its similarity is not as great as that of sulindac's structure. This agent usually will not produce significant gastrointestinal blood loss but it can affect coagulation and bleeding times (12). Tolmetin sodium can interact with aspirin and indomethacin and the concurrent use of these medications should be avoided. Like indomethacin and sulindac, tolmetin sodium tends to have

a greater incidence of gastro-intestinal side effects than do the proprionic acid derivatives. About 10% of the patients receiving this drug will have side effects sufficiently severe to warrant its discontinuation. About 15% will have central nervous system side effects, although they tend to be less severe than those seen with indomethacin (13).

Ibuprofen (Motrin, Rufen, Nuprin, Advil)

Although ibuprofen can prolong bleeding time, it shows less platelet inhibition than is demonstrated by aspirin. This manifestation of the drug has not been noted remarkably to affect bleeding times of those patients receiving concurrent anticoagulants. Appropriate monitoring of such patients should, however, be carried out. This agent is remarkably effective as a postoperative analgesic and is one of the safest and most commonly prescribed nonsteroidal antiinflammatory agents. Side effects include potentially severe gastrointestinal and hepatic disturbances, visual alterations (e.g. blurred vision, diminished vision, and alterations in color perception), and fluid retention. As with all other nonsteroidal antiinflammatory medications elevation of liver enzymes (especially serum glutamic-oxaloxcetic transaminase (SGOT) or serum glutamic-pyrodic transaminase (SGPI)) will be noted in up to 15% of those taking this medication (14). Advil and Nuprin are recently introduced over-the-counter 200 mg doses of this drug. They are marketed for the analgesic potency of the drug and have dosages that are probably insufficient to provide any substantial antiinflammatory capability for the average patient taking them.

Fenoprofen (Nalfon)

Fenoprofen is similar in structure, efficacy, analgesic potential, side effects, and safety to ibuprofen. Its tight binding to plasma proteins causes displacement of concurrently used anticoagulants and oral antihyperglycemic drugs. Its rate of excretion is accelerated by concurrent use of aspirin, making such concurrent use inadvisable. Although rare, severe renal side effects including dysuria, cystitis, hematuria, interstitial nephritis, and even nephrotic syndrome may be noted with use of fenoprofen. These side effects are usually preceded by fever, rash, and generalized arthralgias. Oliguria, azotemia, and anuria may herald the onset of associated severe renal side effects (15). Any significant renal or hepatic side effect is sufficient cause to warrant immediate discontinuation of the drug. Concurrent use of phenobarbital will dramatically decrease the plasma half-life and clinical effectiveness of fenoprofen. The author's observations have indicated that this agent has the least gastrointestinal side effects.

Naproxen (Naprosyn, Anaprox)

Anaprox is the sodium salt of naproxen, has a relatively short duration of activity, and is mainly used for its analgesic properties. In acute gout a loading dose of 750 mg of Naprosyn followed by 250 mg every eight hours (initial daily dose of 1250 mg followed by daily doses of 750 mg) may be given. The drug is quite similar in most aspects to ibuprofen and fenoprofen. Its relatively tight binding to plasma proteins makes twice daily dosing quite effective. Although naproxen has been used effectively in children, as of the date of this writing it was not yet approved for pediatric use. Naproxen has recently been reported to be an effective and relatively safe postoperative analgesic in foot surgery (16).

Mefenamid Acid (Ponstel)

Mefenamid acid is marketed as an analgesic even though it has substantial antiinflammatory efficacy. The frequency and severity of side effects associated with this drug's use dictate that it should not be used for periods of greater than seven days. Gastrointestinal side effects are similar to those noted with the propionic acid derivatives, except that up to 15% of those receiving this drug develop bothersome diarrhea. A reversible, autoimmune, Coomb's positive, hemolytic anemia has been noted with use of this drug for greater than 12 months' duration. Mefenamid acid can interfere with oral anticoagulants and oral antihyperglycemic agents. It can also give a false positive diazo test for bile in urine (17). The availability of safer antiinflammatory agents for long-term use precludes the widespread use of this drug in most rheumatic patients.

Meclofenamate (Meclomen)

Meclofenamate is similar in structure and side effects to mefenamid acid, although hemolytic anemia has not been associated with its use. Besides a substantial number of patients receiving this drug getting diarrhea, other side effects can include Stevens-Johnson syndrome, exfoliative dermatitis, and lupus and serum sickness type symptoms in addition to the gastrointestinal, hepatic, and renal side effects potentially noted with any of the nonsteroidal antiinflammatory drugs. Although use of this agent remains a viable choice for patients who have failed sufficiently to respond to other antiinflammatory drugs, the frequency and severity of side effects associated with its use prevent it from being a "first line" drug in rheumatic patients (18).

Piroxicam (Feldene)

Piroxicam has the longest effective dose duration of any of the drugs in this class. This allows for the convenience of once daily dosing but precludes its effective use as an analgesic for acute problems. Concurrent use of aspirin lowers piroxicam blood levels by about 20%, making concurrent use of these two drugs inadvisable (19). Although this drug shares most of the potential side effects of the other drugs of this group it has a rather high incidence of gastrointestinal side effects. The latter side effects can be noted in almost a third of the patients receiving this drug.

GLUCOCORTICOIDS

Many rheumatic candidates for foot surgery will present with histories of ongoing or previous use of glucocorticoid (steroid) medication. The antiinflammatory and immunosuppresive activity of these drugs can provide remarkable relief of rheumatic symptoms. Disabling symptoms and disease activity unresponsive to other medications will occasionally respond quite well to glucocorticoids in ankylosing spondylitis, hemophilic arthropathy, relapsing polychondritis, systemic sclerosis (scleroderma), and Behçet's disease. These drugs can offer dramatic relief where other agents have failed in rheumatoid arthritis, Reiter's syndrome, psoriatic arthritis, enteropathic arthritis, polymyalgia rheumatica, and sarcoid arthropathy. They can prevent blindness in complications of some rheumatic diseases. Use of glucocorticoids can even reduce or eliminate life-threatening disease processes in lupus nephritis, polymyositis, and periarteritis (20).

Glucocorticoids used in the treatment of rheumatic disease include several derivatives of cortisone. Prednisone is usually the drug of choice. Its oral format and suppression of appetite tend to be quite advantageous. Triamcinolone and dexamethasone are occasionally used but the magnitude of their side effects is potentially much greater. The minimum effective dose will vary depending on the individual patient, the specific disease, and the manifestations of that disease requiring treatment with glucocorticoids. Doses as low as 1 or 2 mg of prednisone per day may be effective for controlling arthralgias, whereas doses of 60 mg or more per day can be required for control of life-threatening disease processes such as lupus nephritis.

When treatment is directed against disease manifestations in one or a few joints judicious use of local glucocorticoid instillations into those joints may prove quite effective and avoid the need for systemic therapy. Required systemic glucocorticoid therapy can be offered on one of three regimens: short-term high dose, long-term high dose, and long-term low dose. Side effects increasing the risk of any surgery to patients and potentially jeopardizing the desired operative result are significantly more common and severe during high dose long-term and short-term therapy.

The use of systemic steroid therapy is associated with adverse reactions and drug interactions that can substantially increase the risks of surgery. These can be noted in those taking the equivalent of 5 mg or more per day of prednisone for periods of longer than five days. The incidence and severity of side effects tend to parallel dose levels and durations of intake. Both increase sharply as doses rise above the equivalent of 15 mg per day.

Preoperative evaluation of any rheumatic patient with a history of significant glucocorticoid intake must include a thorough search for and assessment of any related adverse reactions. Appropriate measures should be taken to minimize surgically related risks posed by any such findings. Glucocorticoids promote sodium retention with potassium and hydrogen ion loss from the kidneys, salivary glands, intestinal mucosa, and sweat glands. Steroid-induced edema, fluid retention, and hypertension can usually be well controlled with a low sodium diet and appropriate use of diuretics. Congestive heart failure associated with similar fluid retention can usually be well managed in the same manner. Potassium supplementation may be necessary especially in patients concurrently using glucocorticoids and digitalis. If these fluid and electrolyte imbalances are not adequately attended to, hypercoagulability and subsequent intraoperative and/or postoperative thromboembolic phenomena can occur.

Additional side effects noted with glucocorticoid use include vasculitis, myopathy, muscle atrophy, osteoporosis, fractures, ocular disorders, and pyschological problems. Vasculitis may be either a result of steroid use or of underlying disease processes. Vasculitis associated with systemic lupus erythematosus may respond to increased doses of glucocorticoids but other forms of vasculitis may respond to reduced doses of these drugs. Vasculitis within muscle tissue combined with the effects of glucocorticoids in promoting muscle tissue (protein) breakdown can produce myopathy and subsequent muscle atrophy. This atrophy is usually most prominent in the proximal musculature of the lower extremities. It is usually reversible when the causative drugs can be discontinued, although repair is a prolonged process. Even with active myopathy muscle enzymes in plasma may be normal, but electromyographical studies and biopsies will reveal abnormalities. The mechanisms that induce muscle protein breakdown can also cause loss of protein in the bone matrix. Subsequent osteoporosis can be associated with pathological fractures and slow healing of osteotomies and traumatic fractures (20). Diets rich in calcium salts and vitamin D can help to reverse and even avoid these effects.

Glucocorticoids can decrease patients' visual acuity because of associated formation of occult posterior subcapsular cataracts. They can produce permanent ocular damage through aggravation of or even induction of glaucoma. Ocular herpes simplex infections can be reactivated with initiation or supplementation of glucocorticoid therapy. Use of these drugs is often associated with psychological euphoria, increased appetite, insomnia, secondary depression, and rarely with induction or reactivation of psychoses. This should be considered in obtaining informed consent from suspect patients. These drugs can also induce gastrointestinal ulceration, associated blood loss, and onset or exacerbation of anemia. Their influence in promoting protein and fat breakdown and hepatic glucose production, as well as their effect in decreasing peripheral glucose uptake by cells, produces hyperglycemia that tends to be resistant to control by insulin (21).

Wound healing is suppressed by glucocorticoids. These drugs inhibit glucose uptake and DNA synthesis in fibroblasts (22). They also inhibit collagen synthesis. These actions lead to the formation of scars with relatively decreased tensile strength. Removal of sutures at standard intervals may risk wound dehiscence. Reinforcement of immature postoperative scars with adhesive strips aids in preventing such dehiscence. Precautions should similarly be taken after tendon lengthening procedures, osteotomies, and other procedures, the results of which will in large part depend on the adequate formation and integrity of collagen produced in the healing process.

Even a short course of oral steroids can increase the risk of postoperative infection. These drugs induce reductions in serum immunoglobulins, decrease white blood cell functional capacity, and decrease the access of these cells to antigens. They create a leukocytosis and concurrent monocytopenia by inducing the premature release of neutrophils and retarding the release of monocytes from bone marrow. In the presence of glucocorticoids monocytes have impaired motility, chemotactic ability, and bacteriocidal activity. The total number of granulocytes reaching an inflammatory focus (e.g. operative site or area of infection) is decreased in spite of the peripheral leukocytosis induced by glucocorticoids because these drugs decrease the motility and chemotactic ability of these cells. They also decrease injured or irritated vascular endothelial stickiness. Such stickiness plays an important role in maintaining white blood cells and platelets in injured and irritated vascular areas. Glucocorticoids additionally decrease vascular permeability to white blood cells. These effects decrease host defenses sufficiently to increase the risk of infection, compromise patients' ability to fight established infection, and slow normal postoperative healing (the initial phase of which is dependent on an inflammatory response) (23). Consideration of the use of perioperative prophylactic antibiotics seems quite valid in these patients.

Many rheumatic patients taking glucocorticoids that may suppress their appetites can have deficiencies in vitamin intake. Others may have gastrointestinal problems resulting from their disease and/or medications(s). The effects on wound healing that steroid medications induce will obviously be more pronouced if vitamins necessary for such healing are insufficiently available. Perioperative dietary supplementation with vitamins A, C, and D can be quite beneficial under such circumstances.

Glucocorticoid intake in insulin-dependent diabetics will raise insulin requirements approximately 20%. In spite of the influence of glucocorticoids on glucose production some authorities believe that if the use of these drugs produces sufficient hyperglycemia in an otherwise normoglycemic patient that the patient most likely had incipient primary diabetes (24). Use of steroids can also increase requirements for antihypertensive and glaucoma medications. It can also alter requirements for sedative, antidepressant, and hypnotic medications. Glucocorticoids may reverse the neuromuscular blockade produced by pancuronium during anesthesia administration (25). These drugs also tend to increase the sensitivity of microcirculation to alpha-adrenergic stimulation (20).

Although use of epinephrine-containing local anesthetics has been proven relatively safe in foot surgery these agents are best avoided in patients taking glucocorticoids, because epinephrine's local vascular effects are mediated through alpha-adrenergic stimulation (26).

The lowest possible effective dose of glucocorticoid should be achieved preoperatively. In planning surgery, reduction in daily intake and even potential withdrawal of these drugs may be possible. Any such reduction in intake must be under the careful scrutiny of a rheumatologist or internist thoroughly familiar with the individual patient, the disease, and the potential signs of adrenal insufficiency and potential flares in disease activity that may accompany such dose reductions. Some patients presenting for surgery may have a history of recent unrelated reduction in steroid intake. Others may be taking medications with steroid components of which they are unaware. Still others may conceal the use of such medication. Occasionally a preoperative inventory of a patient's current and past medications can reveal glucocorticoid intake of which the patient was unaware. Some rheumatic patients receiving steroid-containing medications from foreign clinics are quite reluctant to admit to the use of such medication. They may even be unaware of steroid components in such medications.

The adrenal cortices produce an average of 16 mg of hydrocortisone (range 12 to 29 mg per day) under normal circumstances. This production can be increased ten-fold under periods of physical and emotional stress (21). Glucocorticoids are necessary for the body to function normally. Additional amounts are required for the body to resist the deleterious effects of physical and emotional stress. During times of such stress the adrenal glands increase the production of glucocorticoids to meet the demands of the body. Exogenous glucocorticoids taken for two weeks or more can severely depress the adrenal glands' ability to produce glucocorticoids. This suppressive effect can continue for up to a year after the drugs are discontinued (27). Inadequate availability of glucocorticoids can result from withdrawal or excessive reduc-

tion of exogenous drugs, failure of the adrenal glands to respond adequately to increased demand for glucocorticoids, and failure adequately to supplement exogenous agents during times of stress. Signs of adrenal or replacement drug insufficiency include fever, nausea, vomiting, fatigue, weakness, tachycardia, hypotension, increased rheumatic symptoms, and emotional instability. If these signs are not recognized and adequately treated, vascular collapse and death can follow.

The judicious use of steroid coverage during periods of emotional and physical stress associated with surgery can avoid the serious and potentially life-threatening sequelae of glucocorticoid insufficiency. On the other hand, the side effects and risks associated with the use of these drugs make the administration of unnecessary quantities inadvisable. Each patient must be individually assessed with regard to the emotional and physical stress anticipated with the specific surgery planned. An emotionally stable patient taking 2 mg of prednisone per day and undergoing excision of a small skin lesion in the office usually should not have the glucocorticoid intake increased. Failure to increase the intake of an emotionally labile patient taking 30 mg of prednisone per day and undergoing a triple arthrodesis with general anesthesia can have fatal consequences. Local and spinal anesthesia require less additional coverage than does general anesthesia. For limited procedures performed using local anesthesia in patients on low chronic doses of steroids (e.g. under 5 mg of prednisone per day) doubling the oral intake on the day of surgery and for one or two days afterwards may be sufficient. For those with chronic intake of higher doses of steroids a wide variety of formats for increased coverage have been proposed. A general outline of perioperative coverage that will suffice in most instances is presented in Table 15.2.

In those foot, ankle, and leg surgeries associated with extensive physical and or mental stress, the regimens of Plumpton and associates (28) and of Kantor (20) as shown in Table 15.2 have withstood the test of time. A wide variety of other steroid cov-

Table 15.2
Variations in Perioperative Glucocorticoid Coverage Depending on the Level of Associated Physical and Mental Stress

	Perioperative Glucocorticoid Coverage Based on Physical and Mental Stress (M = Daily Maintenance Dose)				
	Minimal Stress	Mild Stress	Moderate Stress	Extensive Stress	
				A	B
Day before surgery	M	M	M × 2	M	50 mg HC
Morning of surgery	M	M	M × 2	100 mg HC	100 mg HC
Intraoperatively	—	—	—	—	100 mg HC/hr
Postoperatively	M	M	M	—	100 mg HC
1st postoperative day	M	M × 2	M × 2	100 mg HC	M + 50 mg HC q8h
2nd postoperative day	M	M × 2	M × 2	100 mg HC	M + 50 mg HC q12h
3rd postoperative day	M	M	M × 2	100 mg HC	M
4th postoperative day	M	M	M	M	M

A—As recommended by Plumpton and associates (28).
B—As recommended by Kantor (20).

erage schedules have been described but none seems to offer significant advantage over these regimens.

In providing additional steroid coverage for surgical patients taking glucocorticoid medications, a number of principles apply. As previously mentioned, excessive amounts should not be administered. Relatively short-acting steroid medication should be used because the effects of any agent given are dependent on both the dose size and how long that dose will be active within the body. Any increased coverage should be withdrawn at the earliest safe opportunity. In many instances glucocorticoids are used in rheumatic patients to lessen significantly but not eliminate the symptoms of their disease. Quantities required to eradicate disease symptoms in such patients are sufficiently high to be associated with grave danger to the patient. Excessive and prolonged steroid coverage for surgical patients may bring a degree of symptom relief that the patient will vehemently desire to maintain. Similarly, increased and excessive coverage may convert a patient from being on the brink of substantial side effects associated with his or her glucocorticoid intake to a point where these side effects become evident. Considering the relative stress associated with most foot, ankle, and leg surgery, these more complex coverage schedules are unwarranted in most instances. Any increased perioperative steroid coverage should be closely monitored by an internist or rheumatologist well-versed with both the individual patient and the regimen used. When psychological stress is a consideration (e.g. with overly apprehensive patients) judicious use of mild tranquilizers (e.g. diazepam or hydroxyzine) can prove quite efficacious in reducing the need for increased steroid coverage.

REMITTIVE DRUGS

Whereas salicylates, nonsteroidal antiinflammatory drugs, and glucocorticoids offer mainly symptomatic relief of rheumatic manifestations, a group of drugs can offer substantial reduction of symptoms, prolonged remissions of disease activity, and even potential cures. These drugs are classified as remittive agents and include antimalarial drugs, gold salts, penicillamine, and immunosuppressive agents. Some rheumatic patients taking these drugs will present for foot surgery. It is essential that these drugs be continued wherever possible during the perioperative period. Intricacies of dosage and potentially severe and life-threatening side effects mandate that administration be carefully supervised by an internist, rheumatologist, or oncologist thoroughly familiar with the specific drug. The surgeon must be aware of the signs and symptoms of side effects that may warrant adjustment of dosage or discontinuation of these drugs. An awareness of these factors is especially important because they may arise many weeks or months after the discontinuation of these drugs. Use of these agents will warrant consideration of modification of standard perioperative routines.

Antimalarial agents are occasionally used in the treatment of rheumatic patients. Although chloroquine was originally used in this regard its side effects tend to be more frequent and severe than those of hydroxychloroquine, which has largely replaced its use. These drugs have a half-life of 73 days in the body and may not be totally excreted for up to one to three years after discontinuation of their use (29). Their side effects can initially present long after withdrawal. These side effects can include partial or complete blindness, dermatitis, flatulence, irritable colon syndrome, and reduced corneal sensitivity. If a patient who is currently taking, or who has taken, one of these agents presents with signs of asymptomatic eye irritation, a thorough search for a foreign body that may not be felt by the patient is warranted. Frequent ophthalmologic examinations should be given during the use of these drugs. If a patient taking one of these drugs has not had such an examination performed for some time before admission the convenience and availability of in-hospital examination may be quite beneficial.

Gold salts are currently the suppressive and remittive drugs of choice in progressive rheumatoid arthritis. They have potentially toxic side effects in almost a third of those patients receiving them. An equal number of patients can develop remissions on use of these drugs (30). Side effects can include urticaria, skin eruptions, mouth ulcers, eosinophilia, leukopenia, and albuminuria. Urinalysis can document substantial protein loss in patients taking these drugs. If the drugs are not withdrawn after the onset of these side effects, severe and potentially life-threatening exfoliative dermatitis, nephritis, and thrombocytopenia can ensue (31). Withdrawal should always be under the close guidance and supervision of a qualified rheumatologist or internist.

Penicillamine is administered to a number of rheumatic patients. This drug has proven useful in many with systemic sclerosis. Early in treatment there tends to be a loss of taste sensation in many patients receiving the drug. This side effect does not usually herald the onset of more severe side effects. Other side effects associated with use of this drug include skin eruptions, gastrointestinal upset, thrombocytopenia, proteinuria, and nephritis. Potentially fatal marrow suppression can also be noted. Cross-sensitivity with penicillin may be noted. Patients presenting with a history of withdrawal of penicillamine because of allergic side effects should receive penicillin only after a thorough search for other alternatives and after careful consideration. This drug affects collagen synthesis and maturation (31). Although there are not as yet definitive studies documenting penicillamine's effect on wound healing, the clinical application of basic research and academic principles indicates potential decreased or slowed wound healing may accompany the use of this drug. Vitamin C supplementation in surgical patients taking this drug may be beneficial.

Immunosuppressive drugs are occasionally used in life-threatening or severe and relentless rheumatic disease. Drugs used are alkylating agents (cyclophosphamide and chlorambucil), purine analogs (6-mercaptopurine and azothioprine), and folic acid antagonists (methotrexate). All of these agents suppress the body's immune response. Treatment with these drugs is neither palliative nor curative and must be closely monitored by a qualified oncologist, rheumatologist, or internist. The side effects of these drugs can include marrow suppression (with increased bleeding time, leukopenia, thrombocytopenia, and potential hemorrhage) and decreased resistance to infection. Hepatic dysfunction can be noted with the purine analogs and folic acid antagonists. Gastrointestinal intolerance can be seen with use of the alkylating agents and folic acid antagonists. Oral ulcerations can occur with the use of folic acid antagonists. All of these agents are potentially cytotoxic.

The increased metabolic demands of cellular elements responsible for healing postoperatively when combined with the presence of these agents can result in delayed healing. The suppressive effects of these drugs on the immune system can dramatically increase the risk of postoperative infection in these patients. When infections do occur they can often result from agents that are rarely pathogens, are difficult to identify, and are resistant to treatment.

Withdrawal or reduction in the dosage of these agents pre-operatively can be accompanied by severe flares in disease activity and symptoms. Some of these can be potentially fatal (e.g. rheumatic pneumonitis or lupus nephritis). Surgical procedures of an elective nature should usually be withheld from these patients except when they are absolutely necessary for functional reasons or for the relief of incapacitating pain. Even under these circumstances procedures should be undertaken with the utmost caution, meticulous planning, and postoperative management. When such procedures are contemplated perioperative antibiotic administration should be considered.

SPECIFIC CONSIDERATIONS IN RHEUMATIC DISEASES

The first two sections of this chapter have dealt with general considerations in rheumatic patients and considerations with regard to medications frequently taken by these patients. This section will deal with specific aspects of rheumatic disease with which the foot surgeon should be cognizant. Many of these can substantially increase surgical risks to the patient's overall well-being and even to his or her life. Others can significantly jeopardize postoperative outcomes.

At the present time there are well over 100 specific rheumatic diseases that are recognized. Almost all of these diseases have extra-articular manifestations. Many such manifestations require careful consideration before undertaking surgical procedures on involved patients. Description in detail of each of these diseases and their specific manifestations that require consideration would necessitate a textbook unto itself. It must be emphasized that most rheumatic diseases can have far-reaching systemic manifestations. Each individual patient with a rheumatic disease is a unique

entity. The following information is intended to demonstrate the extent and degree of extrapedal rheumatic manifestations in a limited number of diseases. An extensive description of potential findings in rheumatoid arthritis is given, because these patients present for foot surgery with a frequency only exceeded by those with degenerative joint disease. Gout is briefly discussed. A limited description of potential findings in the seronegative arthropathies and systemic lupus erythematosus is also presented, because patients with these disorders are probably the next most common groups presenting for foot surgery. It is incumbent on any foot surgeon that he or she maintain a comprehensive text on rheumatology within his or her library. The safety of rheumatic patients treated by any such surgeon will depend in large part on the willingness to review the appropriate sections of such a text as part of the preparation for surgery on any patient with significant rheumatic disease.

Rheumatoid Arthritis

Extrapedal joint involvement in the rheumatoid arthritis patient can involve any synovial joint or combination of synovial joints. If assistive devices are going to be required postoperatively, pre-operative evaluation of the status of those joints used with and affected by those devices is mandatory. In some patients wrist surgery or fusion of the first carpometacarpal joint will be a prerequisite to the successful use of crutches or similar assistive devices. The assessment of potential benefits from any given foot surgery will also depend in great measure on the degree of involvement and functional capacity of other weight-bearing joints. Temporomandibular joint involvement can make intubation difficult and at times impossible. Lower spinal involvement can make the use of spinal anesthetics difficult and even unwise.

Usually asymptomatic, unknown, and potentially hazardous cervical spinal involvement may be noted in 30% to 40% of rheumatoid arthritis patients (32). Five separate types of cervical involvement can be seen. The joint between the first cervical vertebra (atlas) and the occipital region of the skull is a synovial joint that allows extension and flexion of the head on the neck. Rheumatoid pannus formation (proliferative capsular changes) can not only destroy the cartilagenous surfaces of this joint, but can also erode and destroy supporting capsular, ligamentous, and osseous structures. If the atlas is sufficiently thinned or destroyed by this disease process the upward projecting bony process (dens) on the anterior portion of the second cervical vertebra can enter the foramen magnum from which the spinal cord exits the skull. Severe and permanent spinal cord and even brain stem damage resulting from such impingement can result in permanent spinal cord damage and even instantaneous death. A ligament and synovial joint binds the dens behind the front of the atlas. The joint thus created allows for most lateral rotation of the head on the neck. Disease activity here can erode and destroy this ligament. If the dens is not similarly destroyed forward flexion of the head on the neck can drive the dens back into the spinal cord causing permanent spinal cord injury and paralysis. Lateral projection radiographs of the head gently flexed on the neck will reveal no greater than a 3 to 4 mm space (average 3 mm in males and 2.5 mm in females) between the anterior border of the dens and the adjacent posterior border of the anterior section of the atlas when this ligament is intact (33). If a greater space is noted periorbital x-ray studies can assess the degree of destruction of the dens. This type of subluxation is usually associated with upper cervical pain.

The apophyseal joints connecting the cervical vertebral arches are synovial joints and may be involved in rheumatoid arthritis. Such involvement usually presents with posterior muscle splinting and localized pain. If destructive changes in these joints are sufficiently severe, supporting soft tissue structures can be destroyed. Resultant forward displacement of one or more cervical vertebrae on inferior vertebrae can be noted in such instances. The C3 to C4 level is the most common site for such subluxations. Even extensive subluxations often present no local neck pain. They can, however, cause spinal cord compression and neurological signs thereof (e.g. upper extremity paresthesias and weakness). Similar upper extremity findings can be seen as a result of significant thinning of the intervertebral discs secondary to rheumatoid disease activity.

The severity of complications associated with improper manipulation and positioning of affected rheumatoid cervical vertebrae warrants a thorough evaluation of the cervical spine in those patients in whom such manipulation is anticipated (e.g. with general anesthesia and associated intubation). In positioning patients for spinal anesthesia they are often instructed to lie on one side with the lower and cervical spine fully flexed. This maneuver can cause extensive damage to the spinal cord in any rheumatoid arthritis patient with extensive subluxation of the cervical spine. Such patients should be carefully assessed preoperatively and instructed to flex the lower back while extending the cervical area.

Almost one half of patients with rheumatoid arthritis will have involvement of the cricoarytenoid joints of the larynx (34). In a limited number of these patients the vocal cords will become fixed in a position of partial closure. This condition clinically presents as hoarseness in many such patients. Intubation during general anesthesia must be meticulously performed if tears in the vocal cords are to be avoided.

A number of potential extra-articular findings in rheumatoid arthritis patients warrant consideration preoperatively. Rheumatoid nodules are noted in about 25% of involved patients. They tend to occur at sites of excessive pressure on skin. Recurrence following excision is common. Early lesions may respond well to local instillation of glucocorticoids and relief of pressure on the involved area. Where these lesions are excised any underlying bony prominences causing excessive pressure on the involved areas should be

excised when feasible. Postoperatively attempts should be made to shield these areas from excessive external pressures.

The majority of rheumatoid arthritis patients with disease of significant duration present with a mild normocytic hypochromic anemia that parallels disease activity. This is an anemia of chronic disease that involves ineffective red blood cell production and is unresponsive to iron supplementation. Hemoglobin values are usually above 10 gm% unless other causes of bleeding or anemia are contributory. Eosinophilia and thrombocytosis may also be noted.

Pleuritis is fairly common in rheumatoid arthritis. It tends to be mild and seldom presents major clinical or anesthetic problems. Pulmonary interstitial fibrosis is commonly noted in chronic rheumatoid arthritis. A diffuse reticular pattern of fibrosis can be noted on chest radiographs. Diffuse fine rales can be heard throughout the lung fields. Gas exchange at the alveolar level can be impaired in these patients. Occasional pulmonary nodules can be found on chest radiographs of patients with chronic rheumatoid arthritis. In rare instances a rapidly progressive and fatal pulmonary pneumonitis can develop in rheumatoid arthritic patients. Pulmonary hypertension can also be noted in these patients secondary to arteritis of the pulmonary vessels. Patients with pulmonary interstitial fibrosis, with or without concurrent anemia, may benefit substantially from perioperative pulmonary therapy and from a few hours of oxygen therapy during periods of rest each day.

Cardiac complications can be found in the rheumatoid arthritis patient. Pericarditis can precede or accompany the disease in a large number of patients. It is rarely of clinical importance. Other rheumatoid arthritis patients may present with rare cardiac problems related to arteritis or granulomatous deposits within the heart tissue. Related problems can include myocarditis, aortic and mitral valve incompetence, conduction defects, coronary arteritis with or without myocardial infarction, and even disease of the base of the aorta. Thorough preoperative cardiac evaluation is warranted before the administration of general anesthetics or anticipated extensive rehabilitation programs in those with clinical symptoms and/or abnormal electrocardiograms (35).

Vasculitis can present in these patients in one or more of five ways. These include digital arteritis with circumscribed subcutaneous hemorrhages and/or gangrene and cutaneous ulcerations, peripheral neuropathy, pericarditis, visceral arteritis, and acro-osteolysis. These problems are almost exclusively found in patients with both chronic and severe disease activity. Their only clinical manifestation may be in the form of a neuropathy. The neuropathy can be either a mild distal sensory one or a severe sensorimotor (mononeuritis multiplex) one. In the former, sharp, dull, vibratory, and joint position sensation may be diminished in an area as limited as that of the toes. A subjective sensation of burning of the soles may also be reported. In the latter, weakness and even footdrop may be noted on manual muscle testing and examination in addition to the sensory findings. The neuropathy may be present in the absence of significant vasculitis or it can be associated with such vasculitis. Cervical myelopathy, entrapment neuropathies, and drug-induced neuropathies can also be seen in association with rheumatoid arthritis. When vasculitis is present in the feet, foot surgery should only be undertaken in the most serious and rare instances, because extensive gangrene will frequently follow such procedures. Claudicatory visceral pain in rheumatoid arthritis patients is often a sign of visceral arteritis. If this type of pain becomes a constant boring pain the possibility of visceral infarction should be immediately investigated. Such infarction represents an acute surgical emergency. If it cannot be immediately attended to, gangrene will rapidly develop in the involved organs.

The neuropathy present in many rheumatic diseases, and especially in rheumatoid arthritis, scleroderma, and dermatomyositis, can affect the gastrointestinal tract. Some patients will have reduced esophageal motility and a few may only be able to swallow with great difficulty. This should be assessed and considered before intubation for general anesthesia. Intestinal motility may also be markedly impaired in such patients. Constipation may prove to be a problem in the postoperative period in spite of the best efforts to avoid it. Incontinence must also be considered and evaluated because it can lead to contamination of postoperative dressings in addition to great embarrassment for the patient.

A relatively small percentage of those with rheumatoid arthritis will present with Felty's syndrome. Some authorities consider this syndrome as a distinct rheumatic entity. Others consider it a manifestation of rheumatoid arthritis. The syndrome consists of enlargement of the spleen and neutropenia in the presence of rheumatoid arthritis. Although there is not as yet incontravertible proof that those with rheumatoid arthritis have drastically increased susceptibility to infection, it does appear that these patients do have an increased risk of becoming infected postoperatively. Those with Felty's syndrome are extremely prone to infection. White blood cell counts noted in this syndrome are often under 3000 mm^3. Other manifestations of the syndrome can include leg ulcerations, cutaneous hyperpigmentation, lymphadenopathy, and weight loss.

A number of ocular manifestations can accompany rheumatoid arthritis. Rheumatoid nodules can infiltrate the sclera. The disease can be associated with inflammation of the sclera and episclera with keratitis. Scleromalacia (thinning of the sclera) can be noted. The sclera can be reduced to paper thinness, giving the area a bluish hue. Subsequent perforation and blindness can result.

Sjogren's syndrome is considered by some authorities to be a potential manifestation of rheumatoid arthritis, whereas others consider it a distinct entity. It involves rheumatoid arthritis in combination with decreased lacrimal and salivary secretions. The dry eyes of these patients can be damaged during perioperative periods if precautions are not taken to keep them moistened. Many involved patients will carry artificial tears with them. They should be left by the bedside for use as needed. The nursing staff should be instructed to use them during any extended periods when the patient is sufficiently obtunded (e.g. following general anesthesia) to prevent his or her inappropriate use of them. This medication can be taken to the operating room for instillation by the anesthesiologist during prolonged or even fairly brief procedures. Patients may also carry artificial saliva with them. The dry sensation in the mouth that accompanies this syndrome can be most disturbing to those involved. Pre-operative regimens requiring npo midnight status should allow for judicious use of ice chips, lemon swabs, or the patient's own artifical saliva wherever possible. These same measures should be used postoperatively in the recovery room and in the patient's room following general anesthesia or intravenous sedation when the patient may be too obtunded to use them adequately.

Seronegative Spondylarthropathies

The spondyloarthropathies include four diseases that primarily affect the spinal column and are related by an increased incidence of the histocompatibility antigen HLA-B27 in those patients with these diseases as compared to the general population. They include ankylosing spondylitis, Reiter's syndrome, psoriatic arthritis, and enteropathic arthritis. All of these diseases can have extraspinal joint involvement. Such involvement is usually noted in the weight-bearing joints of the lower extremities. Each of these diseases can have extra-articular manifestations that warrant the foot surgeon's consideration.

Fixed flexion of the cervical vertebrae in ankylosing spondylitis can make intubation difficult. Excessive manipulation associated with such intubation can pose a danger to the integrity of the spinal cord. Decreased chest expansion can increase the risk of postoperative respiratory complications. Use of pre-operative and postoperative respiratory therapy when general anesthesia is used, and even the avoidance of general anesthesia when possible, can aid in preventing these complications. Involvement of the lower spine can make the administration of spinal anesthesia quite difficult. Chronic prostatitis, pulmonary, ocular, and cardiovascular extra-articular manifestations in this disease may be noted. When present they warrant appropriate consideration by the surgeon.

Reiter's syndrome can be associated with chronic eye, cardiovascular, pulmonary, and neurological extra-articular manifestations. Extra-articular ocular disease can also be noted in psoriatic arthritis. Patients with psoriatic arthritis have an increased incidence of hyperuricemia and gout. Surgical incisions in patients with Reiter's syndrome, psoriatic arthritis, and enteropathic arthritis should be planned so as to avoid the various skin lesions that may be encountered in these diseases. Enteropathic arthropathy can be associated with malabsorption and corticosteroid induced osteoporosis and dietary deficiencies. Ocular inflammation, amyloidosis, periostitis, chronic hepatitis, pyoderma gangrenosum, and erythema nodosum can also be noted with this disorder. Most of these symptoms and disorders will wax and wane with primary disease activity. The foot surgeon should also anticipate excessive para-articular fibrosis and stiffness following joint surgeries in these patients, as well as in juvenile rheumatoid arthritis patients.

Gout

Patients with a history of gout will have substantially increased risks of postoperative gout attacks in involved joints. Those likely to have such attacks should have meticulous preoperative control of serum urate levels achieved when feasible. Uricosurric agents taken preoperatively should be continued postoperatively. Nonsteroidal antiinflammatory drugs, especially diflunisal (Dolobid), can be used postoperatively to decrease the likelihood of an attack. They can similarly be used to treat any attack that might develop. When an attack develops at a site distant from the surgical area differentiation from septic arthritis is significantly easier than when one develops at the surgical site. The rapid destruction of joint tissue associated with septic arthritis makes consideration of an early joint aspiration mandatory in cases where there is significant difficulty in differentiating the two conditions. Colchicine can be used in treating these attacks. The associated diarrhea that accompanies use of this drug significantly limits its value in postoperative, as well as other, situations.

Intravenous administration of colchicine can be used to avoid the gastrointestinal side effects noted with the oral administration of this drug. Such administration is difficult and potentially dangerous. If any colchicine should leak from the interior of the vein being used into surrounding tissue a quite severe reaction will be noted in that tissue. If the colchicine is administered too quickly phlebitis may develop in the involved vessel. To treat an acute attack of gout 2 mg (4 ml) is administered, followed as necessary by 0.5 mg (1 ml) every six hours. Prophylaxis can be obtained with a dose of 0.5 to 1.0 mg (1 to 2 ml). The drug should not be administered with, or diluted with, 5% dextrose in water or with any solution containing any bacteriostatic agent. If dilution is desired 0.9% sodium chloride solution should be used. Except when a fresh intravenous line has been established preoperatively intravenous use of colchicine is generally not recommended.

Systemic Lupus Erythematosus

Systemic lupus erythematosus (SLE) is a relatively rare rheumatic disease found in less than 0.1% of the population. It is usually associated with a nondeforming arthritis. Vasculitis (as seen in rheumatoid arthritis) and skin lesions are commonly noted in patients with this disorder. When vasculitis does accompany this disease it warrants all of the considerations previously mentioned with regard to that seen in rheumatoid arthritis. These patients are exceedingly prone to infection because of substantially decreased host defenses. Renal disease can be a severe and life-threatening accompaniment to the disease.

Raynaud's phenomenon is frequently noted in this disease. Its presence is a relative contraindication to the use of epinephrine in foot surgery performed on these patients. Gastrointestinal, hepatic, splenic, and ocular manifestations can be noted in SLE. Parotid glands can become unilaterally or bilaterally involved with the disease. Neurological manifestations can include peripheral neuropathies, paralysis, organic brain syndrome, and, rarely, psychosis. Cephalgia can also be a prominent symptom, as can alterations in mood. Depressive episodes are fairly common. Pericarditis, pulmonary manifestations, and hematological abnormalities that can accompany this disease will warrant careful consideration in planning any potential foot surgery. Concurrent care during the perioperative period with a rheumatologist or internist familiar with the individual patients and their disease is mandatory in working with these patients. Myositis can also accompany the disease.

CONCLUSION

Throughout the medical literature dealing with the care of foot disorders the relationship of the foot as an integral part of the body is stressed. Actions taken during the planning, surgical care, and follow-up of these problems can have far-reaching and pronounced local, regional, and systemic effects. In few instances is this more true than in the surgical treatment of rheumatic patients' foot disorders. Appropriate and judicious care must be based on a thorough understanding of the individual patient, the disease, its many clinical and occult manifestations, the drugs being taken to control the signs and symptoms of that disease, and the reasonable functional capabilities of the patient. Carefully planned and executed foot surgery on these patients can provide substantial benefits. Injudiciously performed care can result in complications including, but surely not limited to, permanent blindness or paralysis, incapacitating and potentially irreversible flares in disease activity, and even death. The benefits and the risks associated with such care should never be underestimated.

References

1. Poss R, Ewald FC, Thomas WH, Sledge CB: Complications of total hip replacement arthroplasty in patients with rheumatoid arthritis. *J Bone Joint Surg* 58A:1130, 1976.
2. Robinson HJ, Phares HF, Graessle OE: Prostaglandin synthetase inhibitors and infection. In Robinson HJ, Vane JR (eds): *Prostaglandin Synthetase Inhibitors.* New York, Raven Press, 1974.
3. Dick CD, DeCevlaer K: Non-steroidal antirheumatic drugs. In Kelly WN, Harris ED, Ruddy S, Sledge CB (eds): *Textbook of Rheumatology.* Philadelphia, WB Saunders Co, 1981.
4. Huskisson EC: Anti-inflammatory drugs. *Semin Arthritis Rheum* 7:1, 1977.

5. Capell HA, Rooney JA, Rooney PJ, Murdock RM, Hole DJ, Dick WC, Buchanan WW: A novel method of testing non-steroidal anti-inflammatory analgesics in rheumatoid arthritis. *J Rheumatol* 6:584, 1979.

6. Jacobs JC: Sudden death in arthritic children receiving large doses of indomethacin. *JAMA* 199:32, 1967.

7. Steelman SL, Cirillo VJ, Tempero KF: The chemistry, pharmacology, and clinical pharmacology of diflunisal. *Curr Med Res Opin* 5:506, 1978.

8. Fowler PD: Indomethacin and phenylbutazone. *Clin Rheum Dis* I:267, 1975.

9. Eade OE, Acheson ED, Cuthbert MF, Hawkes CH. Peripheral neuropathy and indomethacin. *Br Med J* 2:266, 1976.

10. Vanarman CG, Risley EA, Noss SW: Pharmacology of sulindac in the treatment of rheumatic disorders. In Hoskisson EC, Franchimont P (eds): *Inflammatory Arthropathies*. New York, Raven Press, 1976

11. *Physicians' Desk Reference*, ed 38. Oradell, NJ, Medical Economics Co, 1984, p 1248.

12. Beirne JA, Bianchine JR, Johnson PC, Wartham GP: Gastrointestinal blood loss caused by tolmetin, aspirin, and indomethacin. *Clin Pharmacol Ther* 16:821, 1974.

13. Ehrlich GE, Roth S: Rheumatoid arthritis: long term treatment with tolmetin sodium. *Orthop Digest* 4:16, 1976.

14. Davies EF, Avery GS: Ibuprofen: a review of its pharmacological properties and therapeutic efficacy in rheumatic disorders. *Drugs* 2:416, 1971.

15. Hill HF, Hill AG, Mowett AG, Ansell B, Mathews JA, Seifert MH, Grumpel JM, Christier GA: Naproxen, a new nonhormonal anti-inflammatory agent. *Ann Rheum Dis* 33:12, 1976.

16. Borovoy M, Holtz P, Kaczander BI: Postoperative analgesia with naproxen in foot surgery. *J Am Podiatry Assoc* 3:125, 1984.

17. Bernardo DE, Currey HL, Mason RM, Fox WR, Weatherall M: Mefanamic and flufenamic acid compared with aspirin and phenylbutazone in rheumatoid arthritis. *Br Med J* 2:342, 1966.

18. *Physicians' Desk Reference*, ed 38. Oradell, NJ, Medical Economics Co, 1984, p 1498.

19. *Physicians' Desk Reference*, ed 38. Oradell, NJ, Medical Economics Co, 1984, p 1557.

20. Kantor TG: Anti-inflammatory and analgesic drugs. In Katz WA(ed): *Rheumatic Diseases: Diagnosis and Management*. Philadelphia, JB Lippincott Co, 1977, p 876.

21. Castles JJ: Clinical pharmacology of glucocorticoids. In McCarty DJ (ed): *Arthritis and Allied Conditions*. Philadelphia, Lea & Febiger, 1979, p 391.

22. Axelrod L: Steroids. In Kelley WN, Harris ED, Ruddy S, Sledge CB (eds): *Textbook of Rheumatology*. Philadelphia, WB Saunders Co, 1981, p 822.

23. Garner RW, Mowat AG, Hazeleman BL: Wound healing after operations in patients with rheumatoid arthritis. *J Bone Joint Surg* 55B:134, 1973.

24. Famacy JP, Brooks PM, Dick WC: Biologic effects of nonsteroidal anti-inflammatory drugs. *Semin Arthritis Rheum* 5:63, 1975.

25. Laflin MJ: Interaction of pancuronium and corticosteroids. *Anesthesia* 47:471, 1977.

26. Roth RD: Utilization of epinephrine containing anesthetic solutions in the toes. *J Am Podiatry Assoc* 71:189, 1981.

27. Gambone VE: Pre-operative evaluation of the surgical patient. In Marcus SA, Block BH (eds): *American College of Foot Surgeons Complications in Foot Surgery, Prevention and Management,* ed 2. Baltimore, Williams & Wilkins, 1984, p 3.

28. Plumpton FS, Besser GM, Cole PV: Corticosteroid treatment and surgery. 2. The management of steroid cover. *Anesthesia* 24:12, 1969.

29. Mackenzie AH: An appraisal of chloroquine. *Arthritis Rheum* 13:280, 1970.

30. Blohm GB: The treatment of rheumatoid arthritis with gold. *Arthritis Rheum* 5:14, 1976.

31. Ehrlich GE: Remittive pharmaceutical agents. In Katz WA (ed): *Rheumatic Diseases, Diagnosis and Management*. Philadelphia, JB Lippincott Co, 1977, p 897.

32. Nakano KK: Neurologic complications in rheumatoid arthritis. *Orthop Clin North Am* 6:861, 1975.

33. Decker JL, Plotz PH: Extracurricular rheumatoid disease. In McCarty DJ (ed) *Arthritis and Allied Conditions,* ed 9. Philadelphia, Lea & Febiger, 1979, p 479.

34. Bienenstock H, Ehrlich GE, Freyberg RH: Rheumatoid arthritis of the cricoarytenoid joint: a clinicopathologic study. *Arthritis Rheum* 6:48, 1963.

35. Harris ED: Rheumatoid arthritis: the clinical spectrum. In Kelley WN, Harris ED, Ruddy S, Sledger CB (eds): *Textbook of Rheumatology*. Philadelphia, WB Saunders Co, 1981, p 953.

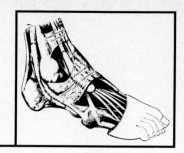

CHAPTER 16

Congenital Disorders

Gary M. Lepow, D.P.M.

Congenital conditions manifesting disorders in the foot and lower extremity can pose special problems for the footcare specialist, particularly when the pathological condition is severe or extensive. Corrective surgery is frequently of significant benefit to the patient in such cases; however, sound surgical judgment and informed participation in a comprehensive health care program are essential. Four major factors must be considered by the podiatric surgeon in determining whether a particular needed surgery is appropriate for a given patient: (a) the patient's life expectancy, (b) the prognosis for ambulation, (c) the patient's mental and physical ability to cope with the stress of surgery, and (d) medical problems associated with the patient's condition that may complicate or contraindicate surgery.

Among the most common congenital conditions that manifest foot disorders are cerebral palsy, spina bifida, muscular dystrophies, and Down's syndrome. Management of each will be discussed in some detail in this chapter.

Other more rare conditions in which foot surgery may be necessary and appropriate include dysautonomia, neurofibromatosis, familial degenerative nerve disease (Friedreich's ataxia, Charcot-Marie-Tooth disease, Roussy-Lévy syndrome), and Marfan's syndrome. Dysautonomia tends to manifest pes planus and indifference to pain. Fibromatosis is characterized by skin, nerve, and intracranial lesions; foot deformities develop secondary to neurological impairment. Familial degenerative nerve disease is frequently associated with cavus deformities. Marfan's syndrome manifests severe pes valgo planus deformity, and tall patients with this type of foot disorder should be screened.

Some conditions, including trisomy 13, trisomy 18, thanatophoric dwarfism, metatrophic dwarfism, Menkes' syndrome, and achondrogenesis II, are so severe that patients rarely survive infancy. Fortunately these conditions are rare, occurring in a ratio of roughly 1 in 4000 to 1 in 10,000 births (1–4).

Surgeons should always be alert to the possibility that a local foot complaint is actually an early manifestation of a more general medical problem. Cerebral palsy and muscular dystrophy in particular present gait disturbances and lower limb disorders as early indications of disease, and some forms of spina bifida may not be apparent until foot or gait problems manifest themselves in childhood or adolescence.

CEREBRAL PALSY

Definition and Classification

Cerebral palsy is a term that describes a wide range of pathological conditions resulting from an intracranial lesion in the central nervous system. The lesion may result from damage occurring in utero, during birth, or in some cases in early infancy. In all cases there is some disturbance of voluntary muscle function and the condition is often associated with some degree of mental impairment. Systems of classification may vary slightly; cerebral palsy is frequently classified according to the tonicity of the primary neuromotor handicap, as spastic paralysis, athetosis, ataxia, rigidity, and tremor (Table 16.l). A lesion affecting several parts of the brain may result in a combination of these conditions.

Spastic paralysis is the most common type of cerebral palsy, comprising roughly 50% of cases identified as such. It results from a lesion at the cerebral cortex. In this type of cerebral palsy a pattern of function is destroyed; there is an irregular distribution of dysfunction and thorough testing is necessary to determine the precise nature and extent of abnormal muscle function. Spasticity manifests an exaggerated stretch reflex, often evidenced by clonus. Although a spastic muscle is usually weaker than a normal one, it tends to overpower its antagonist because it does not relax normally. On palpation muscles of the extremities may be flaccid. Atonia or hypotonia, a condition in which muscles do not respond to volitional stimulation, is often associated with spastic paralysis.

Spastic paralysis may be further identified according to the number of limbs involved. Hemiplegia denotes the involvement of two limbs on the same side, paraplegia the involvement of two legs, and quad-

Table 16.1
Summary of Findings in Children with Cerebral Palsy

Diagnosis	Spastic Hemiplegia	Spastic Paraplegia	Spastic Quadriplegia	Atonic	Athetosis and Tremor	Rigidity	Ataxic
History							
Family				Consanguinity, Genetic disorder, Maternal illness			Genetic disorder
Prenatal							
1st Trimester			Rubella				
3rd Trimester	Toxemia		Toxemia pregnancy		Anoxia, Placenta praevia		
Obstetrical	Trauma	Breech	Trauma, Precipitate Delivery, Caesarean		Placenta abruptio, Breech, Anoxia	Precipitate Delivery Caesarean	Precipitate Delivery Caesarean
Postnatal	Prematurity				Hemolytic anemia, Kernicterus		
Infancy	Meningitis						
Physical findings							
General		Hydrocephaly, Average weight	Microcephaly	Undersized	Underweight		
Cranial nerves	Strabismus						
Deep reflexes	Increased unilateral	Increased bilateral, both legs	Increased, all extremities especially legs		Normal		Hypotonic
Pathologic reflexes	Babinski, Stretch, Clonus } unilateral	Stretch, Babinski, Clonus } both legs	Stretch, Babinski, Clonus, Abdominal		Babinski		
Movement					Abnormal	Pipe stem	
Tonus	Hypertonic, especially upper extremity	Hypertonic, both legs	Hypertonic, especially legs	Hypotonic, all extremities			Hypotonic
Gait	Spastic	Spastic	Spastic	None	Uncoordinated		Ataxic
Associated disorders	O Behavior, Visual/perceptual/motor	Mental, Retardation, Convulsions	Mental, Retardation, Convulsions	Mental, Retardation, Convulsions	Hearing, Vision, Behavior		Variable

riplegia the involvement of four limbs. Diplegia is a term sometimes used to describe a symmetrical paralysis that is more severe in the lower limbs than in the upper limbs.

Spasticity tends to afflict specific muscle groups. In the lower extremity, for instance, congenital spastic paralysis is likely to produce flexion, adduction, and medial rotational disorders. A "scissors" gait, resulting from these disorders, is characteristic of spastic paralysis.

In athetosis the primary lesion is at the base of the brain. It is characterized by involuntary motions of any or all of the extremities and the face. Such motion may make the patient appear to be mentally retarded or emotionally disturbed, but cerebral palsy does not always affect mental capacity. Muscle tension frequently develops as a mechanism by which the patient attempts to control involuntary motions but does not constitute true spasticity. The absence of an exaggerated stretch reflex distinguishes so-called tension athetoids from true spastics.

Ataxia is caused by lesions at the cerebellum that result in impairment or destruction of the kinesthetic sense. Loss of balance, a lurching "drunken" gait, hypermobility of the joints, and slow acquisition of ambulatory skill are characteristic of patients afflicted with ataxia. Such patients can learn balance control and often show spontaneous improvement. A short tendo achillis frequently is associated with this condition as a consequence of delayed walking.

In rigidity the lesion may be at the base of the brain or it may be diffuse. There is a loss of muscle elasticity and rigidity may be either intermittent or constant. When constant rigidity is present considerable mental impairment is likely.

Tremor is also caused by a lesion at the base of the brain. Tremor caused by such a lesion is usually not congenital but is secondary to encephalitis and generally responds to medication (5–9).

Considerations for the Podiatric Surgeon

Surgery may be indicated to correct foot disorders associated with cerebral palsy. The following factors, however, must be taken into account when surgery is considered. First, the severity of the handicap as determined by the nature and extent of brain damage. Some cerebral palsy patients have a good prognosis for ambulation, with or without mechanical aids, but some do not; the prognosis for an individual depends primarily on the patient's neuromuscular condition rather than specific correctible deformities of the lower extremities. Comparison of the neurological and chronological age on the basis of primitive motor activity patterns gives a reliable indication of the prognosis for ambulation. Second, associated cerebral handicaps, such as convulsive disorders, may contraindicate surgery designed to promote ambulation. Third, the patient and parents or guardians must be able to cooperate in postoperative care and rehabilitation if surgery is to be effective. They should be informed that the postoperative phase may be lengthy

and that it will be some time before the foot can be used for weight bearing or shoes can be fitted. Fourth, the patient's mental capacity should always be considered, although many patients are not mentally impaired and diminished mental capacity does not of itself necessarily contraindicate surgery (5,10).

Principles of Surgical Management

Foot disorders in cerebral palsy patients can often be managed conservatively. Surgery, however, can play an important role in correcting local deformities that do not respond to conservative treatment. Podiatric surgery has the following general goals: (a) to correct static or dynamic deformity, (b) to stabilize joints, and (c) to balance muscle power. The latter may be particularly problematic.

Early surgery is advisable although repetition may be necessary to achieve or maintain correction. Surgery is primarily useful in treating disorders related to spastic paralysis. Its use in managing athetosis is increasing and it is sometimes used to treat postural contractures. Surgery is rarely indicated in cases of rigidity. Thorough muscle testing is essential when planning surgery for any type of foot disorder secondary to cerebral palsy. Moreover, specific foot deformities may be secondary to flexion/adduction deformities of the hip and knee, and in this case correction at the hip is essential if foot surgery is to be effective.

Equinus deformities are the most common foot disorders associated with cerebral palsy and are caused by one of the following mechanisms: spastic triceps surae versus spastic, normal, or flaccid dorsiflexors; normal triceps surae versus flaccid dorsiflexors; or flaccid triceps surae versus flaccid dorsiflexors. Conservative management is often successful if initiated early. An equinus deformity, however, tends to recur as the patient grows. A rocker-bottom deformity may result from the heel being forced into valgus to make ground contact; the talus, losing support from the sustenaculum tali, takes a vertical position and the forefoot dorsiflexes on the rearfoot. Lengthening of the tendo calcaneus, or the tendon of m. gastrocnemius, neurectomy of one or more branches of the tibial nerve to the m. gastrocnemius or m. soleus, or a Silferskiold gastrocnemius recession may be appropriate procedures for the correction of equinus, depending on which abnormal mechanism is causing the deformity. In rigid deformities extra-articular subtalar arthrodesis may be indicated for children, triple arthrodesis for adults.

Varus deformities usually result from an imbalance of evertors and invertors, particularly m. tibialis posterior and the peronei. Equinovarus tends to be seen in conjunction with hemiplegia. Several types of surgery are possible to correct the condition, including the following: (a) anterolateral transfer of the tendon of m. tibialis posterior through the interosseous membrane, (b) transfer of the tendons of m. extensor hallucis longus and tibialis anterior to the dorsum of the foot (indicated in treating equinovarus), (c) lengthening—but not a total resection and release—

of m. tibialis posterior, (d) anterior rerouting of m. tibialis posterior (anterior to the medial malleolus), and (e) calcaneal osteotomies.

Valgus deformities are caused by contracture of the triceps surae or overactivity of m. peroneus brevis and other evertors in the presence of weak invertors. Equinovalgus is often associated with diplegia. Conservative management is usually indicated in early childhood. If the valgus persists a subtalar extraarticular arthrodesis may be indicated. Other corrective procedures may include calcaneal osteotomy and/or a sliding tendo achillis lengthening with fractional lengthening of the peronei. A valgus rearfoot in cerebral palsy is often accompanied by a hallux valgus deformity, which can be corrected by standard procedures.

Clawtoes, caused by an imbalance of intrinsic muscles, are often associated with spastic paralysis. Burman's neurectomy (12) is usually the procedure of choice for correction of this deformity. If flexion contractures of the digits are caused by spastic toe flexors it is important to release these by tenotomies in the proximal phalanges before any lengthening of the tendo achillis is performed.

An adduction deformity of the forefoot may be caused by spasticity at the m. abductor hallucis following surgical lengthening of the triceps surae. The condition can be corrected by a resection of a 2.5 cm segment of the m. abductor hallucis muscle and its tendon (5, 8–12).

SPINA BIFIDA

Definition and Classification

Spina bifida is a defect of the spinal column consisting in an absence of or failure of fusion between vertebral arches. In spina bifida occulta there is no protrusion of intraspinal contents and no external cyst; this is a relatively common condition that does not present significant neurological or musculo-skeletal abnormality and rarely requires surgical management. In meningocele a visible meningeal sac is presented along the spinal axia but myelodysplasia is absent and the sac contains no nerve tissue. In myelomeningocele cystic distension of the meninges is present along with myelodysplasia and the presence of nerve tissue in or adherent to the sac. Myelomeningocele is frequently associated with Arnold-Chiari syndrome, a congenital neurological defect characterized by hindbrain abnormalities and hydrocephalus. Myelomeningocele occurs in about 0.5 to 2 births per 1000 in the United States. It causes significant neurologic impairment and multiple handicaps. The pattern of deformity and paralysis depends largely on the level of the primary lesion (Table 16.2). Ethical questions have been raised concerning the advisability of aggressive treatment for severely handicapped infants. The patient with myelomeningocele can, however, lead a useful and satisfying life. Children who survive infancy often have the potential for independent locomotion; thus the podiatric surgeon has a significant

role to play on the interdisciplinary medical team responsible for patient care (8, 13, 14).

Special Considerations for the Podiatric Surgeon

Consultation with other specialists, leading to a plan for comprehensive treatment, should be initiated in early infancy when spina bifida is presented. Nearly all children afflicted with myelomeningocele will be found to require some form of podiatric attention. Foot deformities secondary to myelomeningocele are complicated by sensory loss and vascular impairment. Necrosis may develop after relatively minor surgery and is sometimes severe enough to make amputation necessary. Any undue pressure on plantar skin can cause serious problems, in part because of sensory and vascular disorders, in part because children with myelomeningocele are likely to be obese and to have small feet; thus the reduced weight bearing surface is likely to be heavily loaded. Pathological fractures are fairly common, because of osteoporotic bones and the patient's inability to sense abnormal stress or trauma. Myelomeningocele tends to present congenital foot disorders that are extremely difficult to manage. Some feet behave as if patterned to a particular deformity and in many cases permanent correction is not obtained by primary surgery. Moreover, given the physiological problems associated with myelomenengocele, surgical procedures can give rise to new disorders requiring further treatment.

Although spina bifida occulta does not commonly present serious problems, neuromuscular complications not evident at birth do occur in some patients. Often the symptoms of neuromuscular abnormality are gait disturbance and foot deformity. These symptoms will usually appear in childhood, but onset may be delayed until the second or third decade and possibly later. Careful neurological testing should be performed when patients present muscle weakness, leg length inequality, decreased sensation and reflex actions, mal perforans, and pes cavus. Tax and associates (16) have reported diagnosing diastematomyelia, a form of spinal dysraphism, on the basis of unilateral atrophy and pes cavus in a six-year-old (8, 10, 14–16).

Principles of Surgical Management

The goals of surgery are to produce a foot that allows maximum function, that will withstand trauma, and that has an acceptable appearance. Paralysis, muscle imbalance, and sensory impairment are the major problems to be addressed. Treatment should aim to prevent or correct deformity, correct or improve muscle imbalance, and compensate for joint instability. In treating deformities secondary to myelomeningocele, exceptions are sometimes made to the general contraindication of procedures in bone before the patient has reached skeletal maturity.

Pes varus or equinovarus is commonly seen in association with myelomeningocele, usually as a result of weak dorsiflexors in the presence of strong plantar-

Table 16.2
Effects of Paralysis Below Various Lesions in Myelomeningocele. (From Mishaline MA, Dockery GL: Spina bifida and its effect on the lower extremities. *J Am Podiatry Assoc* 70:84–88, 1980, Table 1, p. 86.)

Paralysis Below	Results In	Appearance of Lower Extremity
T_{12}	Complete lower limb paralysis; position of limbs due to gravity.	
L_1	Weak flexor power at hip due to the sartorius and iliopsoas; upper limb flexed and externally rotated at the hip.	
L_2	Strong hip flexors, adductors and lateral rotaters, limb is flexed, abducted, and laterally rotated; hip dislocation likely; feet equinovarus.	
L_3	Same as above and good power in the quadriceps, limb extended, adducted, laterally rotated with limited knee flexion, hip dislocation likely.	
L_4	Normal hip flexors, adductors, and quadriceps; knee in recurvatum, foot in calcaneovarus; severe deformity of flexion, adduction and lateral rotation of the hip, hip dislocation at birth.	
L_5	All above muscles normal plus gluteus medius, minimus, and extensors compartment of leg; mild flexion and adduction deformity of the hips but no dislocation, foot in calcaneus.	
S_1	Only deformity is in the foot; talipes calcaneus.	
S_2	Only weakness is in the intrinsics of the feet; pes cavus and claw toes.	

flexors and invertors. Frequently a severe, rigid form of the disorder is present at birth. The deformity may be related to a lesion at L3 or L4, and may also be associated with Arnold-Chiari malformations. Conservative management may be effective in obtaining a plantigrade foot and passive stretching exercises are recommended in milder cases. If casts are used special care must be taken to avoid ulceration. It is prudent to assume that the foot is partially or totally anesthetic. If the varus or equinovarus condition does not respond to conservative treatment surgery may be indicated.

For infants and children the following soft tissue procedures may be effective: lengthening of the tendo achillis, release of posterior tibial and long toe flexor muscles, release of plantar toe flexors, tenotomy of the tendo achillis, posterior medial capsular release, and/or split tibialis anterior tendon transfer to the third cuneiform. Older patients in whom skeletal maturity is complete may benefit from tarsometatarsal capsulotomies, cuboid decancellation, metatarsal osteotomy, midtarsal osteotomy, calcaneal osteotomy, excision of the talus, or triple arthrodesis.

Pes calcaneus is sometimes caused by the muscle imbalance secondary to myelomeningocele, particularly by the combination of weak calf muscles and strong anterior leg muscles. An imbalance between m. tibialis posterior and m. tibialis anterior may result in a calcaneovarus deformity. Calcaneovalgus may be caused by the displacement of the peronei anterior to the lateral malleoli. These deformities may be related to a lesion at the fifth lumbar level. Although calcaneovalgus deformities may respond to passive stretching and casting appropriate tendon transfer is usually indicated at an early age. After surgery, casts, splints, and passive stretching exercises may be used to maintain normal alignment.

Paralytic convex pes valgus (vertical talus) is occasionally present. The specific pathogenesis of this disorder in the patient with myelomeningocele is unclear. Clinically the foot presents a plantarflexed talus, a subluxated or dislocated talonavicular joint, and forefoot abduction and dorsiflexion. Early surgical correction is often indicated and may include reduction of the talonavicular dislocation, maintained by a Kirschner wire, and appropriate tendon transfers.

Pes cavus and clawtoes can result from paralytic muscle imbalance associated with myelomeningocele. This disorder may be related to a lesion at the first two sacral neurosegments. Appropriate treatment for these disorders depends on the severity and precise nature of the abnormality; cavus deformities are discussed elsewhere in the text. Special care should be given to deformities of the toes and forefoot associated with myelomeningocele because of a tendency for pressure sores to develop (5, 8, 10–15).

MUSCULAR DYSTROPHY

Definition and Classification

Motor unit diseases, which encompass the muscular dystrophies, affect the lower motor neuron and muscle fibers innervated by it. Table 16.3 indicates differential diagnosis for the principal forms of muscular dystrophy. Duchenne's muscular dystrophy, with which this chapter will primarily be concerned, is a relatively common, progressive, debilitating type of motor unit disease; it is classified as a myopathy, indicating that the primary disorder is in the muscle tissue itself.

Progressive muscular dystrophy occurs in roughly 4 out of 100,000 children. Duchenne's dystrophy is an autosomal sex-linked recessive disorder that occurs only in boys. Clinical symptoms are pseudohypertrophy, weakness, atrophy, loss of reflexes, secondary contractures and deformities, and mental impairment. Leg weakness, an early symptom, begins at three to four years of age. The disease progresses rapidly and walking ceases at about 12 years of age; death usually occurs in the late twenties or early thirties, often because of cardiopulmonary failure. Muscle weakness is not uniform. In the lower extremity ankle plantar flexors are generally stronger than dorsiflexors and invertors are stronger than evertors. Imbalances at the hip, knee, ankle, and subtalar joint tend to cause soft tissue contractures(8, 17).

Principles of Surgical Management

All treatment of progessive muscular dystrophy is directed toward the management of secondary problems to retain maximum functional ability. There is no cure or definitive treatment for the disease itself. The primary goal of podiatric surgery is to keep the patient ambulatory for as long as possible, although surgery may also be beneficial to wheelchair patients in some cases. Because the disease is rapidly progressive appropriate treatment varies according to the stage of the disease and the corresponding biomechanical pathology.

In the early ambulatory stage muscle imbalance is caused by hypertrophy of the calf muscles and weakness of the quadriceps and m. tibialis anterior. This leads to a strong gastrocnemius pull that favors the development of equinus. Treatment is generally conservative at this stage. Heel cord stretching, which may be performed by the parents, is indicated, as is the use of long-leg night splints.

In the late ambulatory stage the foot presents dynamic deformities due to increasing muscular imbalance. Varus deformities are caused by the pull of a strong m. tibialis anterior in the presence of weak peronei. Equinus contractures, which throw weight onto the forefoot, lead to a shortened and unstable gait pattern. Fixed deformities will appear if the deforming forces are allowed to persist. Hence corrective surgery is generally indicated at this stage. Bracing may be an important adjunct to surgical procedures but bracing alone is not recommended because bracing a deformed limb may lead to painful complications in the ambulatory patient. Lengthening of the tendo achillis is indicated for equinus contracture deformities. The procedure is often followed by subcutaneous release of anterior and posterior tibial tendons and plantar fasciotomy. Other appropriate procedures are tendo achillis lengthening in conjunction with posterior tibial tendon transfer and soft tissue release.

In the early wheelchair stage preexisting deformities persist and muscle imbalance progresses. The action of a strong posterior tibial muscle favors the development of equinovarus. The forefoot often dangles from the footrest; although this can be useful to the patient in propelling the chair, the force of gravity and abnormal muscle pull favor the development of equinocavovarus. At this stage conservative treatment is indicated. Daily range of motion exercises of the feet and ankles improves circulation and night or positioning splints may be useful.

In the late wheelchair stage the foot presents well-established deformities. The symptomology includes

Table 16.3
Differential Diagnosis of the Principal Types of Muscular Dystrophy

Clinical Features	Duchenne Type Muscular Dystrophy	Limb Girdle Muscular Dystrophy	Facioscapulo-humeral Muscular Dystrophy	Distal Muscular Dystrophy	Progressive Dystrophia Ophthalmoplegia	Congenital or Infantile Muscular Dystrophy
Incidence	Commonest	Less common, but not infrequent	Not common	Rare	Rare	Rare
Age at onset	Usually prior to 3 yr., some between 3 and 6 yr.	Variable (usually by second decade, occasionally later)	Variable (usually in second decade)	20–77 yr. (mean 47 yr.)	At any age (infancy to over 50 yr.)	At or soon after birth
Sex preponderence	Male	Either sex	Male and female equally affected	Either sex	Either sex	Not yet determined
Inheritance	Sex-linked recessive, autosomal less than 10 per cent	Autosomal recessive, on rare occasions autosomal dominant	Autosomal dominant usually, autosomal recessive very rarely	Autosomal dominant	Simple dominant or simple recessive	Unknown
Pattern of muscle involvement	Proximal (pelvic and shoulder girdle muscles affected early, spreads so periphery of limbs late in course)	Proximal (shoulder and pelvic girdle, spreads to periphery late)	Face and shoulder girdle; later spreads to pelvic girdle	Distal (hand first, anterior tibial, and calf in leg)	Usually limited to external ocular muscles	Generalized
Muscles spared until late	Gastrocnemius, toe flexors posterior tibial, hamstrings, hand muscles, upper trapezius, biceps, triceps, face, jaw pharyngeal, laryngeal, and ocular	In upper extremity brachioradialis and hand, calf muscles	Back extensors, iliopsoas, hip abductors, quadriceps	Proximal until late	See above	— — — —
Pseudohypertrophy	8 per cent of cases (calf muscles)	Less than 33 per cent of cases	Rare	Not seen	Not seen	Not seen
Myotonia	Absent	Absent	Absent	Absent	Absent	Absent
Contractural deformities	Common	Develop late in course, less severe than Duchenne	Mild, occur late	Mild, late	— — —	Severe
Scoliosis and kyphoscoliosis	Common in late stage	Mild, in late stage	Mild, occur late	— — —	— — —	?
Heart involvement	Hypertrophy and tachycardia common; in late stages widespread degeneration, fibrosis, and fatty infiltration	Very rare	Very rare	Very rare	Not seen	Not observed
Endocrine changes	Not seen	Not seen	Not seen	Not seen	Not seen	?
Intellectual level	Commonly decreased	Normal	Normal	Normal	Normal	?
Course	Steady rapid progression	Slow progression, considerable variation in pace of disease	Progresses insidiously	Comparatively benign	Slow progression	Steady progression

pain and pressure sores at bony prominences or points of contact with the chair. Although the foot is now nonfunctional, palliative surgery may be indicated to alleviate pain and/or to correct deformities that make it difficult to position the foot on the footrest or to obtain suitable footwear. Appropriate procedures include tendo achillis lengthening, plantar fasciotomy, and medial release. Medical evaluation before surgery is essential, as is consultation with the anesthesiolo-gist. Anesthesia should be minimal in terms of depth and time. The potential benefits to the patient should be considered in relation to surgical risks, keeping in mind the patient's limited life expectancy (17).

Related Diseases

Becker's muscular dystrophy is a less common, milder, and less rapidly progressive disease than Duchenne's muscular dystrophy. Patients generally have a longer life expectancy. The disease manifests itself in the second decade of life. The first stage includes the development of an equinus gait, often at age 13 or 14. Conservative management is indicated at this stage. The patient becomes wheelchair dependent by the late twenties or early thirties. Soft tissue releases, followed by bracing, may be indicated.

Myotonic dystrophy is a progressive familial myopathy with associated myotonia. Onset usually occurs in late adolescence or early adulthood; in second generation patients the disease usually begins in childhood and is more severe. Most patients are wheelchair-dependent within 20 years of the onset of symptoms and have a shortened life expectancy. There is a distal distribution of muscle weakness and an early involvement of m. tibialis anterior and the peronei. Equinocavovarus is the most frequent severe foot disorder. Podiatric surgery is not often indicated because correctible deformities of the foot are usually not severe. Although the foot is still functional the shoe may be modified to correct gait and relieve pain. Later, orthoses and braces may be helpful in alleviating footdrop.

Spinal muscular atrophy includes a variety of syndromes that produce varying degrees of muscle wasting and weakness, such as Werdnig-Hoffman disease. Surgery may be indicated for patients who are not generally and severely handicapped (8, 17).

DOWN'S SYNDROME
Definition and Description

Down's syndrome, or trisomy 21, is an autosomal chromosome abnormality. It is the most common chromosomal abnormality, occuring in roughly 1 in 700 births. Clinically Down's syndrome presents hypotonia, short broad hands with a simian crease on the palm, short legs, hyperflexibility of the joints, upward slanting of the eyes, epicanthic folds, a furrowed and protruding tongue, a flat broad face, and a widely spaced first and second toe with a plantar furrow proceeding from this cleft. Patients are mentally retarded; IQs range from 25 to 70 and tend to decline with age. Associated medical problems include congenital heart disease, pulmonary and respiratory tract infections, and leukemia. Life expectancy varies considerably depending on the nature and severity of associated medical problems.

There is a 40% first-year mortality rate if congenital heart disease is present. Fifteen percent of infants without heart disease do not survive the first year. Of infants without heart disease who do survive the first year 75% survive the next 10 years. The 10-year survival rate for males with heart disease is 44.9%, for females with heart disease, 32%. Life expectancy studies on institutionalized patients show that death usually occurs at age 30 to 35 years, although some patients reach the fifth decade, and evidence suggests that, in the absence of heart disease, patients who receive appropriate medical care can have normal life spans.

Many patients have considerable social and educational potential. This depends of course on the degree of mental impairment but the majority can learn basic self-care skills and can live in the community with moderate supervision. Many, if adequately supervised, can work outside of special institutions. Down's syndrome patients have poor communications skills but the mean social age is three years, four months above mental age. They are generally affectionate, sociable people who have a good capacity for social adjustment. Recent studies indicate that home care is preferable to institutionalization, but because physical and mental disturbances may vary greatly from one patient to another, all treatment must be directed to the individual case. From 1950 to the present there has been a strong emphasis on the concept of habilitation in treating Down's syndrome patients; the term implies the use of a variety of professional services aimed at helping the patient function as effectively as possible, making maximal use of his or her potential (2, 4, 18, 19).

Podiatric Care

Robert Collette has noted that, in his capacity as medical director at a school for children with Down's syndrome, there is some foot pathology in 100% of the patients he sees (20). The most common foot disorder is pes plano valgus deformity with juvenile hallux valgus. Other disorders sometimes associated with Down's syndrome are retroposition of the fourth toe, syndactyly, and pes cavus. Down's does not, however, manifest specific major foot deformities. Patients may present such conditions at a frequency consistent with what the surgeon would see in general practice.

In recent years there has been a significant movement in the United States toward Special Olympics for the mentally retarded, a large percentage of whom are Down's syndrome patients. As a result a number of sports-related injuries are now being seen in these patients, who are not always adequately trained for competitive physical activities. The establishment of a rigorous training program is obviously problematic for such persons. Injuries then can result when tasks are attempted for which the patient is unprepared.

Mental age and life status will generally determine whether a patient can tolerate the emotional stress of surgery and postoperative care. If the mental age is that of an adolescent the patient should be able to tolerate surgery well; patients whose mental ages are less than adolescent will need much closer supervision, such as that provided by a home environment. Surgery may be helpful to patients both in relieving symptoms and in improving self-image by correcting a deformity. In general good podiatric care may promote the Down's syndrome patient's ability to live independently and to contribute to society.

References
1. Epps CR, Diamond LS: Generalized genetic disturbances involving the foot. In Jahss MH: *Disorders of the Foot*, vol 1.

Philadelphia, WB Saunders Co, 1982.
2. Darter CH: *Handbook of Mental Retardation Syndromes*, ed 3. Springfield, Il, Charles C Thomas, 1975.
3. Memolascina FJ, Egger ML: *Medical Dimensions of Mental Retardation*. Lincoln, University of Nebraska Press, 1978.
4. Scarsrough PR, Finley WH, Finley SC: A review of trisomies 21, 18, and 13. *Ala J Med Sci* 19:174–188, 1982.
5. Ingram AJ: Miscellaneous afflictions of the nervous system. In Crenshaw AH (ed): *Campbell's Operative Orthopaedics*, ed 5, vol 2. St Louis, The CV Mosby Co, 1971.
6. Moncton G: Signs and symptoms of neurologic disease affecting gait and locomotion. In Weinstein F (ed): *Principles and Practice of Podiatry*. Philadelphia, Lea & Febiger, 1968.
7. Denhoff E: Medical aspects of cerebral palsy. In Cruickshank WM (ed): *Cerebral Palsy: A Developmental Disability*, ed 3. Syracuse, Syracuse University Press, 1976.
8. Tachdjian MO: *Pediatric Orthopedics*, vol 2. Philadelphia, WB Saunders Co, 1982.
9. Schlefman BS, McGlamry ED, Bodamer PE: Severe pes valgus in spastic diplegia. *J Am Podiatry Assoc* 73:133–140, 1981.
10. Walker G: Neurologic conditions of the foot in childhood. In Helfet AJ, Gruebel Lee DM (eds): *Disorders of the Foot*. Philadelphia, JB Lippincott Co, 1980.
11. Silferskiold N: Reduction of the uncrossed two-joint muscles of the leg to one-joint muscles in spastic conditions. *Acta Chir Scand* 56:315, 1923–1924.
12. Burman BS: Spastic intrinsic-muscle imbalance of the foot. *J Bone Joint Surg* 20:145, 1938.
13. Brill LR, Lepow GM: The Arnold-Chiari malformation with associated pes equinovarus deformity. *J Am Podiatry Assoc* 71:307–310, 1981.
14. Mishaline MA, Dockery GL: Spina bifida and its effect on the lower extremities. *J Am Podiatry Assoc* 70:84–88, 1980.
15. Duckworth T: Management of the feet in spinal dysraphism and myelodysplasia. In Jahss MH (ed): *Disorders of the Foot*, vol 1. Philadelphia, WB Saunders Co, 1982.
16. Tax HR, Person V, Tuccio M: A podiatric presentation of diastematomyelia. *J Am Podiatry Assoc* 72:337–341, 1982.

CHAPTER 17

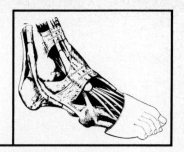

Medical Complications in the Podiatric Patient

John M. Schuberth, D.P.M.

INTRODUCTION

This chapter focuses on the important complications seen in the postoperative podiatric patient. Serious complications are uncommon but when present may be responsible for disabling, or at worst, fatal situations. The podiatric surgeon must be thoroughly familiar with the signs and symptoms of these medical complications and realize the steps necessary to institute the appropriate diagnostic modalities to ensure early recognition and prevention of the catastrophic sequelae. The podiatric surgeon should also be able and willing to request appropriate consultation for diagnosis and treatment. This most commonly involves referral to an internal medicine specialist but may also include other medical or surgical specialists. It is often appropriate for the consultant to assume care of the patient with regard to the specific complication.

This chapter's scope is confined to complications of the pulmonary and vascular systems. The discussion of the immediate postoperative complications that are categorized as postanesthetic complications are thoroughly covered in standard textbooks of anesthesiology and surgery and are beyond the scope of this chapter. These problems include but are not limited to postoperative vomiting, nausea, myocardial infarction, cardiac arrythmias, and thyroid storm. However, it is important for the podiatric practitioner to be aware of these situations to seek the appropriate consultation as needed.

PULMONARY COMPLICATIONS

Impairment of pulmonary function occurring postoperatively is one of the most frequent postsurgical complications. Several circumstances during and after surgery account for this finding. These complications to a large extent are an accentuation of the pulmonary physiological changes as a result of inhalation anesthesia. A summary by Latimer and associates (1) of 19 surgical series showed that although the incidence of postoperative pulmonary complications varied widely (29% to 70%) the highest rates were for upper abdominal and thoracic procedures, and the lowest rates were for nonabdominal, nonthoracic surgery. Podiatric surgery falls into this latter category. Postoperative pulmonary pathological changes are not restricted to patients with preexisting pulmonary disease. They often occur in otherwise healthy patients.

Identifying the Risk Factors

It is the responsibility of the admitting podiatric physician, the attending physician, and the anesthesiologist to identify those risk factors responsible for an increased incidence of pulmonary complications. If this responsibility is left to the anesthesiologist at the time of admission it is often too late to reduce some of the risk factors. A diligent preoperative pulmonary history is invaluable in the preoperative assessment of the podiatric surgical patient. Particular attention should be paid to any history of dyspnea, either at rest or on exertion, wheezing, chest pain, medications, cough, or previous pulmonary disease. A smoking history should also be obtained. A thorough medical history may enable the physician to recommend preoperative pulmonary therapy well in advance of the proposed operation.

The physical examination can also provide valuable information. Although a complete physical examination in the office is seldom indicated, simple observation of the patient during the routine office visit can provide valuable information. Labored breathing, audible wheezing, clubbed nails, and pedal or facial cyanosis are easily observed. In the hospital the patient should be evaluated for diminution of breath sounds, wheezes, rales, and hyperresonance or dullness to percussion. Cardiac size should be assessed. General nutritional status should be evaluated. Patients should be weighed preoperatively.

Specific Risk Factors

Age

Age has been shown to be associated with an increased risk of postoperative morbidity and mortality (2, 3). The specific physiological changes include a decrease in vital capacity, an increase in residual volume and lung compliance, and a decrease in maximum breathing capacity. Arterial oxygen tension also declines progressively with age.

Obesity

Obesity constitutes a major general risk of postoperative pulmonary complications (1, 4). Obese patients without intrinsic lung disease still have potential abnormalities in pulmonary function. There is a progressive reduction in functional reserve capacity correlating directly with weight (5).

The abdomen and chest wall both may alter pulmonary function in obese patients. The effect of the subcutaneous fat is accentuated by recumbency in overweight patients. At any lung volume the compliance of the obese or mass-loaded individual is roughly one half of the normal compliance. The most common abnormal blood gas finding in the obese patient is hypoxemia. Arterial O^2 tensions in the obese patient breathing room air frequently are in the 60 to 80 mm Hg range. Because of these physiological disturbances such patients are susceptible to ineffective cough, basilar atelectasis, progressive hypoxemia, and resultant infections (6).

Pulmonary function tests will help to determine the extent of impairment of pulmonary function, as well as the presence of chronic lung disease. Knowing the level of oxygenation and alveolar ventilation facilitates the preoperative and postoperative management of the obese patient.

Smoking

The extent of respiratory dysfunction is related to the total number of cigarettes smoked and the number of years of habitual smoking. Chronic cigarette smoke inhalation is associated with obstructive pulmonary disease, progressing to emphysema. The ratio of FEV^1/FVC is significantly reduced in smokers. The acute effects of smoking one cigarette are an increased airway resistance of approximately 30% and a decreased dynamic compliance of 20%. Cigarette smoking causes ciliary paralysis acutely and loss of ciliated cells with chronic smoking. This results in a reduction in the tracheobronchial mucociliary clearance rate so that after three months of smoking clearance rates are only 10% of presmoking values.

A history of current smoking increases the frequency of postoperative complications six to seven times that of a nonsmoking control (7). The effects of smoking are partially reversible. Therefore smoking should be minimized before a surgical procedure.

Preexisting Pulmonary Disease

The presence of preexisting pulmonary disease will most likely be discovered during the history taking and the physical examination. The presence of the disease is not in itself a risk factor; rather it is the degree of pulmonary dysfunction caused by that specific disease entity. The process can be classified as obstructive, restrictive, large airway, small airway disease, and others. The physiological parameters are best measured by pulmonary function testing.

Extrinsic Skeletal Disease

The presence of external skeletal disease which might affect pulmonary function and ventilation must be considered. This includes anklylosing spondylitis and kyphoscoliosis. Again, the pulmonary function tests will demonstrate the degree of impairment.

PULMONARY FUNCTION TESTING

Preoperative pulmonary function testing quantifies the degree of preoperative respiratory dysfunction (8, 9). A higher incidence of postoperative pulmonary complications correlates with increasing degrees of preoperative respiratory dysfunction, regardless of the type of surgery performed (10). Any patient who has one or more of the risk factors just discussed, and who is a possible candidate for general anesthesia, should have preoperative pulmonary function evaluation. Initial identification of patients in these groups should be accomplished by history, physical examination, and chest radiography. The information gathered from pulmonary testing will enable the surgeon and the anesthesiologist to make more informed decisions and recommendations to the patient. If the tests are clearly abnormal the patient may be placed on aggressive preoperative pulmonary therapy or another alternative to general anesthesia may be considered.

It is both impractical and unnecessary to perform the entire gamut of respiratory function tests on all patients having elective lower extremity surgery. However, in most cases a simple battery of the most informative tests will provide the surgical team with the data necessary to tailor a perioperative plan to deal adequately with the vast majority of patients.

Forced Vital Capacity (FVC)

Forced vital capacity (FVC) is the total volume of air exhaled after a full inspiration and a forced expiration. This simple and inexpensive spirometric test is a good predictor of total lung capacity and should be routinely performed as part of the pulmonary evaluation.

Forced Expiratory Volume (FEV_1), FEV_1/FVC Ratio

The forced expiratory volume (FEV) is the amount of air forcibly expelled from the total lung capacity in 1 second. The simple calculation of FEV_1/FVC will give one a ratio. Normally a person will be able to expel 80% of the FVC in 1 second. With the three parameters of FEV_1, FVC, and the resultant ratio, lung function can be categorized into normal, obstructive, or restrictive disease. In obstructive lung disease the patient is unable to breathe out full and therefore the FVC and the FEV_1 are reduced, thereby reducing the FEV_1/FVC ratio. In restrictive disease airway resistance is normal but the chest cannot fully expand. Therefore vital capacity is low and FEV_1 is normal giving an increased ratio (Fig. 17.1).

Arterial Blood Gases

In those patients with moderate to advanced disease as revealed with spirometric testing, arterial blood gas and blood pH tests should be obtained. These provide an additional assessment of lung function and offer a baseline from which postoperative values can be compared. When arterial hypoxemia is found in the preoperative patient an attempt should be made to identify the cause.

The ultimate goal of preoperative pulmonary function testing is to identify patients at an increased risk of morbidity. The institution of prophylactic measures or alternate forms of anesthesia in patients in the higher risk group may substantially decrease postoperative complications.

Preoperative Prophylaxis of Pulmonary Complications

Patient education remains the most critical prophylactic measure. Preoperative discussion of the perioperative events and the explanation of those functions the patient is responsible for postoperatively will greatly facilitate the implementation of prophylaxis. The patient should be taught how to use the incentive spirometer, deep breathing and coughing exercises, and the position he or she is expected to assume postoperatively (11).

A wide variety of physical measures has been developed to enhance the expectoration and clearance of sputum and to retrain breathing patterns. The application of these techniques to patients with underlying pulmonary disorders and other individuals at risk for respiratory complications has been found significantly to improve their postoperative morbidity and mortality. The specific goals of the various techniques include the prevention or reversal of mechanical airway obstruction and/or atelectasis by preserving an adequate depth of ventilation, assisting the removal of secretions from the tracheobronchial tree, and

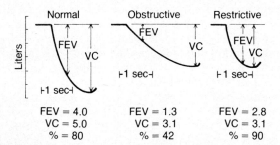

Figure 17.1. Measurement of FEV_1/FVC. Patterns of airflow are shown for normal, obstructive, and restrictive pulmonary circumstances. (From West JB: Disturbances of respiratory function. In Thorn GW, Adams RD (eds): *Harrison's Principles of Internal Medicine*, ed 8. New York: McGraw-Hill, 1977, p 1340.)

maintaining mobility of the chest wall, shoulder, spine, and abdomen (7).

When significant bronchospasm is identified by physical examination or pulmonary function testing it should be treated preoperatively via the use of bonchodilators. Frequently bronchodilators are administered at the time of pulmonary function testing to assess their effect. If a positive response is noted with improvement of pulmonary function then there is ample evidence for preoperative bronchodilator therapy. Ideally this is instituted one month before surgery. Optimized dilation of the airways will assist in the clearance of mucus and minimize the likelihood of the perioperative development of complicating bronchospasm.

Hydration

Water is almost universally present in therapeutic regimens designed to treat abnormalities of the respiratory tract. Dramatic changes in the viscosity of mucus and ciliary action in the absence of water point out the importance of maintaining a normal state of hydration (7). Mild to moderate dehydration must occur before significant respiratory abnormalities are noted. All ambulatory patients with difficulties in the clearance of secretions are encouraged to drink at least 1500 ml of fluids per day.

Postoperative Pulmonary Therapy

Immediately postoperative patients who received a general anesthetic or any procedure with a prolonged period of limited ventilation are likely to have substantial microatelectasis. Aggressive treatment is indicated when the chest x-ray studies and arterial blood gases are abnormal. Patients at risk for pulmonary complications may benefit from treatment for presumed atelectasis even if the pulmonary parameters are stable.

Narcotic analgesics are used frequently for pain management in the postoperative podiatric patient (12). The respiratory depressant effects of these drugs are well known (13). Every attempt to reduce narcotic requirements through patient education and rapport should be made. In addition the institution of other measures to reduce pain such as nonsteroidal antiinflammatory medications (14) and transcutaneous electrical nerve stimulation (TENS) (15) units may greatly decrease the dependency on narcotics for pain control. The use of butorphanol and nalbuphine is known to produce less respiratory depression than meperidine at higher dosage levels. These drugs may be indicated in those patients requiring above average amounts of narcotic analgesics or in those patients at risk for complications.

The horizontal position of the thorax for postoperative care may be desirable for purposes of cardiac output but may not be an ideal position for maximizing lung function. In the supine attitude the diaphragm is elevated relative to lung volume and tidal volumes are smaller. Ideally the patient should be positioned postoperatively in a semireclining or upright manner for maximal lung volume, especially if the patient is obese. Frequent repositioning from side to side may be an effective alternative if the horizontal position seems necessary.

As with the preoperative situation, adequate hydration of the postoperative patient is essential for the same physiological reasons. Fluid replacement postoperatively may be underestimated. Postoperative fluid administration should be vigorous especially in patients at risk of pulmonary complications. The standards of fluid therapy should be familiar to the operating surgeon. (See Chapter 9, Postoperative Management.)

Ideal ventilatory therapy based on the observation of normal breathing patterns should facilitate a deep breath every 5 to 10 minutes to reverse or prevent alveolar collapse. A maneuver that meets this requirement and is generally recognized as being efficacious in the treatment of postoperative pulmonary complications is sustained maximal inspiration. Important aspects are the inspired volume and the duration of end inspiratory hold. Incentive breathing devices have been developed to encourage patient performance. The incentive spirometer best meets these objectives. The expiratory maneuvers are counterproductive and in all likelihood predisposes patients to the very problems the therapy is allegedly designed to prevent (16).

ATELECTASIS

Atelectasis is the most frequently occurring postoperative pulmonary complication despite the advances of modern medicine. Some evidence suggests that much of the atelectasis or at least its earlier stages may occur during surgery (7). It may be defined as closure of the lung units. Such closure covers the spectrum from being diffuse and at sublobular levels that are not visible roentgenographically (microatelectasis), to localized collapse of a segment, lobe, or lung that is apparent radiographically. Microatelectasis is exceedingly common (6). It is a clinical mistake to restrict the diagnosis of atelectasis to that apparent on the chest radiograph. Atelectasis can and does present in the presence of a normal chest x-ray radiograph.

Atelectasis occurs commonly in patients without increased secretions and all too often in patients with normal lungs. The trapped secretions in these occluded lung units are a ripe medium for bacterial growth and can set the stage for a pneumonitis or pneumonia. A decrease in the tidal volume and loss of the sigh mechanism are implicated as pathophysiological causes of atelectasis. These changes in ventilatory patterns have been shown to produce airway closure and a decrease in pulmonary compliance.

The incidence of postoperative atelectasis falls dramatically after the fifth postoperative day. It is considerably more common in the first 24 to 48 hours postoperatively and should be suspected in any patient with a postoperative fever in the first 48 to 72 hours. The patient will usually have a tachycardia and a tachypnea. Reduced breath sounds, dullness to percussion, moist rales, and an asymmetrical limitation of pulmonary excursion are typical signs and symptoms. These are more prevalent in the posterior lung bases. In microatelectasis some or all of these findings may be the only positive clinical finding, and if present presumptive treatment should commence. Dyspnea is present sporadically.

Radiological findings in postoperative pulmonary collapse can range from absent to distinct, depending on the degree of collapse. The radiographic appearance of collapsed tissue is influenced by the presence of preexisting disease, the relative stability of the mediastinum and chest wall, and the presence of pleural adhesions. The specific radiologic interpretations are beyond the scope of this chapter; however, the reader is referred to the standard textbooks of radiology.

Treatment

The treatment of postoperative atelectasis is directed toward removing the obstructing mucus and reexpanding the involved pulmonary parenchyma before bacterial infection supervenes (7). In addition removal of the risk factors, if possible, is paramount to therapy. The reversal of microatelectasis can ordinarily be accomplished with careful hyperinflation that has become a common practice during operation. However, the superimposition of other factors leading to atelectasis such as those found in individuals with a high risk of atelectasis may make the routine techniques for reversal insufficient and larger degrees of atelectasis may occur.

Minor degrees of atelectasis respond to any number of techniques that produce deep breaths. Despite many opinions few objective data document the uniform superiority of any particular technique in comparison to others provided that technique results in frequent and repetitive deep inspirations (7).

Incentive spirometry requires a voluntary effort on the part of the patient. Tri-flow and other devices facilitate maximal inspiratory effort. A poorly motivated patient may not receive maximal benefit and may need intermittent positive pressure breathing (IPPB), chest physiotherapy, or both. Rarely, even more aggressive therapy is necessary.

INFECTIOUS COMPLICATIONS

The range of infectious complications can cover the spectrum of an exacerbation of bronchitis to pneumonia. They arise in patients both with and without chronic airway disease, although the former group has a much higher incidence of these complications. Dehydration, decreased coughing ability, microatelectasis and macroatelectasis, decreased mucociliary clearance of inhaled particles and microbes, analgesia, and supplemental oxygen are all conditions that can predispose a patient to complications (10). Interruption of mucociliary clearance leads to a rapid proliferation of bacteria distal to the site of obstruction (17). The particular bacterial species responsible for the infectious event almost invariably begins from the bacterial population harbored by the patient.

Establishing a diagnosis of pneumonia in the postoperative patient is difficult at times, mainly because of signs and symptoms that may be caused by other conditions. It should be based on a combination of findings in the postoperative patient. Three of the following criteria should be present: fever, rales and/or dullness to percussion, x-ray signs of pulmonary infiltrate, purulent sputum, and leukocytosis (18).

ASPIRATIONS

Aspiration of foreign materials into the lungs can cause considerable postoperative morbidity. Although this is usually an immediate postanesthetic complication its occurrence can lead to the complications discussed specifically in this chapter. In the perioperative period aspiration may occur as a result of chemically or mechanically induced malfunction of the normal glottic and pharangeal protective mechanisms. Diabetics may be at particular risk if vagus nerve autonomic neuropathy causes delayed emptying of the gastric contents. These patients may have full stomachs at the time of surgery even though they have not eaten since dinner the night before (7).

Prevention remains the best form of treatment. This depends on the awareness of the possibility. The long-term complications of pneumonia, sepsis, pulmonary abcesses, and empyema may be seen in up to one third of all patients with aspiration.

BRONCHOSPASM

Postoperative bronchospasm can be precipitated by many exogenous insults. Patients with preexisting airway irritability are at a greater risk. Infection may cause a bronchospastic pattern in asthmatic or bronchitic patients. Allergic individuals may have bronchospasm when exposed to the allergen or to cigarette smoke. Aspirin, other salicylates, or nonsteroidal medications may trigger an asthmatic attach. Environmental stress, coughing, or laughing may be precipitating factors. The former is common enough that a psychotherapeutical approach is used for therapy where a predominately emotional component is responsible. Pulmonary embolism and aspiration are also known to cause postoperative bronchospasm (7).

VENOUS THROMBOEMBOLIC DISEASE
Deep Venous Thrombosis

Deep venous thrombosis is an occasional complication in the postoperative podiatric patient. It can account for a great deal of morbidity in the postoperative patient and a considerable number of mortalities (19) when pulmonary embolism, the most fearful complication of this disorder, ensues (20).

The incidence of deep venous thrombosis is clearly underestimated. In one study 80% of the deep thrombi detected were small and asymptomatic and presumably insignificant clinically (21). Asymptomatic disease undoubtedly occurs but its actual frequency is unknown. Symptomatic patients usually have more clinically significant venous thrombi. The

clinically important situations arising from deep venous thrombosis are deaths from pulmonary embolism, morbidity from the event itself, postphlebitic syndrome, the cost, and prolonged hospitalization.

PATHOPHYSIOLOGY OF THROMBOSIS

Thrombosis is described as the pathological manifestation of those functions normally responsible for the arrest of hemorrhage. These functions include platelet adhesion, platelet aggregation, and fibrin coagulation.

Thrombosis, like hemostasis, may be a reparative process inasmuch as thrombi seal intimal defects and avert hemorrhage. Whereas an inciting incident in a vessel wall is usually sufficient stimulus to elicit the formation of a hemostatic plug, several additional factors contribute to the development of a thrombus. Among these factors are disturbances in blood flow (22, 23) and hypercoagulability (24).

Many of the pathological consequences of venous thrombosis are related to excessive proliferation of the thrombus beyond normal reparative and hemostatic responses. Stable thrombi may persist permanently to disrupt vessel wall integrity, whereas unstable lesions may embolize and create additional injury at distant sites.

Activated platelets in the coagulum can release aggregants and fibrinogen to help create a suitable surface to attach to other platelets. It is this critical stage in thrombus formation that may be suppressed by drugs that inhibit the platelet release reaction (25, 26).

Thrombi proliferate into the lumen toward the opposing vessel wall, as well as along the length of the vessel. These propagated venous thrombi, like those in large superficial and deep leg veins, usually are quite loosely attached to the vessel wall and become even further loosened by retraction. This sets the stage for fragmentation or complete detachment and massive embolization. Thrombi in general are not static structures. They are constantly adapting by resolution, organization, and at times continued growth. The association of slow flow with the development of thrombosis of deep leg veins is so constant that retarded flow might be considered a prerequisite. The combination of trauma to tissues, retarded flow, and probable release of thrombogenic substances poses an especially susceptible situation (24, 27).

Obstruction of a vessel consequent to an intrinsic lesion or some extrinsic cause can promote local and remote hemodynamic disturbances. When a large venous trunk is compressed by a tumor or other external means flow may be slowed in the tributary veins. In the left leg veins slowing of flow from any cause may be intensified by the natural progression of the left common iliac vein as it courses under the right common iliac artery. An above knee cast can compress and occlude the popliteal vein.

In the immediate postoperative period, while the patient is still on bed rest, a decrease in flow becomes an important issue. Careful attention to the positioning of the patient in bed will minimize the loss of the musculovenous pump that is afforded by ambulation. In addition care must be taken not to place pillows injudiciously that may compress a segment of the venous tree. A common error is to place a pillow directly in the popliteal fossa. Hyperextension should also be avoided at the knee. Ideally the patient should be positioned in the so-called antiembolic position. The upper torso is flat or very slightly inclined while the hips and knees are in moderate flexion (Fig. 17.2). Return of blood flow to the right heart should at all times be assisted by gravity if possible.

Hyperviscosity

Viscous blood may augment the slowing of flow and lead to the development of thrombi in the microcirculation, but its significance in contributing to the retardation of flow and thrombosis is less certain. Polycythemia vera and hyperfibrinogenemia are frequent causes of hyperviscosity commonly found in thrombotic conditions (28, 29). In infants hemoconcentration resulting from dehydration is an important thrombogenic factor.

Hypercoagulability

One might consider hypercoagulability as a potentially thrombotic state of the blood whereby the capacity for an increased or an accelerated production of thrombin exists. Thrombi may form locally at any given point in the circulation so that the concept of local hypercoagulability may depend on the actual amount of thrombus produced relative to its removal or neutralization by the circulating blood. Certain hereditary hemorrhagic diseases may be related to the reduction or absence of a single coagulation factor but the converse relationship does not necessarily hold true in regard to thrombosis. Nonetheless cases have been reported that strongly suggest a relationship between an alteration in a single factor and thrombotic disease (30, 31). Of particular interest are the reports of familial thrombosis in cases with decreased levels of the naturally circulating anticoagulant, antithrombin III (32).

Alterations in serum lipids have been shown to influence platelet function and coagulation. Alimentary hyperlipidemia alone may create hypercoagulability through the presence of phosphatidyletholamine in chylomicrons (33). A similar association between lipids and coagulability has been noted in ischemic

heart disease (34), diabetes mellitus (35), and familial hyperlipoproteinemia (36). Recently it has been recognized that two widely used contemporary products effect coagulability of the blood. Activation of factor XII by tobacco glycoproteins may be related to thrombosis (37) along with the possibility of the injurious effect of smoking on the endothelium consequent to the production of carboxyhemoglobin.

Estrogen-containing contraceptives have been linked with thrombogenesis (38) through retardation of factor Xa inhibitory activity (39). Levels of procoagulant factors are substantially raised in women taking oral contraceptives.

Risk Factors

Several clinical conditions may predispose a patient to deep venous thrombosis. These conditions will be discussed individually as they relate to lower extremity procedures.

Surgical Trauma

The relative risk of postoperative thromboembolism is related to the severity, site, and extent of surgical trauma. The risk of thromboembolism becomes proportional to the operative time in procedures lasting over 30 minutes. A large majority of the venous thromboembolic complications occur with major orthopedic surgery above the ankle joint (40). Unfortunately there are no published reports of large series of patients with elective podiatric surgery that demonstrate the actual incidence of postoperative deep thrombophlebitis. However, Simon and associates (41) did show that operations on the forefoot did produce less (0% of 101 patients) than published reports considering other orthopedic operations.

Age

The frequency of deep venous thrombosis and subsequent pulmonary embolism increases with age. The reason for this phenomenon is uncertain. Venous dilation is definitely increased in the elderly. Vascular stasis caused by the resultant valvular incompetence and the relative immobility of the elderly also contribute to this observation. Lastly, the fibrinolytic response to venous occlusion of the legs is significantly lower in persons over the age of 65 compared to people under this age (10).

Immobility

As it relates to podiatric surgery, immobility is probably the most important risk factor. The incidence of deep venous thrombosis rises sharply in patients confined to bed for more than a week. Postoperative patients remain at risk during the entire period of immobility. Postoperative deep venous thrombosis is not prevented in patients who have had anticoagulant prophylaxis and who are immobile beyond that one-week period.

Immobility of the limb itself is significant enough to cause an increase in the frequency of thromboembolic incidents. The lack of the pumping action of the

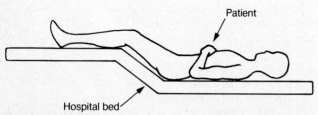

Figure 17.2. Antiembolic position: hips and knees are flexed approximately 30°. Legs are elevated higher than level of heart.

leg muscles enhances venous stasis. This can be observed in the monoplegic lower limb patient, as well as in the limb encompassed in a cast.

Miscellaneous Factors

Although less commonly appreciated, inflammatory bowel disease, Behcet's syndrome, and some gramnegative septicemias are associated with a high risk of deep venous thrombosis (42).

DIAGNOSIS OF DEEP VENOUS THROMBOSIS

Accurate clinical diagnosis of deep venous thrombosis is a time-honored enigma. It is considerably inaccurate because it is both insensitive and nonspecific (20). The presenting signs and symptoms may be completely contrary to the actual clinical problem. Many patients with relatively minor symptoms may have extensive venous thrombosis whereas other patients with suggestive signs frequently have no objective evidence of thrombosis. The low sensitivity of clinical diagnosis occurs because complete obstruction of venous outflow and inflammation of the vessel wall frequently do not occur. Therefore there are no obvious clinical manifestations. Diagnosis is also nonspecific because none of the signs and symptoms are unique to this condition and all can be signs of other nonthrombotic disorders. Most patients who present clinically with a probable deep venous thrombosis usually have less overt signs and symptoms, which require extensive diagnostic workup to rule out the diagnosis. When the thrombus is demonstrated by venography there is usually a poor correlation between the clinical manifestations and the size of the thrombosis (20).

The appearance of a deep venous thrombosis in the postoperative course is quite variable. Classical teaching suggests that deep venous thrombosis is most prevalent in the early postoperative period, approximately three to five days postoperatively. Although most of the studies cite total hip replacement as the index procedure many patients with a developing or acute deep thrombophlebitis will not present for up to two weeks postoperatively (43). However, it should be noted that the time of presentation is highly variable and should not be regarded as a major criterion for diagnosis.

Pain and tenderness are the most common presenting symptoms in a patient with a developing thrombosis. The location and degree of symptoms bears little relationship to the size, extent, or location of the thrombosis. Patients describe the quality of pain in a wide variety of ways. They may present with an ache, cramp, sharp, dull, severe, or mild symptoms. It may be persistent or intermittent and is usually aggravated by weight bearing. Frequently the patient improves with self-initiated bed rest, however, once ambulation resumes the symptomatology returns.

Swelling may be anywhere around the continuum from gross pitting edema to a mild increase in calf tissue turgor. The latter may be appreciated best by comparison to the contralateral limb. When the edema is caused by complete obstruction of a large proximal vein the swelling is usually distal to that point and is frequently painless. On the other hand, swelling caused by perivascular inflammation is usually located about that site and is most often tender (20).

Uncommonly, when a relatively superficial vessel becomes thrombosed it may be palpated as an obvious cord. This is a result of complete thrombosis of the vessel with subsequent inflammation. This may occur at any point along the course of the lower extremity, where the deep vessels course relatively close to the skin. With extensive thrombosis and inflammation this palpable cord may be present for several years.

The color of the affected limb may be a source of clinical confusion. The leg may present as being pale, cyanotic, reddishpurple, or in rare cases palorous. It is important to realize the variability in color presentation and the clinician should not be steered away from the suspicion of a deep venous thrombosis based on this parameter.

Phlegmasia cerulea dolens is the term used to describe the condition of marked swelling and cyanosis occurring with an obstructive iliofemoral vein thrombosis (20). The obstruction to flow caused by venous occlusion and subsequent edema may impair arterial flow enough to produce marked tissue ischemia. Usually the thrombosis includes most of the deep veins of the leg, including the iliofemoral, superficial femoral, and popliteal veins. Occasionally it may also encompass the long saphenous and other superficial tributaries. These patients must be monitored closely for hypotension.

The differential diagnosis in patients who present with signs and symptoms suggestive of a deep venous thrombosis include a ruptured Baker's cyst, muscle tear, muscle cramp, cellulitis, hematoma, external compression by tumor or hematoma, lymphedema, congestive heart failure, and postphlebitic syndrome (20). Further diagnostic workup with reliable objective testing is always necessary to solidify the diagnosis. It is on the basis of these tests, and not on the clinical signs and symptoms, that decisions for therapy are based.

OBJECTIVE DIAGNOSTIC TESTING

Once sufficient clinical evidence is present and suspicion of deep venous thrombophlebitis is aroused the clinician is faced with the task of formulating a diagnostic strategy to confirm or discard the diagnosis. There are numerous diagnostic protocols published, and each clinician should be familiar with the principles, pitfalls, and limitations of each of the diagnostic modalities. In addition local availability, trained technicians, and equipment may also influence the diagnostic strategy to a degree.

It is generally accepted that in those patients who deserve further workup a noninvasive test is indicated initially, unless venography is the only available method. If the noninvasive test is negative it can be either regarded as accurate or it can be confirmed by another noninvasive test. If the noninvasive test is distinctly positive then treatment should be started. With equivocal findings an invasive test should probably be ordered. Again, the limitations of each test, especially in regard to the suspected anatomical location, should be considered, as well as the clinical picture and history. As a general rule, however, there is no noninvasive test that is as accurate as venography.

Doppler

The Doppler ultrasound venous examination is a simple noninvasive technique for the detection of deep venous thrombosis. The rationale for using the Doppler ultrasound for the diagnosis of deep venous thrombosis is quite simple: thrombotic obstruction of the underlying vein distorts the venous flow pattern and these perturbations are readily detected transcutaneously. These differences in flow rates are converted to an audible signal.

Doppler examination has a sensitivity of 94% and a specificity of 90% for detecting acute thrombi in the popliteal or more proximal veins. Below knee thrombi are detected with a sensitivity of 91% and a specificity of 84% (44). Its major drawback is that its interpretation is purely subjective and requires skill and experience to perform reliably. The actual technique and interpretation of this test is well described (44, 45).

Plethysmography

By definition plethysmography is the measurement of changes in blood volume in the extremity. It can be used to measure the extent of calf volume increase that occurs when a pneumatic cuff placed around the thigh is inflated to a level exceeding the underlying venous pressure. When the thigh cuff is suddenly released venous blood trapped in the calf rushes out of the leg. In cases of deep venous thrombosis the outflow resistance is variably elevated depending on which veins are involved and the extent of the thrombotic process.

Again, this technique is extremely useful for proximal thrombi but less reliable in distal thrombosis. A normal result essentially excludes a diagnosis of proximal deep vein thrombosis but does not exclude a diagnosis of calf vein thrombosis. As collateral circulation develops or as partial canalization occurs the plethysmograph may become normal.

False positive results are seen in clinical disorders that interfere with arterial inflow or venous outflow. This includes congestive heart failure, severe arterial insufficiency, hypotension, and external compression of veins (19, 46).

I^{125}-labeled Fibrinogen Leg Scanning

The previous noninvasive modalities are highly sensitive for proximal deep venous thromboses, but unreliable in the diagnosis of calf vein thrombosis. I^{125}-labeled fibrinogen leg scanning can accurately detect calf vein thrombi and lower thigh thrombi. This semiinvasive technique is only applicable at a time when a thrombus is actually forming. Although the result is frequently positive in 24 hours it may not become positive for three days. This delay is unacceptable from a therapeutical standpoint and therefore this technique should not be employed as the sole diagnostic test. Its clinical application is most valuable in confirming or establishing lower leg thrombi in equivocal or negative noninvasive testing especially when the clinical picture strongly suggests such a thrombotic condition.

This type of scan is inaccurate in the upper thigh and pelvis because of the large muscle mass and the increase in background counts. It is also unreliable and gives false positive results in areas of hematoma, a large surgical wound, and in inflamed or edematous areas. This would preclude the use of such scanning in patients who have had tendon transfers, leg surgery, or ankle fractures. The positive scan is based on an increase in radioactivity of more than 20% at any one point compared with the readings over adjacent points in the same leg, or over the same point compared with the previous day, or a corresponding point in the opposite leg (47).

Several protocols are available that incorporate I^{125}-labeled fibrinogen leg scanning as an expectant measure in patients who have had one or more of the risk factors. The test is performed preoperatively and postoperative scanning is then done periodically. The clinical significance of a positive scan is currently being debated because of the dilemma of whether those patients with calf vein thrombosis should be anticoagulated. If there is any contraindication to heparin then this test may be valuable in ruling out the presence of a calf vein deep venous thrombosis.

Venography

Venography is the reference method for the diagnosis of deep venous thrombosis. This technique has been refined but clearly is becoming more and more indicated as the deficiency in clinical diagnosis is being realized. It is the most reliable method for establishment of the diagnosis when performed correctly. However, like all of the other methods, it requires skill and knowledge in the performance and interpretation. Accurate interpretation is based on the thorough knowledge of the venous anatomy and its frequent variations.

A goal of ascending venography is to delineate the anatomy of the deep venous system of the lower extremity. This is done by accurately opacifying the structures. Even though there are numerous variations on technique and attempts at visualization of unconventional anatomical sites, from a practical standpoint this technique provides adequate visualization of the deep calf veins, the popliteal, the femoral, and the external and common iliac veins (Fig. 17.3, A–D).

The pitfalls of venography center around the interpretation and performance of this technique. Oc-

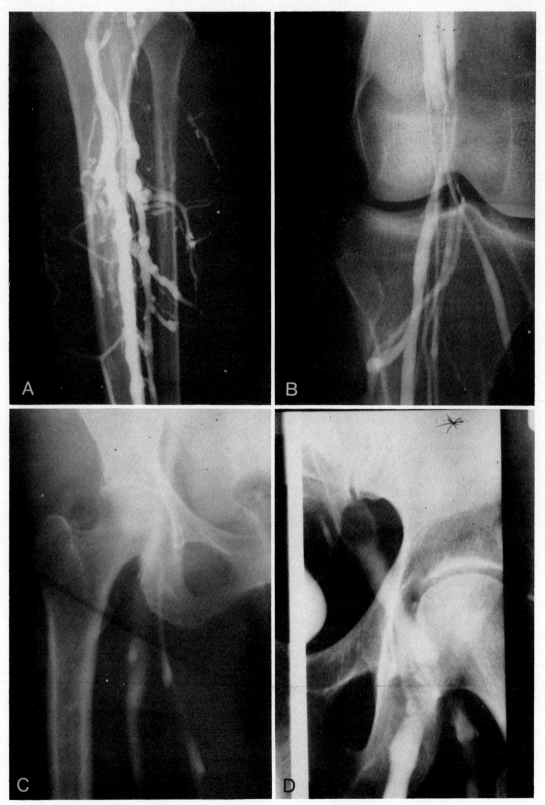

Figure 17.3. (A) Normal filling of deep posterior tibial veins. Note numerous bulging areas consistent with valve pockets. (B) Popliteal vein with filling defect just inferior to inferior pole of patella. (C) Early filling of femoral vein. No thrombus is evident. (D) Large occlusive thrombus seen in external iliac vein.

casionally proximal, nonobstructive thrombi in the common femoral veins may be overlooked because of inadequate filling of the vessel with contrast medium.

In addition overdiagnosis of deep venous thrombosis may be caused by a streaming effect of the medium, again caused by suboptimal opacification.

TREATMENT OF DEEP VENOUS THROMBOSIS

The goals of treatment of a deep venous thrombosis are aimed primarily at preventing the disasterous complications that often ensue. The most catastrophic complication that must be avoided is pulmonary embolism. Prompt recognition and treatment is of paramount importance in the prevention of pulmonary embolism.

Physical Measures

Treatment of a patient with an identifiable deep venous thrombosis begins with the establishment of an environment that minimizes the chance of complications. Because of the fragility of the venous thrombi and the propensity to break and embolize the patients should be kept on bed rest in the antiembolic position. This prevents the patient from assuming the dependent position, which not only stresses an incompetent valvular system but also favors stasis. The added force of gravity on the column of blood in the extremity could potentiate the valvular incompetency and predispose the patient to postphlebitic syndrome. On the other hand, strenous activity may increase turbulence in the vessel lumen and could increase the probability of dislodging an existing clot.

Warm, moist heat may be applied to promote venous dilation, increased capacitance, and thus increased flow around the thrombotic area. Adequate hydration should be ensured either through intravenous or oral fluid administration so that blood viscosity is not compromised or a transient hypovolemic thrombocystosis does not evolve. Analgesics may also be necessary for pain control. Care should be taken to administer those preparations that do not interfere with other pharmacological therapy that is being employed.

Pharmaceutical Treatment

Pharmacological management of a deep venous thrombosis remains the sine quo non of therapy. With the advent and development of the thrombolytic agents treatment of the active deep venous thrombosis has become complex yet much more effective especially in regard to the prevention of the complications. Heparin, however, remains the standard anticoagulant in the management of deep venous thrombosis. These and other pharmaceutical therapies are best managed by specialists in internal medicine.

Anticoagulants do not dissolve existing clots. However, by inhibiting subsequent clotting they may shift the balance between endogenous thrombosis and thrombolysis so as to favor fibrinolysis by the body's own mechanisms.

In general anticoagulants are used to arrest an existing thrombotic process or prophylactically to prevent a thrombus from developing. They have little effect on platelets.

Heparin

Heparin is available as an aqueous solution in concentrations ranging from 1000 to 40,000 units per ml. For intravenous injection a dilute solution is preferable to minimize irritation of the venous intima. The onset of heparin given intravenously is immediate with a dose-dependent duration of action. The half-life in the usual dosages employed is one to two hours. When given by subcutaneous injection the onset of action is delayed but the effect is more prolonged and erratic. Heparin should never be given intramuscularly.

If heparin is used for the initial management of a deep venous thrombosis the intravenous route of administration is preferred. Although there have been conflicting views on the preferred timing and technique of administration, clinical practice is evolving toward continuous intravenous infusion rather than intermittent infusion. Studies indicate that this is a safer method but no more efficacious (48). Although heparin can be administered on a unit/kg of body weight basis it is prudent to evaluate its effect via the laboratory to ensure that proper dosage is obtained. Laboratory control of heparin is based on the activated partial thromboplastin time (PTT). Traditionally the therapeutic range has been defined as being one and a half to two and a half times the normal value for the whole blood clotting time or the activated PTT. Laboratory testing is of less value in predicting bleeding.

Heparin therapy for acute thrombosis should be continued for approximately 7 to 10 days to ensure stabilization of the vessel wall. Oral anticoagulants should be initiated before the heparin is discontinued.

Complications of Heparin Therapy

Bleeding is the major side effect of heparin treatment. It is not directly correlated with the heparin dose and its causes are incompletely understood. Women have a slightly higher incidence of hemorrhagic complications than men. Women over 60 have been shown to have an exceptionally high risk (49). Drugs with platelet-inhibiting properties are to be considered strictly contraindicated in heparinized patients.

Because the half-life of heparin is short antidotes are rarely necessary. Protamine sulfate on a milligram for milligram basis remains the antidote of choice. One hundred units of heparin is roughly equivalent to 1 mg of protamine sulfate.

Thrombolytic Therapy

Abundant documentation of the beneficial effects of thrombolytic agents in certain types of thrombotic conditions is contained in the literature. Equally represented are data that reflect the problems and risks associated with such therapy (50–52).

A proper choice of patient is critical in assuring both a satisfactory degree of lysis of the thrombis or embolus and a clinical course uncomplicated by serious hemorrhage. The ideal patient to treat is one who has a serious or potentially life-threatening thrombosis without an anatomical lesion that may bleed excessively.

Two agents are currently approved by the FDA for clinical use. Streptokinase is indicated for pulmonary embolism, deep vein thrombosis, arterial thrombosis and embolism, arteriovenous cannulae, occlusion, and coronary artery thrombosis. Urokinase is clinically indicated only for the treatment of pulmonary embolism. Both agents occasionally produce pyrogenic side effects, more frequently with streptokinase, which can also produce allergic reactions and occasional anaphylaxis (53).

A decision to initiate streptokinase for the treatment of a deep venous thrombosis requires careful consideration of the evidence for and the extent of the thrombotic disease. This usually means venographic demonstration of such a thrombus. The most discriminate use of streptokinase would be in those patients with thrombi in the popliteal or more proximal veins or extensive thrombosis of the entire deep calf venous plexus. If the diagnosis of thrombotic disease has been established adequately then the physician should consider two clinical aspects regarding patient selection. First, patients with a high likelihood of hemorrhagic complications should be excluded. Second, patients for whom thrombolytic therapy is not likely to be better than that resulting from heparin alone should also be excluded.

The absolute contraindications for streptokinase therapy are: (a) active internal bleeding, (b) recent (two months) cerebrovascular accident, (c) intracranial or intraspinal surgery, and (d) intracranial neoplasm. Those patients within 10 days of previous major surgery, the postpartum state, external cardiac massage, or biopsy of an inaccessible site should be given streptokinase only in extremely rare clinical situations. The patient with recent foot or ankle surgery probably does not need the entire 10-day waiting period. Most of the bleeding here can probably be controlled with local, noninvasive measures, except when the procedure involves the major compartments of the leg. Here thrombolytic therapy would best be avoided until 10 days postoperatively.

When streptokinase has been compared to heparin for the treatment of deep venous thrombosis, better salvage of valvular function and the prevention of postphlebitic syndrome was observed in those patients receiving streptokinase and heparin versus heparin alone (53–55). Most instances of postphlebitic syndrome occur in patients with previous thrombosis in the iliofemoral but not the calf veins (56). These potential benefits are only realized if thrombolytic therapy is initiated relatively early in the acute thrombotic course and not after waiting to observe the effect of heparin (57–59).

After the cessation of the thrombolytic agent anticoagulation is begun. Current practice is intravenous heparin administered at a dosage that maintains the PTT at one and a half to two times the control.

Oral Anticoagulants

The oral anticoagulants are important adjuncts in the management of deep venous thrombosis. Although not used in the acute setting they are uniformly employed following heparinization. These drugs are easily used on an outpatient basis and once the initial dosage adjustments are stabilized laboratory monitoring is performed on an infrequent basis.

The coumarin-like drugs function as anticoagulants by decreasing the amount of the four vitamin K dependent coagulation factors: II, VII, IX, X. After administration of the drug an abnormal prothrombin is produced that lacks coagulant activity.

These drugs require about 24 hours or more to produce their maximal effect. A daily prothrombin time (PT) should be obtained until the dosage adjustments give a result that is one and a half to two and a half times the control level. Spontaneous bleeding rarely occurs when the PT is less than two times the control but rises precipitously when it is above two and a half times the control.

Once adequate dosing levels are attained patients should be continued on oral anticoagulation for at least three months following the acute thrombotic episode. This allows for optimal recanalization of the occluded vessels and minimizes the possibility of a recurrence of the thrombotic episode. When the process occurred distal to the popliteal vessels the period of oral anticoagulation can be reduced. This is because the chance of postphlebitic syndrome is markedly decreased.

The side effects of oral anticoagulation are similar to those with heparin especially in regard to hemorrhage. If excessive bleeding does occur the administration of 250 to 500 ml of plasma becomes the treatment of choice. This results in immediate restoration of factors II, VII, IX, and X. Most cases of minor bleeding do not require this type of treatment and usually respond to withholding the anticoagulants, as well as local treatment.

SURGICAL INTERVENTION FOR DEEP VENOUS THROMBOSIS

Surgical intervention may in some cases be indicated especially when anticoagulation or thrombosis is ineffective or unsafe. Those cases include patients who may have serious hemorrhagic complications as a result of anticoagulation. Vascular surgical consultation should be obtained to determine the most optimal surgical procedure. This can range from ligation of a proximal vein to compartmentalization of the vena cava to prevent recurrent pulmonary embolization. Venous thrombectomy is reserved for the treatment of phlegmasia cerulea dolens, in which limb viability is jeopardized by extensive venous obstruction (60, 61).

PREOPERATIVE PROPHYLAXIS

A discussion of the diagnosis and treatment of deep venous thrombosis would be superfluous if there were a totally reliable regimen of prophylaxis. Unfortunately this is not the case. Even though the treatment of deep venous thrombosis is highly successful one cannot rely on the treatment of pulmonary embolism to save lives. Two thirds of all patients who ultimately succumb to pulmonary embolus are dead within 30 minutes after the acute event.

Standard textbooks of surgery universally fail to define those patients undergoing elective foot or ankle surgery as at risk. Little attention is even given to nonelective or traumatic surgery in this regard. Simon, and associates (41) reported no incidents of deep venous thrombosis after operations on the forefoot in elective surgical procedures in 101 patients. This paper did not consider other parameters that might be considered risk factors for the general population. Therefore, until further studies are done, data from existing literature must be extrapolated to the typical podiatric patient. Many of these patients may have all of the known risk factors and the probability of deep venous thrombosis is not to be taken lightly.

The identification of these patients with the attendant risk factors is the first step in prophylaxis. Most preventive measures have either complications, are inconvenient, or add considerably to the medical cost. Ideally one would prefer to restrict prophylaxis to these patients at higher risk, but because prediction is imperfect many patients must be treated to protect a few. Even this philosophy will not protect all patients.

Prophylactic measures should be free from serious side effects and must be used in the context of the proposed operation. They should also be cost effective. As will be seen, all of these prophylactic measures either eliminate the risk factor or combat the pathophysiological processes responsible for thrombosis.

Physical Measures

The simplest forms of prophylaxis are also the least expensive and have the least number of complications. Ambulation of the postoperative podiatric patient is probably the single most important measure in the prevention of deep venous thrombosis. Although not clearly documented, weight-bearing ambulation is probably superior to crutch ambulation. Even though both modalities get the patient out of bed, the latter form of ambulation is done without the benefit of the musculovenous pump on the operated extremity. This situation of reduced muscular activity is compounded with the use of a cast or other immobilization device. However, some active muscular contraction is afforded even when the leg is non-weight-bearing. The precise benefit of weight-bearing ambulation versus non-weight-bearing ambulation needs to be elucidated.

Intermittent pneumatic compression of the legs increases the rate of venous flow in the lower extremity. It should be employed until the patient is ambulant. This technique is at least as effective as low-dose heparin (62). It is particularly useful in patients where anticoagulation is contraindicated. It has a theoretical risk of dislodging an already formed thrombus but has not been established definitively.

Pharmaceutical Agents

Heparin prophylaxis is a well-established practice (63–65). Typically it is administered in dosages much smaller than those necessary for full anticoagulation. This takes advantage of the amplification implicit in the coagulation cascade. Present clinical practice dictates subcutaneous administration of 5000 units every 8 to 12 hours starting about two hours before surgery. It is continued for the duration of time that the patient is not ambulating. For purposes of podiatric surgery this regimen is probably sufficient although the situation may change as investigators begin to challenge the validity of the indosing protocol. Several authors have suggested that increasing the dose of heparin might make this concept more efficacious (66–68).

Major hemorrhagic side effects of low-dose heparin are uncommon. The thrice daily dosage may be associated with a higher incidence of bleeding. It should be noted that the incidence of bleeding complications arises precipitously if platelets are stunned by the concurrent administration of aspirin or other nonsteroidal antiinflammatory agents.

Laboratory monitoring of minidose heparin is unnecessary but a simple set of screening laboratory tests for hemostatic competence should be obtained because of the possibility of hemorrhagic diathesis from other causes.

Antiplatelet Drugs

The basic theory behind the prophylactic use of antiplatelet drugs is based on the premise that platelets are intimately involved in the initiation of thrombus formation. The use of these agents is therefore rational because prevention of the initial clot might be expected to decrease subsequent progression to frank thrombus.

Aspirin is the most commonly used antiplatelet drug and is the standard. However, most of the clinical trials and demonstrated efficacy are in hip or knee reconstruction. In addition it has been suggested that it is much less effective in women. To dispose of these uncertainties aspirin probably has no place in the prevention of deep venous thrombosis for podiatric surgical patients at the present time. The use of dextrans is also controversial and cannot be recommended for podiatric surgery.

Oral Anticoagulants

Oral anticoagulants have been established as the most effective form of preoperative prophylaxis in the prevention of deep venous thrombosis. The guidelines for their use postoperatively are the same for heparin: until the patient is ambulatory. The suggested level of anticoagulation is one that attains the PT of about two times control. Because of the much higher propensity for bleeding with oral anticoagulants their use should be restricted to the high-risk patient when other methods are known to be ineffective. This virtually excludes all podiatric surgical patients.

PULMONARY EMBOLISM

Pulmonary embolism is the third most frequent cause of death in the United States (69). It is said to occur about 750,000 times per year. The incidence is continuing to rise although the percentage of mortalities is on the decline because of advances in diagnosis and treatment. Nevertheless an unacceptable number of deaths occur every year because of pulmonary embolism, of which 50% could have been prevented with prompt recognition and appropriate management.

Those patients at risk for pulmonary embolism are essentially those at risk for developing deep venous thrombosis. The incidence of fatal pulmonary embolism rises dramatically in the aged because of diminished pulmonary reserve, probable decreased cardiac status, and poor general health. All of these factors, considered by themselves, affect the rate of mortality of pulmonary embolism.

The specific anatomical site of origin of most pulmonary emboli is unknown because many of these are undetected and clinically silent. Autopsy studies are helpful but not completely informative because these are preselected patients. Nevertheless it is established that thrombi originating from the calf have less of a chance of causing a clinically significant pulmonary embolism, unless multiple thrombi are thrown, than those larger thrombi originating more proximally. The larger the thrombus the more potential for occlusion of the larger portion of the pulmonary vasculature. This correlates well with the morbidity and mortality.

The consequences of pulmonary embolism are influenced by a number of factors including the size of the embolus, its location, the condition of the cardiorespiratory reserve, and the rate of lysis of the clots. In patients with normal cardiopulmonary reserve approximately 60% or more of the pulmonary vasculature must be obstructed before significant hemodynamic changes are seen. The long-term sequelae in those patients who survive the event, as far as the cardiopulmonary system is concerned, are usually minimal.

Diagnosis

The clinical diagnosis of pulmonary embolism, like that of deep venous thrombosis, must be made with a high index of suspicion. The signs and symptoms are subtle and the disease is often clinically silent. When clinical manifestations occur they can be divided into a number of syndromes among which there is considerable overlap. The time within the postoperative course that a pulmonary embolism occurs is quite variable. The temporal association of an embolus following a symptomatic venous thrombosis is not a prerequisite because many deep thrombi are detected after the diagnosis of pulmonary embolism is made, even though they are almost always a prodromal

event. When the presentation is typical the diagnosis is readily suspected, however; the classical presentation is uncommon. Familiarity with the risk factors coupled with the clinical setting should keen one's suspicion to the diagnosis.

Signs and Symptoms

The clinical signs and symptoms must be interpreted in view of the patient's preexisting medical condition. As with the deep venous thrombosis once the diagnosis is suspected objective testing should substantiate it before therapeutical intervention.

Dyspnea is the most frequently reported symptom, occurring in over 80% of patients with clinical manifestations. This may be accompanied by tachypnea. Pain can be present as two types. The most common and characteristic is the pleuritic pain caused by inflammation of the pleura overlying the areas of pulmonary infarct or atelectasis. This type of pleuritic pain usually occurs in the low to mid zones of the lung corresponding to the usual sites of embolization. It is usually sudden in onset and aggravated by breathing. The second type of chest pain, which is less common, is that simulating a myocardial infarction. It is described as an aching or compressing type of pain and may be seen in patients with a massive pulmonary embolism.

The presence of hemoptysis indicates that pulmonary infarction has occurred and has produced alveolar hemorrhage. This is an infrequent clinical finding of this condition.

Syncope may be the first and most prominent manifestation of pulmonary embolism. It occurs only in massive pulmonary embolism and is secondary to a reduction in cardiac output. This is usually associated with dyspnea and right-sided heart failure.

The patient's mental status may also be altered ranging from anxiety to actual coma. Other signs and symptoms that are less commonly seen include cyanosis, tachycardia, and pleural friction rub. Fever is occasionally present and is rarely above 101° F.

As can be seen from these signs and symptoms many other clinical entities can be represented by a similar set of symptoms. Pleuritic chest pain and dyspnea may be manifestations of atelectasis. In addition many patients who have recently learned to use crutches for ambulation may complain of unilateral or bilateral chest wall pain. This is frequently aggravated by deep breathing but astute clinical examination will usually differentiate chest wall muscular pain from pleuritic pain. Overall the classical triad of dyspnea, hemoptysis, and pleuritic pain is present in only about 28% of all patients with proven pulmonary embolization. Internal medicine consultation is essential in obtaining a detailed physical examination of the cardiopulmonary system.

Laboratory Studies

Arterial blood gases are seldom very helpful in establishing the diagnosis of pulmonary embolism.

This is because the decreased arterial oxygen content occurs in a large proportion of patients (especially the elderly) without embolic phenomena. However, any patient with a pO_2 of over 90 can be virtually excluded from the pulmonary embolism group.

Other laboratory tests may be helpful in separating the diagnosis of pulmonary embolism from other situations with similar presenting symptoms. This includes the determination of serum CPK, which would be clearly elevated in myocardial infarction but not with pulmonary embolization alone.

Electrocardiographic changes occur in a high percentage of patients with pulmonary embolism. These are most often ST-T changes. However, electrocardiographic changes are also characterized as refinements and are not absolute determinants in the diagnosis. This may also be used to exclude the possibility of an acute myocardial infarction when the clinical presentation is indistinguishable.

Chest X-Ray Studies

The plain chest radiograph is another adjunctive clinical study that provides relatively scant diagnostic findings. Most of the radiographic changes in pulmonary embolism are subtle and nonspecific and therefore need careful scrutiny. Previous chest radiographs of the same patient are helpful, as is a complete history of that patient's cardiopulmonary system. Normal chest radiographs do not rule out pulmonary embolism.

Ventilation Perfusion Scanning

Radioactive tracer techniques are easily applied to the study of both the ventilation and perfusion of the pulmonary tissue. The results of this test when distinctly positive or negative can have immediate impact on the therapeutic course that is to be undertaken. A normal ventilation perfusion scan virtually excludes clinically detectable pulmonary embolism. When the scan is abnormal the likelihood of pulmonary embolism depends more specifically on the nature of the scan defects observed.

The ventilation perfusion scan is highly sensitive in detection of either a ventilation or perfusion defect. It is, however, nonspecific in establishing a diagnosis of embolism. Therefore false negative scans are virtually nonexistent. On the contrary false positive scans for pulmonary embolism are quite common. When this situation is encountered then further diagnostic workup is probably indicated. Many pulmonary diseases can cause abnormalities in a ventilation perfusion scan. Interpretations of the patterns produced by specific pulmonary diseases can be difficult and subjective. A positive diagnosis for pulmonary embolism is based on the attainment of what is called a mismatched ventilation perfusion scan. A mismatch of the perfusion defect with the normal ventilation scan is virtually diagnostic of pulmonary embolism. On the other hand, in a patient with an abnormal perfusion lung scan and a matching abnormal ventilation study pulmonary embolism cannot be absolutely excluded but is less likely. Approximately 10% to 15% of patients will have ventilation perfusion scans that still leave the diagnosis of pulmonary embolism in doubt. Because of the morbidity and mortality associated with both pulmonary embolism and its therapy, further evaluation is indicated.

Pulmonary Angiography

Pulmonary angiography is the most definitive means of making the diagnosis of pulmonary emboli short of a postmortem examination. Pulmonary angiography is usually performed by the passage of a catheter from the femoral or basilic vein through the right heart and into the main pulmonary artery. Once the catheter is in place hemodynamic studies are performed.

There are few if any absolute contraindications to pulmonary angiography. The obvious consequences of an untreated pulmonary embolism far outweigh any serious complication that may result from this procedure.

The interpretation of pulmonary angiography is fairly straightforward although there are remote clinical situations when the diagnosis can still be in doubt. These cases are usually the result of technical or clinical difficulties. In these particular situations clinical judgment and a repetition of previously performed tests may be the ultimate criteria on which the therapeutic decision is based. In some cases venography of the lower extremities, if not already performed, would be indicated because of the high association of deep venous thrombosis and pulmonary embolism.

A normal pulmonary angiogram with selective injection of areas abnormal on the lung scan virtually rules out the diagnosis of pulmonary embolism.

Treatment

Treatment of pulmonary embolism essentially follows the treatment scheme for deep venous thrombosis with several exceptions. The urgency of treatment cannot be underestimated. Again, the patient's clinical condition will dictate whether thrombolytic or anticoagulation therapy is initially indicated. In addition to streptokinase, urokinase is also indicated for the lysis of an acute pulmonary embolus. Definite favorable physiological and anatomical changes have been reported with the use of a thrombolytic agent combined with heparin versus the use of heparin alone. Urokinase is usually administered for a 12-hour course and then is promptly followed by full heparinization. When streptokinase is employed it is usually only necessary for 24 hours. This is in contradistinction to its use in deep venous thrombosis, where 72 hours of therapy may be necessary.

When heparin is used as the initial pharmacological agent for the treatment of pulmonary embolism the duration is usually somewhat shorter than recommended for deep venous thrombosis. Heparinization usually is continued for at least five days before commencing treatment with oral anticoagulants.

Surgical removal of pulmonary emboli is rarely indicated because of the advent of thrombolytic therapy.

References

1. Latimer G, Dickman M, Clinton Day W, Gunn ML, DuWayne Schmidt C: Ventilatory patterns and pulmonary complications after upper abdominal surgery determined by preoperative and postoperative computerized spirometry and blood gas analysis. *Am J Surg* 122:622, 1971.
2. Zeffren SE, Hartford CE: Comparative mortality for various surgical operations in older versus younger age groups. *J Am Geriatr Soc* 20:485, 1972.
3. Klug TJ, McPherson RC: Postoperative complications in the elderly surgical patients. *Am J Surg* 97:713, 1959.
4. Putnam H, Jenicek JA, Cellan CA, Wilson RD: Anesthesia in the morbidly obese. *South Med J* 67:1411, 1974.
5. Morris JF, Koski A, Johnson LC: Spirometric standards for healthy nonsmoking adults. *Am Rev Respir Dis* 103:57, 1971.
6. Laver MB, Bendixen HH: Atelectasis in the surgical patient: recent conceptual advances. *Prog Surg* 5:1, 1966.
7. Urbanetti JS, Fanburg BL: Pulmonary diseases. In Molitch ME (ed): *Management of Medical Problems in Surgical Patients.* Philadelphia, FA Davis Co, 1983.
8. Curry JJ, Ashburn FS: Pulmonary function studies in surgery. *Postgrad Med* 8:220, 1950.
9. Berath G, Crawford C: Function tests in pulmonary surgery. *J Thorac Cardiovasc Surg* 22:414, 1951.
10. Tisi GM: Preoperative evaluation of pulmonary function. Validity, indications, and benefits. *Am Rev Respir Dis* 119:293, 1979.
11. Thoren L: Postoperative pulmonary complications: observations on their prevention by means of physiotherapy. *Acta Chir Scand* 107:193, 1954.
12. Lanham RH, Ramroth D: Hospital drug study. *J Am Podiatry Assoc* 74:611, 1984.
13. Hedley-White J, Burgess GE III, Feeley TW, Miller MG: Critical analysis of preoperative measures. In *Applied Physiology of Respiratory Care.* Boston, Little, Brown and Co, 1976.
14. Borovoy M, Holtz P, Kaczander BI: Postoperative analgesia with naproxen in foot surgery. *J Am Podiatry Assoc* 74:125, 1984.
15. Alm WA, Gold ML, Weil LS: Evaluation of trancutaneous electrical nerve stimulation (TENS) in podiatric surgery. *J Am Podiatry Assoc* 69:537, 1979.
16. Smith RA: Respiratory care. In Miller RD (ed): *Anesthesia.* New York, Churchill-Livingstone, 1981.
17. Lansing AM, Jamilson WG: Mechanism of fever in atelectasis. *Arch Surg* 87:168, 1963.
18. Butler T, Tally FP, Gorbach SL: Infectious diseases. In Molitch ME (ed): *Management of Medical Problems in Surgical Patients.* Philadelphia, FA Davis Co, 1983.
19. Settlemire WE, Benson DE: Deep venous thrombosis and pulmonary embolism. *J Am Podiatry Assoc* 74:268, 1984.
20. Hirsh J, Genton E, Hull R: *Venous Thromboembolism.* New York, Grune and Stratton, 1981.
21. Hirsh J, Hull R: Natural history and clinical features of venous thrombosis. In Colman RW, Hirsh J, Marder VJ, Salzman EW (eds): *Hemostasis and Thrombosis.* Philadelphia, JB Lippincott Co, 1982.
22. Eberth CJ, Schimmelbusch C: *Die Thrombose nach Versuchen und Leichenbefunden.* Stuttgart, V. Enke, 1888.
23. Mustard JR, Rowsell HC, Murphy EA: Thrombosis. *Am J Med Sci* 284:469, 1964.
24. Wessler S: The role of hypercoaguability in venous and arterial thrombosis. *Cardiovasc Clin* 3:1, 1971.
25. Weiss HJ: Antiplatelet drugs. A new pharmacologic approach to the prevention of thrombosis. *Am Heart J* 92:86, 1976.
26. Evans G, Mustard JF: Platelet surface reaction and thrombosis. *Surgery* 64:273, 1968.
27. Field ES, Nicolaides AN, Kakkar VV: Deep vein thrombosis in patients with fractures of the femoral neck. *Br J Surg* 59:377, 1972.

28. Dawson AA, Ogston D: The influence of the platelet count on the incidence of thrombotic and hemorrhagic complications in polycythemia vera. *Postgrad Med* 46:76, 1970.
29. Fulton RM, Duckett K: Plasma fibrinogen and thromboemboli after myocardial infarction. *Lancet* 11:1161, 1976.
30. Easton LW: Studies on a family with an elevated plasma level of factor V and a tendency to thrombosis. *J Pediatr* 68:367, 1966.
31. Penick GD, DeJanov II, Redick RL: Predisposition to intravascular coagulation. *Thromb Haemost* 21(Suppl):543, 1966.
32. Egeberg O: Inherited antithrombin deficiency causing thrombophilia. *Thromb Haemost* 13:516, 1965.
33. Poole JCF: Effect of diet and lipemia on coagulation and thrombosis. *Fed Proc* 21:20, 1962.
34. Nordoy A, Rodset JM: Platelet phospholipids and their function in patients with ischemic heart disease. *Acta Med Scand* 188:133, 1970.
35. Norday A, Rodset JM: Platelet phospholipids and their function in patients with juvenile diabetes and maturity onset diabetes. *Diabetes* 19:698, 1970.
36. Norday A, Rodset JM: Platelet function and platelet phospholipids in patients with hyperbetalipoproteinemia. *Acta Med Scand* 189:385, 1971.
37. Becker CG, Dubin T: Activation of factor XII by tobacco glycoprotein. *J Exp Med* 146:457, 1977.
38. Bouche RT, Medawar SJ, Dockery GL: Oral contraceptives and deep venous thrombosis with pulmonary embolism. *J Foot Surg* 21:297, 1982.
39. Wessler S, Gitel SN, Wan LS: Estrogen-containing oral contraceptive agents. A basis for their thrombogenicity. *JAMA* 236:2179, 1976.
40. Harris WH, Salzman EW, DeSanctis RW: Prevention of venous thromboembolism following total hip replacement. *JAMA* 220:1319, 1972.
41. Simon MA, Mass DP, Zarins CK: The effect of a thigh tourniquet on the incidence of deep venous thrombosis after operations on the fore part of the foot. *J Bone Joint Surg* 64A:188, 1982.
42. Rosenthal T, Halkin H, Shani M: Occlusion of the great veins in the Behcet syndrome. *Angiology* 23:600, 1972.
43. Morris GK, Mitchell JRA: Prevention and diagnosis of venous thrombosis in patients with hip fractures: a survey of current practice. *Lancet* 2:867, 1976.
44. Strandness DE, Jr., Ward K, Krugmire RJ: The present status of acute deep venous thrombosis. *Surg Gyn Obst* 145:433, 1977.
45. Sumner DS, Lambwith A: Reliability of Doppler ultrasound in the diagnosis of acute venous thrombosis both above and below the knee. *Am J Surg* 138:205, 1979.
46. Hull R, VanAken WG, Hirsh J: Impedence plethysmography using the occlusive cuff technique in the diagnosis of venous thrombosis. *Circulation* 53:696, 1976.
47. Hobbs JT, Davies JWL: Detection of venous thrombosis with I^{131}-labelled fibrinogen in the rabbit. *Lancet* 2:134, 1960.
48. Glazier RL, Crowell EB: Randomized prospective trial of continuous vs. intermittent heparin therapy. *JAMA* 236:1365, 1976.
49. Jick H, Stone D, Borda I: Efficacy and toxicity of heparin in relation to age and sex. *N Engl J Med* 279:284, 1968.
50. Fratantoni JC, Ness P, Simon TL: Thrombolytic therapy: Current status. *N Engl J Med* 293:1073, 1975.
51. Sharma, GVRK, Cella G, Panisi AF: Thrombolytic therapy. *N Engl J Med* 306:1268, 1982.
52. Bell WR, Meek AG: Guidelines for the use of the thrombolytic agents. *N Engl J Med* 301:1266, 1979.
53. Marder VJ, Soulen RL, Atichartakarn V: Quantitative venographic assessment of deep venous thrombosis in the evaluation of streptokinase and heparin therapy. *J Lab Clin Med* 89:1018, 1977.
54. Common HH, Seaman AJ, Rosch J: Deep vein thrombosis treated with streptokinase or heparin. Follow up of a randomized study. *Angiology* 27:645, 1976.
55. Johansson L, Nylander G, Hedner U: Comparison of streptokinase and heparin: late results in the treatment of deep venous thrombosis. *Acta Med Scand* 206:93, 1979.
56. Bieger R, Boekhout-Mussert RJ, Hohmann F: Is streptokinase useful in the treatment of deep venous thrombosis? *Acta Med*

Scand 199:81, 1976.

57. Sherry S, Bell WR, Duckert FH: Thrombolytic therapy in thrombosis. *Ann Intern Med* 93:141, 1980.
58. Urokinase-streptokinase embolism trial phase 2 results. A cooperative study. *JAMA* 229:1606, 1974.
59. Duckert FH, Muller G, Nyman D: Treatment of deep venous thrombosis with streptokinase. *Br J Med* 1:479, 1975.
60. Greenfield LJ, McCurdy JR, Brown PP: A new intracaval filter promoting continued flow and resolutaion of emboli. *Surgery* 73:599, 1973.
61. Wingerd M, Bernherd VM, Maddison F: Comparison of caval filters in the management of thromboembolism. *Arch Surg* 113:1264, 1978.
62. Knight MTN, Dawson R: Effect of intermittent compression of the arms on deep venous thrombosis in the legs. *Lancet* 2:1265, 1976.
63. Hatch DJ, Mahnusson PG, DiGiovanni JE: Mini-dose heparin prophylaxis for high risk patients in podiatric surgery. *J Am Podiatry Assoc* 70:73, 1980.
64. Simon TL, Stengle JM: Antithrombotic practice in orthopedic surgery. Results of a survey. *Clin Orthop* 102:181, 1974.
65. Gallus AJ, Hirsh J, Tuttle RJ: Small subcutaneous doses of heparin in prevention of venous thrombosis. *N Engl J Med* 288:545, 1973.
66. DeTakats G: Heparin prophylaxis: room for improvement. *Am J Surg* 143:711, 1982.
67. Salzman EW: Progress in preventing venous thromboembolism. *N Engl J Med* 309:980, 1983.
68. Leyvraz PF, Richard J, Bachmann F: Adjusted versus fixed-dose subcutaneous heparin in the prevention of deep vein thrombosis after total hip replacement. *N Engl J Med* 309:954, 1983.
69. Dalen JE, Alpert JE: Natural history of pulmonary embolism. *Prog Cardiovasc Dis* 17:259, 1975.

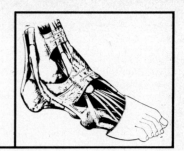

CHAPTER 18

The Geriatric Patient

Kinley W. Howard, C.R.N.A., D.P.M.

The word "geriatric" is derived from the Greek words *geras* (old age) and *iatrike* (surgery, medicine) meaning that branch of medicine that treats all problems peculiar to old age and the aging (1, 2). Podogeriatrics is that medical specialty concerned with the medical and surgical treatment of foot problems in the elderly patient (3).

Foot care has become a major concern in the total care of the geriatric patient. With the increased awareness of foot and ankle problems associated with the total well-being of the patient, and with new and advanced surgical techniques, much attention is now focused on the correction and alleviation of foot deformities in the elderly.

In the United States 82% of women and 67% of men will reach the age of 65. Aged Americans (65 years and older) constitute 11.3% of the total population of 226,505,000 (1980 census) (4–6) but their expenditures for health care account for 28% (approximately $14,000/patient/year) of the total medical care expenses (7, 8).

Seventy-five percent of patients age 65 and older complain of painful feet that interfere with or prevent normal ambulation (9, 10). In this age group orthopedic problems of the knees, hips, or back may cause maldistribution of the weight on the foot. Similarly, foot deformities can lead to difficulties in the knees, hips, or back.

Estimates indicate that by the year 2000 12.2% of the population will be age 65 or older (Table 18.1). By 2020 15.6% and by the year 2035 18.3% of the population will be age 65 or older (5, 6). Based on current projected population growth figures and the need of foot care, by the year 2000 24 million Americans 65 years of age and older will be in need of foot care. It is essential that the podiatric surgeon develop and maintain a strong foundation for surgical correction of geriatric foot deformities.

GENERAL CONSIDERATIONS

Age alone is not a reason to shy away from the surgical correction of a painful or disfiguring foot or ankle deformity in the geriatric patient. Many progressive foot deformities remain asymptomatic for years only to become fixed, rigid, and painful in the senior years. When conservative therapy is inadequate surgical intervention is often required.

Most procedures on geriatric patients should be performed in the hospital or in a well-equipped office. Regardless of the choice of anesthesia the patient will need to be carefully evaluated preoperatively and receive close monitoring by the anesthesiology department intraoperatively. A good general rule to follow is to use the physical status categories published by the American Society of Anesthesiologists (Table 18.2). If the patient is classified in any category other than class 1 or 2, hospitilization is often advisable even for minor procedures such as removing nails or warts. An alternative would be to have an anesthesiologist or anesthetist monitor the patient in the office during the procedure. Even with careful monitoring the geriatric patient may be at increased risk. Regardless of whether the surgery is performed in the office or hospital the podiatric surgeon should obtain a careful history and pay close attention to the cardiovascular and respiratory status. Auscultation of the chest with a stethoscope may detect an abnormality that requires consultation before surgery.

Cardiovascular

Coronary atherosclerosis is the largest cause of death among the geriatric population in the United States (11). The disease is responsible for one third of all deaths and two thirds of fatalities from cardiovascular disease. Symptoms of cardiovascular disease do not appear in 75% of patients until multivessel obstruction develops. Most patients over age 50 have varying degrees of impaired cardiac function. Increased collagen, altered elastin, and increased calcium result in arterial rigidity with elevation of systolic pressure, accelerated pulse wave velocity, and a loss of 10% in cardiac efficiency. Peripheral resistance is increased and diastolic pressure is slightly elevated.

Table 18.1.
Estimates and Projections of Persons 65 and over (in thousands)

Year	Number	Percent of Total
1900	3100	4.1
1940	9036	6.8
1950	12,397	8.2
1960	16,675	9.0
1970	20,087	9.8
1980	24,824	11.2
1990	29,824	12.2
2000	31,822	12.2

Source: U.S. Bureau of the Census, Current Population Reports, Series P-25, No. 704, Projections of the Population of the U.S. (Washington, DC: Government Printing Office, 1977). (From Palmore E: *International Handbook on Aging*. Westport CT, Greenwood Press, 1980, p 436.)

Table 18.2.
Preoperative Physical Status Category

Class 1. Normally healthy patient.
Class 2. Patient with mild systemic disease.
Class 3. Patient with severe systemic disease that is not incapacitating.
Class 4. Patient with an incapacitating systemic disease that is a constant threat to life.
Class 5. Moribund patient who is not expected to survive for 24 hours with or without operation.
E—Added to the above classification to designate emergency surgery

Source: The American Society of Anesthesiologists. (From Dodd RB: Anesthesia. In Stainberg PU (ed): *Care of the Geriatric Patient*, ed 6. St Louis, The CV Mosby Co, 1983, p 327.)

Capillary basement membrane thickness increases from 700 to 1100 between youth and old age (1).

Resting heart rate does not change with age. However, resting cardiac output decreases approximately 25% by age 71 when compared with the young adult (1). With increased age cardiac output and stroke volume decrease during exercise. The maximum attainable heart rate declines in a linear fashion roughly 220 minus the age in years (12). There may be some prolongation in ventricular ejection: however, age-associated electrocardiogram (EKG) changes are minor and of questionable significance (1).

Many elderly patients are on one or more cardiac drugs for the treatment of heart disease. As of this writing no drug commonly used to treat heart disease needs be withdrawn before surgery.

It is desirable for the patient to have a 12-lead EKG recorded before surgery, in addition to a chest x-ray study. If the patient experiences postoperative chest pain the surgeon has a baseline recording for comparison. Any suspicious changes noted should alert one to request an immediate cardiology consult.

Peripheral Vascular Disease

Peripheral vascular disease involves virtually every patient in the geriatric age group (13). The disease is generally classified as arterial or venous, being further subdivided as acute or chronic. Both conditions are commonly found simultaneously in the geriatric patient. Studies by Reichle and associates (14) reported that elderly patients with occlusive arterial disease of the lower extremities had organic heart disease more than 40% of the time.

Physiologically, blood pressure in the lower extremity is normally 20 mm Hg higher than the upper extremity (13). Theoretically a cause and effect relationship between this regional hypertension and a preponderance of localized arteriosclerosis has some validity.

Many factors have been implicated as the cause of chronic peripheral arterial occlusive disease. These include emotional stress, physical inactivity, obesity, smoking hypercoagulability, and hyperlipidemia (13). Martinez and associates (15) reported the following incidence of specific risk increase factors: smoking 87%, hypertension 30%, hyperlipidemia 27%, and diabetes mellitus 24%.

Arterial disease may be suspected when Monckeberg's sclerosis (middle-layer arterial wall calcification) is observed on routine foot x-ray studies. However, the most common symptom in the geriatric patient with peripheral arterial disease is intermittent claudication (13). This is usually described by the patient as a cramping type pain especially in the calf after exercise or ambulation. After resting several minutes, and allowing arterial blood flow to deliver sufficient oxygen to reverse the anaerobic metabolic process, the pain disappears and the patient is able to ambulate once again.

Rest pain is a distinct entity usually consisting of deep, lancinating discomfort in the metatarsal heads (16). With more advanced ischemia rest pain is experienced proximally in the tarsus and ankle. This type of vascular insult is considered pregangrenous.

Hair loss is commonly observed on the lower leg and foot. The hair follicle is one of the first organs to suffer from diminished arterial blood flow. In addition ankle edema is common because of the generalized poor condition of the vessels.

Palpating peripheral pulses is the most important single test in establishing the diagnosis of occlusive arterial disease (17) (Table 18.3). With moderate to severe ischemia the feet will blanch when elevated (pallor) and become excessively red or cyanotic (rubor) when left in a dependent position. A delay of more than 15 to 30 seconds for the dorsal foot veins to fill after the legs have been placed in a dependent position from the elevated position usually indicates ischemia.

An ankle arm index obtained by measuring the systolic arm and ankle pressures with a cuff is an easy and additional diagnostic test (18) (Table 18.4). Normal results (greater than or equal to 1) are obtained by dividing the ankle systolic pressure by the arm systolic pressure. Elective surgery should not proceed without further studies with values of 0.6 or less. If in doubt, Doppler, ultrasound, and/or arteriography should be completed before surgery. If arteriography is requested it is imperative to obtain both left and

Table 18.3.
Grading Scale for Peripheral Pulses

0—Complete Absence
1+—Marked Impairment of Pulsation
2+—Moderate Impairment of Pulsation
3+—Slight Impairment of Pulsation
4+—Normal Pulsation

(From Fairbairn JF II: Clinical manifestations of peripheral vascular disease. In Juergens JL, Spittell JA Jr, Fairbairn JF II (eds): *Allen-Barker-Hines Peripheral Vascular Diseases.* Philadelphia, WB Saunders Co, 1980, p 16.)

Table 18.4.
Ankle Arm Index Scale Chart (Grading System for Occlusive Arterial Disease)

1.00 – 0.9 = Normal
0.89 – 0.7 = Mild, Stable
0.69 – 0.5 = Moderately, Severe
0.49 – 0.3 = Impending Gangrene
0.29 – 0.0 = Distal Necrosis

(From Block BH: Vascular considerations. In Marcus SA, Block BH (eds): *Complications of Foot Surgery*, ed 2. Baltimore, Williams & Wilkins, 1984, p 26.)

right extremities for comparison. Anteroposterior, lateral, and oblique views are necessary because the conventional anteroposterior and lateral views almost invariably underestimate the severity of the disease (16). The percutaneous (Seldinger) technique is performed by most institutions. Because morbidity and mortality risks of 1% to 2% exist arteriography is seldom ordered unless a revascularization procedure is being seriously considered.

In patients with peripheral arterial disease who have rest pain, zinc sulfate has been used in an attempt to preserve the integrity of the skin and soft tissues with some benefit. Whether it affects the arteriosclerotic process is yet to be determined.

Although zinc blood levels are not routinely tested preoperatively additional perioperative intake in the form of vitamins with zinc probably aid wound healing and strength.

The effect of muscular exercise in the treatment of claudication has been studied by Okun (19). He reported that exercise produced widening of collateral vessels and that rhythmic muscular exercise seemed to be the most physiological procedure to enhance blood flows in extremities with vascular occlusion.

If podiatric surgery is contemplated in geriatric patients with established peripheral vascular disease the deformity should be treated conservatively for four to six months if practical. A vascular workup is obtained and the patient placed on a walking program combined with one of the peripheral dilator drugs. After this period of time the patient is reevaluated for surgery.

Acute Arterial Occlusion

Acute arterial occlusion is a rare postoperative complication of which the podiatric surgeon should be aware, especially in the geriatric patient. Within minutes after acute occlusion of the major arterial supply the foot becomes painful and pale. Immediately on examination the pulses are absent. The diagnosis is not a difficult one to make and the clinical manifestations can be simply remembered by the "Five P's: Pain, Pallor, Pulselessness, Paresthesia and Paralysis" (13).

Over 90% of arterial emboli are derived from the heart (13, 18, 20). They may be from the atrium in fibrillation, the ventricle after infarction, a diseased valve, or from a myxoma. The emboli most commonly lodge in the lower extremity.

Controversy exists over immediate systemic heparinization of the patient. However, embolectomy with a Fogarty catheter is usually necessary.

Another type of acute arterial embolization known as livedo reticularis is occasionally seen in the geriatric patient after foot surgery (13). Focal infarcts involving the skin on the distal aspects of the toes and commonly the entire lower extremity is seen. These infarcts initially appear as tiny purplish spots that may be confused with a number of other conditions. A fishnet mottled pattern may be observed on the lower extremity. In the geriatric patient these emboli are usually caused by embolization of cholesterol crystals or fragments of atheromata most often arising from plaques in the aorta; however, the origin may occur from the larger femoral vessels.

Caution must be exercised in using an intraoperative tourniquet on elderly obese patients with elevated serum cholesterol and/or triglyceride levels, and in patients with cardiac and peripheral vascular disease. Careful monitoring of digital color and capillary fill time postoperatively will alert the surgeon to impending complications.

Venous Disease

More than 8 million Americans suffer from varicose veins (17). Heredity is the most important factor in the development of varices but they can develop in elderly patients because the veins tend to lose their elasticity with aging and the muscles supporting them weaken.

Chronic venous insufficiency is the end result of incompetent and damaged valves. The damaged valves are the result of deep vein thrombosis or long-standing varicose veins. The chronic edema, venous pooling, and dermatological changes associated with the disease increase the potential for postoperative complications. Every effort should be made to control and reduce the edema and venous pooling preoperatively.

Elastic custom-fitted stockings (Jobst) that supply 20 to 50 mm Hg per square inch of compression is the simplest and best way to control the deformity and prevent complications (16, 17). Ace wraps or Redigrip may be used as a substitute. The geriatric patient with moderate to severe varicosities should be fitted with Jobst stockings at least two weeks before podiatric surgery. The surgical procedure should be accomplished without a tourniquet if at all possible.

Elastic wraps should be applied postoperatively over the bandage before the patient leaves the operating room. Early ambulation (within 24 hours) after surgery is encouraged if possible.

If prolonged bed rest is required the foot of the bed should be elevated with the patient's knees flexed approximately 30°. The patient must continue to wear elastic support during bed rest and ambulation. Active or passive range of motion exercises should be performed, preferably by a physical therapist, several times a day until the patient becomes ambulatory. One should avoid the use of drugs, such as the phenothiazines, that promote peripheral dilation. The patient is to be observed closely for any sign of deep vein thrombosis or venous ulcer formation. Minidose heparin (5000 units every 12 hours) should be considered if the patient is a high-risk patient, especially if prolonged immobilization and bed rest are required after surgery.

Thrombophlebitis

Thrombophlebitis is a common postoperative problem with a higher than normal incidence in the geriatric population. The incidence is 30% to 35% of all patients operated on and is much more frequent in the 70 and over age group (21). The overall occurrence of postoperative thrombophlebitis in geriatric patients following podiatric surgery is probably less than 5% and the lower rate can be attributed to the early ambulation postoperatively.

Superficial thrombophlebitis usually presents as a red, warm, and tender area under the skin along the course of a vein (17). Edema may not present to a great extent. In the podiatric surgical patient the condition is more often encountered in the upper extremity, especially in patients on intravenous antibiotics. If circumstances necessitate continuation of intravenous therapy for more than 24 hours postoperatively the infusion site is rotated every 48 to 72 hours until discontinued.

Because emboli do not result from superficial thrombophlebitis anticoagulation is not required or recommended. Treatment consists of heat, usually as warm, moist packs with a K-pad held in place about the extremity with Kling gauze. Rest and elevation of the extremity until the pain and tenderness subsides are also helpful. If secondary cellulitis is present appropriate antibiotic coverage is indicated.

Deep vein thrombosis may yield minimal physical findings especially in the geriatric patient (17). These usually consist of edema, distended superficial veins, a reddish cyanotic color, and pain and tenderness that may be confused with other entities. The key to early diagnosis is a high index of suspicion. The diagnosis can be confirmed by venography but is rarely necessary because of new, improved, and accurate diagnostic studies. These include radioactive fibrinogen studies that are much more comfortable for the patient. Noninvasive studies such as impedance phlebography ultrasound (Sonicaid) and Doppler ultrasound are valuable and accurate diagnostic aids.

Once the diagnosis is established the initial treatment includes elevation of the limb and anticoagulation therapy (16, 17, 22–24). Heparin is the most effective drug and an initial subcutaneous or intravenous dose of 10,000 to 20,000 units should be given to the patient, followed by 5000 to 10,000 units every 6 to 12 hours. Regulation of the dosage should be correlated with the partial thromboplastin time (PTT) and/or clotting time. The heparin dosage should be adjusted to maintain the PTT at one to one and one half times the base ine value or normal value.

The nonsteroidal antiinflammatory drugs are helpful in relieving the pain associated with the condition and may help to reduce the inflammation. Antibiotics are given if secondary cellulitis is present.

With improvement warfarin (Coumadin) is usually initiated orally on the seventh to tenth day with the IV heparin (16, 17, 22, 24). The prothrombin time (PT) and the PTT are monitored daily. After 10 days of oral Coumadin the heparin is discontinued and the patient continues the warfarin. The dosage is 25 to 30 mg as a loading dose, 10 to 15 mg the second day, and 5 mg the third day and each day thereafter, depending on the PT.

Heparin and warfarin are difficult drugs to control in the geriatric patient. Difficulty in control correlates with increasing age, debility, liver disease, renal failure, and changing concomitant drug therapy.

Prevention of deep vein thrombosis can best be accomplished by support hose. For a hospitalized geriatric patient undergoing foot surgery, especially one requiring prolonged bed rest for several days postoperatively, the surgeon should consider preoperative support hose and an IV or subcutaneous dose of 2000 to 3000 units of heparin two hours before surgery (22). This is especially critical if the patient has a prior history of thrombophlebitis. Postoperatively the patient is given 5000 units of heparin every 6 to 12 hours until ambulation is established. There is less chance of deep vein thrombosis and minimal increased risk of intraoperative hemorrhage.

Another prophylactic treatment is the use of aspirin, dipyridamole (Persantin), or some other nonsteroidal antiinflammatory drug with the exception of piroxicam (Feldene), which does not affect platelet aggregation. Starting one day before surgery one of these drugs is administered orally. The treatment is aimed at preventing the formation of platelet-thrombin complexes that adhere to the venous endothelium and initiate the thrombotic process. Aspirin and dipyridamole taken together has resulted in a reduction greater than 50% in the incidence of deep vein thrombus formation following surgery (24). A well-hydrated geriatric patient ambulated early postoperatively is at a small risk for deep vein thrombosis.

Pulmonary Embolism

Pulmonary embolism with its high mortality is a constant threat from thrombophlebitis whether the primary peripheral condition is recognized or not. An estimated 50,000 to 100,000 persons die from pulmonary embolism in the United States each year (22). Autopsy studies reveal only 25% to 50% of pulmonary emboli are recognized clinically before death. A surgically compromised geriatric patient who suffers a pulmonary embolism carries an extremely high mortality risk.

The following factors have been recognized as etiological factors in thromboembolism: infection, chronic venous disease, heart disease, immobilization, cancer, trauma, pregnancy, blood coagulation abnormalities, tobacco, dehydration, obesity, anemia, and emphysema (22). When thrombophlebitis is recognized, the following danger signals pose strong suspicion of embolism (22):

1. A sudden stabbing pain in the chest usually on one side or the other.
2. Thereafter the pain may be constant or intermittent but is frequently aggravated by deep breathing.
3. The patient may appear startled, frightened, may clutch the chest, break out in a cold sweat, or appear ashen or cyanotic. Tachycardia is almost always present.
4. Blood pressure may go up because of fright, or if the embolus is large, drop rapidly because of shock. At this point death is usually imminent.
5. If the patient survives the first few hours the chances of survival rapidly improve.

The EKG changes vary and are largely nonspecific, but if ST wave elevation or depression is newly present, it is a helpful finding (22). Chest x-ray studies show atelectatic shadows, frequently V shaped, that are usually multiple. The lung scan shows similar filling defects and is the most useful diagnostic approach available. Pulmonary angiography is rarely necessary to establish the diagnosis.

The prevention of postinjury or postoperative thrombosis or embolism is of special importance in the geriatric patient. The vessel walls are usually rougher and invite easy clotting, thrombosis, and embolism. Three important steps should be taken to prevent thromboembolic complications in the postoperative geriatric patient. These are exercised while immobilized and wearing of knee-length elastic stockings or Ace wraps when in bed, early ambulation, and the use of low-dose heparin or non-steroidal antiinflammatory drugs to prevent thrombus formation.

Ulcers

The podiatric surgeon will occasionally encounter an elderly patient with painful pedal deformities who presents with an open ulcer secondary to arterial or venous circulatory embarrassment or perhaps caused by trauma.

Elective surgery, even if adequate pulses are present, should not proceed. An open ulcer is considered contaminated and is a prime source for seeding bacteria into a fresh surgical wound, creating disastrous postoperative complications and destroying the corrective surgical procedure.

If emergency surgery is required such as open reduction of a fracture, the wound should be gram stained and cultured for aerobic and anaerobic organisms. The patient should be placed on immediate intravenous antibiotics, preferably a first generation cephalosporin such as Ancef, or a beta-lactamase-resistant penicillin such as Nafcillin. Use of an intraoperative tourniquet is inadvisable. The ulcer is prepped, then draped separately with Opsite or some other fluid impermeable material. The proposed surgical site is then prepped separately and draped accordingly.

The elderly patient should be maintained on intravenous antibiotics postoperatively while febrile and hospitalized and discharged on appropriate antibiotics until the surgical wounds are well sealed.

Respiratory

Respiratory tract infections are usually less frequent in the geriatric patient because of immunological experience (1). However, anteroposterior chest diameter is increased, compliance is decreased, and work needed to overcome the elastic forces of the chest and wall is 20% greater in the elderly patient. Total lung capacity is unchanged but residual volume is doubled and vital capacity is reduced. Maximum breathing capacity decreases about 50% between the third and ninth decades. Pulmonary blood flow remains unchanged; therefore blood flows through relatively unaerated portions of the lungs, creating a physiological shunt. There is decreased cough efficiency, decreased ciliary activity of the bronchial epithelium, and increased dead space that enhances the potential for infections.

Whenever possible local anesthesia with intravenous sedation is desirable. Local anesthesia will decrease the postoperative pulmonary complications from anesthesia by 50% especially in a compromised geriatric patient. If general or spinal anesthesia is necessary, incentive spirometry preoperatively and postoperatively is recommended.

If the patient relates a history of severe chronic obstructive pulmonary disease and spinal or general anesthesia is necessary, preoperative arterial blood gases while breathing room air is encouraged. If the patient develops postoperative pulmonary complications the surgeon will have a preoperative baseline arterial blood gas for comparison. A consultation with the anesthesia department and pulmonary medicine is most valuable.

MUSCULOSKELETAL SYSTEM

Muscle loss and disorganization cause a progressive reduction in muscle strength (1). Poor repair characteristics lead to deterioration with progressive loss of joint spaces and resultant degenerative arthritis in the geriatric patient. Bone is continuously remodeled throughout life by reabsorption of internal surfaces and formation on exterior surfaces. In the elderly patient reabsorption exceeds bone formation. Both protein matrix and bone material are involved and clinical osteoporosis often results. In the aged female patient 25% of bone is lost (1, 25). Senile osteoporosis and malnutrition are common in geriatric patients.

Collagen constitutes approximately 40% of the body protein (26). It serves as a matrix on which minerals are deposited to give bones their characteristic hardness. Perhaps more importantly collagen is essential in the healing of soft tissues that surround the bones and joints. In the geriatric patient collagen fibers are increased in size and become irregular in shape because of the development of crosslinkages between their constituent tropocollagen molecules. Elasticity of the collagen fibers is diminished and they become thickened and less mobile. This characteristic change demonstrates the importance of the mobilization of joints as soon as possible postoperatively.

Osteoporosis

Osteoporosis has been found in skeletons dating 2000 BC, and was first described in the sixth century AD by Paulus Aeginata. However, the term "osteoporosis" was coined in 1885 by Pommer. It is the most commonly seen metabolic osseous disease and is found in all geriatric patients to some degree (25). Age, sex, and race must be considered. Blacks show less tendency toward the disease. The condition is characterized by an absolute decrease in the amount of bone per unit volume of tissue. Bone that is present has normal mineralization. Twenty-five percent of the bone mass must be lost before radiographic evidence of the disease is apparent (25, 27).

X-ray studies reveal increased bone lucency with a loss of trabecular pattern. Bone mass may be measured with a photon absorptiometer (bone densiometry), which measures bone absorption of radioactive iodine-125 via a scintillation detector (25). Radiation exposure is minimal and the technique works best in the bones of the feet and hands. Bone calipers may be used to measure the cortical thickness of the bone. However, this method is not totally accurate because cortical thickness may be maintained with the loss of cortical density. The clinician with experience at interpreting radiographs is the best judge of the amount and significance of osteoporosis present.

Modification in the podiatric procedure may be necessary in the geriatric patient with a moderate degree of osteoporosis present who has a painful hallux abducto valgus deformity in need of surgical correction. One would be reluctant to do a closing base wedge osteotomy of the first metatarsal and cast the patient for a prolonged period of time postoperatively when the deformity could be corrected with a head osteotomy and soft tissue correction, which in most cases allows earlier postoperative ambulation.

Calcium supplement perioperatively, especially if osteotomies are performed, seems helpful in speeding bony healing and slowing the osteoporotic process. Likewise, bivalving a cast and lining the edges with moleskin so the patient can remove the cast at intervals for range of motion exercises significantly reduces cast disease in this age group.

Degenerative Joint Disease

After the age of 60, 80% of patients show radiographic evidence of osteoarthritis. Fifteen percent of males and 25% of females have symptomatic osteoarthritis (29).

The disease is characterized by splitting, fragmentation and fissuring of the articular cartilage (28). Histological changes of smaller and less well-organized collagen fibers accompanied by radiographically evident subchondral bone sclerosis without demineralization is present. In addition, juxta-articular subchondral bone cysts, asymmetrical narrowing of the joint spaces, and osteophytic outgrowth of cortical and cancellous bone (hallmark) at joint margins is seen on x-ray films. Pain from chronic degenerative osteoarthritis is thought to be caused by the interruption of nerves that accompany subchondral bone blood vessels. Acute pain may result from traumatic synovitis. In the foot the first metatarsophalangeal joint is most often affected and may be the only joint involved.

The disease is classified as primary or secondary (29). No apparent cause is identified in primary osteoarthritis whereas in the secondary type a cause is recognized. Examples of primary forms include Heberden's nodes (distal interphalangeal) joints, Bouchard's nodes (proximal interphalangeal joints), and generalized osteoarthrosis. This type is found primarily in women over the age of 50. In addition erosive osteoarthritis affects small joints of the feet and hands and may mimic rheumatoid arthritis (RA) although the metatarsals and more proximal joints are not involved.

Secondary forms usually follow trauma, endocrine disorders such as acromegaly, metabolic disease such as hemochromatosis, and other medical problems such as avascular necrosis and hemophilia.

Pain on ambulation is associated with friction in the joints and from shoe pressure or areas of hypertrophied osseous formation. Exacerbation of nonambulatory pain is usually associated with the deposition of calcium hydroxyapatite crystals in the joint spaces. When the elderly patient's pain can no longer be controlled with nonsteroidal antiinflammatory drugs, orthoses, and other conservative measures, surgical intervention is required. The geriatric patient is maintained on the nonsteroidal medication throughout the perioperative period. Good physical therapy and the continuation of orthoses with modifications postoperatively helps the patient return to normal pain-free ambulation in conventional shoegear.

Gout and Pseudogout

Gout and pseudogout are conditions of crystal synovitis that are common, affecting approximately 3% of the geriatric population (1, 28, 29). The diagnosis of gout depends on visualization of bisodium urate crystals in the joint, most commonly the first metatarsophalangeal joint, with males showing a preponderance (1, 28).

Gout is a metabolic disorder of purine metabolism and is classified as primary or secondary (1). Primary gout is inherited as an autosomal recessive disorder. Ninety percent of patients classified as having primary gout are males (28). Secondary gout is an acquired form of the disorder and is usually caused by an excessive breakdown of nuclear protein. It may be seen in such diseases as polycythemia, leukemia, multiple myeloma, sickle cell anemia, chronic renal disease, and the use of thiazide diuretics. Thirty percent of patients affected with secondary gout are female.

Patients are usually classified as overproducers or undersecretors. The pathogenesis of excessive urate accumulation is attributed to increased dietary absorption of purines, endogenous overproduction, decreased gastrointestinal or renal excretion, decreased endogenous destruction, or a combination of these. The normal geriatric patient excretes 250 to 600 mg of urates per day. One fourth of gouty patients excrete excessive amounts of urate.

The pathognomonic lesion of primary gout is the tophus (1, 28). It is a deposition of urate surrounded by inflammatory and foreign body reaction. These urates may be deposited in cartilage, epiphyseal bone, periarticular structures, and the kidney. Early in the disease the deposits occur on the surface of the articular cartilage and synovial membranes. This results in the degeneration of the cartilage, synovial proliferation, and pannus formation. Subchondral bone destruction follows with proliferation of the marginal bone. Before the advent of modern drugs approximately 50% of patients developed tophi (28).

Fifteen percent of patients with chronic gout develop uric acid stones (29). Renal function in general is decreased in these patients because of tophaceous deposits in the kidneys. Intake and output is monitored during the perioperative period. Careful use of nephrotoxic drugs must be exercised to prevent additional kidney damage. Pseudogout is diagnosed by visualization of calcium pyrophosphate dihydrate crystals in the joint, most commonly the knee, although the condition may occur in the ankle and other joints (1, 28, 29).

A geriatric patient with hyperuricemia and nonspecific joint pain probably does not have gout (1, 28, 29). The majority of elderly patients with increased uric acid levels never develop gout and patients with laboratory proven gout may have a normal serum uric acid level, especially if they are taking uricosuric drugs or allopurinal.

The radiologic changes with the characteristic juxta-articular erosions with overhanging margins occur late and should not be relied on for diagnosis (1, 27, 28). Initial radiographic changes reveal periarticular soft tissue swelling similar to rheumatoid arthritis. However, unlike rheumatoid arthritis, the lesions are not symmetrical and there is a lack of osteoporosis. Additionally there is no evidence of subluxation or mal-alignment.

X-ray studies are indicated usually to rule out other pathological conditions, and are more valuable in diagnosing pseudogout because chondrocalcinosis (calcium deposition in hyaline and fibrocartilage) is almost invariably present. The reverse is not true because chondrocalcinosis is present in 10% of geriatric patients who never develop pseudogout (29). The two conditions are compared in Table 18.5.

Podagra should be ruled out in a geriatric patient presenting with first metatarsophalangeal joint pain who has a hallux abducto valgus deformity. However, proposed foot surgery is not contraindicated in the elderly patient with a history of gout or pseudogout. If the elderly surgical candidate has a history of frequent attacks, intravenous colchicine perioperatively should be considered to decrease the chance of an acute flareup. If the patient is on a nonsteroidal agent the drug should be continued through the preoperative and postoperative period because surgical intervention may precipitate a gouty or pseudogouty attack. A postoperative gouty attack with the increased temperature and edema may mimic an infection and/or cause unnecessary tension on the suture line and perhaps dehisence.

The effects of local anesthetics, injected to decrease postoperative pain, would be reduced because of the lower pH in the surrounding tissues.

A delay in ambulation and prolonged convalescence could be expected. Measures taken to prevent an acute attack are desirable; however, the podiatric surgeon should consider gout as a possible differential diagnosis in a postoperative patient who complains of increased pain over the metatarsophalangeal joint after a bunionectomy.

If an acute gouty attack should occur the conventional regime of intravenous or oral colchicine or nonsteroidal drugs such as phenylbutazone or indomethacin is indicated. Colchicine is given intravenously in a dosage of 1 to 2 mg diluted in 250 ml of normal saline, or orally 0.6 mg every hour until abdominal cramps or diarrhea develops. The diarrhea may be controlled with Lomotil. Caution must be used because the intravenous extravasation of colchicine causes intense pain as a result of its tissue irritating capability.

Phenylbutazone 300 to 400 mg orally initially then 100 to 200 mg every six hours for a maximum of seven days may be used. After the initial attack has subsided, allopurinol 200 to 400 mg per day may be prescribed for the overproducers. Caution must be used if the patient is on immunosuppressive drugs such as 6-mercaptopurine and azathioprine because of the potential fatal interaction of the drugs (29). Hypersensitive hepatotoxic reactions have been reported; however, the most common reaction is a pruritic rash. The drug is not recommended preoperatively because it too may precipitate a gouty attack. Uricosuric drugs such as probenecid (Benemid) and sulfinpyrazone (Anturane) are used for long-term therapy to reduce the miscible urate pool, retard urate deposition, and promote resorption of urate deposits. Attacks of pseudogout respond well to the nonsteroidal drugs. Rest is helpful until the acute attack subsides.

Rheumatoid Arthritis

The term "rheumatoid arthritis" was introduced in 1858 by Sir Alfred Garrod for a syndrome that he

Table 18.5.
Distinguishing Features of Gout and Pseudogout.

Feature	Gout	Pseudogout
Sex incidence	Male > Female	Equal
Age	>35 years	>55 years
Typical first joint	Great toe	Knee
Typical joint for subsequent attack	Knee, ankle, tarsus, great toe	Knee, shoulder, hip
Precipitating factors	Surgery, trauma, diet, or alcohol excess	Surgery
Associated conditions	Hyperuicemia, obesity, hypertriglyceridemia, alcohol abuse, hypertension	Diabetes mellitus Hemochromatosis Hyperparathyroidism Wilson's disease Osteoarthrosis
Duration of attack	Self-limiting: 3–10 days	Usually self-limiting: 1–30 days
Serum	Usually elevated uric acid	Usually no positive findings
Radiology	Usually normal	Chondrocalcinosis
Crystals	Sodium urate	Calcium pyrophosphate
Shape	needle	rhomboidal
Number	++++	+
Polarizing light	strong negative birefringence	weak positive birefringence
Unicase	dissolves	resistant
Treatment		
Acute	Indomethacin Phenylbutazone Colchicine	Indomethacin Phenylbutazone Intra-articular steroid
Intercritical	Uricosurics and Indomethacin/colchicine; rarely, allopurinol	None
Chronic disease	Tophaceous gout	Pseudorheumatoid arthritis Pseudo-osteoarthritis Pseudo-Charcot joint

(From Calin A: Gerontologic aspects of rheumatology. In Ebaugh FG (ed): *Clinical Aspects of Aging*, ed 2. Baltimore, Williams & Wilkins, 1983, p 64.)

recognized as distinct from gout and acute rheumatic fever (1).

The disease and joint inflammation is a systemic connective tissue disorder with the actual cause unknown, but is probably related to heredity and hypersensitivity (28). It is chronic and progressive in nature with many patients experiencing remissions and exacerbations. There is a 1% to 3% prevalence and the incidence is two to three times more common in females with the onset most common in the spring and after the fourth decade (1). Two percent of patients experience onset of the disease after age 65 (29). The disease is rare in tropical climates.

Fifty percent of patients will fail to respond to medical management and more than one half of these will require surgical intervention to continue pain-free ambulation in conventional shoegear (29).

The elderly patient often presents with advanced pedal deformities (30). The tendency is symmetrical polyarticular involvement of the feet with fibular deviation of the toes at the metatarsophalangeal and proximal interphalangeal joints (1, 27, 29). The joints may be ankylosed because of fibrous adhesions from pannus formation on opposing surfaces. The deformity is painful and the patient cannot wear normal shoegear.

Radiographs reveal advanced osteoporotic subchondral bone that may prevent the surgeon from using conventional silicone implants to realign the digits.

Twenty-five percent of geriatric patients will demonstrate pedal rheumatoid nodules. Surgical excision, although controversial, is indicated and may be combined with other corrective procedures, if the proper fit of normal shoegear is impossible. The primary goal in these elderly patients is continued pain free ambulation in conventional shoegear.

The traditional Hoffman-Clayton procedure combined with joint implants, tendon transfers, arthrodesis, and arthroplasties as indicated, supported with postoperative orthoses and physical therapy will keep the patient pain free and ambulatory in the majority of cases.

NERVE AND SENSORY ORGANS

Nerve cells are postmitotic and when destroyed are not replaced (1). The weight of the brain remains constant but some studies show significant loss of cortical cells in approximately 45% of aged patients and more importantly a loss of cellular integrity and cellular interconnections (1). By the age of 80, cerebral blood flow decreases from 79 to 46 ml per 100 gm of brain tissue. Oxygen consumption decreases from 3.6 to 2.7 ml per 100 gm of brain. The mean arterial pressure usually remains constant around 90 to 100 mm Hg but the cerebrovascular resistance increases from 1.3 to 2.1 mm Hg per ml of blood per 100 gm of brain tissue.

By age 95 motor nerve conduction velocity has

decreased some 15% to 20% and sensory conduction some 30% (1). Pain fibers appear to be intact but pain threshold and sleep levels 3 and 4 become less prominent and brief arousals become frequent with increasing age. However, total sleep time is not significantly affected. The reciprocal increase of monamine oxidase and the decrease in the amount of norepinephrine in brain tissue may have a related effect on the depression and apathy associated with many elderly patients.

Active involvement in self-care will help to reduce the postoperative aged patient's apathy and convalesence. Instructions should be brief, simple, and may need to be repeated. Requiring the patient to perform active or passive range of motion exercises will enhance self-esteem and develop a sense of need while improving the outcome of the overall surgical procedure.

Decreased visual acuity with increasing age is primarily caused by a decreased transparency of the cortical portion of the system.

Proprioception and balance may be decreased making ambulation postoperatively hazardous. Careful preoperative and postoperative gait training is imperative for the geriatric patient.

SKIN AND INTEGUMENT

Wrinkling and sagging of the skin are hallmarks of aging. The epidermis thins, contains less melanin, and cell replacement slows, resulting in delayed healing (1, 31). Epidermal glands are reduced in number and function resulting in dry skin (xerosis). There is reduced subcutaneous fat and collagen and fragmented inelastic elastin cause the skin to wrinkle. Complaints of metatarsal head pain are common, especially on ambulation, because of the decreased fat pad protection enjoyed in youth (32–36). Blood supply is reduced and with the increased capillary fragility subcutaneous senile purpura are commonly observed.

Reduced tissue viability and increased wound healing time mandates atraumatic surgical technique to decrease the possibility of prolonged postoperaive healing and/or complications. Care should be taken to avoid "grabbing" skin edges with instruments that may cause bruising, wound dehisence, or skin sloughing. Unnecessary pressure from retractors should be avoided to prevent tearing the delicate aged skin; it is better to lengthen the skin incision. Interrupted external skin or running subcuticular sutures are desirable to prevent strangulation of skin margins. Excessively tight sutures invite unwanted ischemic or necrotic skin edges.

Surgical scars usually present good aesthetic results. Aged wrinkled skin reduces tension on skin edges and if postoperative edema is controlled the scar remains narrow.

Ulceration is very likely if pins are poorly padded with a postoperative dressing or a poorly padded cast. Kling gauze used to secure wound dressings should be well padded. Indiscriminate application, especially in the web spaces of the digits across the dorsum of the foot and around the malleoli of the ankle, may cause ischemia with ulceration, abrasions, or lacerations of the fragile aged skin. Application of 2 by 2 or 4 by 4 inch gauze or kerlix squares next to the skin is preferable, with the Kling gauze applied over this in a firm but gentle compressive manner. Large infected ulcers carry a high morbidity and mortality rate in the aged patient.

EXCRETORY SYSTEMS

The number of nephrons in the kidneys decreases 30% to 40% by age 85 (1). Glomerular filtration rate, renal blood flow, and tubular filtration are decreased proportionately although the serum creatinine and blood urea nitrogen (BUN) levels are maintained because of a reduced release of these waste products, reflecting a reduction in the overall muscle mass. The kidney must be damaged approximately 80% before BUN levels increase (1).

Discrimination must be exercised with usage of nephrotoxic drugs. Serum peak and trough levels must be closely monitored with prolonged use of aminoglycoside antibiotics or other nephrotoxic drugs.

Kidney infections are frequently found on routine urinalysis examination in geriatric patients hospitalized for podiatric surgery. A urological consult should be obtained and the patient begun on appropriate antibiotic therapy preoperatively and the surgery proceed as scheduled.

With careless urination and contamination of surgical bandages an increased chance of infection occurs.

Gastric and intestinal motility is often disorganized. Constipation is a common problem in the postoperative patient, causing an elevated temperature, that may mimic an infection (1). A gastrointestinal prep is recommended if the patient is required to maintain complete bed rest postoperatively. A good bowel prep preoperatively is preferable to a postoperative enema with possible contamination of surgical bandages. If solid intake is good the elderly patient would be expected to have a bowel movement the second or third postoperative day. Prune juice or soy bean nuts with meals may be all that is required. Defecation should be monitored closely and constipation ruled out as the cause of a low grade postoperative temperature if no other signs of infection are present. Postoperative digestion and absorption are generally adequate although iron and calcium absorption may be reduced. Calcium supplements are often indicated to aid in healing and strengthening osteotomy sites.

The liver shows the characteristic atrophic changes in the elderly patient (1). Albumin production is decreased approximately 20%. Drugs normally bound to albumin should be decreased from the normal dosage accordingly to prevent toxic effects from increased blood levels (5, 38, 39).

DIABETES MELLITUS

The incidence of diabetes mellitus in the United States is about 5% of the total population with an estimated number of the now 10 million diabetics increasing at a rate of 6% per year, doubling the diabetic population every 15 years (40). Glucose tolerance decreases with age and 50% of patients age 70 and over have diabetes mellitus. With an increasing geriatric population, the increased impairment of glucose tolerance, and the associated foot complications, the podiatric surgeon will be required to treat an increasing number of elderly diabetic patients with pedal deformities.

There is no contraindication to performing podiatric surgery on the aged diabetic patient (17, 41). Blood glucose levels, however, should be well controlled with either diet or insulin, and good circulation should be present in the lower extremities.

The elderly patient with diabetes mellitus and its associated accelerated aging process, with the average being 10 years more than the chronological age, presents a great challenge to the podiatric surgeon (40). The associated increased incidence of vascular problems in the elderly diabetic patient requires careful attention to the circulatory status preoperatively.

Peripheral vascular diseases of the small arteries and arterioles is 50 to 70 times more common in elderly diabetics, and the surgical risk factor is 13% greater in the long-standing diabetic patient (40).

With accelerated cross linking of collagen and connective tissues and thickened capillary basement membranes in the elderly diabetic, delivery of required nutrients to surgical wound sites is delayed, prolonging normal healing time. Estimates indicate a one and one half to three time increase in healing time for poorly controlled geriatric diabetic patients.

NEUROPATHY

Neuropathy in the geriatric diabetic patient ranges from 13% to 62% (40). Evidence suggests that excessive blood sugar levels lead to accumulation through the polyol pathway, or sorbitol and fructose within the myelin sheath cause degeneration of the sheath. Onset is from 5 to 30 years after diabetes is diagnosed, and is most common in the lower extremities. The classic "stocking and glove effect" is most often found. Paresthesias and end-stage anesthesia is common.

Careful preoperative evaluation of epicritic senses is essential. Pressure from improperly padded Kirschner wires or poorly padded casts may cause ischemia and ulceration without causing pain to the patient. A below-knee cast extending beyond the end of the digits for protection, until healing is well advanced, may be indicated. The cast may be bivalved and the edges sealed with moleskin, thereby facilitating easy accesibility to the foot for dressing changes, wound examination, and range of motion exercises. The bivalved cast is easily held in place with an Ace wrap.

Regardless of the podiatric procedure performed the postoperative care should include efforts to improve the neuropathy or slow the progression (40). Vitamin B^{12} injections and large doses of vitamin E have produced poor results. Phenytoin (Dilantin) has

been reported to be effective in some cases and has been used for many years. Results have been more effective in diabetic females than males. Carbamazepine (Tegretol) has been helpful for geriatric patients with painful neuropathy. Caution must be used because of the high frequency of side effects. Probably the most effective therapy in treating painful neuropathic paresthesias and pain is a combination of amitriptyline (Amitril) and fluphenazine (Prolixin) hydrochloride. Pain and paresthesia are diminished and sometimes totally eliminated within only a few days, suggesting the effects of these medicines are not the result of psychic effects that take much longer to occur. Caution must be observed in prescribing these drugs to elderly patients because of the cardiac problems that may be caused. Careful consultation with the diabetologist is encouraged.

PRESCRIBING DRUGS

Reports released in 1981 by the World Health Organization (WHO) reported geriatric patients take an average of 3.2 to 8 drugs per day (42). The report recommended reduction of dosages for the following commonly used drugs: aminoglycosides, benzodiazepines, and meperidine (Demerol). The report also suggested avoiding the following drugs: chlorpropamide, nitrofurantoin, pentazocine, and phenylbutazone.

Adverse drug reactions (Table 18.6) occur more commonly in geriatric white women than men (38). Guidelines for drug prescribing are largely clinical judgment and based on the podiatric surgeon's experience and preference. When prescribing for the elderly patient postoperatively a general rule of thumb is to reduce the recommended dosage by one fourth to one half the recommended adult dosage. One should consider the basic overall health and other drug regimens of the patient. Rarely will oral postoperative pain medication fail to relieve podiatric discomfort. Occasionally no pain medicine is required other than aspirin or Tylenol. The use of oral nonsteroidal drugs and ice applied locally to the surgical site greatly reduce postoperative pain by controlling inflammation and discouraging edema.

Patient compliance must be considered. The senile geriatric patient is more compliant taking one medication per day than one three or four times per day.

The doctor must also consider the economic capabilities of the patient and prescribe the cheapest and least amount of a drug that will accomplish the desired goal. It has been estimated that more than 50% of prescriptions are not filled or consistently used by the patient (38, 39).

Only meticulous attention to the details and careful prescribing habits of the podiatric surgeon will serve to reduce the hazards of chemotherapy in the geriatric patient.

REHABILITATION

The surgeon must be aware of the labile homeostatic balance and diminished learning ability that is

Table 18.6.
Possible Adverse Reactions to Antibiotics[a]

Antibiotics	Adverse reactions
Penicillins	
Penicillin G potassium	Hyperkalemia in patients with renal insufficiency
Penicillin G sodium	Sodium retention, volume overload
Carbenicillin	Pulmonary edema, hypokalemia associated with serious arrhythmias, neurotoxicity, postoperative hororrhage
Ticarcillin	Pulmonary edema, neurotoxicity
Tetracyclines	Exacerbation of pre-existing abnormal renal function; catabolic state leading to azotemia, acidosis, and death; hepatotoxicity
Minocycline	Vestibular disorders (nausea, vomiting, dizziness, vertigo, ataxia)
Cephalosporins	
Cephalothin	Nephrotoxicity, acute renal failure, anaphylaxis in patients hypersensitive to penicillin
Cephalothin and cefazolin	Pain on intramuscular administration, chemical phlebitis following intravenous infusion
Aminoglycosides	Nephrotoxicity, ototoxicity
Clindamycin	Pseudomembranous colitis
Chloramphenicol	Bone marrow suppression, aplastic anemia, neuropsychiatic symptoms
Trimethoprin-sulfamethoxazole	Blood dyscrasias in patients with borderline folate stores, hypersensitivity reactions in azotemic patients

[a] Reprinted with permission from: Gleckman, R. A. and A. L. Esposito, 1980. Antibiotics in the elderly: skating on thin ice. Geriatrics, *35*, 26. (From Lamy PP: Drug prescribing for the elderly. In Reichel W (ed): *Clinical Aspects of Aging*, ed 2. Baltimore, Williams & Wilkins, 1983, p 64.)

commonly present in the geriatric patient population. This and other systemic disabilities that may compromise the patient's ability to ambulate with crutches or a walker must be considered before surgery.

Most older patients ambulate better with a walker. If the patient's home environment requires going up and down stairs the patient should master crutches before discharge from the hospital or office. Perhaps it is wiser to cast the surgical foot with a below knee cast for protection and allow partial weight bearing than to ambulate the unsteady elderly patient with crutches. If in doubt prescribe a wheelchair.

Gait training preoperatively by the physical therapist or nursing staff will help to ensure early ambulation and independence postoperatively.

With major podiatric surgery the rehabilitation time is one and one half to two times that of a young patient. The surgeon should consider this and make appropriate allowances.

Postoperative infections increase in incidence with age and prevention involves the use of good aseptic technique (43). Cephalosporins are commonly used as prophylaxis, and first generation cephalosporins are still the best. Prophylaxis should be considered preoperatively and postoperatively in the compromised geriatric patient.

An infection may be present in aged patients without clinical evidence of an increased temperature. They may run a low normal temperature and a degree of elevation may be carelessly ignored. Elderly patients with tachycardia should be carefully evaluated to rule out infection even if no fever is present. Chills are less common in response to infections.

If the patient is to have a prosthetic implant inserted, or has a previously inserted prosthesis in the body, prophylactic antibiotics are strongly recommended. The patient should be instructed to inform other surgeons of implanted prostheses for future surgery. Minor surgical procedures have been known hematogenously to seed an implant in the foot with bacteria.

Fifty percent of infections occur in the first five to six months postoperatively but late infections with prosthetic joints may appear up to two years later (18, 43). Early and late infections are usually caused by *Staphylococcus aureus*, *Staphylococcus epidermidis*, or *Peptococcus*.

Geriatric patients sometimes have a poor white blood cell (WBC) response to infections (43). Definite changes are observed in the immunological response of the elderly patient. There is a reduced immunoglobulin M (IgM) level, an increased complement 3 (C3) level, and a slightly increased properdin level. There is also evidence to relate changes in a delayed hypersensitivity and reaction to disease and infection.

The most important infection in elderly diabetics relates to gangrene of the foot. In diabetics white blood cells will not migrate normally to an area of infection, will not phagocytose, and will not kill bacteria if they do happen to phagocytose them (43). If the patient develops an infection aggressive intravenous antibiotic therapy should be initiated after gram stain and aerobic and anaerobic cultures are taken. The infection should be treated as polymicrobial and appropriate antibiotic therapy begun. When the sensitivity report is obtained, changes or additions of drugs are made as indicated.

Local wound care with irrigations and topical antibiotics are useful. If there is any doubt regarding the circulatory status of the foot an ingress and egress drainage system may be indicated (44). The system allows high concentrations of antibiotics to be delivered directly to the affected area without subjecting the entire body to large doses of antimicrobial drugs and their secondary toxicity.

SUMMARY

The average life expectancy of the population of the United States will increase over the next 25 years. The geriatric patient populations' increased need for podiatric care must be met by the podiatric physician.

The successful application of care and podiatric surgical techniques in this age group present a challenge to the podiatrist. The natural effects of aging, often compounded by multidisease processes, requires greater emphasis on individualized evaluation and treatment. A detailed systemic evaluation, careful diagnostic workup, and consultation are essential.

Close postoperative monitoring and extensive rehabilitation are essential. The establishment of good rapport and communication with the patient is needed to ensure that treatments, medications, and follow-up care are appropriately used.

References

1. Wyngaarden JB, Smith LH (eds): *Cecil Textbook of Medicine*, ed 16.Philadelphia, WB Saunders Co, 1982.
2. Friel JP (ed): *Dorland's Illustrated Medical Dictionary*, ed 25. Philadelphia, WB Saunders Co, 1974.
3. Conforti JA: On humanistic podogeriatrics. *J Am Podiatry Assoc* 72:102–103, 1982.
4. Bureau of Census, Current Population Reports: *Projections of the Population of the United States*. Washington DC, US Government Printing Office, 1977.
5. Hollister LE: Prescribing drugs for the elderly. In Ebaugh FG Jr (ed): *Management of Common Problems in Geriatric Medicine*. Menlo Park, CA, Addison-Wesley, 1981, pp 82–102.
6. Reichel W: Care of the elderly patient: evaluation, diagnosis and management. In Reichel W (ed): *Clinical Aspects of Aging*, ed 2. Baltimore, Williams & Wilkins, 1983, p 1.
7. Jahnigen DW, LaForce FM: Little things. In Shrier RW (ed): *Clinical Internal Medicine in the Aged*. Philadelphia, WB Saunders Co, 1982, pp 313–315.
8. Rodstein M: Accidents among the aged. In Reichel W (ed): *Clinical Aspects of Aging*, ed 2. Baltimore, Williams & Wilkins, 1983, p 600.
9. Helfand AE: At the foot of south mountain, a five year longitudinal study of foot problems and screening in an elderly population. *J Am Podiatry Assoc* 63:512, 1973.
10. Helfand AE: Guide to a methodological approach for community health foot study for the chronically ill and the aged. *J Am Podiatry Assoc* 54:465, 1964.
11. Dodd RB: Anesthesia. In Steinberg FU (ed): *Care of the Geriatric Patient*, ed 6. St Louis, The CV Mosby Co, 1983, p 327.
12. Harris R: Exercise and physical fitness for the elderly. In Reichel W (ed): *Clinical Aspects of Aging*, ed 2. Baltimore, Williams & Wilkins, 1983, p 90.
13. Ferris PJ: Peripheral arterial disease in the geriatric patient. In Reichel W. (ed) *Clinical Aspects of Aging*, ed 2. Baltimore, Williams & Wilkins, 1983, p 117.
14. Reichle FA, Rankin KP, Shuman CR, Finestone AJ: The elderly patient with severe arterial insufficiency of the lower extremity. *Circulation* 60:1–24, 1979.
15. Martinez BD, Hertzer NR, Beven EG: Influence of distal arterial occlusive disease on prognosis following aorta bifemoral bypass. *Surgery* 88:795, 1980.
16. Miller DC: Diagnosis and management of peripheral vascular disease. In Ebaugh FG (ed): *Management of Common Problems in Geriatric Medicine*. Menlo Park, CA, Addison-Wesley, 1981, pp 286–305.
17. Young JR: Peripheral vascular disease. In Steinberg F (ed): *Care of the Geriatric Patient*, ed 6. St Louis, The CV Mosby Co, 1983, p 373.
18. Block BH: Vascular considerations. In Marcus SA, Block BH (eds): *Complications in Foot Surgery*, ed 2. Baltimore, Williams & Wilkins, 1984, pp 25–26.
19. Okun R: Treatment of claudication in obliterative arterial disease. *Drug Ther* 4:24, 1974.
20. Fairbairn JF II, Joyce JW, Pairolero DC. In Juergens JL, Spittell JA, Fairbairn JF II(eds): *Allen-Barker-Hines Peripheral Vascular Diseases*. Philadelphia, WB Saunders Co, 1980, pp 381–384.
21. Charlesworth D, Baker RH: Surgery in old age. In Brocklehurst JC (ed): *Textbook of Geriatric Medicine and Gerontology*, ed 2. New York, Churchill-Livingstone, 1978, p 718.
22. Wright IS: Venous thrombosis and pulmonary embolism in the elderly. In Reichel W (ed): *Clinical Aspects of Aging*, ed 2. Baltimore, Williams & Wilkins, 1983, p 96.
23. Elkowitz EB: *Geriatric Medicine for the Primary Care Practitioner*. New York, Springer Publishing, 1981, p 185.
24. Coni N, Davidson W, Webster S: *Lecture Notes on Geriatrics*, ed 2. Boston, Blackwell Scientific Publications, 1980, pp 326–327.
25. Pont A: Management of osteoporosis. In Ebaugh FG (ed): *Management of Common Problems in Geriatric Medicine*. Menlo Park, CA, Addison-Wesley, 1981, pp 82–102.
26. Freehafer AA: Injuries to the skeletal system of older persons. In Reichel W (ed): *Clinical Aspects of Aging*, ed 2. Baltimore, Williams & Wilkins, 1983, p 371.
27. Weissman SD: *Radiology of the Foot*. Baltimore, Williams & Wilkins, 1983, p 344.
28. Grob D: Prevalent joint diseases in older persons. In Reichel W (ed): *Clinical Aspects of Aging*, ed 2. Baltimore, Williams & Wilkins, 1983,p 344.
29. Calin A: Gerontologic aspects of rheumatology. In Ebaugh FG (ed): *Management of Common Problems in Geriatric Medicine*. Menlo Park, CA, Addison-Wesley, 1981, p 258.
30. Baum J: Rehabilitation aspects of arthritis in the elderly. In Williams TF (ed): *Rehabilitation in the Aging*. New York, Raven Press, 1984, p 177.
31. Price NM: Cutaneous disease in geriatric patients. In Ebaugh FG (ed): *Management of Common Problems in Geriatric Medicine*. Menlo Park, CA, Addison-Wesley, 1981, pp 194–231.
32. Laine W: Foot problems in the elderly patient. In Ebaugh FG (ed): *Management of Common Problems in Geriatric Medicine*. Menlo Park, CA, Addison-Wesley, 1981, pp 329–352.
33. Werter H, Helfand AE, Margolis E: Disorders of the foot. In Libow LS, Sherman FT (eds): *The Core of Geriatric Medicine* St. Louis, The CV Mosby Co, 1981, p 330.
34. Helfand AE: Foot health for the elderly patient. In Reichel W (ed): *Clinical Aspects of Aging*, ed 2. Baltimore, Williams & Wilkins, 1983, p 384.
35. Helfand AE: Care of the foot. In Steinberg F (ed): *Care of the Geriatric Patient*, ed 6. St Louis, The CV Mosby Co, 1983, p 406.
36. Helfand AE: Common foot problems in the aged and rehabilitative management. In Williams TF (ed): *Rehabilitation in the Aging*. New York, Raven Press, 1984, p 291.
37. Lindeman RD: Application of fluid and electrolyte balance principles to the older patient. In Reichel W (ed): *Clinical Aspects of Aging*, ed 2. Baltimore, Williams & Wilkins, 1983, p 286.
38. Lamy PP: Drug prescribing for the elderly. In Reichel W (ed): *Clinical Aspects of Aging*, ed 2. Baltimore, Williams & Wilkins, 1983, p 21.
39. Myers-Robfogel MW, Bossman HB: Clinical pharmacology in the aged: aspects of pharmacokinetics and drug sensitivity. In Williams TF (ed): *Rehabilitation in the Aging*. New York, Raven Press, 1984, p 23.
40. Levin ME: Diabetes mellitus. In Steinberg F (ed) *Care of the Geriatric Patient*, ed 6. St Louis, The CV Mosby Co, 1983, p 154.
41. Frykberg RG: Podiatric problems in diabetes. In Kozak GP, Hoar GS Jr, Rowbotham JL, Wheelcock FL, Gibbons GW, Campbell D (eds): *Management of Diabetic Foot Problems*. Philadelphia, WB Saunders Co, 1984, p 45.

42. World Health Organization: Health care in the elderly. *Drugs* 22:279, 1980.

43. Smith IM: Infections in the elderly. In Steinberg F (ed): *Care of the Geriatric Patient*, ed 6. St Louis, The CV Mosby Co, 1983, p 231.

44. Marcinko D, Schwartz N: Suction irrigation in podiatric surgery—a dependable closed system. *J Am Podiatry Assoc* 74:216, 1984.

Additional References

Bates B (ed): *Physical Examination*, ed 2. Philadelphia, JP Lippincott Co, 1979.

Beattie LB, Louie VY: Nutrition and health in the elderly. In Reichel W (ed): *Clinical Aspects of Aging*, ed 2. Baltimore, Williams & Wilkins, 1983, p 248.

Clark GS, Bray GP: Development of a rehabilitation plan. In Williams TF (ed): *Rehabilitation in the Aging*. New York, Raven Press, 1984, p 125.

Department of Surgery, University of Louisville School of Medicine: Approaches to revascularization of the ischemic foot. *J Ky Med Assoc* January:31–35, 1981.

Fenton CF, III, McGlamry ED: Reverse bucking to reduce metatarsus primus varus. *J Am Podiatry Assoc* 72:342–346, 1982.

Freiberg TA, Staton R, Bornstein B: Isolated symptomatic deep vein phlebothrombosis in a digit. *J Foot Surg* 23:60–62, 1984.

Friedman LW, Capulong ES: Specific assistive aids. In Williams TF (ed): *Rehabilitation in the Aging*. New York, Raven Press, 1984, p 322.

Gamble JG, Edwards CC, Stephen RM: Enzymatic adaptation in ligaments during immobilization. *Am J Sports Med* 12:221–227, 1984.

Gibbons GW, Eliopoulos GM: Infections of the diabetic foot. In Kozak GP, Hoar GS, Jr, Rowbotham JL, Wheelcock FC, Gibbons GW, Campbell D (eds): *Management of Foot Problems*. Philadelphia, WB Saunders Co, 1984, p 97.

Gohil P, Haynie RL, Spencer AM, Clark TH: Vitamin B-12 neuropathy with pernicious anemia: description and case report. *J Am Podiatry Assoc* 72:73–78, 1982.

Gould N, Schneider W, Ashikaga T: Epidemiological survey of foot problems in the continental United States 1978–1979. *Foot Ankle* 1:8–10, 1980.

Greenberg AJ: Rheumatoid Nodules. *J Am Podiatry Assoc* 72:84–88, 1982.

Hallock GG: The skin graft. *Contemp Orthop* 9:61–63, 1984.

Harris CM: Joint replacement in the elderly. In Williams TF (ed): *Rehabilitation in the Aging*. New York, Raven Press, 1984, p 199.

Hunt TK, Dunphy JE (eds): *Fundamentals of Wound Management*. New York, Appelton-Century-Crofts, 1979.

Johnson RM: Considerations in the determination of the amputation level of the diabetic foot. *J Am Podiatry Assoc* 72:192–194, 1982.

Knight S: Evaluation of the geriatric patient. In Reichel W (ed): *Clinical Aspects of Aging*, ed 2. Baltimore, Williams & Wilkins, 1983, p 11.

Levy LA: Who are the aged? A challenge to podiatric medicine. *J Am Podiatry Assoc* 72:163–165, 1982.

Lombardo M, Aquino JM: Local flaps for resurfacing foot defects: a vascular perspective. *J Foot Surg* 21:302–304, 1982.

Martin SM, Gastwirth CM: Surgical management of tophaceous gout: a literature review and case report. *J Am Podiatry Assoc* 72:195–199, 1982.

Mauro G, Yudkoff N, Resnick M, Sharon S, Knudsen HA: Arteriovenous fistula of the lower extremity: a case study. *J Am Podiatry Assoc* 70:614–618, 1980.

Mellors RC, Jr: Other arthritic disorders in the foot. In Kozak GP, Hoar CS, Jr., Rowbotham JL, Wheelcock FC, Gibbons GW, Campbell D (eds): *Management of Diabetic Foot Problems*. Philadelphia, WB Saunders Co, 1984, p 68.

Miller WA: Postoperative wound infection in foot and ankle surgery. *Foot Ankle* 4:102–104, 1983.

Okun S, Mehl S, DellaCorte M, Shechter D, Esposito F: The use of prophylactic antibiotics in clean podiatric surgery. *J Foot Surg* 23:402–405, 1984.

O'Mara CS, Flinn WR, Neiman HL, Bergan JJ, Yao JST: Correlation of foot arterial anatomy with early tibial bypass patency. *Surgery* 89:743–751, 1981.

Palmore E: *International Handbook on Aging*. Westport, CT, Greenwood Press, 1980.

Ratner SW, Reilly CH, Gudas CJ: Percutaneous transluminal angioplasty in the treatment of ischemic disease of the lower extremity. *J Foot Surg* 22:86–91, 1983.

Reichel J: Pulmonary problems in the elderly. In Reichel W (ed): *Clinical Aspects of Aging*, ed 2. Baltimore, Williams & Wilkins, 1983, p 111.

Riegelhaupt RW, French SM, Toren DJ, Reinherz RP, Naumoff NSR: Lower extremity circulatory studies utilizing radioisotopes. *J Foot Surg* 21:86–90, 1982.

Rosenkranz L, Cataletto MM: Metatarsalgia caused by an increase in circulating platelets: a case report. *Foot Ankle* 4:216–217, 1984.

Rude T, Bunkis J, Walton RL: Hypertensive leg ulcers. *J Foot Surg* 22:134–138, 1983.

Samitz MH (ed): *Cutaneous Disorders of the Lower Extremities*, ed 2. Philadelphia, JP Lippincott Co, 1981.

Sengpiehl KE: Improved salvage of the foot with arterial reconstruction. *J Foot Surg* 23:370–376, 1984.

Silberman J, Kanat IO: Total joint replacement in digits of the foot. *J Foot Surg* 23:207–212, 1984.

Spittel JA: Rehabilitative aspects of peripheral vascular disorders in the elderly. In Williams FF (ed): *Rehabilitation in the Aging*. New York, Raven Press, 1984, p 283.

Till KE, Solomon MG, Kerman BL: Indications and uses of prophylactic antibiotics in podiatric surgery. *J Foot Surg* 23:166–172, 1984.

Waife SO (ed): *Diabetes Mellitus*, ed 8. Indianapolis, IN, Eli Lilly, 1980.

Williams HTG, Fenna D, MacBeth RA: Alpha tocopherol in the treatment of intermittent claudication. *Surg Gynecol Obstet* 132:662, 1971.

Wolcott LE: Rehabilitation and the aged. In Reichel W (ed): *Clinical Aspects of Aging*, ed 2. Baltimore, Williams & Wilkins, 1983, p 182.

Wright JR: Cardiovascular and pulmonary pathology of the aged. In Reichel W (ed): *Clinical Aspects of Aging*, ed 2. Baltimore, Williams & Wilkins, 1983, p 102.

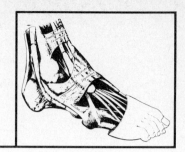

CHAPTER 19

The Insensitive Foot

Vincent J. Hetherington, D.P.M., M.S.

The insensitive foot is best defined as an extremity without a warning mechanism for intricate external and internal environmental changes. The external environment includes the home or workplace, occupation, floor surfaces, and shoegear. The internal environment encompasses altered musculoskeletal function, deformity, vascular modifications, and skin dysfunction. The primary deficit is a lack of appropriate neural function. The alterations in neural function affect sensory, motor, and vascular elements to varying degrees. Pathology results through a combination of external and internal factors. In certain disease processes the homeostatic mechanism of the body is changed such as to pose a greater danger to the denervated limb. This is the case in diabetes mellitus.

The purpose of this chapter is to discuss the role of internal changes, their relationship to external factors, the development of pathological conditions, and their management.

Diseases that result in an insensitive foot are varied in their presentation and etiology. Table 19.1 is a compilation of diseases resulting in insensitivity. The exact mechanism of each individual disease process is beyond the scope of this chapter. The pathology with which the author deals represents the pedal manifestations of these diseases. The conditions most commonly seen by the average clinician are those associated with diabetes mellitus.

PATHOGENESIS OF SOFT TISSUE LESIONS AND THE INSENSITIVE FOOT

Soft Tissue Biomechanics

The pathogenesis of soft tissue lesions in the insensitive foot is closely related to the biomechanical properties of the skin. The skin serves various functions because of its complex constituents. Among these functions are adaptability and the absorption and dissipation of energy.

To function properly the skin must have adequate sensibility and vascularity. The skin can be regarded as a series of networks as described by Gibson and Kenedi (1).

The collagen fiber network functions so that if stretched in any direction most of the fibers will orient parallel along the lines of stretch. At low loads few fibers may be involved. As the load increases the amount of fibers will also increase to resist further tissue extension. The elastic fiber network is intimately related to the collagen fibers. The elastic fibers act as an energy storage device or spring to return the collagen to its relaxed position.

The interstitial fluid that surrounds the network acts to lubricate the mechanical mechanism and serves as a buffer against sudden changes. The interstitial fluid is also important in the dissipation of heat. An increase in the amount of interstitial fluid increases the resistance of skin to deformity. The skin therefore possesses viscoelastic properties. Fluid is forced out of the tissue during deformation and returns during a recovery period (2). The function of the interstitial fluid has been compared to that of a shock absorber.

Mechanism in the Development of Neurotrophic Ulceration

The mechanisms or pathogenesis of the development of plantar ulcers have been discussed by Brand (3) and Brand and Hall (4), and are listed as follows:(a) continuous pressure, (b) concentrated high pressure, (c) repetitive mechanical stress, and (d) excessive heat or cold.

Skin defects that are a result of continuous pressure are caused by a lack of blood supply. Kosiak (5) points out that intense pressures of short duration are as detrimental as low pressures applied for extended periods. Regardless of the type of mechanism necrosis results from ischemia. The result of ischemia is irreversible tissue damage. The normal capillary blood pressure ranges from 13 to 33 mm of Hg. At pressures above this blockage in capillary flow will occur. The extent of tissue involvement because of continuous pressure is dependent on time and pressure and can extend from skin to bone.

Defects caused by concentrated high pressure are usually the result of a sudden trauma such as stepping on a piece of glass or a nail. The force supplied exceeds

Table 19.1
Outline of Diseases and Processes Resulting in an Insensitive Foot

I. Neuropathy Associated with Systemic Disease
    Diabetes mellitus
    Uremia
    Amyloidosis

II. Neuropathy Associated with Nutritional Disturbances
    Alcoholism
    Pernicious Anemia

III. Neuropathy Associated with Infectious Diseases
    Leprosy
    Syphilis
    Poliomyelitis

IV. Neuropathy on a Vascular Basis
    Cerebral vascular accident
    Spinal cord infarction
    Diabetic mononeuropathy
    Arteritis
    Peripheral vascular disease

V. Hereditary Motor and Sensory Neuropathy (HMSN)
    Roussy-Lévy syndrome
    Charcot-Marie-Tooth disease

VI. Hereditary Sensory and Autonomic Neuropathy (HSAN)
    Hereditary sensory neuropathy
    Congenital sensory neuropathy
    Dysautonomia (Riley-Day syndrome)

VII. Cerebellar Degeneration
    Friedreich's ataxia

VIII. Motor Neuron Disease
    Amyotrophic lateral sclerosis

IX. Diseases of the Spinal Cord
    Spina bifida
    Syringomyelia

X. Trauma
    Spinal cord injury
    Peripheral nerve injury
    Spinal root trauma

XI. Compressive Neuropathy
    Spinal cord tumor
    Peripheral nerve compression

XII. Toxic Neuropathy
    Lead poisoning

XIII. Other
    Cerebral palsy

the sheer stress of the skin resulting in tissue tearing. The force required to cause such a break is approximately 600 to 700 pounds per square inch (3).

Active patients develop tissue necrosis as a result of repetitive mechanical stress. The events that lead to ulceration are inflammation and autolysis. Brand (3) relates that the part of the foot that ulcerates most

commonly is exposed to pressures between 1 and 5 kg/cm^2 at every step. Traumatic inflammation occurs and with repeated trauma inflammation gives way to necrosis. Part of the necrosis is caused by the enzymes of inflammatory cells from one episode of trauma that are stimulated to release their enzymes during a second episode. Manley and Darby (6) in their research of mechanical stress and the development of foot ulcerations in rats, made the following conclusions:

1. Repetitive mechanical stress of a magnitude and repetition rate within physiological limits can stimulate the formation of foot ulcers, if the foot is subjected to a significant number of stress repetitions.
2. With the increase in the daily number of repetitions a shorter time period is required for ulcer formation.
3. Denervation predisposes the formation of plantar ulcers.

They also pointed out the role of sympathectomy in the neurectomized animals as contributing to the development of ulceration and necrosis. The presence of edema interferes with the delivery of nutrients to the area because of an increased distance from the capillary to the cell and a decrease in the rate of diffusion proportional to this distance. The removal of metabolites and cell debris and edema would also be impaired. These findings are also supported by the work of Beach and Thompson (7) and that of Bergtholdt (8, 9).

The mechanism of tissue necrosis secondary to thermal injury will not be elaborated on at this time.

THE ROLE OF VASCULAR CHANGES
Autonomic Neuropathy

The role of vascular changes in the development of foot ulcerations are the result of three mechanisms: (a) autonomic neuropathy, (b) microvascular insufficiency, and (c) occlusive peripheral vascular disease.

The role of autonomic neuropathy in the development of complications in the insensitive foot has received much attention in recent years (10–17). This sympathectomy can occur in varying degrees in all forms of the insensitive foot. The role that diabetic autonomic neuropathy plays in the surgical management of the patient with diabetic foot pathology has been reviewed extensively by Schustek and Jacobs (18). Systemic complications that warrant attention are painless myocardial infarction, postural hypotension, and hypoglycemic unawareness.

The local manifestations of the autonomic neuropathy in the insensitive foot can be manifested as: (a) medial vascular calcifications, (b) increased peripheral blood flow contributing to neuropathic edema, and (c) formation of edema, ulcerations, and the development of a painful neuropathy.

The edema present in patients with peripheral neuropathy besides interfering with the mechanical function of the skin also leads to physiological changes in the ability of the skin to respond to injury. Wound healing may be more difficult and require greater care and effort to obtain healing. All attempts should be made to control the edema before any form of surgical intervention.

Watkins and Edmonds (19) found sympathetic denervation may cause structural damage to peripheral arteries. Sympathectomy has been shown to cause atrophy of the smooth muscle cells and long term sympathetic denervation also leads to structural changes in arterial smooth muscle. Watkins and Edmonds point out that substantial calcification best seen in lateral radiographs of the foot and ankle was seen in 16 of 20 patients with severe neuropathy between 22 and 50 years of age. The finding of long-term denervation associated with structural changes has also been confirmed by other authors (20–22).

Increase in blood flow associated with altered vasomotor control may have an effect in the development of Charcot joints and the development of pedal ulcerations. Boulten and associates (23) found that the mean venous PO_2 in the feet of subjects with neuropathy and foot ulcerations was significantly higher than in controls or in diabetic groups without ulceration or evidence of autonomic neuropathy. Their results provide further evidence of abnormal blood flow in the diabetic neuropathic foot that is consistent with those seen in arteriovenous shunting. Shunting has also been demonstrated in animal models with ulcerative change (24). Watkins and Edmonds (19) also found by the use of isotope scans that bone blood flow of the neurotrophic foot is considerably increased. It was their belief that although the isotope uptake reflected osteoblastic activity, as well as blood flow, the increased early uptake probably indicates that the bone blood flow is raised. They postulated that demineralization of the bone is a likely consequence as it is in other cases with increased flow. They suggest that the evolution of destructive bony changes is as follows:

Sympathetic denervation of arterioles causes an increase of blood flow which in turn causes rarefaction of bone making it prone to damage even after mild trauma. This coupled with loss of sensation from the neuropathy, in particular reduction of pain sensation, permits abnormal stresses which would normally be prevented by pain. Therefore, relatively minor trauma causes major destructive changes in susceptable bones" (19).

An abnormally high blood flow, vasodilation, and arteriovenous shunting could result from sympathetic denervation and lead to abnormal venous pooling and cause edema. The edema would interfere with the normal mechanical functions of the skin and predispose the patient to the development of pedal ulcerations. There is also evidence that sympathetic denervation is necessary for ulceration to occur (25).

Other aspects of the autonomic neuropathy that can complicate the insensitive foot include the development of anhydrosis and dyshydrosis, which lead to the development of skin cracking and pedal ulcerations. Ozeran and associates (26) believe that the diabetic neuropathy involving the sympathetic nervous system can be evaluated and two abnormalities

recognized: the hyperactive or vasospastic disorders, and complete autosympathectomy. Operative sympathectomy may be useful in the treatment of the hyperactive form of this process.

VASCULAR OCCLUSIVE DISEASE

Diabetics appear to have a greater and more significant degree of peripheral vascular disease than the normal patient. Various theories have been put forth for the vascular status of the diabetic foot. The literature supports the belief that arterial sclerosis in the diabetic may be different from that in the nondiabetic individual (17, 27). The existence of a true diabetic microangiopathy is still surrounded by a great deal of controversy.

Conrad (27) performed an extensive comparison of large and small vessel disease in diabetic and nondiabetic individuals. One of the major conclusions was that the variation and pattern of obstruction differs in diabetics compared to nondiabetics. In diabetics there appears to be an increase of disease in the calf vasculature. Arterial sclerosis in the diabetic appears to occur distally and progresses in a distal to proximal fashion. In addition in diabetics one usually sees a medial linear calcification as opposed to the splotchy calcification seen in nondiabetics. As a result of this more distal origin of the arterial sclerosis and the progression in a distal to a proximal direction, a less effective collateral circulation appears to develop. However, Conrad believed the existence of a diabetic small artery disease and that capillary permeability could not be backed up by any conclusive evidence. The decrease in blood flow to the digits may be explained by an increase in resistance of the more proximal calf arteries and is not evidence of distal arterial disease. Poor collateralization often occurs because of involvement of the genicular circulation that is affected by diabetes.

However, Colwell (28) and others (29, 30) attribute microvascular insufficiency in the diabetic to a combination of factors. Various aspects of these factors have been investigated by other authors. These factors include: (a) functional changes in the endothelium, (b) endothelial injury (31), (c) platelet adhesion and aggregation (32, 33), (d) basement membrane thickening (34–38), (e) increased plasma viscosity, (f) red blood cell aggregation and microthrombosis (40), (g) microaneurysm (29, 39), and (h) altered fibrinolysis (40).

A dermal microangiopathy has been identified in the toes of diabetics by both light and electron microscopy as a thickening of the capillary basement membrane (37, 38). Williamson and Kilo (36) believed that normalization of blood glucose levels reduces or prevents the progression of vascular disease caused by basement membrane thickening. In the previous section the author referred to the contribution of autonomic dysfunction to the development of vascular disease in the diabetic.

Hyperglycemia in the diabetic appears to lead directly to increased enzymatic incorporation of carbohydrate into the basement membrane. There is an increased ability of the red blood cells to aggregate and a hyperviscosity of the plasma. Diabetics also appear to have a decreased fibrolytic activity of the blood, as well as an increased ability of the platelets to aggregate. It is on the basis of these changes that diabetic microvascular insufficiency is believed to exist.

CLINICAL ENTITIES

The clinical entities involved in the development of soft tissue lesions in the patient with an insensitive foot are the result of continuous pressure, high concentrated pressure, repetitive mechanical stress, thermal injury, ischemia, the origination of sinuses, fissuring, and a final category entitled traumatic vascular.

The ulcerations that arise from continuous pressure are those in the nature of an ischemic bed sore or decubitous ulcer. In the foot this occurs commonly on the heel. Another area of occurrence of this type of lesion is over a bony prominence such as the first metatarsophalangeal joint in a shoe that is excessively tight for a patient. The constant pressure exerted by the shoe over the bony prominence causes compression of the capillary blood flow leading to necrosis. The eventual outcome for this type of lesion is often related to the patient's underlying blood supply. Should a pressure ulcer develop over the first metatarsophalangeal joint in a diabetic with peripheral neuropathy but with adequate circulation, healing will follow quite unremarkably provided there is no infection. However, if this type of ulceration occurs in a patient with compromised circulation it may be the initiation of a progressive ischemic ulceration (Fig. 19.1 A).

With concentrated high pressures such as a penetration injury by perhaps stepping on a thorn or nail the initial break in the skin can act as a focus for

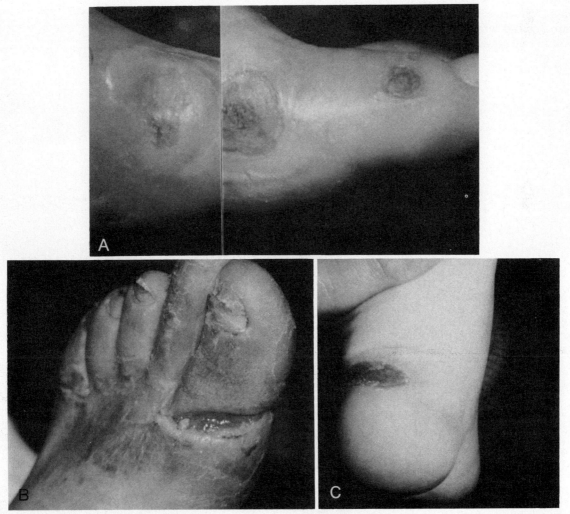

Figure 19.1.   (A) Small skin irritation developed in diabetic with advanced peripheral vascular disease. Lesions were progressive as illustrated in right hand portion of picture. Patient's vascular disease was not amenable to reconstruction, infection ensued, and amputation was required. (B) Neurotrophic ulceration caused by continuous pressure developed as result of home shoe modification. Patient has peripheral neuropathy secondary to chronic ethanol abuse. Ulcer was caused by a shoelace. (C) Painless ulcer developed on posterior portion of heel in two-and-one-half-year-old child with spina bifida because of improper shoe fitting. Seam in shoe rested directly over ulcer site.

increased tissue necrosis and ulceration or be the initiation of infection.

Repetitive mechanical stress is multifactoral in the development of ulcerations. Ulceration may develop as a result of cyclical biomechanical trauma under areas of weight bearing or under areas of bony prominence. Resulting ulcers are usually located on the plantar surface of the foot and are frequently referred to as the mal perforans type of ulcer. Such lesions are a result of inflammation caused by repetitive mechanical stress that exceeds the mechanical limits of the skin and subcutaneous tissue. Inflammation occurs and if rest is not provided the inflammation will become severe. Following the inflammation, autolysis of the soft tissues will occur. A seroma or hematoma occurs within the deeper layers of the subcutaneous tissue and the dermis. Dissection of the subcutaneous tissues occurs with pressures and shear from walking. Continued pressure and injury eventually leads to breakdown of the skin and rupture through the plantar surface of the foot. Continued aggravation of the lesion enlarges the lesion and deepening of the lesion and subsequent infection readily occurs. Factors contributing to the development of these types of ulcers are listed in Table 19.2.

This type of ulceration, although occurring predominantly on weight-bearing surfaces, can occur on dorsal digital surfaces in association with hammertoe deformity (Fig. 19.2).

A healed ulcer can contribute to the formation of further ulceration because the healed ulcer binds the skin to the fascia and ultimately to the bone. The skin is placed at a mechanical disadvantage because the collagen network is replaced with fibrous scar tissue.

Table 19.2
Factors Contributing to the Formation of Neurotrophic Ulceration as a Result of Repetitive Cyclical Biomechanical Trauma (Moderate Repetitive Mechanical Stress)

Unawareness of pain
Hyperkeratosis
Muscle weakness
Fat pad and soft tissue atrophy
Deformity
Stress exceeds mechanical limits of skin
Autolysis
Soft tissue dissection by fluid, blood, or pus
Autonomic neuropathy
Microvascular insufficiency

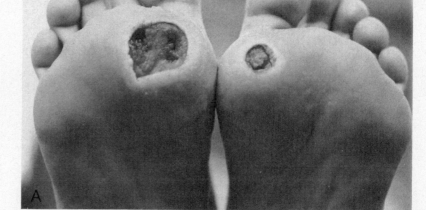
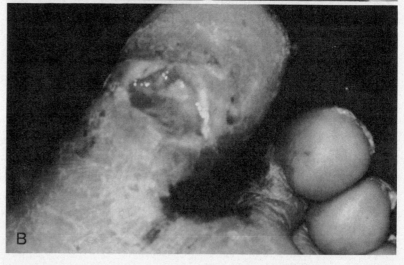

Figure 19.2.   (A) Typical plantar ulcers in diabetic as result of repetitive mechanical stress. (B) Diabetic patient with hallux rigidus developed neurotrophic ulceration beneath great toe as result of altered foot biomechanics.

This tissue is then at a mechanical disadvantage in its attempts to adapt and dissipate energy.

Thermal injuries such as burns or frostbite are common in insensitive feet. Patients who sustain such injury and who are unaware of the injury can often, because of unintentional neglect, convert a partial thickness tissue loss to full-thickness loss by continued ambulation on the foot with the subsequent development of infection (Fig. 19.3).

Ischemic ulceration occurs quite frequently in the diabetic with peripheral neuropathy. Clinical presentation is often seen with gangrene of the digits or the appearance of small ischemic punched-out ulcers.

An insidious type of lesion causing ulceration and infection in the insensitive foot is that of sinus formation. This commonly originates between the fourth and fifth digits under a heloma molle. Fissuring especially about the heel can occur in these patients because of dyshydrosis (Fig. 19.4).

The last clinical entity is a traumatic vascular type of injury that results in an inflammatory thrombosis. This can be seen in diabetics with advanced microvascular insufficiency. After some minor traumatic episode, such as stubbing the toe, inflammation is set up that will lead to thrombosis of the small vessels and ultimately gangrene.

Neurotrophic ulcers have been classified by various methods. The most widely used is that of Wagner (4) which uses a six-grade classification:

Grade 0: The skin is intact, however, there may be some osseous deformity
Grade 1: Localized superficial ulcer
Grade 2: Deep ulcer with extension to bone and ligaments with possible joint involvement
Grade 3: Deep abscess with osteomyelitis
Grade 4: Gangrene of the toes or forefoot
Grade 5: Gangrene of the whole foot

ALTERATIONS IN FOOT BIOMECHANICS

Weight bearing studies have been performed by various authors on the neurotrophic foot. Stokes and associates (42, 43) found that in diabetics peak loads were shifted laterally on the foot and increasing abnormalities in loading occurred consistent with an increase in peripheral neuropathy. They believed their most striking finding was the reduction of load of the toes, which is significant in the diabetic even without evidence of ulceration. Position of maximum load was found in each case to correspond to the position of the ulcer in patients who did develop neuropathic ulcers. Callosities did occur at sites of heavy loading. They theorized that lateral shifting and weight bearing could be the result of weakness of the muscles or loss of coordination caused by a loss of physiological impulses from the tendon receptors and denervation of the intrinsic muscles.

Barrett and Mooney (44) found that lesions of the plantar aspect of the forefoot showed high pressure in areas of ulcer formation. This was also confirmed by Sabato and associates (45) in patients with Hansen's disease. In the analysis of vertical forces acting on the diabetic patient with neurotrophic ulcerations Ctercteko and associates (46) found that toe loading was significantly reduced in diabetics both with ulceration and without ulceration. Their findings differed from those of the Stokes group and they found a medial shift in loading in the metatarsal region. They also found significantly greater forces acting on the first ray area in diabetics both with and without ulceration. One difference noted between ulcerated and nonulcerated diabetics was that in the group of ulcerated diabetics the heel was less heavily loaded. They did, however, concur with the Stokes study in that all ulcers in the metatarsal region occurred at the sites of maximum force and that the peak force was also significantly greater in the ulcerated feet. No significant correlation between contact time and severity of the neuropathy was demonstrated.

The anterior displacement of body weight was also not noted by Burman and Perls (47) in 1958. Ellenberg in 1968 (48) attributed the hammering and

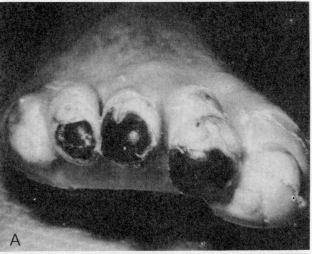

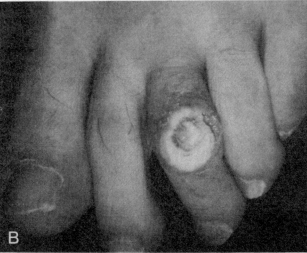

Figure 19.3. (A) Full-thickness chemical burns in diabetic with peripheral neuropathy caused by home remedy. (B) Full-thickness skin loss with exposure of underlying bone caused by commercially available "corn remover" used by diabetic.

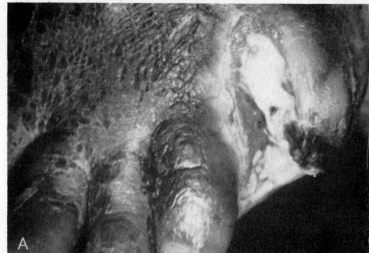
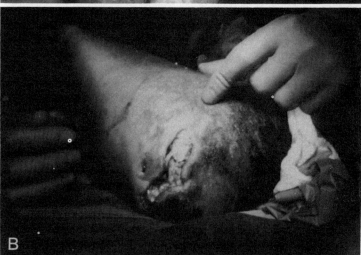

Figure 19.4. (A) Massive soft tissue and plantar space infections of left foot that originated as sinus tract forming between fourth and fifth digits. (B) Result of untreated heel fissure.

contracture of the digits in the diabetic with neuropathy to imbalances and weakness of the intrinsic muscles of the foot. Pati and Behera (49) found clawing of the toes in 50 of 57 cases of ulceration beneath the metatarsal head in leprosy patients. Amputation of the toe was an associated finding in the remaining seven.

Thus a diabetic patient with a short first metatarsal and hypermobility of the first ray may develop a subsecond metatarsal head lesion because of biomechanical trauma inflicted on the area. Intrinsic muscle weakness leads to poor function and hammering of the digits with excess of loading of the metatarsophalangeal joint. However, the question arises as to why only the neurotrophic patient will ulcerate and the normal patient does not. One explanation is that patients who lack sensation of the foot fail to accomodate to the trauma and continue to traumatize the area. The repetitive stress produces injury with resultant inflammation. In normal individuals associated discomfort would perhaps cause limping and alteration in weight bearing. Because of the inability of the patient with neuropathy to perceive this he or she continues to walk on the area without obtaining relief.

Another explanation is that part of the problem may be the result of changes in vascularity. When healing occurs in a neurotrophic foot following any trauma this predisposes the skin to easier breakdown and ulceration.

From this one can see that the biomechanics of the foot, the functional adaptions, and changes secondary to muscle imbalance, and biochemical and other changes in the skin may all lead to the development of neurotrophic ulceration. One must be aware of the possibility of coexistent vascular and neurotrophic changes that may present a diagnostic and therapeutic dilemma in the diabetic. The approach in evaluating the lower extremity requires certain special considerations of both the vascular and neurological examinations.

OSSEOUS AND RADIOGRAPHIC CHANGES ASSOCIATED WITH THE INSENSITIVE FOOT

Osseous changes associated with the insensitive foot can be of two types: an atrophic and a hypertrophic arthropathy.

The atrophic arthropathy exhibits radiographic osteoporosis, atrophy, destruction, and the disappearance of bone substance (33, 50–59). Dislocation of the joints has also been noted to occur. The joints are usually free of osteophytes, sclerosis, or eburnation and fragmentation, which is seen with the hypertrophic arthropathy.

Pogonowska and associates (54) discuss the bone absorption patterns of diabetes. The pattern is described as initially affecting the forefoot in diabetic patients. The metatarsals and phalanges are usually affected first. They summarize the changes as follows: (a) osteoporosis, (b) juxta-articular cortical bone defects, (c) osteolysis, (d) apparent destruction of the entire bone, (e) reconstruction occurring, (f) slight periosteal reaction, and (g) sclerosis of the shaft of the bone.

Many of these changes, which were related to diabetic osteopathy, also occur in other types of neuropathic osteopathy. An example is seen in alcoholic neuropathy (57, 59) and in the distal absorption seen in the bones of the foot in leprosy (56, 58).

Kraft (60), in discussing the diabetic foot, stated that in the absorption type, the bone becomes sclerotic, simulating the appearance of osteomyelitis. Schwarz and associates (53) postulated that the absorption type is caused by autosympathectomy in addition to impaired sensation. Friedman and Rakow (55) believed that both types were etiologically related to increased blood flow. Radiographically osteomyelitis often resembles the changes seen in the neurotrophic foot. In patients with vascular insufficiency the bone may appear radiographically normal even when osteomyelitis is present. The presence of a mottled lytic lesion can be the most frequent and sometimes the only positive finding. The soft tissues should be examined for the presence of air or gas, arterial calcification, and soft tissue swelling.

Radiographically the bones may appear to exhibit penciling or a sucked candy deformity. The pathological process is usually gradual reabsorption of the metatarsal and phalanges of the foot commencing at the distal end progressing gradually towards the base and terminating with a distal pointed deformity. The epiphyseal ends are lost and the remaining points may tend to become sclerotic. The joints may take the appearance of the described mortar and pestle deformity (Fig. 19.5). Absorption of the small long bones in the foot manifest in one of three ways (61) (Fig. 19.6): distal absorption, concentric absorption, or a combination of the two.

Instability and contracture of the toes and cavus foot type will develop.

In contrast hypertrophic neuropathy may present with a pes valgo planus type deformity. The radiographic presentation has been discussed by numerous authors (62–67). Frykberg (68) points out that in every case the primary factor is loss of joint sensation. The joint is subjected to extreme ranges of motion that result in capsule and ligament stretching and joint laxity and instability. Further weight bearing in this unprotected extremity leads to subluxations, dislocations, and osteochondral fragmentation. A continual trauma develops a vicious cycle. Normal inflammatory mechanisms produce joint swelling and hyperemia that leads to further instability and reabsorption (Table 19.3). Untreated continued destruction occurs creating more fragmentation dislocation and deformity (Fig. 19.7). Forgacs (69, 70) classified the changes in three stages:

Stage 1: The initiation of symptoms occurs, there is subluxation of the joints, osteoporosis occurs, and cortical defects become obvious.

Stage 2: The deformity progresses with osteolysis, fracture, and periosteal elevation or new subperiosteal bone formation occur.

Stage 3: First healing stage occurs with the subsiding of swelling, reorganization of cortical defects, and ankylosis of the joints may occur.

Destruction of the tarsus occurs by mechanisms described by Harris and Brand (71). This was divided into the following five patterns of degeneration (Fig. 19.8).

Pattern 1 involves the posterior pillar in which the calcaneus is injured most frequently. The resulting fracture may not be clear cut but is the result of internal trabecular breakdown with flattening of the bone. An incongruity of the subtalar joint may be associated with an ulcer of the heel. The patient also may present with a swollen heel and vague pain and local warmth. Once the damage has occurred there is a tendency for progressive change of shape. With progressive destruction the Achilles tendon loses its leverage and the body weight is transmitted straight down through the center of the foot.

Pattern 2 shows destruction of the body of the talus. It is common for the talus to be the primary focus of disintegration. When the body of the talus is lost, stability of the foot is also lost with the result that the tibia may be resting directly on the ground.

Pattern 3 shows destruction of the anterior pillar of the medial arch. This is described as a common and consistent pattern. This can progress to complete collapse of the medial arch and disintegration of the navicular bone with involvement of the head of the talus. Once the fracture of the navicular occurs continued walking forces the head of the talus into the navicular. With continued weight bearing the navicular will fragment and disintegrate completely. The medial arch loses its continuity and tends to flatten with a plantar declination of the head of the talus.

Pattern 4 shows the anterior pillar and the lateral arch destruction and is described by Brand as dominated by sepsis. Perforating ulcers can occur under the base of the fifth metatarsal and cuboid. The destruction of the portion of the midtarsal joint involved interferes with the stability of the foot. The pull of the Achilles tendon eventually leads to the collapse of the bony architecture of the foot. The calcaneus will tend to be drawn backwards and upwards thrusting the head of the talus downward to complete subluxation of the talonavicular joint (Fig. 19.9).

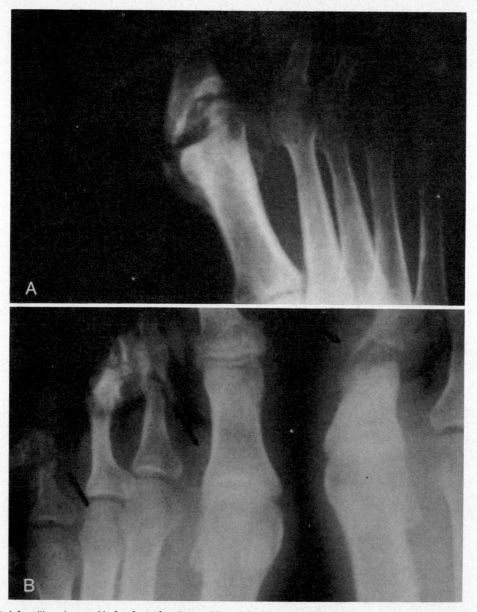

Figure 19.5.   Joint deformities observed in forefoot of patients with peripheral neuropathy. (A) Destruction of first metatarsophalangeal joint in diabetic. (B) Mortar and pestlel appearance of the lesser digits of the left foot caused by chronic alcohol abuse. Osteomyelitis was confirmed by biopsy of right great toe. (B from Weissman SD: *Radiology of the Foot.* Baltimore, Williams & Wilkins, 1983, p 450.)

Pattern 5 shows disruption of the cuneometatarsal joints and appears to be related to trauma.

The etiology of the development of Charcot joints is multifactoral. It occurs in the presence of a denervated foot and appears to have a higher incidence in those with pronounced autonomic neuropathy. Repetitive trauma of this foot type leads to continued destruction and gross foot deformity.

The diagnosis of osteomyelitis in previously diseased bone is difficult.

Radiologic distinction between osteomyelitis and bone changes caused by neuropathy is difficult (72) (Table 19.4). Radioisotopic evaluation of the neurotrophic foot can be somewhat misleading (73–81). Some difficulty occurs with the interpretation of the technetium scan of the neurotrophic foot in that the

bone has been previously diseased by neurotrophic destruction and focal uptake is not a reflection of its osteomyelitis but is actually the repair process for the earlier destruction. An infection of adjacent soft tissue with an underlying neurotrophic bone disease process can provide the radiographic appearance of acute osteomyelitis when in fact one is dealing with soft tissue ulceration with infection and underlying neurotrophic bone disease.

In patients without neurological disease a matched defect on both the technetium and gallium scan could be indicative of acute osteomyelitis. One must be careful in intrepreting technetium scans when dealing with the neurotrophic foot. A positive technetium scan results from basic physiological changes seen in various disease and infectious processes. A

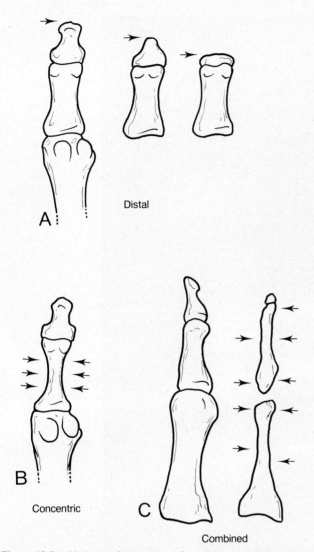

A

Distal

B

Concentric

C

Combined

Figure 19.6. Methods of absorption of small bones. (Modified from Enna CD: The foot in leprosy. In McDowell F, Ena CD (eds): *Surgical Rehabilitation in Leprosy*. Baltimore, Williams Y Wilkins, 1974, p 299.)

Table 19.3

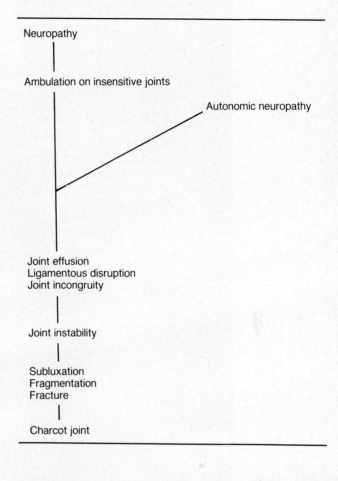

Neuropathy

Ambulation on insensitive joints

Autonomic neuropathy

Joint effusion
Ligamentous disruption
Joint incongruity

Joint instability

Subluxation
Fragmentation
Fracture

Charcot joint

positive technetium scan reflects a hyperemia or an increase in blood supply to the affected bone. Bone injury regardless of the initiating factor will lead to increased blood supply to the site. This is true in fractures, infection, and in neurotrophic disease as the body attempts to initiate repair.

Prolonged increases are the consequences of new vessel formation. Increased uptake has also been attributed to the autonomic neuropathy that increases the blood flow to the extremity. This would affect both the technetium and initially the gallium scans. Gallium scanning is used predominately for the detection of acute inflammatory infected lesions. Gallium accumulates at the site of inflammation because of its relationship to inflammatory proteins and its possible incorporation into the neutrophils. Autoradiographic studies suggest that the intracellular sites localizing gallium are lysozomes or places of lysozomal activity.

Hoffer (82) describes four methods of gallium localization. These are increased permeability, leuko-cyte localization, lactoburn binding at the infected site, and direct bacterial uptake. However, with neurotrophic changes reparative processes require the presence of white blood cells and lysozomal activity in the repair area.

The increased permeability of the blood vessels surrounding the bone may also contribute to an increased uptake of gallium in the area. Glynn (83) noted a marked accumulation of gallium in neuroarthropathy. Although radioisotopic studies can be helpful in evaluating the neurotrophic foot, care must be given to their interpretation and occasionally a bone biopsy is required to make a definitive diagnosis of osteomyelitis (84). Future methods of radioisotopic detection of infection such as the white blood cell scan (85) may prove valuable.

Bergtholdt (8) recommends temperature assessment as a program to demonstrate changes in temperature pattern. Increased physical activity or ill-fitting footwear can be detected by increased temperature at local areas of stress. Bergtholdt terms this method a "pain substitute" that can detect areas sensitive to ulceration. Thermography is also useful in the early diagnosis of Charcot joints because of increased heat in the area of the involved joints (86–88).

Thermography in the management of the insensitive foot can prove invaluable in detecting areas of

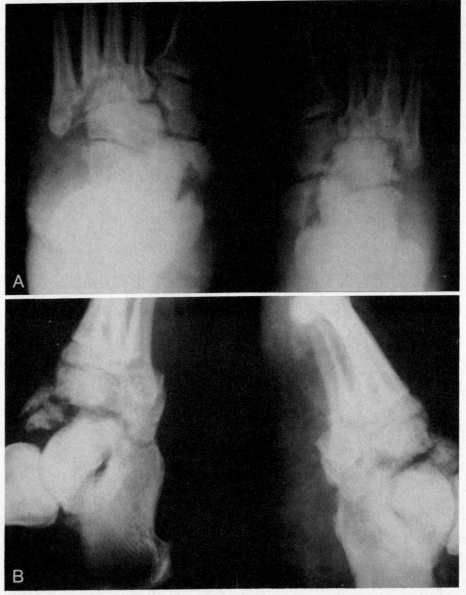

Figure 19.7. Dorsoplantar (A) and lateral (B) projections of hypertrophic neuroarthropathy.

inflammation before the time at which ulceration will occur. Liquid crystal thermography is a convenient method for in-office evaluation (87, 89).

Xeroradiography may also be helpful in the evaluation of the soft tissue in this foot type (90). Arterial calcifications, induration of small arteries, as well as intra-articular bone fragments and periosteal reactions in osteoarthropathy are easily identified by xeroradiology. Sinography may also be of benefit in evaluation of the patient with a sinus tract (91).

Painless fractures and fracture dislocations of the lower extremity involving the calcaneus, midtarsal joint, tarsometatarsal joint, leg, and knee have been reported (85, 92–97). Epiphyseal separation may occur in children (97). These injuries may go unrecognized and lead to severe disability in susceptible individuals (98).

EVALUATION OF A PATIENT WITH INSENSITIVITY

In evaluating a chief complaint a history of paresthesia, anesthesia, hyperesthesia, or change in function should be elicited (99). Patients complaining with paresthesias or pins and needles and a sensation of swollen feet or burning feet are in this category. Burning feet may be the primary indication of an inherited peripheral neuropathy (100). Patients complaining of difficulty climbing stairs, dragging of the toes, or frequent tripping may also be candidates for an evaluation of neurological dysfunction. In this experience the presentation of a patient with paresthesias can precede the diagnosis of the cause of the insensitivity. This is frequently the case of foot discomfort in patients with undiagnosed diabetes mellitus.

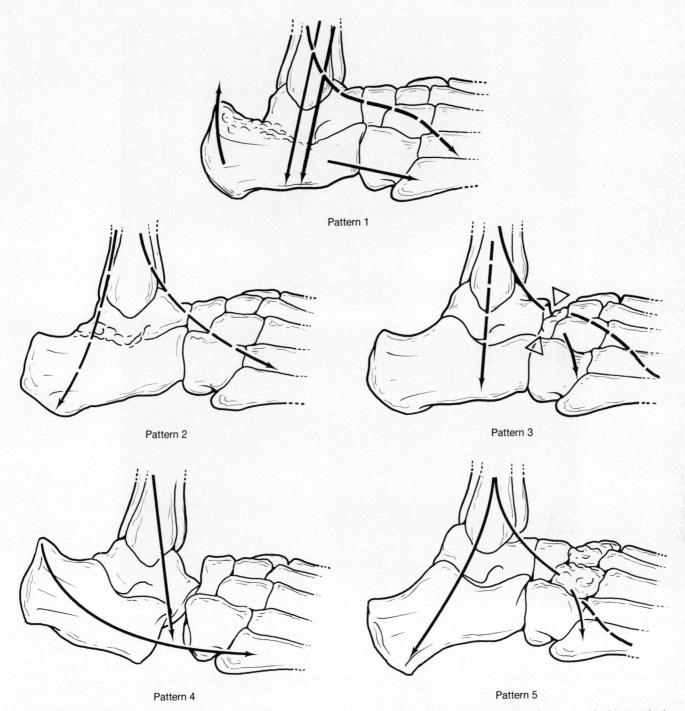

Pattern 1

Pattern 2

Pattern 3

Pattern 4

Pattern 5

Figure 19.8. Patterns of tarsal degeneration. (Modified from Harris JR, Brand PW: Patterns of disintegration of the tarsus in the anesthetic foot. *J Bone Joint Surg* 48A:14–16, 1966.)

From close examination, telltale signs such as loss of vibratory sensation at the level of the forefoot and ankle is also indicative of neuropathy. The author recently examined a young woman who sought attention because of some difficulty walking and lateral ankle instability. Her chief complaint was that of a high arched foot. The patient did have a cavus foot deformity and gave a history of a similar foot deformity in her mother and grandmother. Examination revealed diminished deep tendon reflexes, absent vibra-

tory sensation, atrophy of the muscles innervated by the peroneal nerves, and a dropfoot with steppage gait. Diagnosis of Charcot-Marie-Tooth disease was confirmed by neurological consultation and electromyography.

It is therefore common for a patient with a form of peripheral neuropathy to present with minor sensory and motor weaknesses with no overt evidence of a neuropathic ulceration or osseous deformity (Table 19.5).

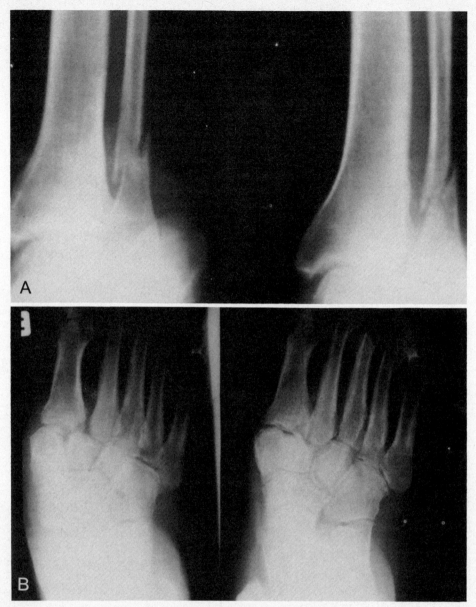

Figure 19.9. Fractures in two diabetic patients caused by insensitivity. (A) Fracture of fibula. (B) Dislocation of tarsometatarsal articulation and metatarsal fractures.

Table 19.4
Comparative Radiographic Appearances in Osteomyelitis Seen in or Mimicked by Neuropathic Bone Disease.

Osteomyelitis	Neuropathic
Bone destruction present	Bone destruction and fragmentation
Increased soft tissue density	Increased soft tissue density
Changes in bone density with early sclerosis and osteo-porosis in later progression	Sclerosis may be present and osteoporosis may present as diabetic osteolysis
Progressive reabsorption of bone occurs	Progressive reabsorption usually is not present
Sequestra formation occurs	Sequestra formation may be mimicked by fragmentation
Subperiosteal new bone formation occurs	Subperiosteal new bone formation occurs

In the patient with a suspected peripheral neuropathy a thorough past medical history needs to be obtained especially with regard to the onset, duration, and progression of the symptoms (Table 19.6). Past medical history should inquire into detail as to the presence of diabetes, peripheral vascular disease, collagen disorder, vitamin deficiencies, anemia, uremia, prolonged illness, infection, trauma to the nervous system, exposure to toxins such as ethanol, and a history of any congenital defect. Family history is

Table 19.5
Signs and Symptoms Associated With the Insensitive Foot

1. Paresthesias
2. Hypoesthesia
3. Anesthesia
4. Nocturnal cramping
5. Diminished or absent deep tendon reflexes
6. Diminished or absent vibratory sensation
7. Diminished or absent temperature or pain sensation
8. Anhydrosis
9. Callous formation
10. Ulceration
11. Intrinsic muscle atrophy
12. Digital deformity
13. Cavus foot deformity or pes valgus deformity
14. Increased skin temperature
15. Edema
16. Change in function (dropfoot)

From Schuster S and Jacobs AM: Diabetic autonomic neuropathy in the surgical management of the diabetic foot. *J Foot Surg* 21(1):16–22, 1982.

Table 19.6
Signs and Symptoms of Neurosteoarthropathy

1. Swelling
2. Warmth
3. Erythema
4. Good vascularity
5. Neurological deficit
6. Joint hypermobility
7. Crepitation
8. Tarsal subluxation (rocker bottom)
9. Digital subluxation
10. Hyperkeratosis
11. Infection and ulceration

extremely important in determining inherited forms of peripheral neuropathy.

A thorough history of current medications and allergies should also be elicited.

The physical examination presented here is directed toward the evaluation of the lower extremity. In general the examination should include inspection, palpation of the muscle mass, and observation of atrophy of the intrinsic muscles. The hand may also be extremely useful in detecting atrophy caused by peripheral neuropathy. In such instances the hand may demonstrate weakness, loss of intrinsic muscle tone and mass, and an increase in noticeable bony prominences.

Vascular examination should include a thorough clinical examination. Special care should be given to the neurological evaluation. Vibratory sensation (101, 102) and light touch evaluation (103) are an important clinical means of determining changes in the patient's sensorium as related to peripheral neuropathy. Recently more sophisticated types of electronic equipment have become available (104) and are useful in the evaluation of more difficult clinical findings. Manual muscle testing is usually included as part of the neurological evaluation. The muscles are evaluated manually on a scale of 0 to 5 as recommended in numerous texts.

The joints of the lower extremity should be evaluated for gross deformity. The range of motion should be evaluated for the presence of crepitation or limited motion. One should also be alert for the presence of swelling and heat that would accompany the development of neuropathic joints (Table 19.6).

Dermatologically the skin should be evaluated for the evidence of ulceration, healed scars, or skin lesions that show no response to pin prick. Such absence of sharp-dull discrimination may be seen in Hansen's disease or in other conditions that produce profound neuropathy.

Gait evaluation plays an integral part in evaluating the extent to which peripheral neuropathy is compromising the patient's normal function.

Biomechanical evaluation should also include measurements of the foot and interaction with the environment. This can be accomplished by various simple methods such as the use of a Harris mat and inked paper (55, 105), or commercially available carbon paper for recording areas of increased weight bearing that would be susceptible to increased tissue damage.

The slipper sock method uses pressure sensitive dyes that have been incorporated into a test sock. The method was developed at the Center for Hansen's Disease in Carville, Louisiana. The Harris mats will measure a direct pressure below the foot while the slipper sock (106, 107) can measure changes in pressure involving dorsal aspects of the toes and the medial and lateral aspects of the foot in relationship to the shoe, as well as the plantar surface.

Electrophysiological findings are used to aid in the diagnosis and extent of the involvement of the patient with peripheral neuropathy. Diagnosis may also require the use of sural nerve biopsy.

Vascular laboratory evaluation is imperative especially in those patients with diabetes mellitus. A simple test such as Doppler ultrasound and the obtaining of an ischemic index (arm-ankle ratio) are usually performed and yield a great deal of information.

The ankle ischemic index is obtained by dividing the ankle pressure by the brachial artery pressure. A normal index is considered 1 or greater. Noting that the pressure at the ankle is usually greater than that at the arm, Walsh (108) used a normal index of 1 or greater with a cut off of 0.9. Vascular disease is felt to be present with an ischemic index of 0.9 or less. The use of ankle pressures can help to differentiate between neurogenic and vascular claudication. If one found an ankle ischemic index to be 0.9 after resting and stabilization and acclimation to the room and then exercised the patient and found the index to remain at 0.9 or increased then the symptoms are not the result of vascular changes. Note that with exercises patients who have a femoral blockage experience claudication. However, occlusion of the calf artery may not lead to claudication, but instead ischemic changes of the skin and digits of the foot may be the first sign.

Diabetic patients complaining of symptomatology

in the legs must be carefully evaluated because the symptoms may also be caused by lumbosacral strain, sciatic neuropathy, arthritis, and obesity. If caused by these problems then they will not manifest themselves with reduced pressure at exercise unless a vascular component is present. A grading system was set up by Aburahma and associates (109) in 1980. They divided patients into four grades. Grade I was considered normal or to have evidence of mild disease. Grade II showed an ischemic index of 0.8 to 0.9 and this is considered mild vascular disease. Grade III has an ischemic index of 0.7 to 0.8 and these patients were considered to have moderate vascular disease. Grade IV included those with an ischemic index of 0.7 or less and were considered to have severe vascular disease.

Wagner (110) found that in nondiabetics with an index as low as 3.5, surgery on an ulcer may obtain healing. In the diabetic, however, surgery on an ulcer should not be attempted with a reading lower than a 4.5.

Baker (111) used the postocclusion reactive hyperemia test with a thigh cuff that was inflated to 100 mm Hg above the systolic pressure for seven minutes to evaluate circulation. The ankle pressure was then measured at 30 seconds, one minute, one minute and 30 seconds, two, three, and four minutes after deflation of the tourniquet.

Failure to return to the normal baseline (preocclusion pressure) in two minutes is abnormal and indicates substantial occlusive disease. The more prolonged the recovery the more advanced the disease. A Doppler ultrasound provides a very convenient and useful method of evaluation of the lower extremities in this foot type.

Photocell plethysmography has also been used in the determination of digital pressure in the dysvascular foot. Barnes (112) used photocell plethysmography in diabetics preoperatively. In diabetics foot amputations failed to heal in two instances with absent digital pulses and 6 of 19 failed with digital pulses. However, in nondiabetics with digital pulses 12 of 13 healed and 4 of 8 healed without digital pulses. Healing of the foot amputation occurred uniformly if the digital pressure was above 10 mm Hg in nondiabetics and above 25 mm Hg in diabetics. They found photocell plethysmography to be more sensitive than strain gauge plethysmography or pneumoplethysmography. One must note though that pneumoplethysmography and strain gauge plethysmography can measure the volume of blood that is passing through the toe. They are quantitative measurements of blood flow whereas photocell plethysmography is qualitative.

Segmental pressures are usually performed using a blood pressure cuff and a Doppler probe. The blood pressure is measured above the knee, below the knee, and at the ankle area. A drop of 20 to 30 mm Hg at any level signifies a significant block in that area.

As mentioned previously, long-term sympathetic denervation leads to arterial calcification in the foot and the ankle. This is significant in the preoperative evaluation of patients in that when performing an ankle pressure or segmental pressure an abnormally high value may be obtained because of the inability of the artery to be compressed. Preoperatively the radiograph should be examined in both anteroposterior and lateral projections for evidence of arterial calcification (113).

More recently radioisotopic flow studies have been used to determine whether healing would occur in an ulcerated extremity. The radioisotope used is thallium 201 (114). Five minutes postinjection a body scan is performed to detect the relative hyperemia. Point counting occurs directly over the ulcer and at three points 2.5 cm from the edge of the ulcer over relatively normal tissue. The counting occurs for 60 seconds at each site. Ten to 15 kcpm were acquired over healing ulcers. A ratio for healing was determined using the activity per unit area of ulcer divided by the activity per unit area of the surrounding tissue. If this was found to be greater than or equal to 1.5, healing occurred. The minimal hyperemic response for healing was 1.5. In their study seven patients with a ratio equal to or greater than 1.5 healed. In those patients with a ratio of less than 1.5, five of six went on to amputation. The study concluded "it appears that healing is not related to the presence or absence of diabetes mellitus and may not be dependent upon a probeable arterial pulse. It is obviously related to the adequacy of the microcirculation and its capacity to produce a hyperemic inflammatory response." Xenon-133 is also used to determine skin perfusion (115).

From the evaluation one basically wants to determine: (a) how much circulation exists in the extremity; (b) if the circulation is adequate to treat the problem; and (c) whether vascular reconstruction surgery is indicated.

A LOGICAL APPROACH TO MANAGEMENT OF INSENSITIVE FEET

For purposes of management the insensitive foot may be classified into three categories (Table 19.7).

The first is the foot with no ulcerations with or without bony deformity and no evidence of active bony destruction.

Second is the foot in which active bony destruction is occurring.

The third category is that of the ulcerated foot with or without a bony deformity. These ulcerations can further be classified as fundamental or complicated.

The first category encompasses the insensitive foot with no ulceration with or without bony deformity and no active bony destruction. Enna (105) in 1982 classified the insensitive foot into four categories as they related to the need for orthotic care. Category one presents with only one deficit, loss of plantar sensation. A soft insole of microcellular rubber, such as Spenco, is provided as a means of prophylaxis.

Category two presents two defects, loss of plantar sensation and deficiency of the subcutaneous soft tissue. This may be present with or without scarring of the plantar skin. In this foot type a molded material

Table 19.7
Logical Approach to Management of The Insensitive Foot

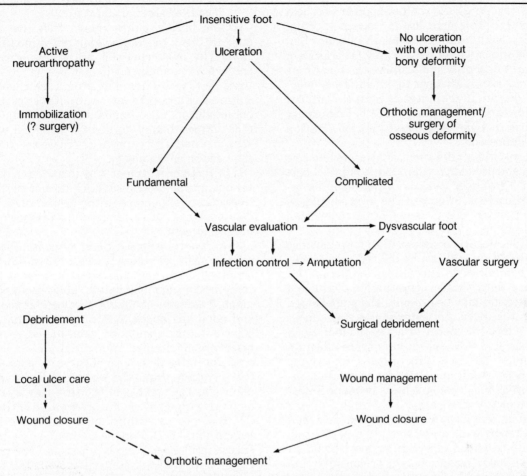

such as plastizote, with or without a layer of microcellular rubber is advantageous to the patient. Any increase in the use of material is accompanied by the use of a shoe that is required to have extra depth to accommodate the thickness of the insole.

Category three includes three deficits. In addition to loss of sensation and the presence of plantar scarring gross deformity is present. Gross deformity may require surgical intervention as recommended by several authors. The surgical intervention may include both resection of prominent osseous structures and in some cases judicious arthrodesis of involved joints. Molded shoes with the appropriate insole materials would be required to manage this type of deformity.

Category four patients present with a short, deformed, and rigid foot. A molded shoe is fabricated to the dimensions of the foot. In this type of deformity the sole of the shoe requires a rocker mechanism to allow a more normal gait and reduce the forces interacting with the insensitive foot.

The use of insoles and shoes as outlined here are also applicable to the follow-up care of patients after they have been successfully treated for superficial or deep ulcerations (116–119). Modifications of shoegear may require application of a rocker-bottom sole, anterior heel, metatarsal bar, or platform shoe.

The second category includes patients who present with active neuroarthropathy (120). Initial treatment after the diagnosis is made depending on the presence of early or late signs. Localized warmth is the cardinal sign of these changes. Rest is required until clinical and radiologic evidence of healing is seen. Lennox (121) advises bed rest followed by non-weight-bearing on crutches followed by partial weight bearing and then the use of gait assistive devices over a period of some weeks until union is achieved. "This sequence is ideal, as it insures an initial period of absolute rest, and then a gradual return to function" (121). As he points out, in practice such ideal treatment may not be feasible. In the latter circumstance the use of plaster immobilization is recommended. "Fixation may be obtained by carefully applying a molded below the knee plaster cast until clinical and radiographic union is achieved." Care must be taken to mold the foot in a good functional position avoiding deviation. He points out the initial basic period of immobilization is three to four months or more and that shorter periods increase the risk of failure.

Return to activity should be gradual and the patient should be followed frequently after the removal of the cast to assess the development of heat and swelling. If incomplete healing occurs, further immobilization is indicated. Arthrodesis of major foot joints may be indicated in select cases. The aims of surgery are (a) to simplify and stabilize the remaining skeleton, (b) to restore the foot to a plantigrade position without deviation, (c) to restore a functional foot for ambulation, and (d) to prevent further deformity (121). The use of bone grafts and internal fixation may also be indicated.

Arthrodesis when performed is at a greater risk for nonunion and pseudarthrosis because of previously diseased bone. Extended periods of time may be required for arthrodesis to occur. The joint should be fixated until radiographic evidence of osseous union has occurred.

The third category of insensitive foot includes those with ulceration and can be divided into fundamental and complicated. The fundamental type includes the foot with simple neurotrophic ulcers and soft tissue infection may be present. The complicated type includes the ulcer that extends past the subcutaneous tissue into the deeper layers of the foot. Such ulcers are associated with deep plantar space infection with involvement of such structures as underlying bone and muscle. Additionally these ulcers are complicated by ischemia, osteomyelitis, systemic infection, or active neuroarthropathy.

In these patients appropriate neurological and vascular laboratory evaluation should be performed. Patients found to have a dysvascular foot should be referred for vascular reconstruction or consideration for amputation. Control of the active infection should be achieved by the use of specific and appropriate parental antibiotics.

In the fundamental uncomplicated ulcer the goal of local care is to remove necrotic tissue, reduce the existing bacterial level, and promote healing.

Management of this type of ulcer consists of the following.

Treatment of a soft tissue skin infection if one is present. This is primarily accomplished with the use of intravenous antibiotics. Colonization of the ulcer must be a consideration. One looks for evidence of systemic infection and deep local infection such as abscess formation. The course of the infection should be followed with regular white blood cell counts and differentials. Systemic antibiotics are not indicated for bacterial colonization.

Topical agents used in the local care of the ulcer can include many modes. Included are topical enzymes such as collaginase (122–124) although they tend to cause tissue maceration and may increase the risk of infection. Betadine (125, 126) can also be used as a topical therapy. Silvadene may be used although it was originally prescribed for use in the treatment of burns (127). Mechanical debridement can be obtained by the use of wet to dry dressings. Debridement may also occur by the use of whirlpool and other methods

of topical therapy such as Debrisan (128). Whirlpool therapy followed by a vigorous rinse has been found to reduce the bacterial count (129).

The literature has shown that the majority of diabetic infections are polymicrobial in etiology (130–133). The most common are gram-positive aerobic cocci. It is recommended that proper anaerobic cultures be taken. There has been a poor correlation of culture findings between swabs of the ulcer and those obtained from uncontaminated deep tissue specimens (131). Much better results are obtained with needle aspirates and with curettage of these specimens rather than swabs of the ulcers.

Although treatment may include the use of intravenous antibiotics, antibiotics do not always appear to eradicate organisms in the deep tissues. A surgical debridement is often required for drainage and definitive treatment.

Appropriate dressing technique is indicated in the management of these ulcers (134). The dressing should provide the following functions: protection, compression, immobilization, and preferably debridement. A dressing should be comfortable to the patient and allow the application of medications as desired. The dressings should be constructed so that three layers are maintained. The initial contact layer should conform to the defect, an absorptive layer should pull the secretions from the wound, and a fixation layer maintains the context of the first two layers. A layer of gauze with an overlying layer of tape is insufficient.

Biological dressings such as porcine may be of benefit (135–137). Porcine cannot be used in the presence of gram negative rod infections. The porcine also may reduce the local bacterial population by creating a healthy environment in which the patient's own defense mechanisms may function. Epithelization of the wound is thus encouraged because of the maintenance of optimum wound conditions. The main property of porcine is its property of adherence to the wound allowing these conditions to be maintained. Usual changes of porcine occur every 48 to 72 hours. Amniotic membrane has also been advocated for management of this type of ulceration (138). Nonbiological dressings have also been used and are reported in the literature.

The key to care of these ulcers is good mechanical debridement. Wet to dry dressings using normal sterile saline have been found to be most beneficial. Such treatment is usually accomplished in conjunction with minimal sharp debridement at bedside. Other types of dressings useful for debridement are dry to dry and wet dressings with Dakin's solution (139). Topical insulin is currently being researched as an adjunct to the management of diabetic foot ulceration (140).

Various supportive measures have been recommended for use in the ulcerated patient. These include overall nutritional support and the use of various vitamin and zinc supplements (141).

One of the keys in allowing patients with complications caused by insensitive feet to return to normal function is total contact weight bearing. This is especially true in patients with neuroarthropathy. Total contact weight bearing allows the weight of the foot to be better and more evenly distributed and can prevent buildup of areas of focal pressure that may lead to ulceration. Casting for the treatment of these types of ulcers has been advocated by various authors. However, there is a risk of potential infection being concealed by a plaster cast.

Although casting is indicated in the treatment of neuroarthropathy and has been advocated for the treatment of plantar ulcers, these patients are prone to cast-related problems. Specifically in the neurotrophic patient a cast may conceal a potential infection and more specifically an ill-fitting cast may lead to the development of pressure type ulcerations further complicating the management of these patients. Frequent cast checks are mandatory. Changing the cast on a frequent basis is preferred as opposed to windowing the cast for the management of pedal ulcerations.

Fundamental ulcerations can be managed by the use of a plastizote sandel that is commercially available. It is an easy appliance to fabricate in the office and is a most helpful adjunct to the management of such ulcer patients.

Management of the complicated ulceration requires precise and accurate surgical treatment (142–145). Debridement and resection of necrotic tissue, including tendon and bone, is required. This is accomplished usually with a radical debridement with a ray resection or amputation of an infected digit. Radical debridement is exactly what the term means, radical excision of all necrotic tissue and infected tissue. It may include bone, tendon, and muscle. All necrotic tissue must be removed to allow healing. A large area may have to be resected and the wound deepened. The guidelines have been established for radical debridement and include: (a) never sacrifice blood supply, (b) allow adequate incisions for drainage, and (c) avoid weight-bearing areas if at all possible. After radical debridement, depending on the amount of exposure that is required, treatment usually consists of local wound management until a healthy granulating base is obtained. Debridement may be required on more than one occasion. Exposed bone will cover spontaneously with granulation tissue followed by epithelium or will sequestrate and then cover providing there is adequate circulation at the wound site (146).

After debridement wound closure may be obtained using various methods such as contracture and reepithelialization, skin grafts, skin flaps, muscle transpositin and in some cases amputation (147–159). Certain cases may be treated as open contaminated wounds. Other methods of wound closure would include the application of a split-thickness skin graft to the sole of the foot. These are generally not preferred in areas required for weight bearing. Other approaches that have been found useful are the application of plantar rotational flaps, or transferring of muscle that is then covered with a split-thickness skin graft.

Amputation is advisable in cases of advanced peripheral vascular disease, life-threatening infection, and unstable osseous deformity. The surgical management of osseous deformity is indicated to correct or prevent deformity. In addition to neurotrophic ulcerations and neuroarthropathy, the patient with an insensitive foot is prone to develop a complex foot deformity such as pes equinovarus, pes cavus, dropfoot, equinus, or an unstable shortened foot. The management of this presentation of the disease requires extensive evaluation and consideration before surgical intervention (160–164) and is addressed in other chapters of this text. The rehabilitation of associated foot deformities such as cavus foot and dropfoot is indicated because this would improve the patient's functional capacity.

References

1. Gibson T, Kenedi RM: Biomechanical properties of skin. *Surg Clin North Am* 47:279–293, 1967.
2. Daly CH: Biomechanical properties of dermis. *J Invest Dermatol* 79:17–20, 1982.
3. Brand PW: Management of the insensitive limb. *Physical Therapy* 59:8–12, 1979.
4. Hall OC, Brand PW: The etiology of the neuropathic plantar ulcer. *J Am Podiatry Assoc* 69:173–177, 1979.
5. Kosiak M: Etiology and pathology of ischemic ulcers. *Arch Phys Med Rehabil* 40:62–69, 1959.
6. Manley MT, Darby T: Repetitive mechanical stress and denervation in plantar ulcer pathogenesis in rats. *Arch Phys Med Rehabil* 61:171–177, 1980.
7. Beach RB, Thompson DE: Selected soft tissue research. *Phys Ther* 59:30–33, 1979.
8. Bergtholdt HT: Temperature assessment of the insensitive foot. *Phys Ther* 59:18–22, 1979.
9. Bergtholdt HT: Measurement in tissue response in rat footpad from repetitive mechanical stress. In Brand PW, Mooney V (ed): *The Effects of Pressure on Human Tissues*. Washington, Rehabilitation Services Administration, Report III, 1977.
10. Edmonds ME, Roberts VC, Watkins PJ: Blood flow in the diabetic neuropathic foot. *Diabetologia* 22:9–15, 1982.
11. Ward JD: The diabetic leg. *Diabetologia* 22:141–147, 1982.
12. Ellenberg M: Diabetic autonomic neuropathy: role in vascular events. *NY State J Med* 78:2214–2217, 1978.
13. Christensen NJ: Spontaneous variations in resting blood flow, postischaemic peak flow and vibratory perception in the feet of diabetics. *Diabetologia* 5:171–178, 1969.
14. Ouayle JB: Diabetic autonomic neuropathy in patients with vascular disease. *Br J Surg* 65:305–307, 1978.
15. Andersson R, Bjerle P: Peripheral circulation, particularly heat regulation reactions in patients with amyloidosis and polyneuropathy. *Acta Med Scand* 199:191–196, 1976.
16. Harrison MJG, Faris IB: The neuropathic factor in the aetiology of diabetic foot ulcers. *J Neurol Sci* 28:217–233, 1976.
17. Barner HB, Kaiser G, Willman V: Blood flow in the diabetic leg. *Circulation* 43:391–394, 1971.
18. Schustek S, Jacobs AM: Diabetic autonomic neuropathy in the surgical management of the diabetic foot. *J Foot Surg* 21:16–22, 1982.
19. Watkins PJ, Edmonds ME: Sympathetic nerve failure in diabetes. *Diabetologia* 25:73–77, 1983.
20. Bevan RD, Tsuru H: Long-term denervation of vascular smooth muscle causes not only functional but structural change. *Blood Vessels* 16:109–112, 1979.
21. Goebel FD, Fuessl HS: Monckeberg's sclerosis after sympathetic denervation in diabetic and nondiabetic subjects. *Diabetologia* 24:347–350, 1983.
22. Edmonds ME, Morrison N, Laws JW, Watkins PJ: Medial arterial calcification and diabetic neuropathy. *Br Med J* 284:928–930, 1982.
23. Boulton AJM, Scarpello JWB, Ward JD: Venous oxygenation

in the diabetic neurotrophic foot: evidence of arteriovenous shunting? *Diabetologia* 22:6–8, 1982.

24. Borkowski M: An experimental study on the role of arteriovenous anastomoses in the pathogenesis of trophic ulcer. *Arch Immunol Ther Exp* 21:363–373, 1973.
25. Deanfield JE, Daggett PR, Harrison MJG: The role of autonomic neuropathy in diabetic foot ulceration. *J Neurol Sci* 47:203–210, 1980.
26. Ozeran RS, Wagner GR, Reimer TR, Hill RA: Neuropathy of the sympathetic nervous system associated with diabetes mellitus. *Surgery* 68:953–958, 1970.
27. Conrad MC: Contributions of large and small vessel disease to severe ischemia of the lower extremities in diabetics and nondiabetics. *Vasc Diag Ther* 2:17–28, 1981.
28. Colwell JA: Studies on the pathogenesis of diabetic vascular disease. *J SC Med Assoc* 77:267–272, 1981.
29. McMillan DE: Deterioration of the microcirculation in diabetes. *Diabetes* 24:944–957, 1975.
30. Arenson DJ, Sherwood CF, Wilson RC: Neuropathy, angiopathy, and sepsis in the diabetic foot (part two: angiopathy). *J Am Podiatry Assoc* 71:661–665, 1981.
31. Janka HU, Standl E, Schramm W, Mehnrt H: Platelet enzyme activities in diabetes mellitus in relation to endothelial damage. *Diabetes* 32:47–51, 1983.
32. Sinziner H, Silberbauer K, Kaliman J, Klein K: Vascular prostacyclin synthesis, platelet sensitivity, plasma factors and platelet function, arteriopathy with and without diabetes mellitus. In Noseda G, Lewis B, Paolett R (eds): *Diet and Drugs in Atherosclerosis*. New York, Raven Press, 1980, pp 93–95.
33. Bern MM: Platelet functions in diabetes mellitus. *Diabetes* 27:342–352, 1978.
34. Williamson JR, Kilo C: Small vessel disease: diabetic microangiopathy. *Angiology* 31:448–454, 1980.
35. Williamson JR, Vogler NJ, Kilo C: Microvascular disease in diabetes. *Med Clin North Am* 55:847–860, 1981.
36. Williamson JR, Kilo C: Capillary basement membranes. *Diabetes* 32:96–100, 1983.
37. Friedericki HHR, Tucker WR, Schwartz TB: Observations on small blood vessels of skin in the normal and in diabetic patients. *Diabetes* 15:233–250, 1966.
38. Banson BB, Lacy PE: Diabetic microangiopathy in human toes. *Am J Pathol* 45:41–50, 1964.
39. Coster AA, Swedlow BL: Ultrastructural morphology of diabetic microangiopathy. *J Am Podiatry Assoc* 66:69–75, 1976.
40. Almer L, Sundvist G, Lilja B: Fibrinolytic activity, autonomic neuropathy and circulation in diabetes mellitus. *Diabetes* 32:4–19, 1983.
41. Wagner FW: The insensitive foot. In Kiene RH, Johnson KA (eds): *AAOS Symposium of the Foot and Ankle*. St. Louis, The CV Mosby Co, 1981, pp 135–158.
42. Stokes IAF, Faris IB, Hutton WC: The neuropathic ulcer and loads on the foot in diabetic patients. *Acta Orthop Scand* 46:839–847, 1975.
43. Stokes IAF, Hutton WC: The effect of the diabetic ulcer on the load bearing function of the foot. In Kenedi RM, Cowden JM (eds): *Bedsore Biomechanics*. Baltimore, University Park Press, 1976, pp 245–247.
44. Barrett JP, Mooney V: Neuropathy and diabetic pressure lesions. *Orthop Clin North Am* 4:43–47, 1973.
45. Sabato S, Yosipovitch Z, Simkin A, Sheskin J: Plantar trophic ulcers in patients with leprosy. *Int Orthop* 6:203–208, 1982.
46. Ctercteko GC, Chanendran M, Hutton WC, Lequesne LP: Vertical forces acting on the feet of diabetic patients with neuropathic ulceration. *Br J Surg* 68:608–614, 1981.
47. Burman M, Perls W: The weight stream in Charcot disease of Joints. *Bull Hosp Joint Dis* 19:31–47, 1958.
48. Ellenberg M: Diabetic neuropathic ulcer. *J Mt Sinai Hosp* 35:585–594, 1968.
49. Pati L, Behera F: Metatarsal head pressure (MHP) sores in leprosy patients. *Lepr India* 53:588–593, 1981.
50. Buchman NH: Bone and joint changes in the diabetic foot. *J Am Podiatry Assoc* 66:211–226, 1976.
51. Geoffroy J, Hoeffel JC, Pointel JP, Drouin P, Debry G, Martin R: The feet in diabetes. *Diagn Imaging* 48:286–293, 1979.
52. Enna CD: Skeletal deformities of the denervated hand in Hansen's disease. *J Hand Surg* 4:227–233, 1979.
53. Schwarz GS, Berenyi MR, Siegal MW: Atrophic arthropathy and diabetic neuritis. *Am J Roentgenol, Rad Ther Nucl Med* 106:523–529, 1969.
54. Pogonowska MJ, Collins LC, Dobson HL: Diabetic osteopathy. *Radiology* 89:265–271, 1967.
55. Friedman SA, Rakow RB: Osseous lesions of the foot in diabetic neuropathy. *Diabetes* 20:302–307, 1971.
56. Riordan DC: The hand in leprosy: a seven year clinical study. *Diabetes* 42A:683–960, 1960.
57. Miller RM, Hunt JA: The radiological features of alcoholic ulceroosteolytic neuropathy in blacks. *S Afr Med J* 54:159–161, 1978.
58. Enna CD, Jacobson RR, Rausch RO: Bone changes in leprosy: a correlation of clinical and radiographic features. *Radiology* 10:295–306, 1971.
59. Thornhill HL, Richter RW, Shelton ML, Johnson CA: Neuropathic arthropathy (Charcot forefeet) in alcoholics. *Orthop Clin North Am* 4:7–20, 1973.
60. Kraft E, Spyropoulos E, Finby N: Neurogenic disorders of the foot in diabetes mellitus. *Am J Roentgenol Rad Ther Nucl Med* 124:17–24, 1975.
61. Enna CD: The foot in leprosy. In McDowell F, Enna CD (eds): *Surgical Rehabilitation in Leprosy and in Other Peripheral Nerve Disorders*. Baltimore, Williams & Wilkins, 1974.
62. Bruckner FE, Howell A: Neuropathic joints. *Semin Arthritis Rheum* 2:47–69, 1972.
63. Wolf DS, Raczka EK, Shevlin AM: Charcot's joint in a juvenile-onset diabetic. *J Am Podiatry Assoc* 67:200–203, 1977.
64. Sella AJ: Diabetic neurosteoarthropathy of the tarsus. *Conn Med* 43:70–74, 1979.
65. McNamara G, Shor RI: Diabetic neuropathic osteoarthropathy. *J Am Podiatry Assoc* 73:485–489, 1983.
66. Newman JH: Non-infective disease of the diabetic foot. *J Bone Joint Surg* 63B:593–596, 1981.
67. Weissman SD, Weiss A: Diabetic neurotrophic osteoarthropathy (Charcot joint). *J Am Podiatry Assoc* 70:196–200, 1980.
68. Frykberg RG: The diabetic Charcot foot. *Arch Podiatr Med Foot Surg* 5:15–27, 1978.
69. Forgacs S: Clinical picture of diabetic osteoarthropathy. *Acta Diabetol Lat* 13:111–115, 1976.
70. Forgacs S: *Bones and Joints in Diabetes Mellitus*. The Hague, Netherlands, Hungary, Martinus Nijhoff Publishers, 1982.
71. Harris JR, Brand PW: Patterns of disintegration of the tarsus in the anaesthetic foot. *J Bone Joint Surg* 48B:4–16, 1966.
72. Defeo WT, Jay RM: Osteomyelitis associated with peripheral vascular disease secondary to diabetes medicine. *J Foot Surg* 15:159–160, 1976.
73. Hetherington VJ: Technetium and combined gallium and technetium scan in the neurotrophic foot. *J Am Podiatry Assoc* 72:458–463, 1982.
74. Park HM, Wheat LJ, Siddiqui AR, Burt RW, Robb JA, Ransburg RC, Kernek CB: Scintigraphic evaluation of diabetic osteomyelitis: concise communication. *J Nucl Med* 23:569–573, 1982.
75. Maurer AH, Chen DCP, Camago EE, Wong DF, Wagner HN, Alderson PO: Utility of three phase skeletal cintiraphy in suspected osteomyelitis. *J Nucl Med* 22: 941–949, 1981.
76. Thrall JH, Geslien GE, Corcoron RJ, Johnson MC: Abnormal radionuclide deposition patterns adjacent to focal skeletal lesions. *Radiology* 15:659–661, 1975.
77. Clark WD, Fann TR, McCrea J, Venson JN: Uses of bone scanning in podiatric medicine. *J Am Podiatry Assoc* 68:621–630, 1978.
78. Deutsch SD, Gandsman EJ, Spraragen SC: Quantitative regional blood flow analysis and its clinical application during routine bone scanning. *J Bone Joint Surg* 63A:295–305, 1981.
79. Eymontt MJ, Alavi A, Dalinka MK, Kyle GC: Bone scintigraphy in diabetic osteoarthropathy. *Radiology* 140:474–477, 1981.
80. Kirchner PT, Simon MA: Current concepts review radioisotopic evaluation of skeletal disease. *J Bone Joint Surg* 63A:673–682, 1981.

81. Lisbona R, Rosenthall L: Observations on the sequential use of 99mTC phosphate complex and 67Ga imaging in ssteomyelitis, cellulitis, and septic arthritis. *Radiology* 123:123–129, 1977.
82. Hoffer P: Gallium mechanisms. *J Nucl Med* 21:282, 1980.
83. Glynn TP: Marked gallium accumulation in neurogenic arthropathy. *J Nucl Med* 22:1016–1017, 1981.
84. Sugarman B, Hawes S, Musher DM, Kilma M, Young EJ, Pircher F: Osteomyelitis beneath pressure sores. *Arch Intern Med* 143:683–688, 1983.
85. Propst-Proctor SL, Dillingham MF, McDougall IR: The white blood cell scan in orthopedics. *Clin Orthop* 168:157–165, 1982.
86. Wilkinson JD: Section of dermatology: ulcerating and mutilating acropathy with thermographic findings. *Proc R Soc Lond* 69:513–515, 1976.
87. Dribbon BS: Application and value of liquid crystal thermography. *J Am Podiatry Assoc* 73:400–404, 1983.
88. Sandrow RE, Torg JS, Lapayowker MS, Resnick EJ: The use of thermography in the early diagnosis of neuropathic arthropathy in the feet of diabetics. *Clin Orthop* 88:31–33, 1972.
89. Matlin SR: Liquid crystal therography. *Arch Podiatr Med Foot Surg* 1:235–264, 1974.
90. Popmynaloua H, Yaneja R, Koev D, Dyankov L, Koeva L: Xeroradiology of the diabetic foot. *Rev Roman Med Endocr* 19:249–251, 1981.
91. Goldman F, Manzi J, Carver A, Torre R, Richter R: Sinography in the diagnosis of foot infections. *J Am Podiatry Assoc* 71:497–502, 1981.
92. Coventry MB, Rothacker GW: Bilateral calcaneal fracture in a diabetic patient. *J Bone Joint Surg* 61A:462–464, 1979.
93. El-Khoury GY, Kathol MH: Neuropathic fractures in patients with diabetes mellitus. *Radiology* 134:313–316, 1980.
94. Giescke SB, Dalinka MK, Kyle GC: Lisfranc's fracture dislocation: a manifestation of peripheral neuropathy. *Am J Roentgenol* 131:139–141, 1978.
95. Williams B: Orthopedic features in the presentation of syringomyelia. *J Bone Joint Surg* 61B:314–323,1979.
96. Fath MA, Hassanein MR, James JIP: Congenital absence of pain. *J Bone Joint Surg* 65B:186–188, 1983.
97. Schneider R, Goldman AB, Bohne WHO: Neuropathic injuries to the lower extremities in children. *Pediatr Radiol* 128:713–718, 1978.
98. Kristiansen B: Ankle and foot fracture in diabetic provoking neuropathic joint changes. *Acta Orthop Scand* 51:975–979, 1980.
99. Dyck PJ, Lambert EH, O'Brien PC: Pain in peripheral neuropathy related to rate and kind of fiber degeneration. *Neurol* 26:466–471, 1976.
100. Dyck PJ, Low PA, Stevens JC: "Burning feet" as the only manifestation of dominantly inherited sensory neuropathy. *Mayo Clin Proc* 58:426–429, 1983.
101. Nielsen NV, Lund FS: Diabetic polyneuropathy, corneal sensitivity, vibratory perception and Achilles tendon reflex in diabetes. *Acta Neurol Scan* 59:15–22, 1979.
102. Christensen NJ: Vibratory perception and blood flow in the feet of diabetics. *Acta Med Scand* 185:553–559, 1969.
103. Dyck PJ, Schultz PW, O'Brien PC: Quantitation of touch-pressure sensation. *Arch Neurol* 26:465–473, 1972.
104. Dellon AL: The vibrometer. *Plast Reconstr Surg* 71:427–431, 1982.
105. Enna CD: Rehabilitation of leprous deformity. *Ann Rev Med* 33:41–45, 1982.
106. Brand PW: Patient monitoring. In Trautman JR (eds): *The Effects of Pressure on Human Tissues* Carville, LA, Northwestern University Publishers, 1977, p 50–51.
107. The Slipper-Sock Footprint Test, U.S. Public Health Service Hospital, Carville, LA 70721.
108. Walsh R, Wolfson P, Haspel U, Smith R, Dunlap S: Leg arterial insufficiency in patients with significant coronary artery disease. *Angiology* 31:185–188, 1980.
109. Aburahma AF, Boland J, Diethrich E: Correlation of the resting and exercise Doppler ankle/arm index to angiographic findings. *Angiology* 31:331–336, 1980.
110. Wagner FW: Transcutaneous Doppler ultrasound in the pre-

diction of healing and the selection of surgical level for dysvascular lesions of the toes and forefoot. *Clin Orthop* 142:110–114, 1979.
111. Baker JD: Poststress Doppler ankle pressures, *Arch Surg* 113:1171–1173, 1978.
112. Barnes RW, Thornhill B, Rittgers SE, Turley G: Prediction of amputation wound healing. *Arch Surg* 116:80–83, 1981.
113. Stanton PE, Rosenthal D, Lamis PA: Differentiation of vascular and neurogenic claudication. *Am Surg* 46:44–49, 1980.
114. Siegel ME, Stewart CA, Wagner W, Sakimura I: A new objective criterion for determining, noninvasively, the healing potential of an ischemic ulcer. *J Nucl Med* 22:187–189, 1981.
115. Daly MJ, Henry RE: Quantitative measurement of skin profusion with Xenon-133. *J Nucl Med* 21:156–160, 1980.
116. Block P: The Diabetic Foot Ulcer: A complex problem with a simple treatment approach. *Milit Med* 146:644–646, 1981.
117. Seder JI: Management of foot problems in diabetics. *J Dermatol Surg Oncol* 4:708–709, 1978.
118. Singleton EE, Cotton RS, Shelman HS: Another approach to the long term management of the diabetic neurotrophic foot ulcer. *J Am Podiatry Assoc* 68:242–244, 1978.
119. Brenner MA: An ambulatory approach to the neuropathic ulceration. *J Am Podiatry Assoc* 64:862–869, 1974.
120. Goldman F: Identification, treatment, and prognosis of Charcot joint in diabetes mellitus. *J Am Podiatry Assoc* 72:485–490, 1982.
121. Lennox WM: Surgical treatment of chronic deformities of the anesthetic foot. In McDowell F, Enna CD (eds) *Surgical Rehabilitation in Leprosy and in Other Peripheral Nerve Disorders.* Baltimore, Williams & Wilkins, 1974, p 350.
122. Scherer PR: An assessment of collagenase therapy for dermal ulcerations of the foot. *J Am Podiatry Assoc* 74:25–30, 1984.
123. Varma AO, Bugatcch E., German FM: Debridement of dermal ulcers with collagenase. *Surg Gynecol Obstet* 136:281–282, 1973.
124. Boxer AM, Gottesman N, Bernstein H, Mandl A: Debridement of dermal ulcers and decubiti with collagenase. *Geriatrics* 24:78–86, 1969.
125. Brenner MA: Another approach to the management of lower extremity ulcerations. *J Am Podiatry Assoc* 72:79–83, 1982.
126. Lee BY, Trainor FS, Thoden WR: Topical application of povidone-iodine in the management of decubitus and stasis ulcers. *J Am Geriatr Soc* 27:302–206, 1979.
127. Stefanides MM, Copeland CE, Kominos SD, Yee RB: In vitro penetration of topical antiseptics through eschar of burn patients. *Am Surg* 183:358–364, 1975.
128. Sawyer PN, Sopie Z, Dowbak G, Cohen L, Feller J: New approaches in the therapy of the peripheral vascular ulcer. *Angiology* 31:666–675, 1980.
129. Bohnannon RW: Whirlpool versus whirlpool and rinse for removal of bacterial from a venous stasis ulcer. *Phys Ther* 62:304–307, 1982.
130. Louie TJ, Bartlett JG, Tally FD, Gorbach SL: Aerobic and anaerobic bacteria in diabetic foot ulcers. *Ann Intern Med* 85:461–463, 1976.
131. Sharp CS, Bessman AN, Wagner FW, Garland D, Reece E: Microbiology of superficial and deep tissues in infected diabetic gangrene. *Surg Obstet Gynecol* 149:217–219, 1979.
132. Sapico FL, Canawati HN, Witte JL, Montgomerie JZ, Wagner FW, Bessman AN: Quantitative aerobic and anaerobic bacteriology of infected diabetic feet. *J Clin Microbiol* 12:413–420, 1980.
133. Walsh CH, Campbell CK: The multiple flora of diabetic foot. *Ir J Med Sci* 149:366–369, 1980.
134. Noe JM, Kalish S: Dressing materials and their selection. In Rudolph R, Noe JM (eds): *Chronic Problem Wounds.* Boston, Little, Brown and Co, 1983, p 37.
135. Axler DA, Terleckyj B, McCarthy D, Kwasnik RE, Novicki D, Culliton P: The efficacy of porcine skin grafts for treating non-healing cutaneous ulcers. Part III. Microbiologic studies. *J Am Podiatry Assoc* 68:141–150, 1978.
136. Culliton P, Kwasnik RE, Novicki D, Corbin P, Patton G, Collins W, Terleckyj B, Axler DA: The efficacy of porcine skin grafts for treating non-healing cutaneous ulcers, Part I. clinical

studies. *J Am Podiatry Assoc* 68:1–10, 1978.

137. McCarthy, DJ, Axler DA: The efficacy of porcine skin grafts for treating non-healing cutaneous ulcers. Part II. Microanatomical studies. *J Am Podiatry Assoc* 68:86–89, 1978.

138. Rudnick SS: The use of amniotic membrane grafting in podiatric office practice. *J Am Podiatry Assoc* 71:679–683, 1981.

139. Rudolph R, Noe JM: Initial treatment of the chronic wound. In Rudolph R, Noe JM (eds): *Chronic Problem Wounds* Boston, Little, Brown and Co, 1983, p 9.

140. Glasser J, Barth A: Diabetic wound healing and the case for supplemental treatment with topical insulin. *J Am Podiatry Assoc* 21:117–121, 1982.

141. Engel ED, Erlick NE, Davis RH: Diabetes mellitus: impaired wound healing from zinc deficiency. *J Am Podiatry Assoc* 71:536–544, 1981.

142. Robson MC, Edstrom LE: Conservative management of the ulcerated diabetic foot. *Plast Reconstr Surg* 59:551–554, 1977.

143. Kritter AE: A technique for salvage of the infected diabetic gangrenous foot. *Orthop Clin North Am* 4:21–30, 1973.

144. Rice JS: Diabetic infection, ulceration and gangrene. *J Am Podiatry Assoc* 64:774–781, 1974.

145. LaPorta GA, Richter KP, Marzzacco JC: Local radical amputation in the foot for arterial insufficiency. *J Am Podiatry Assoc* 67:192–197, 1977.

146. Brown PW: The fate of exposed bone. *Am J Surg* 137:464–468, 1979.

147. Singer A: Surgical treatment of mal perforans. *Arch Surg* 111:964–968, 1976.

148. Wexler MR, Barlev A, Peled IJ: Plantar split-thickness skin grafts for coverage of superficial pressure ulcers of the foot. *J Dermatol Surg Oncol* 9:162–164, 1983.

149. Kipp LJ: Hynes reverse dermal skin graft. *J Foot Surg* 15:26–

28, 1976.

150. Shapiro GD, Brownstein M, Coulter KR, Woodcox LH: Nondiabetic neurotrophic ulcer of the heel. *J Foot Surg* 21:285–291, 1982.

151. Morain WD: Island toe flaps in neurotrophic ulcers of the foot and ankle. *Ann Plast Surg* 13:1–8, 1984.

152. Hartwell SW: Local flaps of the foot and leg. In Grabb WC, Myers MB (eds): *Skin Flaps*. Boston, Little, Brown and Co, 1975, p 497.

153. Curtin JW: Functional surgery for intractable conditions of the sole of the foot. *Plast Reconstr Surg* 59:806–811, 1977.

154. Colem LB, Buncke HJ: Neurovascular island flaps from the plantar vessels and nerves for foot reconstruction. *Ann Plast Surg* 12:327–332, 1984.

155. Snyder GB, Edgerton MT: The principle of the island neurovascular flap in the management of ulcerated anesthetic weightbearing areas of the lower extremity. *Plast Reconstr Surg* 36:518–528, 1965.

156. Ger R: Newer concepts in the surgical management of lesions of the foot in patients with diabetes. *Surg Gynecol Obstet* 158:213–215, 1984.

157. Nelson EW, Scurran B, Tuerk D, Silvani SH, Karlin JM: Reconstruction of plantar heel defects. *J Am Podiatry Assoc* 73:235–239, 1983.

158. Scheflan M, Nahai F: Reconstruction. In Mathes JJ, Nahai F (eds): *Clinical Applications for Muscle and Musculocutaneous Flaps*. St Louis, The CV Mosby Co, 1982, pp 585–809.

159. Mathes SJ, Nanai F: A systemic approach to flap selection. In Mathes SJ, Nahai F (eds): *Clinical Applications for Muscle and Musculocutaneous Flaps*. St Louis, The CV Mosby Co, 1982, pp 3–15.

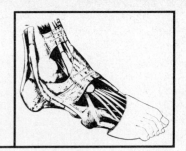

CHAPTER 20

Limb Salvage

Louis G. Pack, D.P.M.

There are currently 10 million diabetics in the United States and most of these have some degree of pedal pathology (1). The most serious and difficult problem that occurs is a severely infected ischemic foot often accompanied with patchy areas of gangrene and osteomyelitis. Patients with these problems require a very thorough clinical evaluation to determine the probability of limb salvage. Infectious disease specialists, vascular surgeons, orthopedists, and diabetologists may all become involved and are usually helpful but the ultimate responsibility for limb salvage often rests with the podiatrist. It has been the experience of this author that a great many lower extremity amputations can be avoided by proper evaluation and treatment.

PEDAL INFECTIONS

Diabetics often develop severe pedal infections because of the pathological changes that occur in the epidermal, vascular, neurological, and osseous structures of the lower extremity. It is the combined effect of this pathology that results in the ominous changes so often seen in the foot.

Epidermal involvement includes trophic skin changes and mycotic and monilial infections. Thinning of the skin and fissuring caused by these cutaneous pathogens cause breaks in the skin often producing a portal of entry for bacterial infections. This is especially serious in the web spaces of the foot where a small fissure may result in a closed-space anaerobic fascial plane infection (Fig. 20.1).

Occlusive vascular disease affecting the tibial and popliteal vessels, as well as the characteristic small vessel disease of the digits, causes lower extremity ischemia. This increases the susceptibility to tissue breakdown and assures slower wound healing. The reduced local vascularity may also decrease the cardinal signs of inflammation and may therefore mask serious underlying infections. In addition significant tissue levels of antibiotics are difficult to obtain in such ischemic areas.

Diabetic peripheral neuropathy results in decreased sensation and proprioceptive ability. Because of the absence of pain, injuries, ulceration, and necrosis may occur and often go unnoticed.

Atrophy of the interosseous muscles occurs and the subsequent muscle imbalance leads to cock-up digital deformities. This causes a retrograde buckling of the metatarsophalangeal joints and in turn produces a thinning and anterior displacement of the plantar fat pad. This type of foot is extremely susceptible to plantar ulceration and subsequent infection.

Osseous abnormalities may include multiple arthritic changes and Charcot joints. This malaligned and inflexible foot further enhances the risk of tissue damage and subsequent infection.

General Medical Evaluation

Because of the prevalance and severe lower extremity pathological conditions that occur in diabetes the podiatrist is often faced with the treatment of a severely infected ischemic foot. The decision of when to amputate and when to attempt limb salvage is one of the most difficult problems confronting those who treat the diabetic foot.

Amputation of the foot or leg that has the ability to heal is a pitifully common occurrence. On the other hand, attempting to salvage a "lost limb" may cause serious medical problems. Besides a higher level of amputation, prolonged futile treatment may cause sepsis, diabetic ketoacidosis, and even death. Patients must therefore be evaluated as to the status of their general health when salvage is attempted. Cardiac and renal problems may contribute to pedal edema. This will result in poor tissue perfusion making overall treatment difficult and delaying wound closure. Congestive heart failure causes anoxia to the local tissues and uremia may decrease leukocyte phagocytic ability (2). Uncontrolled hyperglycemia may make salvage impossible because of massive resistant infection and decreased oxygenization to the tissues. Diuretics may additionally increase the blood sugar levels. Elevated sedimentation rates, white blood cell counts, and temperature further signal an unfavorable prognosis.

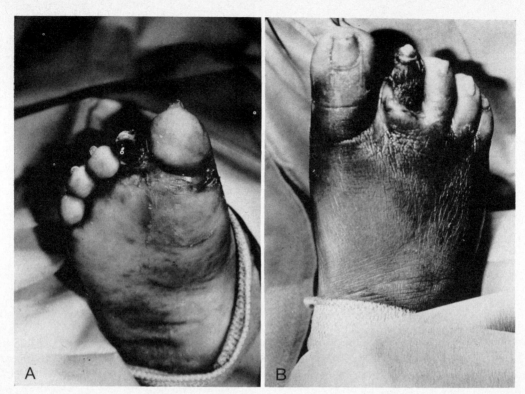

Figure 20.1. (A, B) 38-year-old female, severe diabetic with fissure in second web space. Treated with elevation. Progressed to closed space fascial plane infection. Note fullness of arch and gangrene of second and third toes. Patient had below knee amputation performed.

Despite this the presence of positive local clinical signs of inflammation may forecast the possibility of salvage. The clinical signs of inflammation are dependent on a good local blood supply. Therefore the presence of these signs indicates adequate underlying vascularity and thus healing potential. Furthermore it has been found that a decreased hemoglobin level is associated with a more favorable prognosis. Lower hemoglobin levels decrease blood viscosity and heighten tissue perfusion.

Consideration must also be given to the effects of the possible amputation. The fitting of an appropriate prosthesis is an important consideration. There will be a significant increased energy expenditure because of the amputation and the use of a prosthesis. Levin (3) states: "The energy cost of walking on two below-the-knee prostheses is about 41 percent higher than normal walking at a rate that is 21 percent slower". In addition there is a significant mortality rate caused by cardiovascular and renal complications after amputation. Fifty-six percent of those who survive a unilateral below-the-knee amputation will lose the other limb in three to five years (3).

Peripheral Vascular Evaluation

Noninvasive Testing

There are many ways of locally evaluating the probability of limb salvage in diabetics with severe pedal infections. Although this author does not feel that there is any substitute for thorough clinical evaluation, noninvasive vascular testing has become quite popular. This consists of Doppler ultrasound, plethysmography, and oscillometry.

Although much more specific and often essential, arteriography carries a far greater risk. According to Levin (3) the indications for its use as a preoperative diagnostic technique are (a) rest pain or night pain not caused by neuropathy, (b) ulcerations that are not healing despite vigorous treatment, and (c) incipient gangrene.

Doppler Ultrasound. Ultrasound allows a quantitative assessment of the severity of the arterial disease. The pressure is expressed as the ratio of ankle to brachial pressure and is known as the ischemic or pressure index. It is generally accepted that an ischemic index of greater than 0.45 is associated with the potential for successful wound healing in 93% of the cases. An index of less than 0.45 indicates the need for revascularization procedures when possible. False positive ankle pressures may be recorded when calcification and neuropathy are present (4, 5).

Plethysmography. Plethysmography records changes in the tissues with each heart beat. A toe systolic pressure of less than 20 mm Hg is found in greater than 70% of the patients with rest pain or ischemic ulcers. Toe pressures less than 20 mm Hg indicate that the chances of healing a lesion of the foot are less than 10% (4). Therefore, from the clinical point of view, the value of data from the digits and the ease with which the information is obtained makes digital plethysmography a useful procedure for the preoperative evaluation of the patient with arterial disease.

Oscillometry. Instruments for the detection of the pulse and for its measurement at various occluding pressures are known as oscillometers. They permit explorations of the artery through several levels and therefore can be very helpful in determining the proximal site of an occlusion. They permit indirect indices of the rate of local arterial inflow through the main arterial channels of the limb. In essence they provide more accurate measures of blood flow into an extremity than can be obtained by palpating pulses. The oscillometer is useful for following the course of arterial disease and the long term effects of therapy.

Local Evaluation

Once a decision has been made to salvage a limb the physician must carefully consider the management of the medical condition of the patient. This entails commitments to time, effort, and cost. It is extremely important to choose salvage patients properly and accurately. The bottom line in evaluation is an assessment of the vascular status and the potential for the patient to respond to therapy. For this there is absolutely no substitute for a thorough clinical evaluation.

History

Duration is an important factor in evaluating salvage probabilty. Although certainly the shorter period of time one has an infection the better, the length of time an infection has been present can be of diagnostic importance. Contrary to logic the longer an infection has been present, often the better the prognosis (6). A diabetic who overnight develops a gangrenous infected foot with little signs of inflammation generally has a very poor prognosis indeed. The rapid development of this type of clinical picture indicates a very virulent organism, an inability to fight infection, and/or serious vascular impairment. On the other hand, the diabetic with a long-standing infection with excellent clinical signs of inflammation usually has very good salvage possibilities. This is true because if the infection were severe or if the vascular status were poor, limb loss would have occurred earlier.

Besides the other general pertinent findings elicited on a history the length of time the diabetes has been present is very significant. Generally with long-standing diabetes there is greater avascularity, neuropathy, and overall peripheral tissue compromise. It should be remembered that because the blood glucose level is "under control" does not eliminate underlying pathological conditions. It should never be assumed that the controlled diabetic has the same healing potential as the normal patient. The pathological mechanisms of the disease place the patient at risk in any stressful situation and ample attention should be given to this special state.

Basic Lower Extremity Examination

Diabetics and other patients with peripheral vascular disease and ischemic infected feet should initially be evaluated in the manner similar to otherwise normal patients. Such a basic examination is completed before beginning a thorough evaluation of the local clinical signs of inflammation.

Dermatological examination is usually nonspecific. Decreased hair growth and atrophy of the skin generally occurs with age and are not specific for ischemia.

Orthopedic evaluation may reveal significant diabetic osteoarthropathy or Charcot joints that may influence the actual surgical repair but is not informative regarding salvage.

Generally neurological deficit indicates the chronicity of diabetes and may show involvement of the vaso nervorum. The patient with impaired pain perception, diminished reflexes, and footdrop is often the long standing diabetic who is unaware of a potentially dangerous pedal situation. It is helpful from the point of view of potential salvage to have a fairly intact neurological status.

Vascular examination is obviously a most important part of the evaluation. It is well known that the diabetic may have severe distal digital ischemic disease in the presence of good pulses. Therefore color changes in the digits, wound healing potentials, skin condition, and presence of paresthesias should be evaluated without regard to pulses. Despite this it is still better prognostically to have palpable pulses. Adequate collateral circulation as a result of the chronicity of the atherosclerotic process and demand permit enough blood flow for tissue nourishment. In this case pulses may be elicited in limbs with proximal occlusive disease. Generally blanching on elevation and rubor on dependency is impressive clinically but of little diagnostic value if the pulses are already known to be absent. In a patient without other overt signs of peripheral vascular insufficiency these manifestations are helpful in its diagnosis. These signs are usually more significant if they are unilateral (3). Diffuse plantar rubor and cyanosis may occur without ischemia and may be associated with many other abnormalities (7). The vascular status is best assessed by evaluation of the local clinical signs of inflammation.

Radiographic Evaluation

Destructive bone changes beneath an infected and/or gangrenous ulcer is a good prognostic sign and indicates good local vascularity (3). One such study was done by Meltzer and associates (8) in which they reviewed foot x-ray films of 32 diabetic patients with soft tissue necrosis. Seventeen of the patients with no radiographic evidence of osseous resorption were put into an ischemic limb category. Only three of these had palpable dorsalis pedis and posterior tibial pulses. All of these patients had soft tissue necrosis but no bony resorption. Yet all of them required major amputation within one week to three months. The other 15 patients were classified as non ischemic but had lesions with underlying bony resorption. Thirteen of these patients had pulses palpable above the ankle and none of these patients required a major amputation.

Clinical Evaluation

As mentioned earlier the best method of evaluating the salvagability of a limb is a detailed assessment of the clinical signs of local inflammation. Patients who have no underlying pathological conditions and develop an infection show all the clinical signs of inflammation: rubor, calor, dolor, and tumor. These signs are present in direct relation to the severity of the infection. They indicate good local vascularity and the ability to respond to the infective organisms. The absence of clinical signs thus indicates an inability of local body response and more specifically suggests absence of local vascularity. As one can well see, this has significant prognostic implications.

Rubor.   Localized rubor is a good indication of superficial vascularity. A more cyanotic hue may indicate impending gangrene and is obviously a poor prognostic sign.

Calor.   Calor (heat) is the single most important prognostic sign in evaluating an ischemic limb. It is the most specific indicator of local vascularity. Traditionally the temperature is assessed by placing the back of the examiner's hand on the involved foot and leg and with a gliding stroke determining any temperature change. A much more valuable determination can be made, however, by laying the palm of one's hand over the infected site and evaluating any heat transmission. Active penetrating heat indicates the fulminating stages of an infection in a patient with adequate circulation (6). Levin (3) adds that healing depends on the adequacy of the microcirculation to produce local hyperemic inflammatory response. More disseminating heat is seen with the subacute stages or a somewhat decreased vascular status. Coolness ac-

companying an infective process usually represents a gross lack of vascular response or infarction. This is especially true in diabetics because they respond to infection by thrombosis and necrosis (6). The author has specifically noted many instances in which there was heightened clinical signs with treatment and the regression of the infection.

Heat assessment is therefore the most important part of the examination and must be closely evaluated. If it is present it will actually "map out" the infected process in the foot and alert the examiner as to the extent and locale of the infection. If the infected foot is hotter than the opposing foot the prognosis is excellent for salvage. If it is the same temperature the prognosis is guarded. A cool, infected foot compared to the contralateral limb is a very poor prognostic sign indeed. Other authors share the opinion that heat is a valuable determinant of the potential for salvage. Bose (9) uses skin temperature gradients as a criterion for the site of amputation and accrues a wide range of acceptance. Siegel and associates (10) found that when the relative hyperemic index was greater than 1.5 all ulcerations healed, and with a lower index, 83% failed and required amputation. Williams and associates (11) predict success in cases of "necrosis in a hot foot" and predict failure in cases of "necrosis in cold feet." They further state that a warm foot is intermediate (Fig. 20.2A, B).

Tumor.   Closely observing the infected foot as compared to the contralateral limb may indicate more involvement than initially thought. Swelling of the digits and narrowing of the web spaces, loss of skin creases, obscurity of prominent tendons and veins, and alterations of foot contours are all indications of the processes of infection. Other than helping to in-

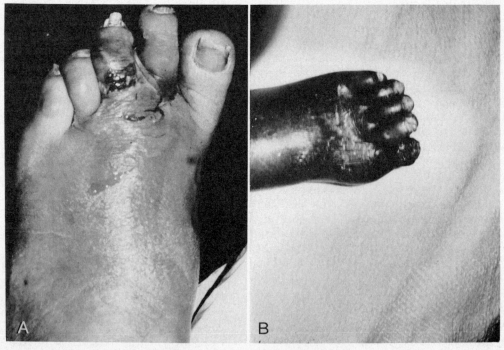

Figure 20.2.   (A) Red, swollen foot. (B) Pale, bluish foot.

dicate the extent of involvement edema does not have a positive or negative prognostic significance for salvage (6). Although edema will decrease tissue perfusion and may delay healing it is the author's opinion that the infected foot should never be elevated despite extensive documentation to the contrary. Elevation of even a superficial digital infection permits enough of a gravitational effect to drain the invasive organism deeper into the tissue planes of the foot. Infection spreading via the tendons of the dorsum of the foot can convert a minor problem into a major cellulitis.

Dolor. Although it will certainly facilitate treatment if pain is diminished or absent dolor will have a negative prognostic significance. The absence of pain usually indicates an under-nourished nerve supply or peripheral nerve damage caused by a malfunctioning vaso nervorum.

After individual assessment the clinical signs of inflammation and the history of duration must all be analyzed together. As mentioned previously, the presence of heightened clinical signs of inflammation present for a long period of time indicate a much better prognosis than the total absence of clinical signs in an ulcer or infected area that developed in a rather short period of time.

Although all of the aspects of the history and physical examination are important, limb salvage is most accurately and easily assessed by determining: (a) clinical signs of inflammation, (b) the duration of inflammation, and (c) underlying osteoporosis.

Treatment

The treatment of a diabetic's severely infected foot is one of the most difficult problems encountered in podiatric practice. It must be reiterated that patients should be thoroughly and carefully evaluated for the long and difficult treatment road towards salvage. Only if the local clinical signs of inflammation are favorable should this course of treatment be attempted. The goal of treatment is to eliminate the infection, permit healing, and establish a structurally sound foot capable of adequate function.

Eliminating infection is the initial priority. Although there is much debate regarding the increase of susceptibility to infection in diabetics there is general accord that once an infection of the foot or lower leg has become established it is generally more severe and refractory in the diabetic patient (3). However, if adequate vascularity is present and incision and drainage are properly established and maintained, infection should resolve despite the presence of diabetes.

The time required for healing will be significantly reduced if a good treatment plan is meticulously followed.

Despite the importance of some increased heat indicating good local vascularity significant increases in temperature cause an increased metabolic demand. Intact skin at 74° F needs 0.8 to 1 ml/100gm per minute of blood to stay viable. At 104° F 11/ml/100gm per minute is required. Resting muscle requires 3 ml/100 gm of tissue per minute and exercising muscle

requires 40 to 50 ml of blood per 100 gm of tissue per minute (12). Infection increases the demand even higher and at the same time increases the infarction and occlusion in the diabetic. If the increased demand cannot be met then tissue necrosis will ensue. Treatment must therefore increase blood supply and decrease tissue demand. Other than vascular surgical repair, treatment of the infection will increase circulation because the diabetic responds to infection by infarction and necrosis. Decreasing tissue inflammation is accomplished by proper incision and drainage and cool evaporating wet dressings.

The final goal of surgical treatment is maintaining a good structural foot capable of adequate ambulation. Whenever a bone is removed because of osteomyelitis or because of a structural deformity that is precipitating an ulceration, careful planning must be done to preserve as much function as possible. Skin loss over the tibia or lower fibula from an operation or chronic ulceration results in a lesion based on bone primarily the result of the lack of muscular covering over such a broad area of bone. This places these areas in a vulnerable situation that invites recurrent breakdown. While primary healing is desirable and is often obtained by applying a split-thickness graft to the area, a scar adherent to bone has a strong tendency to break down. Filling of the defect with transposed muscle is often most suitable in this circumstance (13).

Basic Treatment Principles

The basic treatment for infections of the foot is no different than treatment of infections elsewhere in the body. Additional special considerations, however, do exist in different anatomical areas.

The single most important aspect in treating any infection is primary wound care. Without proper local treatment including adequate incision and drainage, debridement of necrotic tissue, thorough cleansing, and periodic dressing changes, antibiotics may be ineffective. In addition the hyperkeratotic ring that forms especially around plantar ulcerations and infections should be debrided because it causes additional pressure on the wound and may further delay healing.

The more frequent a wound is cleansed, debrided, and basically attended to, the greater the chance of salvage. The author recommends four to five treatments daily when possible to decrease bacterial growth and to enhance healing. The advantages of repetitive wound care become very obvious to the attending physician who has inspected a wound after it has been cleansed three or four times before examination. This is in marked contrast to the appearance of the wound in the early morning hours after an entire night without any wound care.

For purulent infections this author uses 10% providone-iodine solution for cleaning. After this solution is flushed clear with sterile saline, an evaporating wet dressing of potassium permanganate is applied. According to Goodman and Gilman (14) most bacteria are killed within one hour by permangenates in a dilution of 1:10,000. Although some organisms are resistant to this dilution, concentrations above 1:10,000 are toxic to the tissues. Warm wet dressings are preferred because they are soothing and prevent further vasoconstriction that cold solutions can cause (6). It is also acceptable to use intermittent isotonic saline solution with Bacitracin, Polymixin B and Neomycin every one to two hours. It is wise to permit air drying between applications. Plain gauze is preferred to enhance drainage when necessary. Care must be taken to place these drains loosely so as to enhance drainage. Tightly packed drains actually act as a plug occluding the wounds and preventing drainage.

Gram stains, cultures, and sensitivity tests, both aerobic and anaerobic, with a mean inhibitory concentration evaluation, are all a necessary part of the treatment protocol. It must be emphasized that this is no replacement for extensive and consistent wound care (Fig. 20.3A–E). Generally 4 to 6 gm of a broad spectrum IV antibiotic (cephalosporin or another in combination with an aminoglycoside) are used initially. These must be carefully monitored for peak and trough levels to prevent renal and otic complications. Cultures must be taken periodically because new and different bacterial growth may occur.

Additional studies consisting of complete blood counts, serum glucose levels, renal function studies, and roentgenograms must also be done periodically. The latter may indicate osteomyelitis, pyogenic arthritis, or gas gangrene.

All of the treatment protocols instituted for lower extremity infections are basic accepted medical principles and apply to most infections elsewhere in the body. There is, however, one basic principle constantly recommended throughout the medical literature for foot infections that this author strongly feels is contraindicated: elevation.

The principle of resting an infected foot is sound. Walking, for example, with an infected foot will cause a muscular pumping action and may spread an infection (3). An infected foot that is constantly dependent becomes edematous decreasing tissue perfusion, increasing pain, and may delay wound closure. Elevation of an infected foot will certainly act to decrease swelling but will more importantly cause the spread of infection by "gravitational pull." Indeed some of the worst infections the author has seen are those that have been treated with bed rest and elevation.

Other medical specialists acknowledge the importance of gravitational drainage. For example, in the treatment of subarachnoid hemorrhage, pulmonary congestion, and liver injuries, patient positioning is extremely important (15–17). Postural drainage is therefore an effective way to enhance wound drainage.

The author feels that no infected foot should ever be elevated. Even without elevation of the limb a patient in the supine position in the hospital bed permits a distal foot infection to spread proximally. It is interesting and quite relevant here to note that Levin (3), throughout his book, mentions that eleva-

tion, among other things, does more to aid in the localization of an infection than does other steps. He adds that the "most important generalizations that relate to an already established infection or incipent gangrene are . . . elevation of the extremity." He further states that "antibiotics alone will fail unless rest and continuous elevation are also included." Levin therefore apparently believes strongly in elevation, as do many other authors. Despite this, he states that "further spread of a central plantar abscess may occur in the proximal part of the central plantar space particularly in bedridden patients because the pus may gravitate." It is exactly because of this point that the author recommends postural drainage as opposed to elevation. The patient is placed so that the apex of the infection is downward, allowing gravity to assist in draining the site (6). Patients with infection of the web spaces, for example, are placed in a prone position to facilitate drainage, whereas elevation of a supine leg in these individuals leads to the proximal spread of the infection through fascial planes (Fig. 20.1).

Special consideration must be given to particular infections in the diabetic or vascularly compromised patient. These categories include infections of the nail, dorsal foot infections, plantar ulcerations, puncture wounds, and web space infections. Bose (9) studied the different types of infections and found that in a study of 300 major foot infections in diabetics, abscesses in the deep spaces of the foot represented 80% of these infections, 8% were cellulitis of the dorsum of the foot, and plantar ulcerations represented 12%.

Nail Infections. Nail infections may occur because of excessive nail length facilitating stubbing, excessive subungual debris resulting in mycotic disease, or because of improper nail trimming. In addition excessive length may cause an infection of an adjacent toe or if the nail is extremely onychogryphotic the combination of excessive length and curvature can puncture the skin. These infections generally stay localized although they may spread dorsally via the lymphatics or may involve the extensor tendon sheath if digital necrosis occurs. Expedient and adequate nail avulsion is the cardinal treatment.

Dorsal Foot Infections. Dorsal infections like infections of the nails, rarely spread with the severity of those with plantar involvement. This is because of the deep plantar fibrosepta that extend from the dermis to the tendon sheath. These fibrous bands seldom permit distal dorsal infections to spread circumferentially around the digit. Such infections are perpetuated, however, by continued use of the foot by the diabetic with neuropathy. This may result in necrosis of the involved skin sections.

Plantar Ulcerations. Plantar ulcerations generally occur deep to chronic callous areas beneath prominent metatarsal heads. Mal perforans implies severe neuropathy in the presence of good blood flow (3). Because adequate blood supply is present these lesions often go through remissions and exacerbations for many years without serious sequelae. They become

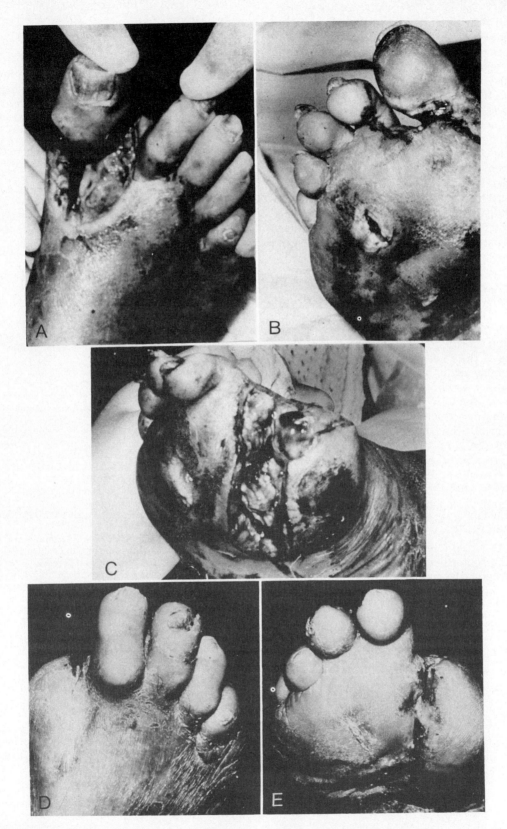

Figure 20.3. (A) Gangrenous hallux. Note pregangrenous dorsal and plantar foot, osteomyelitic first, second, and third metatarsals. Patient is 56-year-old insulin-dependent diabetic. (B) Same patient. Plantar view of infected ulceration. (C) Same patient 10 days after toe amputation. Note patchy gangrenous stump. (D) Same patient 53 days later showing complete limb salvage after aggressive local tissue treatment. No reconstructive vascular surgery was performed. Note skin color difference in (A) versus (D) (E) Same patient, plantar aspect.

serious surgical considerations when deep flexor tendons become involved or osteomyelitis develops. Conservative treatment or localized surgical treatment consisting of removal of the prominent metatarsal head often causes total resolution.

Puncture Wounds. Puncture wounds produce one of the most serious infections that occur in the foot. Often unnoticed until quite some time after the initial injury they may seem innocuous because of the lack of clinical signs of inflammation. A puncture wound may occur when a nail or other foreign object impregnates debris into the plantar space. An anaerobic closed space fascial plane infection may develop and may rapidly result in limb loss. Initially this seemingly innocuous wound should be opened to allow adequate cleaning, debridement, and aeration. Tetanus and antibiotic therapy should also be instituted.

Web Space Infections. Web space infections are by far the most serious of all pedal conditions affecting the diabetic. Without any previous anatomical deformity a fissure or minor break in the skin can result in entire limb loss. Levin (3) states: "infections beginning in the interdigital webs are especially dangerous because of the closeness of the digital arteries and because of the ready access to the deeper structures of the foot by way of the lumbrical tendons." He further suggests that "in the inexpansatile plantar space, infections can quickly obliterate the plantar metatarsal arterial arch and its branches to be followed by necrosis not only of the tissues in the central plantar space but also of the second, third, and fourth toes which receive most of their blood supply from the plantar arch" (Fig. 20.1). Treatment consists of extensive incision and drainage sometimes involving the entire length of the foot from the web space to the distal aspect of the heel pad. Postural drainage is critical with the patient instructed to lay prone (not supine with the foot elevated). Thick gauze may be placed distally between the toes to prevent interdigital occlusion and maceration. Adequate drainage is perhaps nowhere more important than in the web space infection.

CONCLUSION

It is the author's sincere belief that the most minor of foot infections should be treated with diligence as soon as they are noted. The author further believes that the diabetic should be regularly counseled as to the importance of the daily inspection of the feet. Beyond any doubt, teamwork involving the patient, the internist, and the podiatrist can do much to prevent the loss of diabetic limbs.

References

1. Bessman AN: Foot problems in the diabetic. *Compr Ther* 8:32–37, 1982.
2. Bagdade JD, Root RK, Bulger RJ: Impaired leukocyte function in patients with poorly controlled diabetes. *Diabetes* 23:9–15, 1974.
3. Levin ME, O'Neal LW: *The Diabetic Foot*, ed 3. St. Louis, The CV Mosby Co, 1983.
4. Farris I: *The Management of the Diabetic Foot*. London, Churchill-Livingstone, 1982.
5. Gibbons GW, Wheelock FC, Siembieda C, Hoar CS, Rowbotham JL, Persson AB: Noninvasive prediction of amputation level in diabetic patients. *Arch Surg* 114:1253–1257, 1979.
6. Pack LG, Lockson SS: Pedal infections in the vascularly compromised, evaluation and treatment. *J Am Podiatry Assoc* 71:24–26, 1981.
7. Pack LG: Burning feet. *Arch Podiatr Med Foot Surg* 2:1, 1974.
8. Meltzer AD, Skuersky N, Ostrum BJ: Radiographic evaluation of soft tissue necrosis in diabetes. *Radiology* 90:300, 1968.
9. Bose K: A surgical approach for the infected diabetic foot. *Int Orthop* 3:177, 1979.
10. Siegel ME, Stuart CA, Wagner W, Sakimura I: A new objective criteria for determining non invasively the healing potential of an ischemic foot. *J Nucl Med* 22:187, 1981.
11. Williams HG, Hutchinson KJ, Brown GD: Gangrene of the feet in diabetes. *Arch Surg* 108:609, 1974.
12. Lippman HI: Rehabilitation and treatment of the diabetic foot. *NY Sate J Med* 79:90, 1979.
13. Ger R: Surgical management of ulcerative lesions of the leg. *Curr Prob Surg* October:15, 1971.
14. Goodman LS, Gilman A: *The Pharmacological Basis of Therapeutics*, ed 4. London, MacMillan, 1983, p 1047.
15. Hayakawa T: Influence of head position on prognosis of experimental subarachnoid hemmorhage. *Neurology* 35:206, 1978.
16. Thacker EW: *Postural Drainage and Respiratory Control*, ed 3. London, Lloyd-Luke, 1971.
17. Schwartz SI: *Principles of Surgery*, ed 2. New York, McGraw-Hill, 1974, p 234.

CHAPTER 21

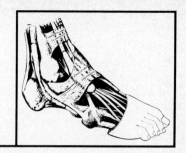

Reflex Sympathetic Dystrophy

John M. Buckholz, D.P.M.

The peripheral autonomic nervous system serves a protective purpose for the extremities by control of trophic mechanisms in response to stimuli received from the external environment. An interpretive overlay modifies this response via the individual's cognition. Occasionally a nonvolitional, abnormal, prolonged autonomic reflex is evoked in a limb in reaction to a traumatic episode. The result is a difficult, often intractable syndrome known as reflex sympathetic dystrophy. This condition is heralded by severe pain, swelling, color changes, temperature variation, and hyperhydrosis manifested distally in the limb. No definite statement can be made, however, on a specific set of symptoms. It seems that in this state the sympathetic system is completely disoriented and the symptoms are only limited in expression by the multitude of effects given to their functional range. Therefore any combination of symptoms may exist. The pattern may change in intensity with time or spontaneously resolve. In essence any statement made on reflex sympathetic dystrophy will apply to some cases but not all. Nevertheless pain dominates the clinical picture.

TERMS

In 1945 DeTakats (1) called for a redefinition of causalgia so that a poorly defined group of causalgic states could be recognized by a greater number of clinicians. The classical causalgia described by Mitchell and associates (2) during the American Civil War was then well known. However, the subtle forms of vasomotor disturbances were being identified under such various titles as minor causalgia, mimo-causalgia, posttraumatic dystrophy, reflex dystrophy, shoulder-hand syndrome, Sudeck's atrophy, Sudeck's osteodystrophy, and posttraumatic osteoporosis. To a large extent the term "reflex sympathetic dystrophy" has satisfied DeTakats's plea by encompassing all of these titles within one concept. Most terms describe a special form of reflex sympathetic dystrophy and cannot be used interchangeably. For example, Sudeck's atrophy is a specific osteolysis, pathognomonic for the second stage of reflex sympathetic dystrophy. Causalgia is a severe form of reflex sympathetic dystrophy represented by burning pain commonly produced by traumatic injury to the nerve trunk.

ETIOLOGY

The pathogenesis of reflex sympathetic dystrophy remains theoretical; however, the initiating factor triggering the clinical response is consistently trauma. This trauma should be interpreted in a general sense. Typical violent injuries of war and industry are obvious causes for initiating reflex sympathetic dystrophy. For the civilian surgeon the traumatic factor is more likely to be irritative in nature and often not so obvious. A listing of all the reported sources initiating reflex sympathetic dystrophy would be unreasonable, but does include such a diverse grouping as ankle sprains, pes valgo planus, neuroma, plantar wart, injections, minor surgical procedures, tourniquet use, thromboses, vasculitis, osteoarthritis, infection, or poliomyelitis.

The severity of injury has little correlation to the severity of symptoms. There does seem to be some correlation to the type of injury, with nerve avulsion or traction more likely to produce experimental reflex sympathetic dystrophy. Nerve contusion is also more likely to produce altered vasomotor response than is a clean severence of a nerve. The greater length of the nerve influences the intensity of reaction to injury, the sciatic and median nerves being more likely to produce a causalgic syndrome (3). A few reports note an emotional diathesis for reflex sympathetic dystrophy. These may be unfair statements for the sufferer of great pain with few objective facts to justify the complaint. Patients become emotionally distraught when a disbelieving family and physicians impose an erroneous diagnosis of psychoneurosis, hysteria, or malingering.

SYMPTOMS

The cruel feature of reflex sympathic dystrophy is pain. The surgeon should appreciate this reality of the patient's experience. Often two types of pain exist together. One (type I) is a deep pain described as tearing, ripping, crushing, stabbing, or bursting. The second pain (type II) occurs on the skin as an exaggerated sensitivity with an extreme tenderness or burning. The deep pain is invariably constant but typically modulates through the course of one or several days often becoming worse at night. Some relief is achieved superficially for type II pain by moist pack application whereas immobilization may provide some relief for either deep or superficial pain.

Both external and emotional stimuli aggravate the pain. When severe pain is already experienced this additive effect provokes the patient to withdraw from possible sensory stimuli, including noises, visual experiences, or even a slight wisp of air across the affected limb. This withdrawal conduct is frequently misinterpreted as a personality change. Response to temperature treatments will vary according to the status of the vascular tone. When vasodilation is present, as is commonly the case, heat will often aggravate the pain. During vasospasm heat lessens the pain. In addition to pain various sensory changes may be experienced such as local or radiating tingling, numbness, or the sensation of bleeding.

Clinical observation of patients with reflex sympathetic dystrophy has established at least three phases of development. The author would include an additional phase that is seen before the classically described first phase. Knowledge of these phases is essential to the surgeon determining the appropriate course to follow for reversing the neurogenic crisis and also evaluating the effectiveness of treatment.

From the author's experience in dealing with cases involving minor ankle sprains, the first response is phase IA, a vasoconstriction with an obvious decrease in the temperature of the affected foot. This symptom borders on coldness. Hyperalgesia is always present and paresthesias may already be present. The skin is typically mottled by patches of pallor on a pinkish-blue background. The nail beds are mild to moderately cyanotic and swelling exceeds the extent justified by the amount of ecchymosis or soft tissue injury. Phase IA exists for a relatively short period of two to six weeks, when the classically described initial phase (phase IB) sets in with the onset of vasodilation, increased warmth to the affected foot, hyperhydrosis, and a change in color of the skin to red.

The swelling in phase IB is softer, more doughy, and slightly reduced. Superficial veins may be dilated and distended in comparison to the opposite foot, especially during dependency. Spontaneous spasms of the foot and leg muscles may occur. Hyperalgesia continues and the patient is now realizing the special circumstances of his or her case, having experienced no improvement in some weeks since the injury. Treatment attempts with ultrasound agitate the pain whereas heat therapy and a whirlpool aggravate the pain. Immobilization of the affected foot may prove to be somewhat effective. During this early phase there is the greatest likelihood of remission. This phase lasts

approximately two to six months. If remission has not occurred phase II develops with its hallmark of Sudeck's osteoporosis seen on x-ray films. Typically the distribution of osteolysis is "spotty." Less often the vascular cages of the metaphyses are affected producing a polar distribution. Sudeck's atrophy is not initiated by disuse as is advanced in some writings. Rather hyperemia, decreased pH, and possibly increased intramedullary bone pressure (IMP) produce osteolysis.

A peculiar fibromatosis may be seen in the plantar fascia or at the aponeurotic insertions of the extrinsic tendons (4). The skin is taut and glossy and the swelling becomes brawny. Pain persists and the patient very often becomes dependent on narcotic analgesics. There is less likelihood of reversing the condition at this phase.

In approximately 6 to 12 months the final phase prevails, and the clinical picture is grim. The foot appears withered, pale, and waxlike. Vasoconstriction has taken over. Stiffness of the joints is marked and Sudeck's atrophy has advanced beyond the spotty appearance to a radiographic ghostlike appearance throughout the entire foot skeleton. The skin is dry. Contrary to the belief that all cases of reflex sympathetic dystrophy spontaneously resolve, the condition can be permanent. The patient in later stages may require institutional care or even attempt suicide after months of agony.

Reflex sympathetic dystrophy affects pediatric patients more often than clinicians realize. There is some evidence that this age group does not manifest the trophic changes of adults in second and third phase reflex sympathetic dystrophy. This should not be misconstrued to mean that children suffer less than adults (5, 6).

DIAGNOSIS

Early diagnosis is essential to the reversal of reflex sympathetic dystrophy and prevention of permanent disability. When the symptoms of the condition present, especially disproportionate pain, hyperesthesia, swelling, discoloration, temperature change, and hyperhydrosis, then a precise paravertebral block of the sympathetic chain should be performed by an experienced clinician, usually an anesthesiologist. Acquiring a vasomotor flush without loss of somatic sensation and relief of pain confirms the diagnosis with one exception. In long-standing cases, after prolonged major sensory inflow from the limb, central effects may develop above the peripheral level, in which case temporary or permanent sympathectomy will fail to relieve pain. Sunderland (3) reports one case where excision of the sensory cortex and chordotomy failed to relieve the pain of sympathetic reflex dystrophy following spinal injury.

When the possibility of malingering or psychoneurosis is in question a sham block can be performed with sterile saline (7, 8). The patient reporting the block's effectiveness may confirm the suspicion.

Other diagnostic methods have been endorsed by various authors; however, these procedures should be viewed as supportive rather than providing proof of reflex sympathetic dystrophy. Included in these tests would be the histamine flare test, the digital skin wrinkling test, plethysmographic blood flow studies of deep muscles, nerve conduction studies, intramedullary bone pressure, x-ray tests, bone scanning, and skin potential responses (9–17). Early sympathetic blockade is of utmost importance in diagnosing reflex sympathetic dystrophy and to proceeding with appropriate treatment modes (7, 8). Recently infrared thermography has been introduced as an alternative diagnostic procedure to paravertebral block. Early indications hold promise for the use of this noninvasive technique (18–20).

DIFFERENTIAL DIAGNOSIS

A diagnostic pitfall to reflex sympathetic dystrophy is tarsal tunnel syndrome. This has not been previously reported in the literature and from the author's experience warrants attention. Apparently, during the second phase the prolonged effects of reflex sympathetic dystrophy will affect the vaso nervorum in the distal nerve trunks to the level of the reflex's abnormal influence, which is often at the ankle. The result is a delayed conduction velocity of the motor nerves, which begins abruptly at the tarsal tunnel and is consistent with the impression of a mechanical compression of the nerve. The neurologist is easily led to believe that the diagnosis is tarsal tunnel syndrome and will probably recommend surgical decompression. An accurate sympathetic block should be accomplished first to avoid unnecessary surgery when clinical symptoms of reflex sympathetic dystrophy are also present. It is also possible that the influence of the sympathetic reflex on the vaso nervorum plays a role in the development of the clinical phases or symptoms.

Other differential diagnoses include those conditions that produce severe pain conditions such as diabetic sensory neuropathy, meralgia paresthetica, ischemic neuropathy, Fabry's disease, myeloma neuropathy, and an exhaustive listing of nearly all neuropathies. Once again sympathetic block is critical to differentiating reflex sympathetic dystrophy from the neuropathic diseases.

TREATMENT

The rebellious nature of reflex sympathetic dystrophy requires a planned treatment directed at the level of pain origin. The initial task is to define the site from which the reflex eminates. Rarely, this might be as simple as a discovery of a focal nerve lesion such as a neuroma, a thrombus, or fascial trigger point. However, the pain source usually stems from the abnormal autonomic reflex long after the initiating factor is gone. Through attempts to explain the pain mechanism authors have offered differing opinions as to which is the level of the neuron at which the reflex begins (1, 3). These neurons are referred to from distal to proximal, as first, second, and third order or postganglionic, preganglionic, and central. Practically, the treatment should depend on whether interruption of the peripheral sympathetic system relieves the pain. If a sympathetic block does not relieve the pain, the reflex can be assumed to be centralized (neurons of the third order) and efforts to treat the condition peripherally will fail (21). This includes treatment by sympathectomy.

Sunderland (3) advises that the reflex can initiate centrally, however, long-term persistence is the usual factor allowing the development of a centrally established reflex. For this reason the earlier the condition is recognized and properly managed the greater the likelihood of a successful resolution to the problem. The sympathetic block is paramount not only to diagnosis but also for determining where the treatment effort is to be directed (22). Thus two categories of treatment methods evolve: peripheral and central.

Probably the simplest treatment for the peripheral reflex is injection of a local anesthetic into trigger points of pain. Serial injections are performed at intervals of three to seven days and can periodically include low doses of steroids. Serial somatic nerve blocks of the limb have been favored by podiatric surgeons as a treatment of choice for years. Omer (7) reports employing continuous nerve blocks by leaving a Vacucath (an indwelling catheter) in situ and reinjecting perineurally when anesthesia begins to dissipate. The block is continued over a several day span under inpatient observation.

Transcutaneous nerve stimulation has more recently been used and probably has its maximum effectiveness as a continuous "block" of a trigger point (23, 24). Perfusion of the affected vascular tree with catecholamine competitors or vasodilators has been advanced as an alternative treatment to peripheral blocks. Two methods of perfusion are reported; direct intra-arterial injection and venipuncture in conjunction with a double cuff perfusion procedure commonly employed for regional anesthesia (25, 26). The intent of using vasodilators such as tolazoline or phenoxybenzamine hydrochloride is to decrease sympathetic activity. Competitors of norepinephrine such as reserpine, guanethidine, or methyl dopa have been used by both vascular routes with apparent success: however, this treatment mode is presently considered observational. For consistent results and the preservation of time the sympathetic block remains the most advantageous form of treatment (27–32). Omer (7) states there are five possible responses to sympathetic blockade: (a) total relief, (b) reduction of pain to tolerance, (c) progressive relief by multiple blocks, (d) diminishing periods of relief by multiple blocks, and (e) relief only during the effective period of the local anesthetic. Although the prognosis for permanent relief of pain by the last two responses is decreased, all five responses can be considered beneficial toward relief of the condition because surgical sympathectomy could be effective in either circumstance of response (d) or (e).

A treatment regimen by Willenegger was effective in reversing a case of 20 years' duration (H. Willenegger, unpublished observations). This treatment consists of a combination of inpatient control, elevation of the affected limb, diuretics, tranquilizers, corticosteroids, and sympathetic blocks. Specifically, prednisolone is given by the descending dosage of 100 to 150 mg the first and second days, 50 mg the third and fourth days, 45 mg the fifth and sixth days, and 40 mg the seventh and eighth days. The dose is lowered by 5 mg every two days thereafter until the 10 mg level is reached. The patient is permitted bathroom privileges with supportive stocking or elastic bandage. Furosemide, lumbar blocks, and tranquilizers are given daily (H. Willenegger, lecture notes and personal communication, 1981).

Surgical sympathectomy may seem an aggressive form of treatment until the alternative consequence of permanent pain and disability is recognized (34–37). In selected cases sensory neurectomy can achieve relief when the focus of pain is highly localized and unrelieved by repeated local blocks. When a known lesion acts as the provoking source for the stimulus of the reflex a direct surgical procedure can be considered, as in the case of a neural tumor.

Supportive measures that can augment the primary treatment or soothe the patient's pain include physical therapy, antiinflammatory drugs, vasodilators, analgesics, strapping, Unna's boot, moist packs, battery-heated socks, and massage. These ancillary procedures should not be employed as primary treatment modes because they generally fail to reverse the condition and waste precious time needed to "catch" the reflex peripherally. An interesting approach employed in European clinics has been the use of calcitonin therapy. Reports of significant improvement during the first phase of reflex sympathetic dystrophy are encouraging (39–41). Glucocorticoid therapy has been endorsed by the rheumatology community (42, 43).

Treatment for those cases where the reflex has centralized presents the most difficult of clinical circumstances. Often the treatment is extreme and even then can fail. Such radical procedures as chordotomy, lobotomy, local excision of sensory cortex, and midbrain sectioning have been reported with failure to relieve the pain (3, 44). These patients deserve to be placed in the care of a pain clinic before any operations have been performed. It is possible in some cases for a pain clinic to control the patient's agony with drug therapy, counseling, and biofeedback. Ideally, there can be a broader recognition during the early symptoms of reflex sympathetic dystrophy by surgeons and clinicians so that these progressive cases with centrally acting reflexes can be less likely to occur or even avoided.

SUMMARY

When a patient complains of severe pain in the distal extremity, which does not coincide with the history or objective finding other than a comparative unilateral color, temperature, perspiration, or swelling change, then reflex sympathetic dystrophy should be highly suspected. Sympathetic blockade should be performed as soon as possible to confirm the diagnosis, in addition to its value in initiating a therapeutical course.

Reflex sympathetic dystrophy is unpredictable. The course can become progressively worse by a series of phases each more resistant to treatment than the preceding phase. Intractable pain and atrophy can result in permanent disability if the abnormal reflex sensitizes central neurons to become the origin for perpetuating the symptoms. For this reason an appropriate course of management includes early diagnosis and treatment by interruption of the dysreflexic peripheral sympathetic system.

References

1. DeTakats G: Causalgic states in peace and war. JAMA 128:699, 1945.
2. Mitchell S, Morehouse CR, Keen W: Gunshot Wounds and Other Injuries of Nerves. Philadelphia, JB Lippincott Co, 1864.
3. Sunderland S: Pain mechanisms in causalgia. J Neurol Neurosurg Psych 39:471, 1976.
4. Lankford L, Thompson J: Reflex sympathetic dystrophy, upper and lower extremity: diagnosis and management. AAOS Instructional Course Lectures 26:163, 1977.
5. Bernstein B, Singsen B, Kent J, Kornreich H, King K, Hicks R, Hanson V: Reflex neurovascular dystrophy in childhood. J Pediatr 93:211, 1978.
6. Ruggeri S, Athereya B, Doughty R, Gregg J, Das M: Reflex sympathetic dystrophy in children. Clin Orthop 163:225, 1982.
7. Omer GE: Management of the painful extremity. Curr Pract Orthop Surg 8:86, 1979.
8. Ghia J, Duncan G, Scott D, Gregg J: Therapeutic nerve blocks for chronic pain. AFP 20:74, 1979.
9. DeTakats G: Causalgic states and neurotrophic lesions of the extremities. AAOS Reconstructive Surgery Extremity Instruction Section 112, 1944.
10. Braham J, Sadeh M, Sarova-Pinhas I: Skin wrinkling on immersion of hands. A test of sympathetic function. Arch Neurol 36:113, 1979.
11. Sylvest J, Jensen EM, Siggaard-Anderson J, Pedersen L: Reflex dystrophy. Resting blood flow and muscle temperature as diagnostic criteria. Scand J Rehabil Med 9:25, 1977.
12. Ficat RP, Arlet J: Ischemia and Necrosis of Bone. Baltimore, Williams & Wilkins, 1980.
13. Kozin F, Genant H, Bekerman C, McCarty D: The reflex sympathetic syndrome. II. Roentgenographic and scintigraphic evidence of bilaterality and of periarticular accentuation. Am J Med 60:322, 1976.
14. Carlson D, Simon H, Wegner W: Bone scanning and diagnosis of sympathetic dystrophy secondary to herniated lumbar discs. Neurol 27:791, 1977.
15. Kozin F, Soin J, Ryan L, Carrera G, Wortmann R: Bone scintigraphy in the reflex sympathetic dystrophy syndrome. Radiology 138:437, 1981.
16. Holder L, Mackinnon S: Reflex sympathetic dystrophy in the hands: clinical and scintigraphic criteria. Radiology 152:517, 1984.
17. Cronin K, Kirsner R: Diagnosis of reflex sympathetic dysfunction. Use of skin potential response. Anaesthesia 37:848, 1982.
18. Uematsu S, Hendler N, Hungerford D, Long D, Ono N: Thermography and electromyography in the differential diagnosis of chronic pain syndromes and reflex sympathetic dystrophy. Electromyogr Clin Neurophysiol 21:165, 1981.
19. Uematsu S: Telethermography in the differential diagnosis of reflex sympathetic dystrophy and chronic pain syndrome. In Pain Therapy. Elsevier Biomedical Press, 1983, p 63.

20. Hendler N, Uematesu S, Long D: Thermographic validation of physical complaints in "psychogenic pain" patients. *Psychosomatics* 23:283, 1982.
21. Buckholz J: Current concepts for the diagnosis and management of Sudeck's dystrophy. *Strides* 22:4, 1985.
22. Erdemir H, Gelman S, Galbraith J: Prediction of the needed level of sympathectomy for posttraumatic reflex sympathetic dystrophy. *Surg Neurol* 17:353–354, 1982.
23. Stilz R, Carron H, Sarcers D: Case history no. 96. Reflex sympathetic dystrophy in a 6 year old, successful treatment by transcutaneous nerve stimulation. *Anesthesia Analgesia Curr Res* 56:438, 1977.
24. Leo K: Use of electrical stimulation of acupuncture points for the treatment of reflex sympathetic dystrophy in a child. *Phys Ther* 63:957, 1983.
25. Hannington-Kiff JG: Relief of Sudeck's atrophy by regional intravenous guanethidine. *Lancet* 1:1132, 1977.
26. McKay N, Woodhouse N, Clarke A: Post-traumatic reflex sympathetic dystrophy syndrome (Sudeck's atrophy): effects of regional guanethidine infusion and salmon calcitonin. *Br Med J* 1:155, 1977.
27. Bonica JJ: Causalgia and other reflex sympathetic dystrophies. *Postgrad Med* 53:143, 1973.
28. Leipzig T, Mullan S: Causalgic pain relieved by prolonged procaine amide sympathetic blockade. *J Neurosurg* 60:1095, 1984.
29. Thompson JE: The diagnosis and management of post-traumatic pain syndromes (causalgia). *Aust NZ J Surg* 49:299–304, 1979.
30. Klaer S: Remarks on the prognosis of the post-traumatic dystrophy of the extremities. *Acta Orthop Scand* 17:3–4, 1947.
31. Rickles J: Ambulatory use of sympathetic nerve blocks: present day clinical indications. *Angiology* 28:394, 1977.
32. Menke HE: Reflex sympathetic dystrophy. *Dermatologica* 147:186, 1973.
33. Pak TJ, Marten G, Magness J, Kavanaugh G: Reflex sympathetic dystrophy. Review of 140 cases. *Minn Med* 53:507, 1970.
34. Barnes R: The role of sympathectomy in the treatment of causalgia. *J Bone Joint Surg* 35B:172, 1953.
35. Evans JA: Reflex sympathetic dystrophy: report on 57 cases. *Ann Intern Med* 26:417, 1947.
36. Mayfield F: Causalgia. *Postgrad Med* 32:436, 1952.
37. Homans J: Minor causalgia: a hyperesthetic neurovascular syndrome. *N Engl J Med* 222:870, 1940.
38. Johnson JB: Post traumatic sympathetic dystrophy: a brief review and a new aid to its treatment. *J Am Podiatry Assoc* 67:870, 1977.
39. Kissing W: Calcitonin in der therapie des Sudeck's syndrons. *Therapiewoche* 29:4774, 1979.
40. Breitenfelder J: Zur therapie des Sudeck syndroms. *Therapiewoche* 29:6578, 1979.
41. Krause W: Die algodystrophie (morbus Sudeck). *Therapiewoche* 30:5919, 1980.
42. Kozin F, McCarty D, Sims J, Genant H: The reflex sympathetic dystrophy syndrome. I. Clinical and histological studies: evidence for bilaterality, response to corticosteroids and articular involvement. *Am J Med* 60:321, 1976.
43. Glick E: Reflex dystrophy (algoneurodystrophy): results of treatment by corticosteroids. *Rheumatol Rehabil* 12:84, 1973.
44. Jaeger R: Causalgia: its etiology and treatment in traumatic conditions of the peripheral nerves and spinal cord. *Pen Med J* 60:977, 1957.

CHAPTER 22

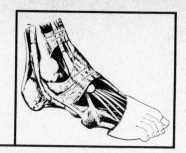

Prostheses Following Lower Extremity Amputations

Richard P. Reinherz, D.P.M. and **Howard R. Reinherz, D.P.M.**

Limb amputations have been performed for centuries. Historically these resulted from rampant diseases (ergotism and leprosy), the effects of war, or gruesome judicial punishments (1). Original prostheses were crudely manufactured and served to replace useless parts, reduce invalidism, or save life. As societies developed peripheral vascular disease became recognized as a primary cause of extremity amputation. Improved techniques in determining the actual level of disease led to more distal amputations (2). Hence greater attention was directed to cosmetic appearance and improved function as opposed to merely replacement.

The literature indicates that Aristophanes, as early as 500 BC, hired an actor with an artificial leg. Hegistratus, during the same era, escaped from prison by cutting off his chained foot and later designed a wooden replacement. Through the Middle Ages battle scars were considered indications of inferiority among warriors. Unless an appropriate alternative could be constructed, metal armor had to be altered to conceal the lost limb (1).

Ambrose Pare is credited for his foresight in identifying the fundamental principles in lower extremity prosthetic design. During the sixteenth century he described the essentials of fixed equinus, knee locks, adjustable sockets, and controls needed for lower limb function. This led to a variety of appliances being developed that continued through the nineteenth century. Prosthetic feet were then constructed from catgut cord and later solid rubber. Brigg in 1885 emphasized the importance of biomechanical alignment of artificial limbs with their body counterparts. He especially referenced the knee joint axis. By the end of that century a pneumatic rubber foot was developed that could overcome abrupt jerking movements (1).

During the twentieth century artificial limb architecture continued to improve. Surgeons recognized that certain operative characteristics predisposed to a better prosthetic fit. The appearance and integrity of a stump are critical. It should be conical, and in the past was covered solely with fascia and skin. Today some muscle tissue is sutured over the distal, rounded bones to provide total contact in the socket of the prosthesis. The incision should be placed transversely rather than vertically. The surgical scar should be freely mobile from underlying tissues and every attempt made to minimize adhesions.

Certain perioperative considerations are also important. Emotional factors can affect successful prosthetic use. Children especially are susceptible to curious gazes or thoughtless comments. Family and professional support are needed. An appliance is best dispensed early in life, or soon after an amputation, to maximize its therapeutic value.

MATERIALS

Various materials are used in constructing artificial limbs. Durability, ease of adjustment, moisture resistance, and weight are the factors that determine product usage. Willow, or balsa wood, is one of the oldest and best known materials. Steel was used for frames but subsequently has been replaced by aluminum. Thermoplastics, recently developed, offer lightweight materials that conform well to many anatomical surfaces and are moisture resistant.

Vulcanized rubber contributes to prosthetic design by its shock-absorbing qualities. Urethanes, or synthetic rubbers, possess a high tensile strength, are inert, resist abrasion, and adhere well to several surfaces. They absorb force by stretching yet return to their original configuration(3).

Leather is common for straps, belts, and sometimes laced cuffs. It is easily managed and may be included as internal lining. However, the material can become hot, heavy, and difficult to clean following perspiration stains. Velcro is a modern material used as a fastener and replaces buckles on some applications.

Methylmethacrylate is a plastic used in dentistry and in podiatry and orthopedics as an internal bone cement. It promotes attachment of prosthetic sockets or replacement of suction valves. This material seals cracks, smooths rough surfaces, and reinforces areas as necessary (4).

Artificial skin cover for prosthetic limbs was introduced in 1974. Lower limb appliances are now available in Caucasian or Negroid colors. The skin is rolled on and secured with glue. This protective covering is applied over a 1/16 inch to 1/8 inch soft foam padding (5).

PROSTHETIC DESIGN

Prostheses may be static or dynamic. Those devices that passively replace a lost part are static. One that is capable of actively expelling energy or determining sensations through electrodes attached to the body is dynamic. Whether static or dynamic the connection between an amputee and the artificial part is important.

The socket of a prosthesis transfers the weight bearing loads to the ground through the distal portion of the prosthesis, transmits power from the body to the artificial device for control, and provides a suspension to the prosthesis when it is not in contact with the ground (6). These connections are known as sockets and appear as cuplike receptacles that enclose the amputated stump. They are often secured proximally by straps, bands, or suction.

No efficient method to measure pressures between a socket and its stump is available. Neither can one predetermine the effect of additional pressure during active movement on the socket. Thermoplastics are available to serve as transparent sockets and afford the advantages of increased strength, less weight, and more flexibility than other materials.

The foundation of all lower limb prostheses is the foot. Most common among pedal connections is the solid ankle cushioned heel (SACH) (Fig. 22.1). The bulk of the foot is constructed from wood or rubber. Varying densities of rubber or polyurethane are laminated into the SACH heel to provide different compressibilities. As the limb is loaded following heel strike the foot passively plantarflexes approximately 15°. During this gait phase shock absorption is nec-

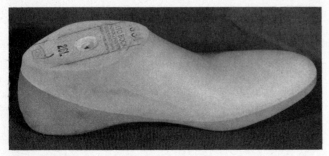

Figure 22.1. SACH foot. Note aperture in dorsal surface where bolt is used to connect ankle portion. Various densities of foam or rubber may be applied in heel to gauge shock absorption.

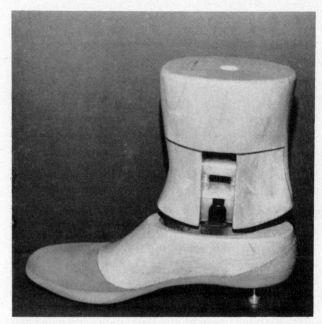

Figure 22.2. The Greissinger Multi-Axis foot, developed in Germany. (Courtesy of Paul Leimkuehler, PEL Supply Company, Cleveland, Ohio.)

essary. Weist and associates (7) examined the effects of various heel designs on rigid ankle-foot orthoses. They investigated four heel modifications in an attempt to determine the most effective shock absorption at heel strike. The SACH heel impaired knee movement the least while still providing very good absorption properties.

Prosthetic feet are constructed in an attempt to duplicate human biomechanics (8). During the early stance phase of gait the leg and foot internally rotate. The leg externally rotates and the foot becomes fixed with respect to the ground later in the stance phase. Extension of the toes creates tension on the plantar fascia allowing the foot to convert into a semirigid lever (the windlass mechanism). This principle is important for dynamic prosthetic design.

The Greissinger Multi-Axis foot and ankle joint come closest to human foot and ankle movements. A universal type of ankle joint and a doughnut-shaped rocker rubber mounted between the foot and ankle block provide good plantarflexion, some dorsiflexion, and lateral, medial, and rotational movements (9) (Fig. 22.2).

The stationary attachment, flexible endoskeleton (SAFE) foot is secured by means of a bolt block to the lower leg. The appliance is constructed entirely of plastic and weighs less than certain foot types although it is heavier than the SACH foot. The design incorporates dome-shaped arches of polyurethane and a flexible keel. The appliance has no mechanical joints (10). A long band attached to the keel tightens during gait and promotes toe-off.

Greater sophistication in prosthetic foot design has been mandated by an increasing popularity of aerobic sports. Burgess and associates (11) reported

61% of 134 limb amputees participated in athletics but only a few wore specifically designed recreational prostheses. The need for an efficient, dynamic appliance thus became evident. This resulted in the development of the Seattle Foot. The appliance stores energy through compression as weight is borne. A series of fiberglass leaf-springs, with a rubber deflection bumper, initiate activity of the triceps surae allowing for both energy storage and release. A cable limits the degree of limb extension.

Amputations through the foot have traditionally been frowned on. This is based on a fear of potential equinus deformity from proximal muscle imbalances and the difficulty in achieving an adequate socket fit (12). Prostheses formerly were bulky with metallic foot plate, toe fillers, and laced leather ankle cuffs. The advantages related to a more distal weight-bearing surface, additional proprioception, and a longer lever arm eventually prevailed.

When a partial foot amputation is performed, one must insure that dynamic function and intrinsic stability within shoegear are both maintained. Engelmeier (13) recently described a technique for the replacement of a lesser digit using dental stone and molten wax. The result was a silicone prosthesis covered with kaolin and tinted by oil paints. Following resection of multiple digits, a toe filler attached to a shoe insert may be all that is needed (Fig. 22.3). A plaster cast is taken of the part. A shoe should also be forwarded to the prosthetist for adequate fit. Any areas of plantar pressure must be identified so as to be accommodated with the appliance (Fig. 22.4). The insole portion may consist of leather or plastazote (Fig. 22.5). The toe filler must be soft enough to avoid irritation and may consist of cork with leather cover-

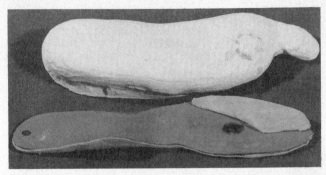

Figure 22.4. Insert with toe filler for lesser digits. Plantar accomodation for second metatarsal lesion is noted.

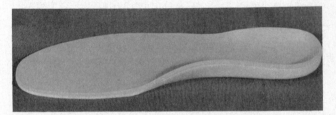

Figure 22.5. Plastozote material used for insoles.

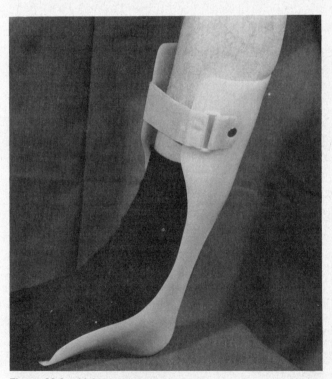

Figure 22.6. Molded plastic insert to protect against equinus deformities.

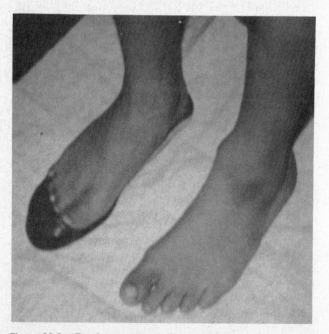

Figure 22.3. Forefoot prosthesis. This case demonstrates child with congenital absence of distal digits of his right foot. Prosthesis was designed because short right foot created functional limb length anomaly and therefore severe intoeing unilaterally.

ing, rubber, or polyurethane foam. When the hallux has been amputated, active propulsion is limited, so a long steel spring should be inserted within the sole of the shoe to assist in push-off.

Amputations proximal to the metatarsal bases usually result in dorsiflexion and plantarflexion muscle imbalances, especially during ambulation (14). A molded plastic lower leg insert (Fig. 22.6) with special shoe (Fig. 22.7), or with toe filler and steel spring (Fig. 22.8), will increase stability by avoiding equinus. A plastic laminated prosthesis for Chopart's amputations, known as the "clamshell," is commonly used (14). For greater stability a double bar aluminum ankle-foot orthosis (AFO) may be ordered (15) (Fig. 22.9). This is also beneficial when swelling or skin irritation precludes use of the thermoplastic device.

Total foot amputation requires the Symes pros-

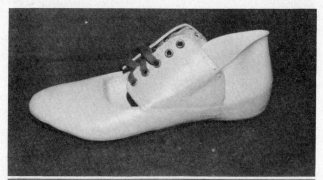

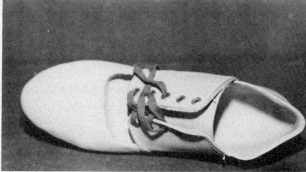

Figure 22.7. Special prosthetic shoe for Chopart's amputee. (Top) Side view. (Bottom) Front view. (Courtesy of Paul Leimkuehler, PEL Supply Company, Cleveland, Ohio)

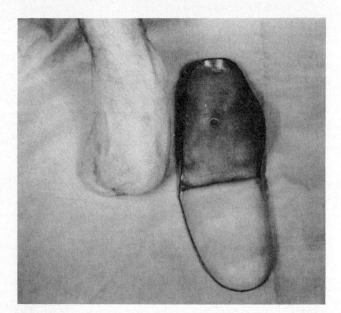

Figure 22.8. Partial foot amputee with accomodative insert prosthesis. The rivet indicates that steel spring is incorporated within leather sole.

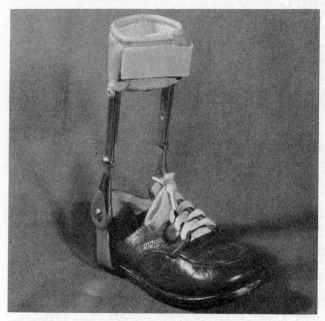

Figure 22.9. Double bar aluminum ankle-foot orthosis.

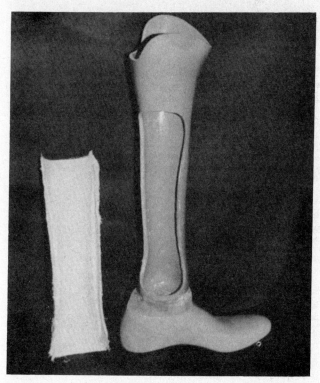

Figure 22.10. Symes prosthesis. (Left) One can visualize how medial opening permits insertion of a bulbous stump. (Courtesy of Richard Selsberg, Orthopedic Braces and Appliances, Kenosha, WI.) (Right) Prosthesis with intact window.

thesis. Disarticulation is performed immediately proximal to the cartilage of the distal tibia. The heel pad is fashioned, inclusive of the remainder of the posterior tibial nerve and vessels, as a weight-bearing stump. Appliances are constructed with a removable posterior or medial opening to permit insertion of the bulbous stump (Fig 22.10). Some inherent strength is

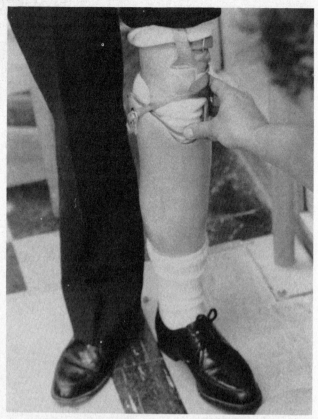

Figure 22.11. Patellar tendon-bearing appliance with supracondylar cuff. (Courtesy of Steven Mersch, Post Rehabilitation, Kenosha, WI)

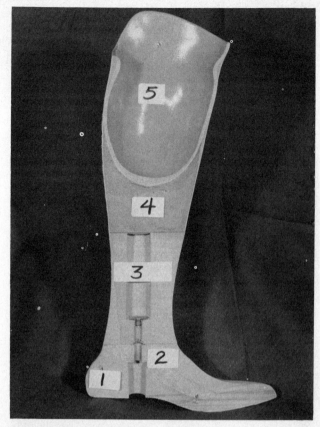

Figure 22.12. Hemisection of a patellatendon-bearing prosthesis. (1) SACH foot. (2) Inflexible keel. (3) Ankle block. (4) Foam cushion. (5) Connection with body part (socket). (Courtesy of Steven Mersch, Post Rehabilitation, Kenosha, WI)

lost with a windowed prosthesis, and one may prefer an appliance with an expandable inner lining instead (16).

Amputations of the rearfoot, or those of the forefoot with an ulcerated plantar surface, where no weight-bearing is desired, are indications for a modification of the patellar tendon-bearing (PTB) appliance (8, 14) (Fig. 22.11). Specific regions of the prosthesis transfer different loads. Vertical load, for example, is carried primarily by the socket near the patellar tendon (17). The PTB prosthesis is usually attached distally to a SACH foot (Fig. 22.12). Stresses can be transmitted between the socket and floor with maximal efficiency. A balsa wood variant is described for less active or lighter patients (18). This allows more efficient energy expenditure.

Lower extremity amputees lack the ability to discriminate sensation distal to the surgical site. This can be particularly devastating in the diabetic, where repetitive stress may lead to stump ulceration (19). Clippinger and associates (20) discuss the feasibility of direct sensory feedback using electrodes sutured to nerves and a receiver embedded within the fascia. A piezoelectrical crystal is placed in the heel of a SACH foot (20). The advantages of this technique include enhancement of tissue healing postoperatively and more efficient discrimination of fine movements. This is especially helpful when walking in the dark with such functions as stair climbing.

Successful management of the lower extremity amputee requires a team approach. This includes the surgeon, prosthetist, rehabilitative therapist, and often a biomedical engineer. Podiatric expertise, especially in the biomechanics of locomotion, dictates that the podiatrist be an active contributor to this important field of health care.

References

1. Thomas A, Habban CC: *Amputation Prosthesis.* Philadelphia, JB Lippincott Co, 1945, pp 1–82.
2. Pritham CH: Suspension of the below-knee prosthesis: an overview. *Orthotics Prosthetics* 33:1–19, 1979.
3. Wilson MP: Clinical application of R.T.V. elastomers. *Orthotics Prosthetics* 33:22–29, 1979.
4. Horndeak S, Boryk RJ, Staats TD: Prosthetic applications of methylmethacrylate acrylic plastic. *Orthotics Prosthetics* 35:49–53, 1981.
5. Lundt J, Staats T: The USMC prosthetic skin. *Orthotics Prosthetics* 37:59–61, 1983.
6. Wilson AB: The connections. *Orthotics and Prosthetics* 34:19–25, 1980.
7. Wiest DR, Waters RL, Bontrager SL, Quigley MJ: The influence of heel design on a rigid ankle-foot orthosis. *Orthotics Prosthetics* 33:3–10, 1979.

8. Rubin G, Fischer E: Selection of components for lower limb amputation prostheses. *Bull Hosp Joint Dis* 1:39–67, 1982.
9. American Academy of Orthopaedic Surgeons: *Atlas of Limb Prosthetics: Surgical and Prosthetic Principles.* St Louis, The CV Mosby Co, 1981, p 9.
10. Campbell JW, Childs CW: The S.A.F.E. foot. *Orthotics Prosthetics* 34:3–16, 1980.
11. Burgess EM, Hittenberger DA, Forsgren SM, Lindh D: The Seattle prosthetic foot—a design for active sports: preliminary studies. *Orthotics Prosthetics* 37:25–31, 1983.
12. Pritham CH: Partial foot amputation—a case study. *Newsletter: Prosthetics Orthotics Clin* 1:5–7, 1977.
13. Engelmeier RL: Technique for prosthetic replacement of missing toes. *J Am Podiatry Assoc* 73:36–38, 1983.
14. Demopoulos JT: Orthotic and prosthetic management of foot disorders. In Jahss MH: *Disorders of the Foot*, vol 2. Philadelphia, WB Saunders Co, 1982, pp 848–854.
15. Reinherz RP, Reinherz HR: Orthopedic bracing for the lower extremities. *J Am Podiatry Assoc* 67:848–854, 1977.
16. Leimkuehler JP: Symes prosthesis—a brief review and a new fabrication technique. *Orthotics Prosthetics* 34:3–12, 1980.
17. Seliktar R, Bar A, Susak Z, Najenson T: A prosthesis for very short below-knee stumps. *Orthotics Prosthetics* 34:25–35, 1980.
18. Leimkuehler JP: A lightweight laminated below-the-knee prosthesis. *Orthotics Prosthetics* 36:46–49, 1982.
19. Lange LR: Prosthetic implication with the diabetic foot. *Orthotics Prosthetics* 36:96–102, 1982.
20. Clippinger FW, Seaber AV, McElhaney JH, Harrelson JM, Maxwell GM: Afferent sensory feedback for lower extremity prosthesis. *Clin Orthop* 169:202–206, 1982.

INDEX

Page numbers in *italics* denote figures; those followed by "t" denote tables